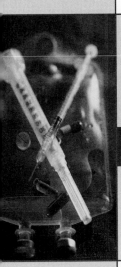

PHARMACOLOGY
FOR THE
PHYSICAL THERAPIST

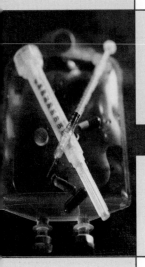

PHARMACOLOGY

FOR THE

PHYSICAL THERAPIST

Peter C. Panus, PhD, PT
Associate Professor
Departments of Pharmaceutical Sciences
and Physical Therapy
Division of Health Sciences
East Tennessee State University, Johnson
City, TN

Erin E. Jobst, PT, PhD
Assistant Professor
School of Physical Therapy
Pacific University, Hillsboro, OR

Susan B. Masters, PhD
Professor and Academy Chair of
Pharmacology Education
Department of Cellular & Molecular
Pharmacology
University of California, San Francisco
San Francisco, CA

Bertram Katzung, MD, PhD
Professor Emeritus of Pharmacology
Department of Cellular & Molecular
Pharmacology
University of California, San Francisco
San Francisco, CA

Suzanne L. Tinsley, PT, PhD
Associate Professor
Program in Physical Therapy
School of Allied Health Professions
Louisiana State University Health
Sciences Center Shreveport
Shreveport, LA

Anthony J. Trevor, PhD
Professor Emeritus of Pharmacology
and Toxicology
Department of Cellular & Molecular
Pharmacology
University of California, San Francisco
San Francisco, CA

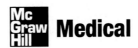 **Medical**

New York Chicago San Francisco Lisbon London Madrid Mexico City
Milan New Delhi San Juan Seoul Singapore Sydney Toronto

Pharmacology for the Physical Therapist

1 2 3 4 5 6 7 8 9 0 DOC/DOC 0 9 8

ISBN 978-0-07-146043-9
MHID 0-07-146043-8

This book was set in AGaramond by International Typesetting & Composition.
The editors were Catherine A. Johnson and Regina Y. Brown.
The production supervisor was Phil Galea.
Project management was provided by International Typesetting & Composition.
The cover designer was The Gazillion Group.
The indexer was Arc Films Inc.
RR Donnelly was printer and binder.

This book is printed on acid-free paper.

Library of Congress Cataloging-in-Publication Data

Pharmacology for the physical therapist / Peter C. Panus ... [et al.].
    p. ; cm.
  Includes bibliographical references and index.
  ISBN-13: 978-0-07-146043-9 (pbk.)
  ISBN-10: 0-07-146043-8 (pbk.)
    1. Pharmacology. 2. Physical therapy. I. Panus, Peter C.
  [DNLM: 1. Pharmacology. 2. Drug Therapy. 3. Pharmaceutical Preparations.
  4. Physical Therapy (Specialty) QV 4 P5365 2008]
  RM300.P5196   2008
  615'.1—dc22
                                                          2008008580

CONTENTS

V. CHEMOTHERAPEUTICS

VI. DRUGS AFFECTING THE MUSCULOSKELETAL SYSTEM

VII. SPECIAL TOPICS

PREFACE

This book is based on what healthcare professionals in rehabilitation need to know about pharmacology. Three licensed physical therapists (Drs. Jobst, Panus, and Tinsley) who are also professional pharmacologists worked together with three authors previously involved in medical pharmacology texts (Drs. Katzung, Masters, and Trevor) to provide a broad base of information. We believe this text offers a complete but focused presentation of pharmacology as it affects patients in rehabilitation and will be useful to all professionals in this field.

The information follows the sequence of traditional pharmacology textbooks and integrated systems based curricula. The initial section is a synopsis of the nature of drugs, basic principles of pharmacodynamics and pharmacokinetics, and an overview of the drug development and approval process in the United States. Subsequent chapters are organized around organ systems and include the autonomic and central nervous systems, cardiovascular and pulmonary systems, endocrine system, and drugs acting on the musculoskeletal system. A separate section discussing anti-infective drugs is included. Finally, a glossary is provided as a student reference for defining many of the terms used in this textbook.

Chapters 21 and 30 are of particular importance to all therapists. Chapter 21 concerns the use of licit drugs such as tobacco and alcohol, and the illicit use of drugs for either mind-altering or bodybuilding effects. The use of these drugs by patients in rehabilitation is often hidden from healthcare professionals. The manifestations and adverse clinical effects resulting from use of these drugs are complicated by the diverse types of drugs being abused by patients. Chapter 30 involves the using of antiseptics and disinfectants to minimize the transfer of pathogens between patients. Their use in rehabilitation should be standard practice due to the extensive equipment utilized by therapists, and the extraordinary potential of therapists to inadvertently facilitate pathogen transmission when equipment is not properly disinfected or sterilized.

Each chapter follows a similar general outline. A brief synopsis of pathophysiology is followed by a discussion focused on the drug classes used clinically, and commonly recognized prototypes for each drug class. Within each drug class, the important chemistry, relevant pharmacokinetics, and mechanism(s) of action, as well as physiologic effects, clinical use, and potential adverse effects are presented. At the end of each chapter are sections designed to emphasize the importance of the drugs in the rehabilitation setting (Rehabilitation Focus) and the effects of drug classes on rehabilitation outcomes (Clinical Relevance for Rehabilitation). A clinical study (Problem Oriented Patient Study – POPS) presenting the rehabilitation process and potential drug interactions is also included. Each chapter also contains a list of many of the available preparations for drugs discussed in the chapter, and those currently available in the

United States (Preparations Available). The authors believe that this format will provide the reader quick access to pertinent information when required.

An accurate medical history for a patient is required prior to a correct clinical diagnosis and effective treatment regimen. An essential component of the medical history is the current medication list for the patient. The drugs a patient takes have the potential to significantly influence medical and functional outcomes, either positively or negatively, regardless of whether the professional currently treating the patient is prescribing the drugs. Thus, all healthcare professionals have a responsibility to determine whether a patient's current medications have the potential to influence any component of the interaction between the professional and the patient. We hope this textbook will assist all healthcare professionals, especially those in physical therapy in that process.

ACKNOWLEDGMENTS

As I have been repeatedly told, the first edition of any textbook is the most time-consuming and difficult to produce. Therefore extra space should be allotted for all the individuals who made this difficult task a reality. First, my co-authors have spent considerable time developing, reviewing, and rewriting the content of this first edition. A special note of appreciation is due to Dr. Bert Katzung, who took special interest and effort to make this book a reality. The professionals at McGraw-Hill also contributed their expertise and knowledge in assisting in the completion of this textbook. In particular, I would like to express my special appreciation to Mr. Michael Brown, who had the foresight to recognize the potential of this concept, and to Ms. Catherine Johnson who continued providing guidance and encouragement. I would also like to acknowledge all of the graduate assistants and tuition scholarship students in the Doctor of Physical Therapy program at East Tennessee State University. These individuals, while obtaining their own professional education, were essential in the background preparatory work responsible for the successful completion of this edition. They typed the tables, obtained the multiple references, scanned figures, developed and maintained the glossary for the textbook, and provided database management of the original sources for all the tables and figures within this textbook. Finally, I would like to express my appreciation to Dr. Leslie Panus, my wife, who has not only assisted me in the development of this book but who over twenty-five years has been both a recognized and unrecognized co-author in all my scholarly activities. To all of these individuals, and those I have undoubtedly forgotten to mention, I express my appreciation.

Peter C. Panus
July 2008

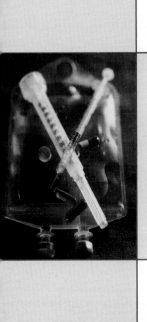

BASIC

PRINCIPLES

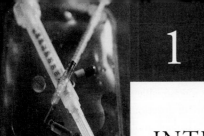

1

INTRODUCTION

Pharmacology may be defined as the study of substances that interact with living systems through chemical processes, especially by binding to regulatory molecules and activating or inhibiting normal body processes. In this book, these substances will be referred to as drugs. Drugs are administered to achieve a beneficial therapeutic effect on some process within the patient or for their toxic effects on regulatory processes in organisms infecting the patient. Such deliberate therapeutic applications may be considered the proper role of pharmacotherapeutics, which is often defined as medical pharmacology (i.e., drugs used to prevent, diagnose, and treat diseases). Pharmacotherapeutics may be further subdivided into pharmacodynamics and pharmacokinetics. Pharmacodynamics evaluates the effect of the substance on biologic processes, and will be discussed in Chapter 2. Pharmacokinetics examines the absorption, distribution, and elimination of substances, and will be discussed in Chapter 3. Toxicology is the branch of pharmacology that deals with the undesirable effects of chemicals on living systems, from individual cells to complex ecosystems.

The use of substances for their medicinal value has occurred throughout history. Prehistoric people undoubtedly recognized the beneficial or toxic effects of many plant and animal materials. The earliest written records from China and Egypt list remedies of many types, including a few still recognized today as useful drugs. Most, however, were of limited clinical value or were actually harmful. Around the end of the 17th century, reliance on observation and experimentation began to replace theorizing in medicine. In the late 18th and early 19th centuries, methods for experimental animal physiology and advances in chemistry further increased the understanding of these chemical substances. This understanding resulted in the concept of drug selectivity, and that drugs may be grouped together into pharmacologic classes based on their physiologic effect or chemical structure. About 50 years ago, there began a major expansion of research efforts in all areas of biology. This expansion coincided with the development of controlled clinical trials that allowed accurate evaluation of the therapeutic value of drugs. As new concepts and new techniques were introduced, information accumulated about the action of drugs on the biologic substrate. During the last half century, many fundamentally new pharmacologic classes and new members of old classes were introduced.

The extension of scientific principles into everyday pharmacotherapeutics is still ongoing. Unfortunately, the drug-consuming public is still exposed to vast amounts of inaccurate, incomplete, or unscientific information regarding the pharmacologic effects of drugs. This has resulted in the faddish use of innumerable expensive, ineffective, and sometimes harmful remedies and the growth of a huge "alternative health-care" industry. Conversely, lack of understanding of basic scientific principles and the investigative process has led to rejection of medical science by a segment of the public, and a common tendency to assume that all adverse drug effects are the result of malpractice. Two general principles should form the basis of understanding for the evidence-based use of drugs. First, *all* substances may, under certain circumstances, be toxic. Second, *all* therapies promoted as health-enhancing should meet the same standards of evidence of efficacy and safety. There should be no artificial separation between scientific medicine and "alternative" or "complementary" medicine.

To learn each pertinent fact about each of the many hundreds of drugs mentioned in this book would be an impractical goal and, fortunately, is unnecessary. Almost all of the several thousand drugs currently available may be arranged in about 70 pharmacologic classes. Many of the drugs within each class are very similar in pharmacodynamic actions and often in their pharmacokinetic properties as well. For most pharmacologic classes, one or more prototypic drugs (bolded in this book) may be identified that typify the most important characteristics of the class. This permits classification of other important drugs in the class as variants of the prototype, so that only the prototype must be learned in detail and for the remaining drugs, only the differences from the prototype learned.

THE NATURE OF DRUGS

In the most general sense, a drug may be defined as any substance that brings about a change in biologic processes through its chemical actions. Drugs in common use include inorganic ions, nonpeptide organic molecules, small peptides and proteins, nucleic acids, lipids, and carbohydrates. *Poisons* may also be used clinically as drugs. A poison is a chemical whose action is detrimental to biologic processes. *Toxins* are usually defined as poisons of biologic origin that are synthesized by plants or animals.

A drug is often administered at a location distant from its intended site of action. For example, a pill is given orally to relieve a headache. Therefore, a useful drug must have the necessary properties to be transported from its site of administration to its site of action. A practical drug should also be inactivated or excreted from the body at a reasonable rate so that its actions will be of appropriate duration. In the great majority of cases, the pharmacologic molecule interacts with a specific molecule in the biologic system that plays a regulatory role. This molecule is called a receptor. In order to interact chemically with its receptor, a pharmacologic molecule must have the appropriate size, electrical charge, shape, and atomic composition.

Because of application requirements, a drug may be a solid, liquid, or gas at room temperature. These physical factors often determine the best route of administration. Many drugs are weak acids or weak bases. Drugs may also vary in size from a small ion (e.g., lithium ion) to a large protein (e.g., tissue-plasminogen activator). The lower limit of this range is probably set by the requirements for specificity of action. In order to have a good "fit" to only one type of receptor, a medicinal molecule must be sufficiently unique in, for example, shape and charge to prevent its binding to other receptors. In contrast, drugs that are too large will not diffuse readily between compartments of the body.

Rational Drug Design

Rational design of drugs implies the ability to predict the appropriate molecular structure of a drug on the basis of information about its biologic receptor. Until recently, no receptor was known in sufficient detail to permit such drug design. Instead, drugs were developed through random testing of chemicals or modification of drugs already known to have some effect. However, during the past three decades, many receptors have been isolated and characterized. A few drugs now in use were developed through molecular design based on knowledge of the three-dimensional structure of the receptor site. As more becomes known about receptor structure, rational drug design will become more feasible.

RESEARCH AND NEW DRUG DEVELOPMENT

Preclinical Development

By law, the safety and efficacy of drugs must be defined before they are marketed in the United States. The development of new drugs is a multistep process

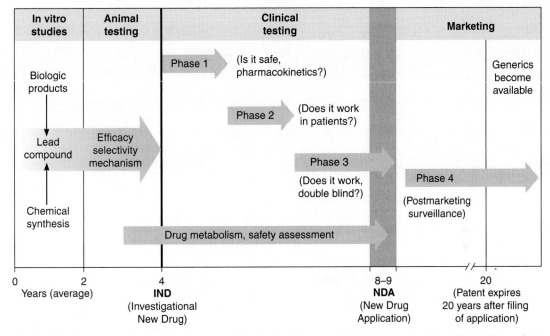

Figure 1–1. The development and testing process required to bring a drug to market in the United States. Some of the requirements may be different for drugs used in life-threatening diseases.

requiring molecular, cellular, animal, and human clinical trials prior to governmental approval and marketing (Figure 1–1). New drugs may be developed through a basic understanding of chemical structure or biologic mechanisms, or based on the actions of previous drugs. Alternatively, drugs may be developed from screening a large number of biologically derived or synthesized substances.

Regardless of the source or the key idea leading to a candidate molecule, testing it involves a sequence of experimentation and characterization called drug *screening*. A variety of biologic assays at the molecular, cellular, organ system, and whole animal levels are used to define the activity and selectivity of the drug. The molecule will be studied for a broad array of actions to establish the mechanism of action and selectivity of the drug. This has the advantage of demonstrating unsuspected toxic effects and occasionally discloses a previously unsuspected therapeutic action. As a result of this research effort, a candidate molecule, called a lead compound, is investigated further. A patent

application may then be filed for a novel compound that is efficacious, or for a new and nonobvious therapeutic use for a previously known drug.

As part of the preclinical investigative process, lead compounds are evaluated for potential toxicity. Several of the toxicity tests are listed in Table 1–1. No drug can be certified as completely free of risk, since every drug is toxic at some dosage. These investigations can estimate the risk associated with exposure to the drug under specified conditions. In addition to the studies shown in Table 1–1, several quantitative estimates are required and are discussed in Chapter 3.

Evaluation in Humans

Less than one-third of the drugs tested in clinical trials reach the marketplace. Federal law in the United States requires that the study of new drugs in humans be conducted in accordance with stringent guidelines. The federal Food and Drug Administration (FDA) is the administrative body that oversees the drug evaluation process in the United States and grants approval

Table 1–1.	Safety tests conducted in animals
Type of Test	**Comment**
Acute Toxicity	Compares single therapeutic dose to that which is lethal in approximately 50% of animals.
Subacute Toxicity	Compares multiple doses at therapeutic and toxic concentrations. Usually 4 weeks to 3 months in duration.
Chronic Toxicity	Compares multiple doses at therapeutic and toxic concentrations. Conducted when intended clinical use is prolonged. Duration 6 months or longer.
Carcinogenic Potential	Two-year duration. Conducted when drug is intended for prolonged clinical use.
Mutagenic Potential	Examines genetic stability and the potential for mutations in prokaryotic and eukaryotic organisms.
Toxicologic Potential	Determines the sequence and mechanisms of toxic actions.

for marketing of new drugs. The FDA's authority to regulate drug marketing is derived from federal legislation. To receive approval by the FDA for marketing, a drug must be demonstrated to be "safe and efficacious" through experimental investigation. Unfortunately, "safe" means different things to the patient, the physician, and society. A complete absence of risk is impossible to demonstrate, but this fact is not well understood by the average member of the public, who assumes that any drug sold with the approval of the FDA must indeed be free of serious "side effects." This confusion continues to be a major cause of litigation and dissatisfaction with medical care. Of course it is impossible to certify that a drug is absolutely safe. Experimental investigation, however, can identify most of the hazards likely to be associated with use of a new drug and to place some statistical limits on frequency of occurrence of such events in the population under study. As a result, an operational and pragmatic definition of "safety" can usually be reached that is based on the nature and incidence of drug-associated hazards compared with the hazard of nontherapy for the target disease.

Clinical Trials

The new drug approval process involves a systematic series of investigations. Once a lead compound is judged ready to be studied in humans, a Notice of Claimed Investigational Exemption for a New Drug (IND) must be filed and approval of the proposed clinical studies obtained from the FDA (Figure 1–1).

In phase 1, the effects of the drug, as a function of dosage, are established in a small number (25 to 50) of healthy volunteers. If the drug is expected to have significant toxicity, as is often the case in cancer and AIDS therapy, volunteer patients with the disease are used in phase 1 rather than normal volunteers. Phase 1 trials are done to determine whether humans and animals show significantly different responses to the drug, and to establish the probable limits of the safe clinical dosage range. Pharmacokinetic parameters (Chapter 3) are often established in phase 1.

In phase 2, the drug is administered for the first time in patients with the target disease to determine its efficacy. A small number of patients (100 to 200) are studied in great detail. The clinical benefits of the drug and a broader range of toxicities can be determined in this phase.

In phase 3, the drug is evaluated in much larger numbers of patients to establish safety and efficacy under conditions of proposed use. Phase 3 studies can be difficult to design and execute, and are usually expensive because of the large numbers of patients involved and the mass of data that must be collected and analyzed.

Often 4 to 6 years of clinical testing are required to accumulate all the data. Chronic safety testing in animals is usually done concurrently with clinical trials.

In each of the three formal phases of clinical trials, volunteers or patients must be informed of the investigational status of the drug as well as possible risks, and must be allowed to decline or to consent to participate and receive the drug. If the clinical and animal investigative results meet expectations, an application is made for permission to market the new drug. The process of applying for marketing approval requires submission of a New Drug Application (NDA) to the FDA (Figure 1–1). The FDA review of this material and a decision on approval can take 3 years or longer. If the FDA approves the NDA, the drug manufacturer in conjunction with the FDA develops a *"label"* for the drug. This label describes the medical condition treated by the drug, adverse effects of the drug and dosages for the drug. After the drug is approved and marketed, the drug may be prescribed for other medical conditions not listed on the label. Such usage is the drug's *"off-label"* use. In cases where an urgent need is perceived, the process of preclinical and clinical testing and FDA review may be greatly accelerated. For serious diseases, the FDA can permit extensive but controlled marketing of a new drug before phase 3 studies are completed.

Once marketing of a drug has commenced, phase 4 begins. This constitutes monitoring the safety of the new drug under actual conditions of use in large numbers of patients. Phase 4 has no fixed duration.

The time from the filing of a patent application to approval for marketing of a new drug can be 5 years or considerably longer. Since the lifetime of a patent is 20 years in the United States, the owner of the patent, usually a pharmaceutical company, has exclusive rights for marketing the product for only a limited time after approval of the NDA. Because the FDA review process can be lengthy, the time consumed by the review process is sometimes added to the patent life. However, the extension (up to 5 years) cannot increase the total life of the patent to more than 14 years after NDA approval. After expiration of the patent, any company may produce and market the drug as a *generic drug*, without paying license fees to the original patent owner. The FDA drug approval process is one of the rate-limiting factors in the time it takes for a drug to be marketed and reach patients.

ADVERSE EVENTS AND DRUGS

Severe adverse reactions to marketed drugs are uncommon, although less dangerous toxic effects, as noted elsewhere in this book, are frequent for some pharmacologic classes. Life-threatening reactions probably occur in less than 2 percent of patients admitted to medical wards. The mechanisms of these adverse reactions fall into two main categories. The first group is often an extension of known pharmacologic effects and thus is predictable. These toxicities are generally discovered during phases 1 through 3 of testing. The second group, which might be immunologic or of unknown mechanism, is frequently unexpected and is often not recognized until a drug has been marketed for some years. These toxicities are therefore usually discovered after marketing has begun (phase 4). Thus, health-care professionals should be aware of the various types of allergic reactions to drugs.

REFERENCES

Berkowitz BA, Sachs G: Life cycle of a block buster: Discovery and development of omeprazole (Prilosec™). *Mol Interv* 2002;2:6.

Billstein SA: How the pharmaceutical industry brings an antibiotic medication to market in the United States. *Antimicrob Agents Chemother* 1994;38:2679.

Chappell WR, Mordenti J: Extrapolation of toxicological and pharmacological data from animals to humans. *Adv Med Res* 1991;20:1.

Collins JM, Grieshaber CK, Chabner BA: Pharmacologically guided phase I clinical trials based upon preclinical medication development. *J Natl Cancer Inst* 1990;82:1321.

DiMasi JA: Success rates for new medications entering clinical testing in the United States. *Clin Pharmacol Ther* 1995;58:1.

DiMasi JA: Risks in new medication development: approval success rates for investigational medications. *Clin Pharmacol Ther* 2001;69:297.

Editor's Page: Code of ethics of the World Medical Association: Declaration of Helsinki. *Clin Res* 1966;14:193.

Guarino RA: New medication approval process. In *Medications and Pharmaceutical Sciences*, Vol.100. New York: Marcel Decker, 2000.

Jelovsek FR, Mattison DR, Chen JJ: Prediction of risk for human developmental toxicity: How important are animal studies? *Obstet Gynecol* 1989;74:624.

Kessler DA: The regulation of investigational medications. *N Engl J Med* 1989;320:281.

Laughren TP: The review of clinical safety data in a new medication application. *Psychopharmacol Bull* 1989;25:5.

McKhann GM: The trials of clinical trials. *Arch Neurol* 1989;46:611.

Moscucci M, et al: Blinding, unblinding, and the placebo effect: An analysis of patients' guesses of treatment assignment in a double-blind clinical trial. *Clin Pharmacol Ther* 1987;41:259.

Sibille M, et al: Adverse events in phase one studies: A study in 430 healthy volunteers. *Eur J Clin Pharmacol* 1992;42:389.

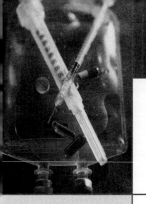

2

DRUG RECEPTOR DYNAMICS

Therapeutic and toxic effects of the majority of drugs result from their interactions with molecular targets, that is, receptors, in the patient. The drug molecule (the ligand) interacts with the receptor and initiates the chain of biochemical and physiologic events leading to the drug's observed effects. This ligand-receptor interaction and its results are denoted as pharmacodynamics.

The receptor concept has important practical consequences for the development of drugs. It forms the basis for understanding the actions and clinical uses of drugs described in almost every chapter of this book. These consequences may be briefly summarized as follows: First, receptors largely determine the quantitative relations between dose or concentration of drug and pharmacologic effects. The receptor's affinity for binding a drug determines the concentration of drug required to form a significant number of ligand-receptor complexes, and the total number of receptors may limit the maximal effect a drug may produce. Second, receptors are responsible for selectivity of drug action. The molecular size, shape, and electrical charge of a drug determine whether the drug will bind to a particular receptor among the vast array of chemically different binding sites available in the patient. Accordingly, changes in the chemical structure of a drug can dramatically increase or decrease its affinities for different classes of receptors, with resulting alterations in therapeutic and toxic effects. Third, receptor activation and blockade play a key role in the mechanisms of many clinical effects of drugs.

▮ DRUG-RECEPTOR BONDS

As previously discussed (Chapter 1), receptors are specific molecules with which drugs interact to produce changes in the function of cells within the patient. Receptors must be selective in their binding characteristics in order to respond to specific chemical stimuli. The receptor site presents a unique three-dimensional configuration for the drug to bind. The complementary configuration of the drug is, in part, what creates the affinity of the drug for the receptor site (Figure 2–1). Drugs that bind to a limited group of receptor types may be classified as specific, whereas drugs binding to a larger number of receptor types may be considered nonspecific.

Drugs interact with receptors by means of chemical bonds. The three major types of bonds are covalent, electrostatic, and hydrophobic. Covalent bonds are strong and, in many cases, not reversible under biologic conditions. Electrostatic bonds are weaker than covalent bonds, more common, and often reversible. Hydrophobic bonds are the weakest and are probably the most important in the interactions of lipid-soluble drugs and in hydrophobic "pockets" of receptors.

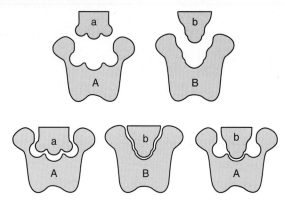

Figure 2–1. Specificity of a drug for the receptor. The structure of drug "a" allows binding only to receptor "A." In contrast, the structure of drug "b" allows binding to either receptor "A" or "B." The conformation of drug "a" is such that this drug would be considered to be specific to receptor "A."

■ DOSE-RESPONSE CURVES

Graded Dose-Response Relationships

In order to initiate a sequence of cellular events that ultimately results in physiologic and clinical responses, almost all drugs, and all endogenous ligands (hormones, neurotransmitters) must bind to specific receptors. When the response of a receptor system is measured against the concentrations of a drug, the graph of the response versus the drug concentration or dose is called a graded dose-response curve (Figure 2–2a). Plotting

the same data with a logarithmic dose axis usually results in a sigmoid curve which simplifies the manipulation of the dose-response data (Figure 2–2b). The concentration of a drug required to achieve 50 percent of the maximal response is called the effective concentration for 50% response (EC_{50}). For some ligands, the EC_{50} also estimates the concentration that binds 50 percent of available receptors. Thus, the dose-response curve relates the binding of the drug to the receptor; that is, the *affinity* of the drug for the receptor. In order to produce a response the drug must demonstrate not only binding to the receptors, but an intrinsic activity or ability to initiate a response. There are drug concentrations below which no clinically beneficial response is observed. The concentration at which lower doses produce no clinical benefit is the minimal effective dose. Additionally, at some point (the maximal effect; E_{max}), no additional clinical response is observed with higher concentrations. The E_{max} may also be defined as the maximal *efficacy* of the drug.

Quantal Dose-Response Relationships

When the minimum dose required to produce an intended magnitude of response is evaluated for a population, a quantal dose-response relationship may be determined. When plotted as the fraction of the population that responds at each dose versus the log of the dose administered, a cumulative quantal dose-response curve is obtained (Figure 2–3). From these curves

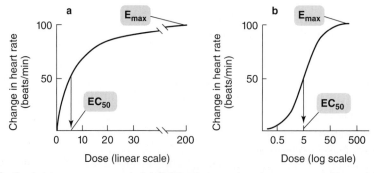

Figure 2–2. Graded dose-response graph. (a). Relation between drug dose or concentration and drug effect. When the dose axis is linear, a hyperbolic curve is commonly obtained. (b). Same data on a logarithmic dose axis.

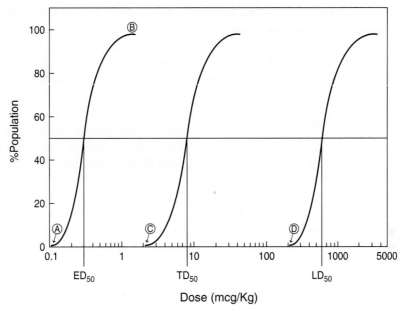

Figure 2–3. Quantal dose-response plot. The curves are generated from the frequency distribution of doses of a hypothetical drug required to produce specified effects. The median effective dose (ED$_{50}$: 0.3 mcg/kg), median toxic dose (TD$_{50}$: 8 mcg/kg) and the median lethal dose (LD$_{50}$: 600 mcg/kg) are depicted. The following abbreviations are used in the graph: A: minimal effective dose (MED: 0.1 mcg/kg), B: maximal effective dose (1.5 mcg/kg), C: minimal toxic dose (MTD: 2 mcg/kg), and D: minimal lethal dose (200 mcg/kg). The therapeutic index is calculated by dividing the TD$_{50}$ value (8 mcg/kg) by the ED$_{50}$ (0.3 mcg/kg) to obtain approximately 27. The therapeutic window is determined by the range between the MED (0.1 mcg/kg) and the MTD (2 mcg/kg) to obtain 0.1-2 mcg/kg.

the median effective dose (ED$_{50}$), median toxic dose (TD$_{50}$) and, in animals, the median lethal dose (LD$_{50}$) can be calculated.

From these quantal dose-response relationships several safety characteristics may be determined for each drug. These variables are the therapeutic index and the therapeutic window. The *therapeutic index* represents an estimate of the safety of a drug, since a very safe drug might be expected to have a very large toxic dose and a much smaller effective dose. The calculation for the therapeutic index is made by dividing the TD$_{50}$, or LD$_{50}$, by the ED$_{50}$ for the drug. Unfortunately, varying slopes for the dose-response plots sometimes make the therapeutic index a poor measure of safety. An alternative safety index is the therapeutic window. The *therapeutic window* describes the dosage

range between the minimal effective dose and the minimal toxic dose. Figure 2–3 depicts dose-response plots for the clinical benefit, toxicity, and lethality for a hypothetical drug. The therapeutic index is calculated to be approximately 27 based on the TD$_{50}$ and the ED$_{50}$. The therapeutic window for this same hypothetical drug is about 0.1 to 2.0 mcg/kg.

Potency

Potency denotes the amount of drug needed to produce a given effect. Potency can be determined from either graded dose-response curves or quantal dose-response curves; however, the values are not identical. In graded dose-response measurements, the potency is characterized by the EC$_{50}$ (Figure 2–2). The smaller the EC$_{50}$, the greater the potency of the drug. In quantal dose-response curves the ED_{50}, TD_{50}, and LD_{50} measurements are identified as the potency variables (Figure 2–3).

DRUG-RECEPTOR DYNAMICS

Full Agonists and Partial Agonists

Some exogenous drugs and many endogenous ligands, such as hormones and neurotransmitters, regulate the function of receptors as full agonists. These agents demonstrate both affinity and maximal efficacy for the receptors that ultimately result in the physiologic response observed in the clinic (Figure 2–4). A partial agonist binds to the receptor at the same location as the full agonist ligand, but log dose-response curves for a partial agonist and full agonist demonstrate that a partial agonist achieves a lower maximal effect, even with full receptor occupancy (Figure 2–4). By

definition, partial agonists have a lower maximal efficacy than full agonists, and in the presence of full agonists, may inhibit the full agonists, decreasing their response.

Not all drugs demonstrate the same affinity for the receptor even if they are able to demonstrate the same maximal efficacy, and some drugs may demonstrate a lower maximal efficacy, yet demonstrate a higher potency. Figure 2–4 presents two full agonists (A and B) that both produce equal maximal efficacy, yet "B" has a lower affinity for the receptor compared to "A." As a result of this binding difference, the full agonist "A" is described as having a higher potency compared to "B." The potency of partial agonists also varies with each medication. The partial agonist "C" demonstrates a lower maximal efficacy than either of the full agonists (A or B), yet has a higher potency than either of the full agonists. Thus, potency and maximal efficacy are not interchangeable. That is, a drug may have a higher potency and a lower maximal efficacy.

Competitive Antagonists

Some drugs may occupy a receptor without activating the signaling mechanism. These drugs are antagonists in that they have affinity for the receptor without efficacy. Competitive antagonists bind reversibly at the same receptor site as the agonist (Figure 2–5a). In the presence of a competitive antagonist, the agonist log dose-response curve is shifted to higher doses; that is, horizontally to the right. Competitive antagonists shift the ED_{50} to higher doses; however, with sufficient agonist concentration, the same E_{max} can still be achieved.

Irreversible or Pseudoirreversible Antagonists

In contrast to competitive antagonists, some antagonists bind to the agonist receptor site with very strong electrostatic and hydrogen bonds or bind covalently. Once bound to the receptor, these antagonists are released slowly. Under such conditions, the binding may be considered irreversible or pseudoirreversible. From a functional viewpoint, this may be considered noncompetitive antagonism. The log dose-response curve for these antagonists results in a decrease in the

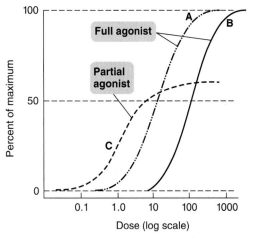

Figure 2–4. Comparison of theoretical log dose-response curves for full agonists (**A** & **B**) and a partial agonist (**C**). Both full agonists demonstrate the same maximal efficacy. Drug "A" is also more potent than drug "B" because the EC_{50} for "A" is approximately 10, whereas for "B" the EC_{50} is approximately 100. The partial agonist acts at the same receptor site as the full agonists and also demonstrates affinity for the receptor. Compared to the full agonists, however, the partial agonist produces a lower maximal effect; i.e., has less efficacy. The EC_{50} for the partial agonist is approximately 1. A partial agonist may be more potent (as depicted), less potent, or equally potent as the full agonist.

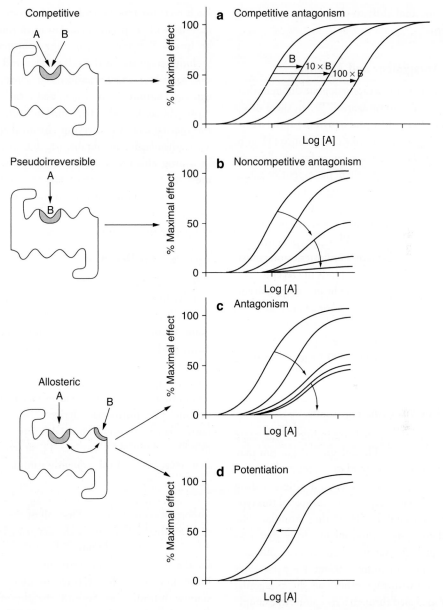

Figure 2–5. Mechanisms of drug receptor interaction. (a) Competitive antagonism occurs when the agonist "A" and competitive antagonist "B" compete for the same binding site on the receptor. Response curves for the agonist are shifted to the right in a concentration-related manner by the antagonist. (b) If the antagonist binds to the same site as the agonist but does so irreversibly, or with a very slow dissociation rate (pseudoir-reversibly), it causes a minimal shift in the dose-response curve to the right, but depresses the maximal response (noncompetitive antagonism [b]). Allosteric effects occur when "B" binds to a different site on the receptor compared to "A." (c) If the binding of "B" decreases the response to "A," this is denoted allosteric antagonism. (d) If the binding of "B" increases the response of "A," this is allosteric potentiation (d). (Reproduced, with permission, from Brunton LL, Lazo JS, Parker KL, eds. Goodman & Gilman's: The Pharmacological Basis of Therapeutics, 11th ed. New York: McGraw-Hill, 2006:36.)

E_{max} and a minimal shift to the right of the ED_{50} (Figure 2–5b).

Allosteric Antagonists and Agonists

Other drugs bind to the receptor at a site different than the endogenous ligand or agonist. When these drugs inhibit the effects of the ligand or agonist at the receptor, they are known as allosteric antagonists (Figure 2–5c). The log dose-response curve for an allosteric antagonist is similar to that of a noncompetitive antagonist with a minimal shift to the right of the ED_{50} and a decrease in the E_{max}. This is due to the fact that allosteric antagonists and the agonist are binding at different sites on the receptor. Thus, no concentration of agonist is going to displace the allosteric antagonist.

Alternatively, when a drug binds the receptor at a site different than the endogenous ligand or agonist, and potentiates the effects of the ligand or agonist, the drug is known as an allosteric potentiator (Figure 2–5d). Allosteric potentiators shift the log dose-response curve to the left, decreasing the ED_{50} and maintaining the E_{max}.

Additional Forms of Antagonism

Antagonism is not restricted to binding to the same receptor as the agonist. Physiologic antagonism may occur by having one drug bind to a receptor that produces an effect opposite to that of a different drug binding at a different receptor. An example of this type of antagonism would be drugs that stimulate the parasympathetic system antagonizing drugs that activate the sympathetic system. Chemical antagonism is a nonreceptor-dependent mechanism. Here the drugs interact directly with each other and the antagonist effect is not mediated through a receptor. An example of this type of antagonism would be a drug that directly binds another drug to prevent its action; for example, digoxin antibodies.

▮ SIGNALING MECHANISMS

Most transmembrane signaling is accomplished by a small number of different molecular mechanisms.

Each receptor type is made up of distinctive protein families with a specific mechanism to transduce one or many different signals. These protein families include receptors on the cell surface and within the cell, as well as enzymes and other components that generate, amplify, coordinate, and terminate postreceptor signaling within the cell. This section discusses the mechanisms for carrying chemical information across the plasma membrane, which ultimately results in a drug effect when an agonist binds. Five basic mechanisms of transmembrane signaling are well understood (Figure 2–6). Each uses a different strategy to circumvent the barrier posed by the lipid bilayer of the plasma membrane.

Intracellular Receptors

The first receptor type responds to a lipid-soluble agonist that crosses the membrane and acts on an intracellular receptor molecule (Figure 2–6a). One example for this class is the gas nitric oxide (NO). Nitric oxide stimulates the intracellular enzyme guanylyl cyclase, which produces cyclic guanosine monophosphate (cGMP), a second messenger. Other classes of agonists that act on intracellular receptors include the hormones derived from cholesterol (adrenocorticosteroids, gonadal hormones, and vitamin D) and thyroid hormones. These agonists bind to their receptors and subsequently stimulate gene transcription. The mechanism used by hormones that act by regulating gene expression has two therapeutically important consequences. First, all of these hormones produce their effects after a characteristic lag period of 30 minutes to several hours. This is the time required for the synthesis of new proteins. Thus, gene-active hormones cannot be expected to alter a pathologic state within minutes. Second, the physiologic effect from stimulation of these receptors may persist for hours or days after the agonist concentration has been reduced to zero. The persistence of the effect is primarily due to the relatively slow turnover of most enzymes and proteins, which can remain active in cells for hours or days after they have been synthesized. Consequently, this means that the beneficial (or toxic) effects of a gene-activated system will usually decrease slowly following termination of the stimulation.

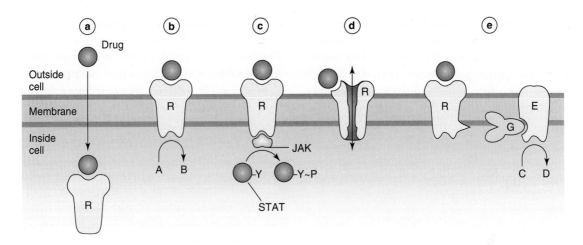

Figure 2–6. Signaling mechanisms for drug effects. Five major signaling mechanisms are recognized: (a) transmembrane diffusion of the ligand to bind to an intracellular receptor; (b) transmembrane enzyme receptors, whose outer domain provides the receptor function and inner domain provides the effector mechanism converting A to B; (c) transmembrane receptors that, after activation by an appropriate ligand, activate separate mobile protein tyrosine kinase molecules (JAKs), which phosphorylate molecules that regulate transcription (STAT); (d) transmembrane channels that are gated open or closed by a ligand at the receptor site; and (e) G protein-coupled receptors, which utilize a coupling protein to activate a separate effector molecule. The following symbols are used in the figure: A, C, substrates; B, D, products; R, receptor; G, G protein; E, effector (enzyme); Y, tyrosine; P, phosphate, JAK, Janus-kinase, STAT, signal transducers and activators of transcription.

Receptors on Transmembrane Proteins

Some transmembrane receptors have intracellular enzymatic activity that is allosterically regulated when an agonist binds to a site on the protein's extracellular domain (Figure 2–6b and c). This class of receptors mediates the first steps in signaling by insulin and various growth factors and trophic hormones. These receptors are polypeptides consisting of an extracellular hormone-binding domain and a cytoplasmic enzyme domain. The cytoplasmic domain may have enzymatic activity directly linked to the receptor, or a separate enzyme molecule may be associated with the cytoplasmic domain. In all these receptors, the two domains are connected by a hydrophobic segment of the polypeptide that crosses the lipid bilayer of the plasma membrane. The receptor kinase signaling pathway is an example and begins with ligand binding to the receptor's extracellular domain. The resulting change in receptor conformation brings together the kinase domains of two adjacent receptors, which become enzymatically active and phosphorylate additional downstream signaling proteins. Activated receptors catalyze phosphorylation of tyrosine residues on different target signaling proteins, thereby allowing a single type of activated receptor to modulate a number of biochemical processes.

Receptors on Transmembrane Ion Channels

Many useful drugs act by mimicking or blocking the actions of endogenous agents that regulate the flow of ions through plasma membrane channels (Figure 2–6d). The endogenous ligands include acetylcholine, serotonin, gamma-aminobutyric acid (GABA), glycine, aspartate, and glutamate. All of these molecules are synaptic transmitters. Each of these receptors transmits its signal across the plasma membrane by increasing transmembrane conductance of the relevant ion (usually sodium, potassium, calcium, or chloride) and thereby altering the electrical potential across the membrane.

G Protein–Linked Receptors

Finally, many extracellular ligands act by increasing the intracellular concentrations of second messengers such as cyclic adenosine-monophosphate (cAMP), calcium ion, or the phosphoinositides (Figures 2–6e). In most cases, they use a transmembrane signaling system with three separate components. First, the extracellular ligand is specifically detected by a cell-surface receptor. Binding to the receptor in turn triggers the activation of a G protein located on the cytoplasmic face of the plasma membrane. The activated G protein then changes the activity of an effector element, usually an enzyme or ion channel. This element then changes the concentration of the intracellular second messenger.

Termination of drug action at the receptor level results from one of several processes. In G protein-linked receptor systems, the second messenger (as exemplified by cAMP) is inactivated by a phosphodiesterase (Figure 2–7). Alternatively, the ion channel opened by the receptor eventually closes, terminating the event. In some cases, the effect lasts only as long as the drug occupies the receptor, so that dissociation of drug from the receptor automatically terminates the effect. In many cases, however, the action may persist after the drug has dissociated because, for example, some coupling molecule is still present in activated form. In the case of drugs that bind covalently to the receptor, the effect may persist until the ligand-receptor complex is destroyed and new receptors are synthesized.

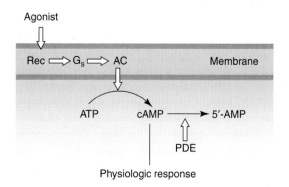

Figure 2–7. The cAMP second-messenger pathway. Key proteins include hormone receptors (Rec), a stimulatory G protein (G_s), catalytic adenylyl cyclase (AC), and phosphodiesterases (PDE) that hydrolyze cAMP. Hydrolysis of cAMP terminates the activity of the second messenger.

RECEPTOR REGULATION

The number of receptors present in a biologic system and available for interaction with a drug is not constant. The ability of the receptor to initiate a signal as a result of the binding of an agonist varies, as does the actual number of receptors available for binding of the agonist. The variables responsible for this receptor regulation may include repeated short-term or long-term activation of the receptors, or other variations in the homeostasis of the cell. Changes in receptor regulation may be the result of pharmacologic therapy, and may have significant adverse effects.

Desensitization and Down-Regulation

Receptor-mediated responses to agonists often decrease with time (desensitization). There are no changes in the number of receptors available for binding; however, the ability of the receptors to initiate the signal diminishes over seconds or minutes in the presence of the agonist. The decreased responsiveness of the receptor system as a result of the repetitive or prolonged stimulation may be the result of chemical alteration of the receptor, depletion of intracellular second messengers, intracellular build-up of extracellular ions, or other limitations in the signaling process. Desensitization of the receptor is usually reversible if longer intervals are provided between the exposures to the agonist.

In contrast, down-regulation is a decrease in the number of receptors available for binding by the agonist (Figure 2–8b). Down-regulation is the result of exposure of the receptors to agonists for periods of hours to days. Down-regulation occurs more slowly and is usually the result of net degradation of receptors exceeding synthesis of new receptors. Both desensitization and down-regulation can result in a decrease in the maximal response when an agonist stimulates the receptors.

Up-Regulation

A prolonged decrease in stimulation of receptors, or chronic blockade of receptors by an antagonist, may result in an increase in the number of receptors available

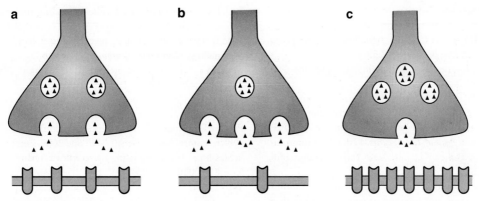

Figure 2–8. This figure represents a typical synapse with neurotransmitter released from the presynaptic membrane and receptors located on the postsynaptic membrane under three different conditions: normal (a), down-regulation (b), and up-regulation (c). In comparison to normal stimulation rates (a), down regulation (b) may be the result of increased neurotransmitter release from the presynaptic side and stimulation of the post-synaptic receptors over a period of hours or days. The result is a decrease in post-synaptic receptor numbers. In contrast, up-regulation is an increase in the number of receptors available for binding compared to normal stimulation rates (a). Up-regulation may result from chronic blockade of the receptors by a competitive receptor antagonist (not shown), or decreased release of neurotransmitter from the presynaptic side and diminished post-synaptic receptor stimulation for a similar period of time (c).

for binding and stimulation. This increase in the number of receptors is denoted up-regulation (Figure 2–8c). Lack of receptor stimulation might decrease the rate of degradation of the receptors, and if synthesis of the receptors is maintained, the result is an increase in the total number of receptors available for stimulation. Similarly, chronic blockade of receptors might lead to decreased receptor degradation with continued receptor synthesis, resulting in an increase in the total number of receptors available for stimulation. Owing to the increase in the total number of receptors available in an up-regulated system, stimulation may result in an enhanced maximal response. This event may occur, for example, when the antagonist for the receptors is abruptly withdrawn.

◼ REHABILITATION FOCUS

The physical therapist should remember that all beneficial clinical effects of drugs occur within specific concentration ranges. These concentration ranges are unique to the different pharmacologic classes and drugs, and for some drugs, to the specific patient. Concentrations below this effective range provide no therapeutic benefit, and concentrations above this range almost always result in adverse effects. As discussed in Chapter 3, a drug's mechanism of action may involve mimicking or inhibiting an endogenous ligand. Further, the mechanism of action may involve direct competition with an endogenous ligand, or the drug may modulate the affinity of the receptor for that ligand. Some drugs may permanently inactivate the receptor to which they bind or stimulate additional cellular homeostatic mechanisms, resulting in their clinical effect lasting after the drug itself is no longer detectable within the patient. Finally, receptor numbers are not static but are in a state of constant flux.

Therapists should know whether a drug is an agonist, antagonist, or partial agonist. This classification scheme is central to the understanding of pharmacology. This determination will also assist the therapist in evaluating the physiologic response of the patient to the drug, potential adverse effects, and drug-drug interactions.

REFERENCES

Bootman MD, et al: Calcium signalling—An overview. *Semin Cell Dev Biol* 2001;12:3.

Bourne HR: How receptors talk to trimeric G proteins. *Curr Opin Cell Biol* 1997;9:134.

Buxton IL: Pharmacokinetics and Pharmacodynamics: The Dynamics of Drug Absorption, Distribution, Action and Elimination. In *Goodman & Gilman's: The Pharmacological Basis of Therapeutics*, 11th ed. Brunton LL, Lazo JS, Parker KL, eds. New York: McGraw-Hill, 2006:36.

Catterall WA: From ionic currents to molecular mechanisms: The structure and function of voltage-gated sodium channels. *Neuron* 2000;26:13.

Farfel Z, Bourne HR, Iiri T: The expanding spectrum of G protein diseases. *N Engl J Med* 1999;340:1012.

Jan LY, Stevens CF: Signalling mechanisms: A decade of signalling. *Curr Opin Neurobiol* 2000;10:625.

Kenakin T: Efficacy at G-protein–coupled receptors. *Nat Rev Drug Discov* 2002;1:103.

Mitlak BH, Cohen FJ: Selective estrogen receptor modulators: A look ahead. *Drugs* 1999;57:653.

Pierce KL, Premont RT, Lefkowitz RJ: Seven-transmembrane receptors. *Nature Rev Mol Cell Biol* 2002;3:639.

Schlessinger J: Cell signaling by receptor tyrosine kinases. *Cell* 2000;103:193.

Tsao P, von Zastrow M: Downregulation of G protein–coupled receptors. *Curr Opin Neurobiol* 2000;10:365.

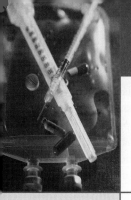

3

PHARMACOKINETICS

The term *pharmacokinetics* denotes the effects of biologic systems on both endogenous ligands and drugs. Almost all drugs, except those delivered directly to the target tissue where the proposed receptors are located, are absorbed from the site of administration, transported by the circulation to various tissues in the body, and then arrive at the target tissue. At the same time, the body attempts to convert these drugs into forms that allow for easier removal from the body. This sequence represents the absorption, distribution, biotransformation, elimination, and excretion of drugs.

◼ PHYSICAL AND CHEMICAL NATURE OF DRUGS

Currently available drugs include inorganic ions, nonpeptide organic molecules, small peptides and proteins, nucleic acids, lipids, and carbohydrates. Drugs may vary in size and molecular weight (MW) from MW 7 for lithium to over MW 50,000 for thrombolytic enzymes. The majority of drugs, however, have molecular weights between 100 and 1,000. They are often found in plants or animals, but many are partially or completely synthetic. Natural drugs, especially herbs, are sometimes thought to be safer than synthesized drugs. This is a popular misconception. The safety of a drug is based on its pharmacodynamic (Chapter 2) and pharmacokinetic properties, not its source.

Aqueous and Lipid Solubility

One of the important properties of a drug is its solubility in various components of the body; for example, the aqueous extracellular and intracellular environments and the lipid membranes of cells. The aqueous solubility of a drug is often a function of the degree of ionization or polarity of the molecule. Water molecules behave as dipoles and are attracted to charged molecules, forming an aqueous shell around them. Conversely, the lipid solubility of a molecule is inversely proportional to its charge. Many drugs are weak bases or weak acids. For such molecules, the pH of the medium determines the fraction of ionized versus nonionized molecules. If the pK_a of the drug and the pH of the medium are known, the fraction of molecules in the ionized state can be predicted from the Henderson-Hasselbalch equation (Equation 1):

$$\text{Log (Protonated form/Unprotonated form)} = pK_a - pH \qquad (1)$$

In Equation 1, "protonated" means associated with a proton; that is, hydrogen ion. This form of the equation applies to both acids and bases. Weak bases are ionized and, therefore, more polar and more water soluble when they are protonated. In contrast, weak acids are not ionized when they are protonated, and so are less water-soluble. The following equations summarize these points for weak bases (Equation 2) and weak acids (Equation 3):

$$\text{Weak Base} \quad \underset{\text{(Protonated)}}{RNH_3^+} \Leftrightarrow \underset{\text{(Unprotonated)}}{RNH_2} + H^+ \quad (2)$$

$$\text{Weak Acid} \quad \underset{\text{(Protonated)}}{RCOOH} \Leftrightarrow \underset{\text{(Unprotonated)}}{RCOO^-} + H^+ \quad (3)$$

The Henderson-Hasselbalch relationship is clinically important in both the absorption of nutrients and drugs from the gastrointestinal (GI) lumen and excretion of metabolites by the kidneys. In the GI tract, weak acids can be passively absorbed in the stomach where the pH is around 1 to 3 and these acids are non-ionized (Figure 3–1a), but weak bases are very poorly absorbed here because they are ionized at this pH. In contrast, weak bases are normally passively absorbed in the small intestine where the pH is approximately 5 to 7 (Figure 3–1b). A similar mechanism can be applied in the kidney to trap bases and acids in the urine by acidifying or alkalinizing the urine, ionizing the molecules, and reducing their reabsorption.

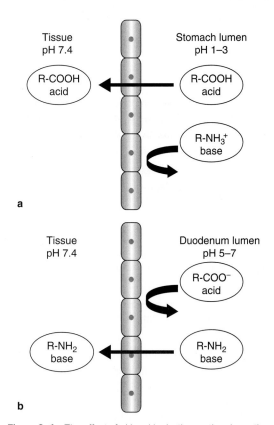

Figure 3–1. The effect of pH and ionization on the absorption of weak acids and bases in the gastrointestinal system. (a) The pH in the stomach allows for the passive absorption of acids, but not weak bases. (b) In contrast, the higher pH in the small intestine allows for the passive absorption of weak bases but not weak acids.

ROUTES OF ADMINISTRATION AND ABSORPTION

When drugs enter the body at sites remote from the target tissue or organ, they require transport by the circulation to the intended site of action. To enter the bloodstream, a drug must be absorbed from its site of administration. Absorption, therefore, describes the entry of the drug into the body. Not all routes of administration result in similar amounts of drug reaching the systemic circulation and the target tissue. In fact, for some drugs and certain routes, the amount absorbed may be only a small fraction of the amount administered. Thus, the rate and efficiency of a drug's absorption differ depending on a drug's route of administration. The two main routes of administration of drugs are enteral and parenteral administration. Enteral routes involve the GI system for administration of the drug. Parenteral routes are all those routes of absorption not associated with the GI system and use the vasculature, musculoskeletal, pulmonary, and integumental systems for sites of administration. Common routes of administration are listed in Table 3–1.

Enteral Administration

Enteral routes of administration include *oral, sublingual* or *buccal,* and *rectal.* Oral administration is defined as the swallowing of the drug and absorption from the GI lumen. The majority of drugs currently prescribed are intended for oral delivery. The oral route offers maximum convenience and is used when chronic drug treatment is required. Absorption using the oral route may be slower and less complete than when some parenteral routes are used. Additionally, when the drug is administered orally and absorbed from the stomach and intestine all of the drug must pass through the liver prior to entering the systemic circulation. As described below,

Table 3–1.	Routes of administration, general characteristics, and bioavailability	
Route	**Characteristics**	**Bioavailability (%)**
Enteral		
PO	Most convenient; first-pass effect may be significant	5 to <100
Sublingual/buccal	Avoids first-pass effect	75 to <100
PR	Less first-pass effect than oral	30 to <100
Parenteral		
IV	Most rapid onset	100 (by definition)
IM	Large volumes often feasible; may be painful	75 to ≤100
SC	Smaller volumes than IM; may be painful	75 to ≤100
Inhalation	Often very rapid onset	5 to <100
Transdermal	Usually very slow absorption; used for lack of first-pass effect; prolonged duration of action	80 to ≤100

PO = oral; PR = rectal; IV = intravenous; IM = intramuscular; SC = subcutaneous.

the liver may transform the drug into an inactive form prior to entering the systemic circulation. This effect of the liver on oral administration of a drug is known as the *first-pass effect*. All parenteral routes avoid the first-pass effect.

The buccal (administration into the pouch between the gums and cheek) and sublingual (administration under the tongue) delivery routes are unusual in that they allow direct absorption of the drug into the systemic circulation without a first-pass effect. This process may be fast or slow depending on the physical formulation of the product. The sublingual route offers the same features as the buccal route. The sublingual and buccal administration routes are utilized clinically for nitroglycerin and several other therapeutic agents. In nicotine users, smokeless tobacco is also placed in the buccal space.

The rectal route also offers partial avoidance of the first-pass effect, although not as completely as the sublingual or buccal routes. Rectal formulations are usually prescribed as suppositories and inserted into the lower rectum, but tend to migrate upward into the upper rectum. The absorption from this higher location results in the drug undergoing the same bioavailability limitations as drugs administered orally. Larger amounts of drug and drugs with unpleasant tastes are better administered rectally than by the buccal or sublingual routes. Some drugs administered rectally may cause significant irritation.

Parenteral Administration

Vascular administration includes the *intravenous* and *intra-arterial* routes. The intravenous route offers instantaneous and complete absorption. This route is potentially more dangerous though because of the high blood levels reached if administration is too rapid. Intra-arterial routes are used less frequently, and are designed to administer a drug to a specific organ or tissue.

Another parenteral route is into the musculoskeletal system, almost always via *intramuscular* injection. Absorption from an intramuscular injection site is often faster with a higher bioavailability than oral administration. Large volumes, such as 5 mL into each buttock, may be administered if the drug is not too irritating. Some drugs may not be administered via this route because of localized adverse events at the site of injection. Parenteral anticoagulants, such as heparin, may cause a hematoma when the drug is injected into the musculature. In contrast, *intra-articular* administration is utilized to achieve high local concentrations of drug in the joint space in conditions such as arthritis or joint infection. Absorption from joints into the blood is usually slow.

Administration into the pulmonary system includes the intranasal and *inhalation* routes. This administration may be for localized or systemic effects. Intranasal administration of nasal decongestants is intended for localized effects in patients with colds or rhinoconjunctivitis. Similarly, inhalation of bronchodilators and steroidal anti-inflammatory drugs is intended for localized effects in the pulmonary airways in patients with asthma or chronic obstructive pulmonary disease. Systemic delivery may also be achieved from these administration sites. Calcitonin and cocaine may be delivered systemically when administered intranasally. Similarly, systemic delivery of nicotine occurs rapidly after inhalation of tobacco smoke.

The skin may also be used to administer drugs. If the intended target tissue is localized to the skin, then administration is *cutaneous*. If the intended target tissue is deeper than the skin or the drug is applied to the skin with the intent of systemic effects, then administration is *transdermal*. Physical therapists utilize transdermal routes to (in theory) deliver anti-inflammatory and analgesic drugs locally to subcutaneous tissues. To enhance the percutaneous delivery of these drugs, mechanical energy (i.e., *phonophoresis*) or direct electrical current (i.e., *iontophoresis*) can be employed. Some controlled clinical investigations report positive outcomes with these administration routes. However, the pharmacokinetic parameters involved in phonophoresis and iontophoresis, such as direct depth of tissue penetration by the drug at the application site, are still under investigation. In *subcutaneous* administration, the drug is injected under the skin, and is intended for systemic delivery. Insulin is the drug most commonly delivered via subcutaneous injection. For all routes of administration involving the skin, absorption usually occurs slowly.

Other administration routes include localized delivery for the ocular or vaginal surfaces and injections into specific compartments such as the intrathecal space surrounding the spinal cord.

Several factors influence absorption from the delivery site and the clinical effect of the drug. The first is blood flow to the site. High blood flow rapidly distributes the drug away from that application site and maintains a high drug depot to blood concentration gradient. The concentration of the drug at the site of administration is also important in determining the gradient between the depot and the blood. (See Box 3–1: Fick's Law of Diffusion).

Box 3–1: Fick's Law of Diffusion

Diffusion is a major determinant of the rate of absorption across a barrier such as the cell membrane, the epidermis, or vascular wall. Fick's law predicts that the rate of movement of molecules (Diffusion Rate) across a barrier is directly proportionate to the concentration gradient ($C_1 - C_2$), the permeability coefficient for the molecule, and the area of diffusion; and inversely proportional to the thickness of the barrier (Equation 4).

This relationship quantifies the observation that drug absorption is faster from organs with large surface areas such as the small intestine compared to organs with smaller surface areas such as the stomach. Furthermore, drug absorption is faster from organs with thin membrane barriers such as the lung compared to those with thick barriers such as the skin.

$$\text{Diffusion Rate} = (C_1 - C_2) \times (\text{Permeability coefficient/Thickness}) \times \text{Area} \qquad (4)$$

▉ DISTRIBUTION

Most drugs must move from a site of administration to a distant target tissue. This movement of the drug in the body is distribution. In order for a drug to be distributed, it must travel through barriers such as capillary walls and cell membranes. This movement within and between biologic compartments is called permeation.

Permeation

Permeation may involve several different processes including diffusion, specific transport carriers, and endocytosis along with exocytosis. Permeation of drugs by diffusion occurs in both aqueous and lipid environments. Other drugs require transport carriers or endocytosis and exocytosis to reach targeted tissues and organs. In the latter case, these drugs may be too large or too lipid insoluble otherwise to reach tissue and organ targets.

Diffusion

Diffusion involves the passive movement of molecules from an area of greater concentration to an area of lower concentration. The magnitude of this diffusion process is predicted by Fick's law (see Box 3–1: Fick's Law of Diffusion). Diffusion may occur in both an aqueous environment or a lipid or hydrophobic environment. Aqueous diffusion takes place through the watery extracellular and intracellular spaces. For example, the membranes of most capillaries have small water-filled pores that permit the aqueous diffusion of molecules up to the size of small proteins between the blood and the extravascular space. Lipid diffusion is involved in the movement of molecules through membranes and other lipid structures.

Transport Carriers

A large number of drugs are transported across barriers by carrier molecules that move similar endogenous substances. In general, these carriers are proteins and may be specific or may transport a wide variety of compounds. Examples of the former include the amino acid carriers in the blood-brain barrier. Examples of the latter include nonspecific acid and base transporters in the renal tubule. Many neoplastic cells are capable of transporting chemotherapeutic drugs

out of these cells via such carriers, thereby achieving considerable resistance to treatment. Unlike aqueous and lipid diffusion, carrier transport is not governed by Fick's law and is capacity limited. These carriers may use several different transport mechanisms. The first is *active transport* that requires the dephosphorylation of adenosine triphosphate to adenosine diphosphate. This type of transport carrier may move a molecule against its diffusion gradient (from an area of lower concentration to one of higher concentration). This mechanism is used to transport sodium from the inside of a cell to the outside of a cell (the sodium pump). Alternatively, *facilitated diffusion* transports molecules *down* a diffusion gradient. This mechanism allows the permeation of polar molecules across lipid barriers, such as cell membranes, that would otherwise occur at an extremely slow rate. Transport of amino acids from the GI lumen into epithelial cells lining the lumen utilizes this technique.

Endocytosis and Exocytosis

Endocytosis, sometimes referred to as pinocytosis, occurs through binding of the permeating molecules to specialized receptors on cell membranes. Following binding, the cell membrane subsequently internalizes the molecule by infolding of that area of the membrane. The contents of the resulting intracellular vesicle are subsequently released into the cytoplasm of the cell. Endocytosis permits very large or very lipid-insoluble chemicals to enter cells. For example, large molecules such as peptides may enter cells by this mechanism. Smaller but highly polar substances such as vitamin B_{12} and iron combine with special proteins—intrinsic factor with B_{12} and transferrin with iron—and the complexes enter cells. Exocytosis is the reverse process; that is, the expulsion of membrane-encapsulated material from cells into the extracellular space.

Volume of Distribution (V_D)

When determining the distribution of drugs, the body is assumed to represent one or more physical volumes in which the drugs are sequestered, separated by barriers. Specific variables may be used to predict these volumes of distribution.

Table 3–2.	Physical volumes in liters (L) of some body compartments into which drugs may be distributed

Compartment and Physical Volume
Water
Total body water (42 L)[1]
Extracellular water (14 L)
Blood (5.6 L)
Plasma (2.8 L)
Fat (14.0–24.5 L)
Bone (4.9 L)

[1]An average figure for a 70-kg individual. Total body water in a young lean man weighing 70 kg might be 49 L; in an obese 70-kg woman, 35 L.

Often the distribution of a drug is not homogenous throughout the body, and the drug may concentrate in one or more tissues (e.g., blood, fat, bone). These tissues are described as "physical compartments" and the volumes for them can be defined (Table 3–2). However, as noted, many drugs do *not* distribute equally in all compartments. Therefore, we say that drugs have an *apparent* (i.e., not equivalent to the physical size) volume of distribution (V_d). The V_d relates the amount of drug in the body to the plasma concentration (Equation 5):

$$V_d = \text{Amount in body/Plasma concentration} \quad (5)$$

Equation 5 is graphically described in Figure 3–2, and examples of drugs and their apparent V_d are presented in Table 3–3. The calculated parameter for the apparent V_d has no direct physical equivalent. If a drug is avidly bound in peripheral tissues, its concentration in plasma may drop to very low values even though the total amount in the body is large. As a result, the calculated volume of distribution may greatly exceed the total volume of the body.

Determinants of V_d
The distribution of drugs to tissues varies and is dependent upon multiple variables including organ mass, blood flow, solubility of the drug, intravascular and extravascular binding, and comorbidities. The size of the organ determines the concentration gradient between blood and the organ. For example, skeletal muscle can take up a large amount of drug because the concentration in the muscle tissue remains low, and the blood to tissue gradient high. This gradient continues even after relatively large amounts of drug have been transferred because skeletal muscle is a very large organ. In contrast, because the brain is smaller, distribution of a smaller amount of drug into it will raise the tissue concentration and reduce the blood to tissue concentration gradient to zero.

Blood flow to the tissue is an important determinant of the *rate* of uptake, although blood flow may not affect the steady-state amount of drug in the tissue. As a result, well-perfused tissues such as the brain, heart, kidneys, and splanchnic organs, will often achieve high tissue concentrations sooner than poorly perfused tissues such as fat, cartilage, and bone. If the drug is rapidly eliminated, the concentration in poorly perfused tissues may never rise significantly.

The solubility of a drug in tissue influences its concentration in the extracellular fluid surrounding the blood vessels. If the drug is very soluble in the cells, the concentration in the perivascular extracellular space will be lower and diffusion from the vessel into the extravascular tissue space will be facilitated. Some organs, including the brain, have high lipid content and thus dissolve a high concentration of lipid-soluble agents. As a result, some psychotropic drugs such as amitriptyline or fluoxetine will transfer out of the blood and into the brain tissue more rapidly and to a greater extent than a drug with a low lipid solubility (Table 3–3).

Binding of a drug to macromolecules in the blood or a tissue compartment will tend to increase the drug's concentration in that compartment. Warfarin is strongly bound to plasma albumin, which restricts the diffusion of warfarin out of the vascular compartment (Table 3–3). Conversely, chloroquine is strongly bound to tissue proteins, which results in a marked reduction in the plasma concentration of chloroquine. As a result, warfarin has a low V_d, whereas chloroquine has a very high V_d (Table 3–3).

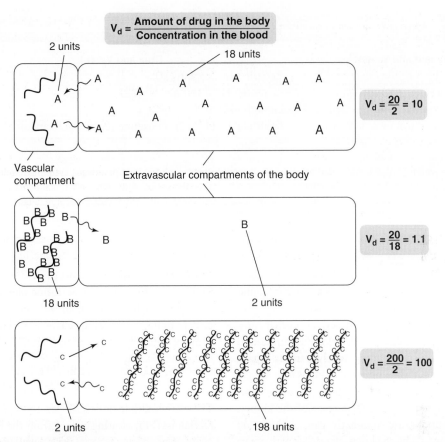

$$V_d = \frac{\text{Amount of drug in the body}}{\text{Concentration in the blood}}$$

Figure 3–2. Effect of drug binding on the apparent volume of distribution. Drug A does not bind to macromolecules (heavy wavy lines) in the vascular or the extravascular compartments of the hypothetical organism in the diagram. Drug A diffuses freely between the two compartments. With 20 units of the drug in the body, the steady-state distribution leaves a blood concentration of 2 units. Drug B, on the other hand, binds avidly to proteins in the blood. Drug B's diffusion is much more limited. At equilibrium, only 2 units of the total have diffused into the extravascular volume, leaving 18 units still in the blood. In each case, the total amount of drug in the body is the same (20 units), but the apparent volume of distribution is very different. Drug C is avidly bound to molecules in peripheral tissues, so that a larger total dose (200 units) is required to achieve measurable plasma concentrations. At equilibrium, 198 units are found in the peripheral tissues and only 2 in the plasma, so that the calculated volume of distribution is greater than the physical volume of the system.

The V_d of drugs may also be altered by comorbidities. Thus, the V_d of drugs that are normally bound to plasma proteins such as albumin may be increased by liver disease owing to reduced albumin synthesis, and by kidney disease through urinary protein loss.

ELIMINATION

Along with the dosage, the rate of elimination determines the duration of action for most drugs. Therefore, knowledge of the time course of the concentration of the drug in plasma is important in predicting the

Table 3–3.   **Apparent volumes of distributions (V$_d$) for several drugs**

Compartment and Volume[1]	Drug and V$_d$[2] (L)
Blood (5.6 L)	Heparin (4), warfarin (10)
Extracellular water (10–20 L)	Ibuprofen (11), gentamicin (22)
Total body water (22–42 L)	Lithium (46), ethanol (42)
Concentrated outside vasculature[2]	Amitriptyline (1,050), fluoxetine (2,450), chloroquine (13,755)

[1]All volumes based on a 70-kg individual.
[2]Many drugs with high V$_d$ are often lipid soluble and concentrate into both the central nervous system and adipose tissue. Chloroquine is the exception above, which concentrates in the skeletal muscles. Although the V$_d$ documents the concentration of the drug outside of the vasculature, it does not allow determination into which tissue the drug is being sequestered.

intensity and duration of effect. Elimination results in the disappearance of the biologically active compound from the body by metabolism or excretion.

Elimination may occur by several mechanisms. Biotransformation (discussed later) of the compound may render it inactive. Alternatively, various organs such as the kidney, skin, GI tract, or lungs may excrete the active compound out of the body. For most compounds, excretion is primarily by way of the kidney. Major exceptions are anesthetic gases, which are excreted primarily by the lungs. For drugs with active metabolites, such as diazepam, elimination of the parent molecule by biotransformation is not synonymous with termination of action. For drugs that are not metabolized, excretion is the mode of elimination. A small number of drugs combine irreversibly with their receptors, so that disappearance from the bloodstream is not equivalent to cessation of drug's action. For example, aspirin is an irreversible inhibitor of cyclooxygenase. Even after the drug is eliminated from the blood, the receptors that were bound while the drug was circulating are still inactivated.

Clearance (CL)

Elimination of a drug is conveniently expressed as its clearance. Clearance is the ratio of the rate of disappearance of the active molecule from the plasma to the plasma concentration. Clearance is dependent upon the extraction ratio ($[C_i - C_o]/C_i$) and the blood flow (Q).

The extraction ratio represents the ability of an organ to remove a drug from the perfusing blood during its passage through the organ, and is expressed as a percentage or fraction. Clearance is expressed in Equation 6, and graphically presented in (Figure 3–3).

$$CL = \frac{\text{Rate of drug elimination}}{\text{Plasma drug concentration}} \qquad (6)$$

There are multiple organs of clearance, and multiple mechanisms for clearing a drug from the blood. The major organs of clearance are the kidney, liver, lung, and

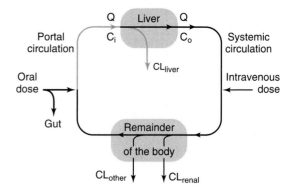

Figure 3–3. The principles of organ extraction (Clearance; CL) effect are illustrated. The volume of blood cleared of drug from the circulation by the liver (CL$_{liver}$) is proportionate to blood flow (Q) times the difference between drug concentration entering (C_i) and leaving (C_o) the liver. Part of the administered oral dose is lost to metabolism in the gut and the liver before it enters the systemic circulation: this is the first-pass effect.

GI tract, although all tissues have some capacity to clear drugs. Mechanisms of clearance include extraction and binding by the tissue, metabolism of the drug to an inactive metabolite as in the liver, or excretion of the active molecule or metabolite as in the kidney. As shown in Figure 3–3, following oral administration, the drug must pass through the GI mucosa and liver prior to entering the systemic circulation. A portion of the drug dose may be extracted and metabolized at these locations prior to reaching the systemic circulation. Drugs administered parenterally also undergo hepatic and renal clearance. After steady-state concentration in plasma has been achieved, the extraction ratio is one measure of the elimination of the drug by that organ.

The magnitudes of clearance for different drugs range from a small fraction of the blood flow to a maximum of the total blood flow to the organ of elimination. Clearance depends on the drug and the condition of the organs of elimination in the patient. The clearance of a drug that is very effectively extracted by an organ is often flow limited; that is, the blood is completely cleared of the drug as it passes through the organ. For such a drug, the total clearance from the body is a function of, and is limited to, the blood flow through the eliminating organ.

Elimination Kinetics

Elimination of drugs is conveniently described as either first-order or zero-order kinetics. The term *first-order elimination* implies that the rate of elimination is proportional to the concentration. That is, the higher the concentration, the greater the amount of drug eliminated per unit time. The result is that the drug's concentration in plasma decreases exponentially with time (Figure 3–4a). Drugs with first-order elimination have a characteristic half-life of elimination (discussed below) that is constant regardless of the amount of drug in the body. The concentration of such a drug in the blood will decrease by 50% for every half-life. Most drugs in clinical use demonstrate first-order kinetics.

The term *zero-order elimination* implies that the rate of elimination is constant regardless of the drug's concentration (Figure 3–4b). This occurs with drugs that saturate their elimination mechanisms at

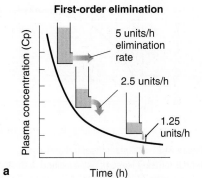

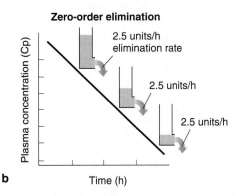

Figure 3–4. Comparison of first-order and zero-order elimination. For drugs with first-order kinetics (a), rate of elimination is proportionate to concentration. First-order elimination is the more common process. In the case of zero-order elimination (b), the rate is constant and independent of concentration.

concentrations of clinical interest. As a result, the concentrations of these drugs in plasma decrease in a linear fashion over time. This is typical of ethanol over most of its plasma concentration range, and of phenytoin and aspirin at high therapeutic or toxic concentrations.

Half-Life

Half-life ($t_{1/2}$) is a parameter determined by the drug's volume of distribution and clearance. Half-life can be determined graphically from a plot of the blood level versus time for a drug (Figure 3–5), or calculated (Equation 7):

$$t_{1/2} = 0.7 \times V_d/CL \qquad (7)$$

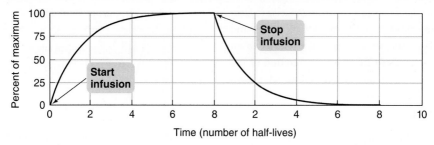

Figure 3–5. Plasma concentration (plotted as percentage of maximum) of a drug given by constant intravenous infusion for eight half-lives and then stopped. The concentration rises smoothly with time and always reaches 50% of steady state after one half-life, 75% after two half-lives, 87.5% after three half-lives, and so on. The decline in concentration after stopping drug administration follows the same type of curve: 50% is left after one half-life, 25% after two half-lives, and so on. The asymptotic approach to steady state on both increasing and decreasing limbs of the curve is characteristic of drugs following first-order kinetics.

One must know both primary variables, V_d and CL, to predict changes in half-life. Disease, age, and other variables usually alter the clearance of a drug much more than they alter its volume of distribution. However, if the volume of distribution decreases at the same time as the clearance, the half-life of a drug may not change. The half-life also determines the rate at which blood concentration rises during a constant infusion and falls after administration is stopped (Figure 3–5). In general, during an infusion, plasma levels of the drug will reach a plateau and equilibrium will be established after four to five half-lives. At this time, the rate of administration and the rate of elimination are equal. Conversely, following the termination of the infusion, the loss of the drug is such that, with first-order elimination kinetics, greater than 95% of the drug will be lost after five half-lives. The concept of a half-life for a drug is essential in developing pharmacokinetic models used to estimate the changes in plasma concentration of a drug over time (see Box 3–2: Pharmacokinetic Models).

Box 3–2: Pharmacokinetic Models

The elimination of drugs from the body may be estimated based on a compartmental model. A model may be based on an assumption of equal distribution of the drug throughout all tissues with the body acting as a single compartment. Alternatively, the drug can be modeled as sequestered in two or more tissues with the body acting as a multicompartment model. A few drugs may behave as if they are distributed to only one compartment, especially if they are restricted to the vascular compartment. Others have more complex distributions that require more than two compartments for construction of accurate mathematical models. After absorption into the circulation, many drugs undergo an early distribution phase followed by a slower elimination phase. Mathematically, this behavior can be modeled by means of a "two-compartment model" (Figure 3–6). Each phase is associated with a characteristic half-life: $t_{1/2\alpha}$ for the distribution phase and $t_{1/2\beta}$ for the elimination phase. When the concentration is plotted on a logarithmic axis, the elimination phase for a first-order drug is a straight line.

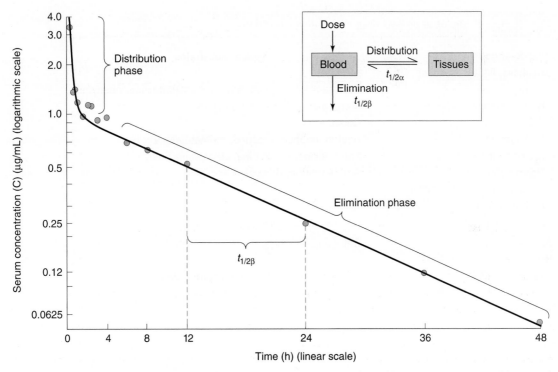

Figure 3–6. Serum concentration-time curve after administration of chlordiazepoxide as an intravenous bolus. The experimental data are plotted on a semilogarithmic scale as filled circles. This drug follows first-order kinetics and appears to occupy two compartments. The initial curvilinear portion of the data represents the distribution phase $t_{(1/2\alpha)}$, with drug equilibrating between the blood compartment and the tissue compartment. The linear portion of the curve represents drug elimination. The elimination half-life ($t_{1/2\beta}$) can be extracted graphically as shown by measuring the time between any two plasma concentration points on the elimination phase that differ by twofold. (Reproduced and modified, with permission, from Greenblatt DJ, Koch-Weser J: Drug therapy: Clinical pharmacokinetics. *N Engl J Med* 1975;293:702.)

BIOTRANSFORMATION

All organisms are exposed to foreign chemical compounds in the air, water, and food. Many tissues act as portals for entry of external molecules into the body. To ensure elimination of pharmacologically active foreign chemicals as well as to terminate the action of many endogenous substances, metabolic pathways are available to alter their activity and increase their susceptibility to excretion. Biotransformation is a metabolic mechanism used to decrease the activity of exogenous and endogenous chemical compounds. The products of biotransformation are therefore called *metabolites*. Most drugs are relatively lipid soluble, a characteristic favorable to absorption across membranes.

This same property would result in very slow removal from the body because the molecule would also be readily reabsorbed from the urine in the renal tubule. The body hastens excretion by transforming many drugs to less lipid-soluble and more readily excreted forms.

Sites of Drug Biotransformation

The most important organ for biotransformation is the liver. The kidneys also play an important role in the metabolism of some drugs. A few drugs, such as esters, are metabolized in many tissues because of the broad distribution of esterases responsible for the metabolism of these molecules.

Table 3–4.	Examples of phase I drug-metabolizing reactions
Reaction Type	**Typical Substrates**
Oxidations, P450 dependent	
Hydroxylation	Barbiturates, amphetamines, phenylbutazone, phenytoin
N-Dealkylation	Morphine, caffeine, theophylline
O-Dealkylation	Codeine
N-Oxidation	Acetaminophen, nicotine, methaqualone
S-Oxidation	Thioridazine, cimetidine, chlorpromazine
Deamination	Amphetamine, diazepam
Oxidations, P450 independent	
Amine oxidation	Epinephrine
Dehydrogenation	Ethanol, chloral hydrate
Reductions	Chloramphenicol, clonazepam, dantrolene, naloxone
Hydrolyses	
Esters	Procaine, succinylcholine, aspirin, clofibrate
Amides	Procainamide, lidocaine, indomethacin

Types of Biotransformation Reactions

Biotransformation may be divided into phase I and phase II reactions. Phase I reactions include oxidation, reduction, deamination, and hydrolysis (Table 3–4). Oxidation is mediated in part by the cytochrome P450 group of enzymes; also called mixed-function oxidases. Phase II reactions involve conjugation of hydrophilic subgroups to specific chemical structures (Table 3–5). These additions occur at hydroxyl (–OH), amine (–NH$_2$), and sulfhydryl (–SH) functions on the substrate molecule. The subgroups that are added include glucuronate, acetate, glutathione, glycine, sulfate, and methyl groups. Most of these subgroups are relatively polar, and increase the aqueous solubility of the metabolite compared to the original drug molecule.

Table 3–5.	Examples of phase II drug-metabolizing reactions
Reaction Type	**Typical Drug Substrates**
Glucuronidation	Acetaminophen, morphine, diazepam, sulfathiazole, digoxin, digitoxin
Acetylation	Sulfonamides, isoniazid, clonazepam, mescaline, dapsone
Glutathione conjugation	Ethacrynic acid, reactive phase I metabolite of acetaminophen
Glycine conjugation	Salicylic acid, nicotinic acid (niacin), deoxycholic acid
Sulfate conjugation	Acetaminophen, methyldopa, estrone
Methylation	Epinephrine, norepinephrine, dopamine, histamine

Determinants of Biotransformation Rate

The rate of biotransformation of a drug may vary markedly among different individuals. This variation is most often due to comorbidities, genetic differences, or drug-drug interactions. For a few drugs, age or disease-related differences in drug metabolism are significant. Hepatic metabolism often decreases with age and liver disease. Gender is important for only a few drugs such as ethanol. (First-pass metabolism of alcohol is lower in women than in men.) Because the rate of biotransformation is often the primary determinant of clearance, variations in drug metabolism must be considered carefully when evaluating a patient and designing their rehabilitation treatment plan. A few examples of genetic-based effects and drug-drug interactions on biotransformation are discussed below.

Genetics

Several drug-metabolizing systems have been shown to differ among families or populations in genetically determined ways. These include hydrolysis of esters, acetylation of amines, and some oxidation reactions.

Succinylcholine is an ester that is metabolized by plasma cholinesterase (pseudocholinesterase or butyrylcholinesterase). In most individuals, this process occurs very rapidly, and a single dose of this neuromuscular blocking drug has a duration of action of about 5 minutes. Approximately 1 person in 2,500 has an abnormal form of this enzyme that metabolizes succinylcholine and similar esters much more slowly. In such individuals, the neuromuscular paralysis produced by a single dose of succinylcholine may last many hours and reduce functional capacity (e.g., ability to breathe) for that period.

The dosage of certain amines, such as isoniazid (used for tuberculosis) and procainamide (used for arrhythmias) is often higher in Native American and Asian individuals due to their higher rates of acetylation. Similarly, the rate of oxidation of metoprolol and some tricyclic antidepressants by certain P450 isozymes has also been shown to be genetically determined.

Drug-Drug Interactions

Coadministration of certain agents may alter the disposition of many drugs. For example, smoking is a common cause of enzyme induction in the liver and lung, and may increase the metabolism of some drugs. Enzyme induction usually results from increased synthesis of cytochrome P450-dependent drug-oxidizing enzymes in the liver. Many isozymes of the P450 family exist and inducers selectively increase subgroups of these isozymes. Common inducers of a few of these isozymes and the drugs whose metabolism is increased are listed in Table 3–6. Several days are usually required to reach maximum induction. A similar amount of time is required to return these metabolizing enzymes to normal levels after withdrawal of the inducer. The most common inducers of drug metabolism that are involved in serious drug interactions are carbamazepine, phenobarbital, phenytoin, and rifampin. In patients comedicated with these and other pharmacologic inducing agents, the half-life of many drugs may be decreased.

In contrast, some drugs inhibit their own metabolism and the metabolism of other agents. Common inhibitors and the drugs whose metabolism is diminished are listed in Table 3–7. The inhibitors of drug metabolism most commonly involved in serious drug interactions are amiodarone, cimetidine, furanocoumarins (present in grapefruit juice), ketoconazole and related antifungal agents, and the human immunodeficiency virus (HIV) protease inhibitor ritonavir.

Suicide inhibitors are drugs that are metabolized to products that irreversibly inhibit the metabolizing enzyme. Such agents include ethinyl estradiol, spironolactone, secobarbital, allopurinol, fluroxene, and propylthiouracil. Metabolism may also be decreased by pharmacodynamic factors such as a reduction in blood flow to the metabolizing organ. For example, propranolol reduces hepatic blood flow.

Intestinal P-Glycoprotein Transporters

P-glycoproteins comprise a family of adenosine triphosphate (ATP)–dependent transporters that expel targeted molecules from the cytoplasm into the extracellular space. The P-glycoprotein transporters have been identified in the epithelium of the gastrointestinal tract, in the blood-brain barrier, and in cancer cells. These transporter proteins are especially important in decreasing absorption of drugs from the GI system by

Table 3–6. A partial list of drugs that significantly induce P450-mediated drug metabolism in humans

CYP Family Induced	Important Inducers	Drugs Whose Metabolism Is Induced
1A2	Benzo(a)pyrene (from tobacco smoke), carbamazepine, phenobarbital, rifampin, omeprazole	Acetaminophen, clozapine, haloperidol, theophylline, tricyclic antidepressants, (R)-warfarin
2C9	Barbiturates,[1] especially phenobarbital, phenytoin, primidone, rifampin	Barbiturates,[1] chloramphenicol, doxorubicin, ibuprofen, phenytoin, chlorpromazine, steroids, tolbutamide, (S)-warfarin
2C19	Carbamazepine, phenobarbital, phenytoin	Tricyclic antidepressants, phenytoin, topiramate, (R)-warfarin
2E1	Ethanol,[1] isoniazid	Acetaminophen, ethanol (minor), halothane
3A4	Barbiturates, carbamazepine, corticosteroids, efavirenz, phenytoin, rifampin, troglitazone	Antiarrhythmics, antidepressants, azole antifungals, benzodiazepines, calcium channel blockers, cyclosporine, delavirdine, doxorubicin, efavirenz, erythromycin, estrogens, HIV protease inhibitors, nefazodone, paclitaxel, proton pump inhibitors, HMG-CoA reductase inhibitors, rifabutin, rifampin, sildenafil, SSRIs, tamoxifen, trazodone, vinca anticancer agents

CYP = cytochrome P450; SSRIs = selective serotonin reuptake inhibitors.
[1]Substrates that also act as inducers.

transporting the drugs back into the GI lumen. In contrast, inhibitors of intestinal P-glycoprotein cause increased absorption and decreased fecal excretion of several drugs and mimic drugs that inhibit hepatic biotransformation. Verapamil and furanocoumarin are inhibitors of these transporters in the GI system. Important drugs that are normally expelled by these GI transporters include digoxin, cyclosporine, and saquinavir. Thus, P-glycoprotein inhibitors may result in toxic plasma concentrations of the latter drugs when given at normally nontoxic dosages.

Biotransformation Metabolites

Metabolism is often thought to result in an inactive metabolite. For example, some drugs, when given orally, are metabolized before they enter the systemic circulation. The actions of many drugs such as the sympathomimetics and phenothiazines are terminated before they are excreted because they are metabolized to biologically inactive derivatives.

Other effects of biotransformation are also important. Alternative outcomes include conversion of an inactive compound, a prodrug, into an active form. Dexamethasone phosphate is inactive as administered, and must be metabolized in the body to become active. Dexamethasone phosphate can be administered transdermally by iontophoresis from the negative electrode because the drug is an anion and negatively charged at pH 7. The phosphorylated prodrug is then metabolized in the body to dexamethasone, the active form of the drug. Metabolites of the biotransformation process may also be active. Several benzodiazepines have bioactive

Table 3–7.	A partial list of drugs that significantly inhibit P450-mediated drug metabolism in humans	
CYP Family Induced	**Inhibitor**	**Drugs Whose Metabolism Is Inhibited**
1A2	Cimetidine, fluoroquinolones, grapefruit juice, macrolides, isoniazid, zileuton	Acetaminophen, clozapine, haloperidol, theophylline, tricyclic antidepressants, (R)-warfarin
2C9	Amiodarone, chloramphenicol,[1] cimetidine, isoniazid, metronidazole, SSRIs, zafirlukast	Barbiturates, chloramphenicol, doxorubicin, ibuprofen, phenytoin, chlorpromazine, steroids, tolbutamide, (S)-warfarin
2C19	Omeprazole, SSRIs	Phenytoin, topiramate, (R)-warfarin
2D6	Amiodarone, cimetidine, quinidine, SSRIs	Antidepressants, flecainide, lidocaine, mexiletine, opioids
3A4	Amiodarone, azole antifungals, cimetidine, clarithromycin, cyclosporine,[1] erythromycin,[1] fluoroquinolones, grapefruit juice, HIV protease inhibitors[1] (e.g., ritonavir), metronidazole, quinine, SSRIs, tacrolimus	Antiarrhythmics, antidepressants, azole antifungals, benzodiazepines, calcium channel blockers, cyclosporine, delavirdine, doxorubicin, efavirenz, erythromycin, estrogens, HIV protease inhibitors, nefazodone, paclitaxel, proton pump inhibitors, HMG-CoA reductase inhibitors, rifabutin, rifampin, sildenafil, SSRIs, tamoxifen, trazodone, vinca anticancer agents

CYP = cytochrome P450; SSRIs = selective serotonin reuptake inhibitors; HMG-CoA = 3-hydroxy-methylglutaryl coenzyme A.
[1]Substrates that also act as inhibitors.

metabolites. Finally, the body does not modify some drugs such as lithium. They continue to act until they are excreted.

Toxic Biotransformation

Metabolites resulting from the biotransformation process may also be toxic. Methanol is metabolized to metabolites such as formaldehyde and formic acid. These metabolites are toxic to multiple organs. Acetaminophen when taken in large overdoses may also result in toxic metabolites. At normal dosage, acetaminophen is conjugated to harmless glucuronide and sulfate metabolites by phase II reactions. If a large overdose is taken, a P450-dependent phase I reaction converts some of the drug to a reactive metabolite. The reactive metabolite may combine with essential hepatic cell proteins, resulting in cell death. In severe liver disease, stores of phase II conjugates may be depleted, making phase I reactions more prominent, and the patient more susceptible to hepatic toxicity with near-normal doses of acetaminophen. Also, enzyme inducers such as ethanol may increase acetaminophen toxicity because they increase phase I metabolism compared to phase II metabolism, resulting in increased production of the reactive acetaminophen metabolites.

BIOAVAILABILITY

The bioavailability of a drug is the fraction (F) of the administered dose that reaches the systemic circulation, and is specific to both the drug and the route of administration (Table 3–1). Bioavailability is defined as unity (or 100%) in the case of intravenous administration. Bioavailability by other routes may be much lower. Mechanisms that account for reduced bioavailability include incomplete absorption from the site of administration, P-glycoprotein-mediated transport back into the lumen of the GI tract, binding in tissues prior to reaching the systemic circulation, or biotransformation at the application site or prior to entering the systemic circulation. The mechanism of reduced bioavailability following oral administration is the first-pass effect, and accounts for the fact that some drugs have low bioavailability when given orally. Even for drugs with equal bioavailabilities, entry into the systemic circulation occurs over varying periods of time depending on the drug formulation and other factors. To account for such factors, the concentration appearing in the plasma is integrated over time to obtain an integrated total area under the plasma concentration curve (AUC) (Figure 3–7). The AUC assists in determining the bioequivalence of different formulations of the drug.

DOSAGE REGIMENS

A dosage regimen is a plan for drug administration over a period of time. The regimen may be divided into *loading* and *maintenance* doses. Ideally, the dosing regimen is based on knowledge of the therapeutic window, discussed in Chapter 2, and the drug's clearance and volume of distribution. An appropriate dosage regimen results in the achievement of therapeutic levels of the drug in the blood while staying within the therapeutic window.

If the therapeutic concentration must be achieved rapidly and the volume of distribution is large, a large loading dose may be needed at the onset of therapy. The loading dose is a function of the volume of distribution for the drug (Equation 8):

$$\text{Loading Dose} = \frac{(V_d \times \text{Desired plasma concentration})}{\text{Bioavailability}} \tag{8}$$

Note that clearance does not enter into this computation. If the V_d is much larger than blood volume and the loading dose is very large, the dose should be given slowly to avoid plasma levels in the toxic dose range during the distribution phase.

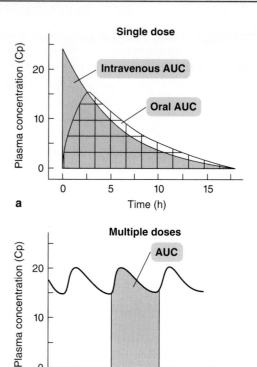

Figure 3–7. The area under the curve (AUC) is used to calculate the bioavailability of a drug. The AUC can be derived from either single-dose studies (panel a) or multiple-dose measurements (panel b). Bioavailability is calculated from $AUC_{(route)}/AUC_{(IV)}$.

During chronic therapy, maintenance dosing is required so that the rate of drug administration is equivalent to the rate of elimination; that is, steady state is maintained. Calculation of the maintenance dosage is a function of clearance (Equation 9).

$$\text{Maintenance Dosage} = \frac{(CL \times \text{Desired plasma concentration})}{\text{Bioavailability}} \tag{9}$$

Note that volume of distribution is not directly involved in the above calculation. The dosing rate computed for maintenance dosage is the average dose per unit time. For chronic therapy, oral administration is desirable. The number of doses to be given per day is usually determined by the half-life of the drug and the therapeutic window. To encourage adherence to the dosing regimen, doses should be given only once or a few times per day. If maintaining a concentration within the therapeutic window is important, either a larger dose may be given at long time intervals or smaller doses at more frequent intervals. If the therapeutic window is narrow, then smaller and more frequent doses must be administered to avoid adverse events.

Theoretical Dosing Regimen

Development of a dosing regimen is exemplified by the following hypothetical scenario, which involves both pharmacodynamics from Chapter 2 and the pharmacokinetic principles in this chapter. The medication for this example (theophylline) has a minimum therapeutic concentration range of 7 to 10 mg/L and a minimum toxic concentration range of 15 to 20 mg/L. The therapeutic window for a given patient might thus be fixed in the range of 7.5 to 15.0 mg/L (Figure 3–8). In Figure 3–8a, a comparison of three dosing regimens is presented: continuous intravenous (IV) infusion, three 224-mg doses at 8-hour intervals, and one 672-mg dose a day. Notice that the continuous infusion achieves the desired plasma concentration with minimal variation. This administration format is impractical for chronic therapy. The once-a-day dosage achieves the desired plasma concentration part of the time, but plasma concentrations spike into the toxic levels and increase the risk of adverse events. This regimen also results in plasma concentrations decreasing below the therapeutic window prior to the next dose. The dosage on an 8-hour interval also achieves the desired average plasma concentration. Furthermore, this plasma concentration is achieved with minimal time spent in either toxic or subtherapeutic ranges. Also note that the time to reach steady-state average plasma levels is approximately 4 to 5 half-lives for theophylline regardless of the frequency of administration. Patient compliance with regular dosing is a significant problem and affects all health-care professionals. Figure 3–8b and c examines the effects of noncompliance on systemic theophylline plasma concentrations. In Figure 3–8b, the patient missed the dose at the 72-hour time point. The plasma concentration continued to fall, and at the 80-hour time point (one half-life later) was 50% below the therapeutic window (at 4 mg/L). At that time, the patient decided to correct the error by taking two 8-hour doses together, a total of 448 mg. Now the systemic plasma concentration increased above the therapeutic window and into the toxic range at 19 mg/L, raising the risk of adverse events. Thus, maintaining regular dosing on a daily basis is required to achieve therapeutic benefits from the medication, and to avoid adverse events. Unfortunately, for some medications, the therapeutic and toxic concentrations vary so greatly among patients that predicting the therapeutic window in a given person is impossible. Such medications must be titrated individually in each patient.

▇ REHABILITATION FOCUS

The *effective* drug concentration is the concentration of a drug at the receptor site. This contrasts with the concentration of the drug in the blood, which is more readily measured. Except for topically applied agents, the effective concentration is usually proportional to the concentration of the drug in the plasma or whole blood. The plasma concentration is a function of the rate of input of the drug through absorption, the rate of distribution to the peripheral tissues including the target tissue, and the rate of elimination from the body. These are all functions of time; but if the delivery rate is known, the remaining processes are well described by V_d and CL. These parameters are unique for a particular drug in a particular patient, but have average values in large populations that can be used to predict drug concentrations. These pharmacokinetic parameters allow the calculation of loading and maintenance doses required for dosage regimens.

The physical therapist should understand that dosage regimens depend on the pharmacokinetics of the drug (discussed in this chapter), its pharmacodynamics (Chapter 2), and the individual patient's specific comorbidities. General guidelines for dosing regimens are available in the literature; however, renal disease or reduced cardiac output often decrease the clearance of drugs that depend on renal function. The decreased clearance will increase the half-life.

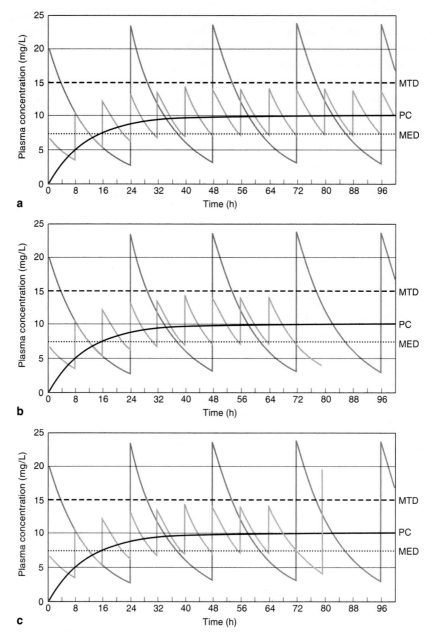

Figure 3–8. The therapeutic window for theophylline in a hypothetical patient, and the relationship between frequency of dosing, minimum effective dose (MED) (dotted line), and minimum toxic dose (MTD) (dashed line) (a). The MED in this patient was found to be 7.5 mg/L; the MTD was found to be 15 mg/L. The half-life of theophylline is approximately 8 hours in this patient. The desired steady-state plasma concentration (PC) was 10 mg/L. The smoothly rising solid black line represents the PC achieved with an intravenous infusion at 28 mg/h. The doses at 8-hour intervals (light gray) are 224 mg, and for 24-hour intervals are 672 mg (dark gray). To maintain the PC within the therapeutic window, the theophylline must be given at least once every half-life because the MED is half the MTD and the PC will decay by 50% in each half-life. In each of the three dosing regimens, the average steady-state PC is 10 mg/L. The effects of missing a maintenance dose (b) and subsequently taking a double 8-hour maintenance dose at the next dosing interval (c) are also presented.

Alteration of clearance by liver disease is less common but can occur, especially if the biotransformation of the drug is reduced. Impairment of hepatic clearance also occurs for high extraction drugs when liver blood flow is reduced, as in heart failure. When clearance of a drug is reduced by such conditions the dosage and possibly the frequency of dosing must be modified appropriately. The therapist should discuss with other health-care professionals whether these comorbidities and drug interactions may affect the dosing regimen and the rehabilitation treatment program for the patient. Finally, the therapist should remember that when a patient is either beginning a new drug or terminating a current drug, the risk of adverse events increases. The most important question to ask the patient is not "Did you take your medicine today?", but "Have you been taking your medicines as prescribed and are you taking any others, such as over-the-counter or herbal medications?".

REFERENCES

Benet LZ, Hoener B: Changes in plasma protein binding have little clinical relevance. *Clin Pharmacol Ther* 2002;71:115.

Evans WE, et al: Conventional compared with individualized chemotherapy for childhood acute lymphoblastic leukemia. *N Engl J Med* 1998;338:499.

Gilmore DA, et al: Age and gender influence the stereoselective pharmacokinetics of propranolol. *J Pharmacol Exp Ther* 1992;261:1181.

Guengerich FP: Role of cytochrome P450 enzymes in drug-drug interactions. *Adv Pharmacol* 1997;43:7.

Ingelman-Sundberg M: Pharmacogenetics: An opportunity for a safer and more efficient pharmacotherapy. *J Intern Med* 2001;250:186.

Kroemer HK, Klotz U: Glucuronidation of drugs: A reevaluation of the pharmacological significance of the conjugates and modulating factors. *Clin Pharmacokinet* 1992;23:292.

Meyer UA: Pharmacogenetics and adverse drug reactions. *Lancet* 2000;356:1667.

Thummel KE, Wilkinson GR: In vitro and in vivo drug interactions involving human CYP3A. *Annu Rev Pharmacol Toxicol* 1998;38:389.

Willson TM, Kliewer SA: PXR, CAR and drug metabolism. *Nat Rev Drug Discov* 2002;1:259.

Xu C, et al: CYP2A6 genetic variation and potential consequences. *Adv Drug Delivery Rev* 2002;54:1245.

Rehabilitation

Banga AK, Panus PC. Clinical applications of iontophoretic devices in rehabilitation medicine. *Crit Rev Phys Rehabil Med* 1998;10:147.

Byl NN. The use of ultrasound as an enhancer for transcutaneous drug delivery: Phonophoresis. *Phys Ther* 1995;75:539.

Henley EJ. Transcutaneous drug delivery: Iontophoresis, Phonophoresis. *Crit Rev Ther Drug Carr Syst* 1991;2:139.

Machet L, Boucaud A. Phonophoresis: Efficiency, mechanisms and skin tolerance. *Int J Pharm* 2002;243:1.

Panus PC, Banga AK. Iontophoresis devices: Clinical applications for topical delivery. *Int J Pharm Compound* 1997;1:420.

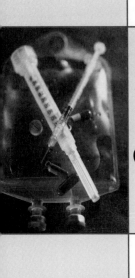

DRUGS AFFECTING THE CARDIOVASCULAR SYSTEM

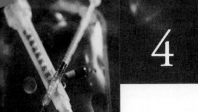

4

INTRODUCTION TO AUTONOMIC PHARMACOLOGY

The motor (efferent) portion of the nervous system can be divided into two major subdivisions: *autonomic* and *somatic.* The *autonomic nervous system* (ANS) is largely autonomous (independent) in that its activities are not under direct conscious control. The ANS is concerned primarily with visceral functions that are necessary for life. The somatic system is largely concerned with consciously controlled functions such as movement and posture. Both systems have important afferent (sensory) inputs that provide sensation and modify motor output through reflex arcs of varying size and complexity.

The nervous system has several properties in common with the endocrine system, which is the other major system for control of bodily functions. These properties include high-level integration in the brain, the ability to influence processes in distant regions of the body, and extensive use of negative feedback. Both systems use chemicals for the transmission of information. In the nervous system, chemical transmission occurs between nerve cells and between nerve cells and their effector cells. Chemical transmission takes place through the release of small amounts of transmitter substances from the nerve terminals into the synaptic space. The transmitter crosses the space by diffusion and activates or inhibits the postsynaptic cells by binding to a specialized receptor molecule.

Drugs that mimic or block the actions of chemical transmitters can selectively modify many autonomic functions. These functions involve a variety of effector tissues, including cardiac muscle, smooth muscle, vascular endothelium, exocrine glands, and presynaptic nerve terminals. Drugs affecting the autonomic nervous system are useful in many clinical conditions. Conversely, a very large number of drugs used for other purposes have unwanted effects on autonomic function.

ANATOMY OF THE AUTONOMIC NERVOUS SYSTEM

The autonomic nervous system lends itself to division on anatomic grounds into two major portions: the *sympathetic (thoracolumbar)* division and the *parasympathetic (craniosacral)* division (Figure 4–1). Both divisions originate in nuclei within the central nervous system and give rise to preganglionic efferent fibers that exit from the brain stem or spinal cord and terminate in motor ganglia. The sympathetic preganglionic fibers leave the central nervous system through the thoracic and lumbar spinal nerves. The parasympathetic preganglionic fibers leave the central nervous system through several of the cranial nerves and the third and fourth sacral spinal roots.

41

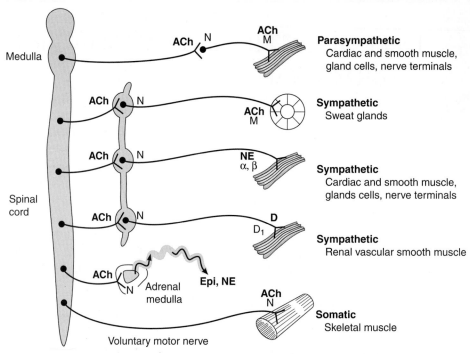

Figure 4–1. Schematic diagram comparing some anatomic and neurotransmitter features of autonomic and somatic motor nerves. Only the primary transmitter substances are shown. Parasympathetic ganglia are not shown as discrete structures because most are in or near the wall of the organ innervated. Note that some sympathetic postganglionic fibers release acetylcholine or dopamine rather than norepinephrine. The adrenal medulla, a modified sympathetic ganglion, receives sympathetic preganglionic fibers and releases mainly epinephrine and some norepinephrine into the blood. (ACh, acetylcholine; D, dopamine; Epi, epinephrine; NE, norepinephrine; N, nicotinic receptors; M, muscarinic receptors. See text.)

Sympathetic preganglionic fibers terminate in ganglia located in the paravertebral chains that lie on either side of the spinal column, or terminate in prevertebral ganglia, which lie in front of the aorta. From these ganglia, postganglionic sympathetic fibers traverse to the innervated tissues. The majority of parasympathetic preganglionic fibers terminate on ganglion cells in the walls of the organs innervated, others terminate in parasympathetic ganglia located outside the innervated organs.

In addition to these clearly defined peripheral motor portions of the autonomic nervous system, there are large numbers of afferent fibers that run from the periphery to integrating centers, including the enteric plexuses in the gut (Chapter 36), the autonomic ganglia, and the central nervous system. Many of the sensory neurons that end in the central nervous system terminate in the integrating centers of the hypothalamus and medulla and evoke reflex motor activity that is carried to the effector cells by the efferent fibers described above.

■ NEUROTRANSMITTER CHEMISTRY OF THE AUTONOMIC NERVOUS SYSTEM

An important traditional classification of autonomic nerves is based on the primary transmitter—acetylcholine or norepinephrine —that is released from the presynaptic terminal. A large number of peripheral autonomic nervous system fibers synthesize and release acetylcholine (Figure 4–1). These are *cholinergic* fibers, and they include all preganglionic efferent autonomic fibers. The somatic motor fibers to skeletal muscles are also cholinergic. Thus, almost all efferent fibers leaving the central nervous system are cholinergic. In addition, most parasympathetic postganglionic and a few sympathetic postganglionic fibers are cholinergic (Figure 4–1). A number of parasympathetic postganglionic neurons also utilize nitric oxide or peptides for transmission (Table 4–1).

Most sympathetic postganglionic fibers release norepinephrine (Figure 4–1). These are *noradrenergic*, and are often referred to as adrenergic fibers. A few sympathetic postganglionic fibers release acetylcholine. Dopamine is a very important transmitter in the central nervous system, and there is evidence that it is released by some peripheral sympathetic fibers in the cardiac, gastrointestinal, and renal systems. Adrenal medullary cells, which are embryologically analogous to postganglionic sympathetic neurons, release a mixture of epinephrine and norepinephrine.

Five key features of neurotransmitter function represent potential targets for pharmacologic therapy: synthesis, storage, release, activation of receptors, and termination of transmitter action.

Cholinergic Transmission

The terminals of cholinergic neurons contain large numbers of small membrane-bound vesicles concentrated near the synaptic portion of the cell membrane (Figure 4–2) as well as a smaller number of large dense-cored vesicles located farther from the synaptic membrane. The latter vesicles contain cotransmitters with or without acetylcholine (Table 4–1). Vesicles are initially synthesized in the neuron's soma and transported to the terminal. They may also be recycled several times within the terminal. Acetylcholine is synthesized in the cytoplasm from acetyl coenzyme A (CoA) and choline (Figure 4–2). The acetyl CoA is synthesized in the mitochondria and the choline is transported into the cell. Once synthesized, acetylcholine is transported from the cytoplasm into the vesicles. Acetylcholine synthesis is a rapid process capable of supporting a very high rate of transmitter release. Storage of acetylcholine is accomplished by the packaging of acetylcholine molecules, usually 1,000 to 50,000 molecules in each vesicle. Release of the transmitter is dependent on extracellular calcium, and occurs when an action potential reaches the terminal and triggers a sufficient influx of calcium ions. The increased intracellular Ca^{2+} concentration allows fusion of the vesicular membranes with the presynaptic terminal membrane. Fusion of the membranes results in release of the contents of the vesicle into the synaptic space. After release from the presynaptic terminal, acetylcholine molecules may bind to and activate an acetylcholine receptor. Eventually all of the acetylcholine released will diffuse within range of an acetylcholinesterase (AChE) molecule, which splits

Table 4–1.	Some of the transmitter substances found in the ANS
ACh	The primary transmitter at ANS ganglia, somatic neuromuscular junction, and at all postganglionic parasympathetic and limited sympathetic nerve endings.
NE	The primary transmitter at most postganglionic sympathetic nerve endings.
D	A possible postganglionic sympathetic transmitter in the renal blood vessels.
ATP	Inhibits release of ACh and NE release from ANS nerve endings.
NPY	A cotransmitter in many parasympathetic postganglionic neurons and sympathetic postganglionic noradrenergic vascular neurons. Causes long-lasting vasoconstriction.
NO	Probable transmitter for parasympathetic vasodilation.

ANS = autonomic nervous system; ACh = acetylcholine; NE = norepinephrine; D = dopamine; ATP = adenosine triphosphate; NPY = neuropeptide Y; NO = nitric oxide.

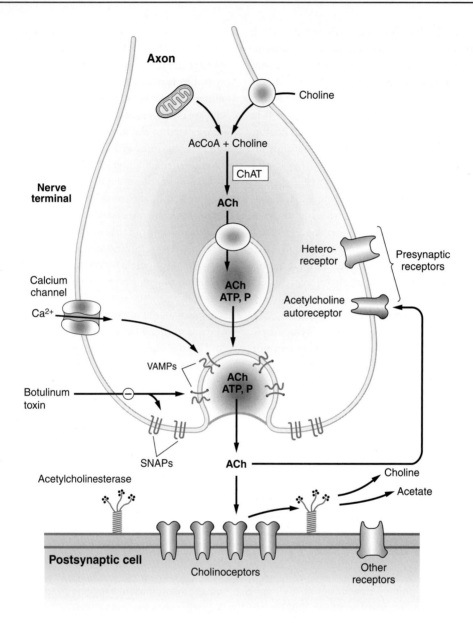

Figure 4–2. Schematic illustration of a generalized cholinergic junction with cholinergic receptors (cholinoceptors) in the postsynaptic membrane (not to scale). Choline is transported into the presynaptic nerve terminal by a sodium-dependent choline transporter. Acetylcholine (ACh) is synthesized from acetyl coenzyme A (AcCoA) and choline by choline acetyltransferase (ChAT) in the cytoplasm, and then transported into the storage vesicle by a second carrier. Release of transmitter occurs when voltage-sensitive calcium channels in the terminal membrane are opened, allowing an influx of calcium. The resulting increase in intracellular calcium causes fusion of vesicle-associated membrane proteins (VAMPs) with synaptosomal nerve associated proteins (SNAPs) on the inner membrane surface and expulsion of ACh and cotransmitters into the synaptic space. Autoreceptors and heteroreceptors depicted on presynaptic terminals regulate additional release of ACh when stimulated. Acetylcholine's action is terminated by metabolism by the enzyme acetylcholinesterase.

acetylcholine into choline and acetate, terminating its action (Figure 4–2). Most cholinergic synapses are richly supplied with acetylcholinesterase; the half-life of acetylcholine in the synapse is therefore very short.

Adrenergic Transmission

Adrenergic neurons also transport a precursor molecule, tyrosine, into the nerve ending, then synthesize the catecholamine transmitter, and finally store it in membrane-bound vesicles (Figure 4–3). Several catecholamine transmitters and cotransmitters are listed in Table 4–1. As indicated in Figure 4–4, the synthesis of the catecholamine transmitters is more complex than that of acetylcholine. In most sympathetic postganglionic neurons, norepinephrine is the final product. In the adrenal medulla and certain areas of the brain, norepinephrine is further converted to epinephrine. Conversely, synthesis terminates with dopamine in the dopaminergic neurons of the central nervous system. Several important processes in these nerve terminals are potential sites of drug action.

Release of transmitters from noradrenergic nerve endings is similar to the calcium-dependent process described above for cholinergic terminals. Various chemicals in the diet, such as tyramine or drugs (amphetamines), are capable of releasing stored transmitter from noradrenergic nerve endings. These compounds are taken up into presynaptic noradrenergic nerve endings, and may displace norepinephrine from storage vesicles, inhibit the enzyme responsible for metabolism and inactivation of the neurotransmitter, or have other effects that result in increased norepinephrine activity in the synapse. Termination of noradrenergic transmission results from simple diffusion of the neurotransmitter away from the receptor site with eventual metabolism in the plasma or liver, or reuptake into presynaptic or postsynaptic locations (Figure 4–3). Metabolism of norepinephrine and epinephrine may occur by several enzymes such as monoamine oxidase (MAO) in the presynaptic terminal or catechol-*O*-methyltransferase (COMT) at other tissue locations (Figure 4–4).

AUTONOMIC RECEPTORS

Historically, careful comparisons of the potency of a series of autonomic agonists and antagonists led to the definition of different autonomic receptor subtypes, including muscarinic and nicotinic receptors, and alpha (α), beta (β), and dopamine (D) receptors (Table 4–2). The primary cholinergic receptor subtypes were named after the alkaloids originally used in their identification: muscarine and nicotine. Both muscarinic and nicotinic receptors are stimulated by acetylcholine. The adrenergic receptors are subdivided into α, β, and D subtypes on the basis of both agonist and antagonist selectivity. The α and β receptor subtypes respond mainly to norepinephrine. The D receptors respond to dopamine. Development of more selective blocking drugs has led to the naming of subclasses within these major subtypes. Within α receptors, both α_1 and α_2 receptors have been characterized, and within β receptors, β_1, β_2, and β_3 receptors have been defined. The tissue locations and physiological actions of these receptors are presented in Table 4–3.

FUNCTIONAL ORGANIZATION OF AUTONOMIC ACTIVITY

A basic understanding of the interactions of autonomic nerves with each other and with their effector organs is essential for an appreciation of the actions of drugs affecting the autonomic nervous system, especially because of the significant reflex, i.e., compensatory, effects that may be evoked by these agents. Autonomic reflexes are particularly important in understanding cardiovascular responses to these drugs. As indicated in Figure 4–5, the primary controlled variable in cardiovascular function is mean arterial pressure. Changes in any variable contributing to mean arterial pressure will evoke powerful secondary homeostatic responses that tend to compensate for the directly evoked change.

Central Integration

Central integration occurs at the highest level in the midbrain and medulla. The two divisions of the autonomic nervous system and the endocrine system are integrated with each other, with sensory input, and

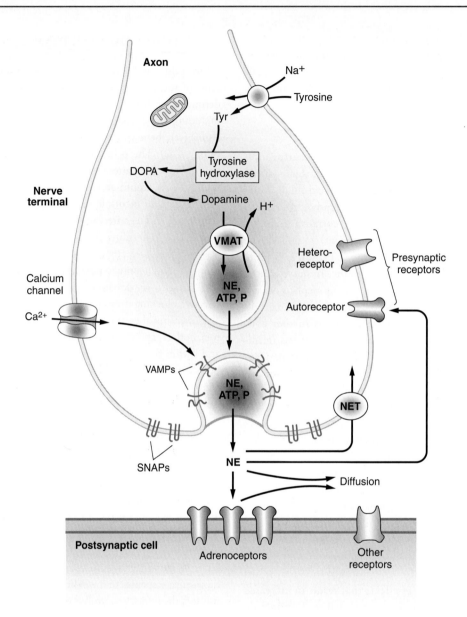

Figure 4–3. Schematic diagram of a generalized noradrenergic junction with adrenergic receptors (adrenoceptors) in the postsynaptic membrane. Tyrosine is transported into the noradrenergic ending. Tyrosine is converted to dopamine, which is transported into the vesicle by the vesicular monoamine transporter (VMAT). The same carrier transports norepinephrine (NE) and several other amines into these vesicles. Dopamine is converted to NE in the vesicle. Release of transmitter occurs when an action potential opens voltage-sensitive calcium channels and increases intracellular calcium. Fusion of vesicles with the surface membrane results in expulsion of norepinephrine into the synaptic space. After release, norepinephrine diffuses out of the space or is transported into the cytoplasm of the presynaptic terminal by the norepinephrine transporter (NET), or into the postsynaptic tissue. The NET may be inhibited by cocaine, resulting in an increase of transmitter activity in the synaptic space. Autoreceptors and heteroreceptors depicted on presynaptic terminals regulate additional release of sympathetic neurotransmitter when stimulated.

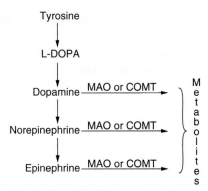

Tyrosine

L-DOPA

Dopamine — MAO or COMT →

Norepinephrine — MAO or COMT →

Epinephrine — MAO or COMT →

} Metabolites

Figure 4–4. Biosynthesis of catecholamines from tyrosine through epinephrine. Metabolism of dopamine, norepinephrine, or epinephrine by either monoamine oxidase (MAO) or catechol-*O*-methyltransferase (COMT) results in inactivation of the neurotransmitter.

with information from higher central nervous system centers. Within the various organ systems of the body, the interactions between the sympathetic and parasympathetic divisions are often in opposition to each other (Table 4–4). Thus, the parasympathetic system is often referred to as a *trophotropic* system, leading to growth, and the sympathetic system is referred to as an *ergotropic* system, leading to energy expenditure. For example, slowing of the heart and stimulation of digestive activity are typical energy-conserving ("rest and digest") actions of the parasympathetic system. In contrast, cardiac stimulation, increased blood sugar, and cutaneous vasoconstriction are responses produced by sympathetic discharge that are suited to fighting or surviving an attack ("fight or flight"). At a more subtle level of interactions in the brain stem, medulla, and

Table 4–2.	Autonomic receptor types with documented or probable effects on effector tissues	
Receptor Name	**Typical Location(s)**	**Results of Receptor Stimulation**
Cholinergic		
M_1	CNS neurons, sympathetic postganglionic neurons, some presynaptic sites	Formation of second messengers and increases in intracellular calcium
M_2	Myocardium, smooth muscle, some presynaptic sites	Opening of potassium channels, inhibition of adenylyl cyclase
M_3	Exocrine glands, vessels (smooth muscle and endothelium)	Formation of second messengers and increases in intracellular calcium
N_N	Postganglionic neurons, some presynaptic cholinergic terminals	Opening Na^+/K^+ channels, depolarization
N_M	Skeletal muscle neuromuscular end plate	Opening Na^+/K^+ channels, depolarization
Adrenergic		
α_1	Postsynaptic effector cells: especially smooth muscle	Formation of second messengers and increases in intracellular calcium
α_2	Presynaptic adrenergic nerve terminals, platelets, adipocytes, smooth muscle, postsynaptic neurons in brainstem and spinal cord	Inhibition of adenylyl cyclase

(*continued*)

Table 4–2.	Autonomic receptor types with documented or probable effects on effector tissues (*continued*)	
Receptor Name	**Typical Location(s)**	**Results of Receptor Stimulation**
β_1	Postsynaptic effector cells: heart, adipocytes, brain, presynaptic adrenergic and cholinergic nerve terminals	Stimulation of adenylyl cyclase
β_2	Postsynaptic effector cells: smooth muscle and cardiac muscle, liver, pancreas	Stimulation of adenylyl cyclase
β_3	Postsynaptic effector cells: adipocytes	Stimulation of adenylyl cyclase
D_1, D_5	Brain, effector tissues: smooth muscle of renal vasculature	Stimulation of adenylyl cyclase
D_2	Brain, effector tissues: smooth muscle, presynaptic nerve terminals	Inhibition of adenylyl cyclase, increased opening K^+ channels
D_3	Brain	Inhibition of adenylyl cyclase
D_4	Brain, cardiovascular system	Inhibition of adenylyl cyclase

CNS = central nervous system; α = alpha; β = beta; D = dopamine; M = Muscarinic; N = Nicotinic receptors.

spinal cord, there are important cooperative interactions between the parasympathetic and sympathetic systems. For some organs, sensory fibers associated with the parasympathetic system exert reflex control over motor outflow in the sympathetic system. Thus, the sensory carotid sinus baroreceptor fibers have a major influence on sympathetic outflow from the vasomotor center. Similarly, parasympathetic sensory fibers in the wall of the urinary bladder significantly influence sympathetic inhibitory outflow to that organ.

Peripheral Integration

In the peripheral tissues, integration may be regulated at either presynaptic or postsynaptic locations. Presynaptic regulation uses the concept of negative or positive feedback control to regulate neurotransmitter release. Important presynaptic inhibitory control mechanisms have been shown to exist at most nerve endings. A well-documented mechanism involves α_2 receptors located on noradrenergic nerve terminals. Norepinephrine and similar molecules activate these receptors; activation diminishes further release of

norepinephrine from the nerve endings. Conversely, a presynaptic β receptor appears to facilitate the release of norepinephrine. Presynaptic receptors that respond to the primary transmitter substances released by the nerve ending are called *autoreceptors* (Figures 4–2 and 4–3). Autoreceptors are usually inhibitory, but many cholinergic fibers, especially somatic motor fibers, have excitatory nicotinic autoreceptors. Control of transmitter release is not limited to modulation by the transmitter itself. Nerve terminals also carry regulatory receptors that respond to many other substances. Such *heteroreceptors* (Figures 4–2 and 4–3) may be activated by substances released from other nerve terminals that synapse with the nerve ending. For example, some vagal fibers in the myocardium synapse on sympathetic noradrenergic nerve terminals and inhibit norepinephrine release. Alternatively, the compounds that influence these receptors may diffuse to the receptors from the blood or from nearby tissues. Presynaptic regulation by a variety of endogenous chemicals probably occurs in all nerve fibers.

Postsynaptic regulation can be considered from two perspectives. The first is modulation by the prior

Table 4–3.	Types of adrenoceptors,[1] some of the peripheral tissues in which they are found, and the major effects of their activation	

Type[2]	Tissue	Action
α_1	Most vascular smooth muscle	Contracts ($\uparrow$ vascular resistance)
	Pupillary dilator muscle	Contracts (mydriasis)
	Pilomotor smooth muscle	Contracts (erects hair)
α_2	Adrenergic and cholinergic nerve terminals	Inhibits transmitter release
	Platelets	Stimulates aggregation
	Some vascular smooth muscle	Contracts
	Adipocytes	Inhibits lipolysis
	Pancreatic beta cells	Inhibits insulin release
β_1	Heart	Stimulates rate and force
	Juxtaglomerular cells	Stimulates renin release
β_2	Respiratory, uterine, and vascular smooth muscle	Relaxes
	Liver (human)	Stimulates glycogenolysis
	Pancreatic beta cells	Stimulates insulin release
	Somatic motor nerve terminals	Causes tremors
β_3 (β_1, β_2 may also contribute)	Adipocytes	Stimulates lipolysis
D_1	Renal and other splanchnic blood vessels	Dilates ($\downarrow$ resistance)
D_2	Nerve terminals	Inhibits adenylyl cyclase

[1]Adrenoceptor distribution in the central nervous system is discussed in Chapter 12.
[2]See Table 4–2 for abbreviations.

history of activity at the primary receptor, that is, receptor up-regulation or down-regulation, or receptor desensitization. Up-regulation occurs in response to decreased activation of the receptors. In contrast, down-regulation and desensitization occurs in response to increased activation of the receptors. For additional information, see Chapter 2. Alternatively, receptor modulation may occur by other temporally associated conditions such as electrolyte levels inside or outside of the effector cell, or circulating hormones.

■ PHARMACOLOGIC MODIFICATION OF AUTONOMIC FUNCTION

Because transmission involves different mechanisms in different segments of the autonomic nervous system, some drugs produce highly specific effects,

whereas others are much less selective in their actions. A summary of the steps in transmission of impulses is presented in Figure 4–6. Modifying any step in this process may increase or decrease the amount of neurotransmitter reacting with appropriate receptors.

Drugs that block action potential propagation are very nonselective in their action, since these drugs act on a process that is common to all neurons. On the other hand, drugs that act on the biochemical processes involved in transmitter release and turnover are more selective. Modulation at this level may either increase or decrease the concentration of transmitters interacting with their receptors. Inhibition of transmitter synthesis, storage, or release may decrease the amount of transmitter interacting with the receptors. These agents are classified as **indirect-acting** antagonists. This is in contrast to agents that have affinity, but no efficacy, and block

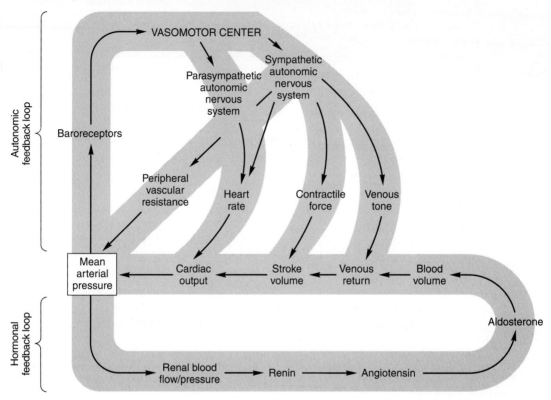

Figure 4–5. Autonomic and hormonal control of cardiovascular function. Note that two feedback loops are present: the autonomic nervous system loop and the hormonal loop. The sympathetic nervous system directly influences four major variables: peripheral vascular resistance, heart rate, contractile force, and venous tone. The sympathetic system also directly modulates renin production (not shown). The parasympathetic nervous system directly influences heart rate. In addition to its role in stimulating aldosterone secretion, angiotensin II directly increases peripheral vascular resistance and facilitates sympathetic effects (not shown). The net feedback effect of each loop is to compensate for changes in arterial blood pressure. Thus, decreased blood pressure due to blood loss would evoke increased sympathetic outflow and renin release. Conversely, elevated pressure due to the administration of a vasoconstrictor drug would cause reduced sympathetic outflow, reduced renin release, and increased parasympathetic (vagal) outflow.

the postsynaptic receptors. These agents are classified as **direct-acting** antagonists. Within the adrenergic drug group, these indirect and direct antagonists are called *sympatholytics*; that is, agents that antagonize the sympathetic system. In contrast, agents that decrease reuptake of the transmitter, or inhibit the enzyme(s) responsible for breakdown of the transmitter, increase the interaction of the transmitter with the receptors. These agents are classified as indirect-acting agonists. Agents that have both affinity and efficacy for the postsynaptic receptors are called direct-acting agonists. Within the adrenergic drug group, these indirect and direct agonists are called *sympathomimetics*; that is, agents that mimic the sympathetic system. Similar direct-acting and indirect-acting classifications exist for agonists and antagonists that interact with the parasympathetic system.

Table 4–4. Direct effects of autonomic nerve activity on some organ systems

	Effect of			
	Sympathetic Activity		**Parasympathetic Activity**	
Organ	**Action[1]**	**Receptor[2]**	**Action**	**Receptor**
Eye				
Iris radial muscle	Contracts	α_1	...	...
Iris circular muscle			Contracts	M_3
Ciliary muscle	[Relaxes]	β	Contracts	M_3
Heart				
Sinoatrial node	Accelerates	β_1, β_2	Decelerates	M_2
Ectopic pacemakers	Accelerates	β_1, β_2	...	
Contractility	Increases	β_1, β_2	Decreases (atria)	M_2
Blood vessels				
Skin, splanchnic vessels	Contracts	α	...	
Skeletal muscle vessels	Relaxes	β_2	...	
	[Contracts]	α	...	
	Relaxes	M^3	...	
Endothelium			Releases EDRF[4]	$M_3, M_5{}^5$
Bronchiolar smooth muscle	Relaxes	β_2	Contracts	M_3
Gastrointestinal tract				
Smooth muscle				
Walls	Relaxes	$\alpha_2, \beta_2{}^6$	Contracts	M_3
Sphincters	Contracts	α_1	Relaxes	M_3
Secretion	...	...	Increases	M_3
Genitourinary smooth muscle				
Bladder wall	Relaxes	β_2	Contracts	M_3
Sphincter	Contracts	α_1	Relaxes	M_3
Uterus, pregnant	Relaxes	β_2	...	
	Contracts	α	Contracts	M_3
Penis, seminal vesicles	Ejaculation	α	Erection	M
Skin				
Pilomotor smooth muscle	Contracts	α	...	
Sweat glands				
Thermoregulatory	Increases	M	...	
Apocrine (stress)	Increases	α	...	
Metabolic functions				
Liver	Gluconeogenesis	β_2, α	...	
Liver	Glycogenolysis	β_2, α	...	
Adipocytes	Lipolysis	β_3	...	
Kidney	Renin release	β_1	...	
Autonomic nerve endings				
Sympathetic	...	...	Decrease NE release	M^7
Parasympathetic	Decreases ACh release	α	...	

NE = norepinephrine.
[1]Less important actions are shown in brackets.
[2]Specific receptor type: α = alpha, β = beta, M = muscarinic.
[3]Vascular smooth muscle in skeletal muscle has sympathetic cholinergic dilator fibers.
[4]The endothelium of most blood vessels releases EDRF (endothelium-derived relaxing factor), which causes marked vasodilation, in response to muscarinic stimuli. However, unlike the receptors innervated by sympathetic cholinergic fibers in skeletal muscle blood vessels, these muscarinic receptors are not innervated and respond only to circulating muscarinic agonists.
[5]Cerebral blood vessels dilate in response to M_5 receptor activation.
[6]Probably through presynaptic inhibition of parasympathetic activity.
[7]Probably through M_1, but M_2 may participate in some locations.

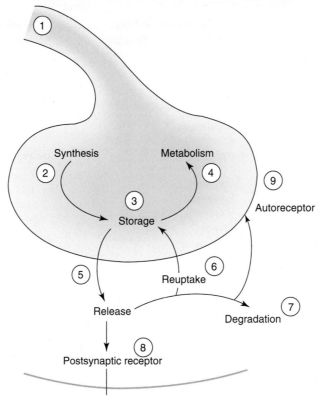

Figure 4–6. Potential sites of pharmacologic modulation at synapses. Electrical impulses progress down the axon. At the presynaptic membrane, an influx of extracellular calcium results in fusion of the vesicle with the presynaptic membrane, and release of the neurotransmitter into the synaptic space. The neurotransmitter may interact with presynaptic autoreceptors or postsynaptic receptors. Eventually, the neurotransmitter may be taken back up into the presynaptic terminal or postsynaptic terminal or migrate from the synaptic space. Metabolism, (i.e., degradation) of the neurotransmitter may occur at any of these locations. Pharmacologic manipulation may occur at any of the previously mentioned locations. Local anesthetics inhibit the action potential in the axon (1). An indirect-acting antagonist may inhibit synthesis, storage, or release of the neurotransmitter (2, 3, 5). Direct-acting antagonists inhibit the postsynaptic receptors (8). In contrast, an indirect-acting agonist may augment neurotransmitter interaction by inhibiting metabolism, reuptake, or degradation of the neurotransmitter (4, 6, 7). Finally, stimulation of presynaptic autoreceptors often leads to a decrease in further neurotransmitter release from the presynaptic nerve terminal (9).

Finally, the biochemistry of adrenergic transmission is very different from that of cholinergic transmission. Owing to these differences, activation or blockade of either adrenergic or cholinergic receptors on effector cells offers maximum flexibility and selectivity of effect. Furthermore, individual subgroups within nicotinic cholinergic receptors or α- and β-adrenergic receptors can often be selectively activated or blocked. The subsequent chapters in this section (Chapter 5 to 10) provide examples of selective receptor activation or blockade in the clinical use of these drugs.

REFERENCES

Bernstein D: Cardiovascular and metabolic alterations in mice lacking beta$_1$- and beta$_2$-adrenergic receptors. *Trends Cardiovasc Med* 2002;12:287.

Burnstock G, Hoyle CHV: *Autonomic Neuroeffector Mechanisms.* Harwood Academic Publishers, 1992.

Chang HY, et al: Musings on the wanderer: What's new in our understanding of the vago-vagal reflex? IV. Current concepts of vagal efferent projections to the gut. *Am J Physiol Gastrointest Liver Physiol* 2003;284:G357.

Docherty JR: Age-related changes in adrenergic neuroeffector transmission. *Auton Neurosci* 2002;96:8.

Fetscher C, et al: M$_3$ muscarinic receptors mediate contraction of human urinary bladder. *Br J Pharmacol* 2002;136:641.

Furchgott RF: Role of endothelium in responses of vascular smooth muscle to drugs. *Annu Rev Pharmacol Toxicol* 1984;24:175.

Goldstein DS, et al: Dysautonomias: Clinical disorders of the autonomic nervous system. *Ann Intern Med* 2002;137:753.

Huikuri HV, Makikallio TH: Heart rate variability in ischemic heart disease. *Auton Neurosci* 2001;90:95.

Jarvis SE, Zamponi GW: Interactions between presynaptic Ca^{2+} channels, cytoplasmic messengers and proteins of the synaptic vesicle complex. *Trends Pharmacol Sci* 2001;22:519.

Lepori M, et al: Interaction between cholinergic and nitrergic vasodilation: A novel mechanism of blood pressure control. *Cardiovasc Res* 2001;51:767.

Lundberg JM: Pharmacology of cotransmission in the autonomic nervous system: Integrative aspects on amines, neuropeptides, adenosine triphosphate, amino acids and nitric oxide. *Pharmacol Rev* 1996;48:113.

Miller RJ: Presynaptic receptors. *Annu Rev Pharmacol Toxicol* 1998;38:201.

Südhof TC: The synaptic vesicle cycle: A cascade of protein-protein interactions. *Nature* 1995;375:645.

Schlicker E, Gothert M: Interactions between the presynaptic alpha$_2$-autoreceptor and the presynaptic inhibitory heteroreceptors on noradrenergic neurons. *Brain Res Bull* 1998;47:129.

Skok VI: Nicotinic acetylcholine receptors in autonomic ganglia. *Auton Neurosci* 2002;97:1.

Toda N, Okamura T: The pharmacology of nitric oxide in the peripheral nervous system of blood vessels. *Pharmacol Rev* 2003;55:271.

Westfall DP, et al: ATP as a cotransmitter in sympathetic nerves and its inactivation by releasable enzymes. *J Pharmacol Exp Ther* 2002;303:439.

Zanzinger J: Role of nitric oxide in the neural control of cardiovascular function. *Cardiovasc Res* 1999;43:639.

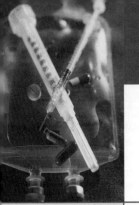

5

DRUGS AFFECTING
THE CHOLINERGIC SYSTEM

When synaptic transmission depends upon acetylcholine as the primary neurotransmitter, it is labeled *cholinergic*. The termination of acetylcholine activity is mediated by the enzyme acetylcholinesterase. There are two subtypes of cholinergic receptors, muscarinic (M) and nicotinic (N). Agonists that mimic the effects of acetylcholine are defined as cholinomimetics. Some drugs are direct-acting agonists for the cholinergic receptors (Figure 5–1). Other drugs function as indirect-acting agonists by preventing the inactivation of acetylcholine. Antagonists that inhibit acetylcholine at muscarinic or nicotinic receptors are defined as *anticholinergics*. Drugs that selectively inhibit muscarinic receptors are called *antimuscarinics* (Figure 5–2), whereas those that selectively inhibit nicotinic receptors are *antinicotinics*.

CHOLINOMIMETIC DRUGS

The subtypes of cholinoreceptors are set forth in Table 5–1. At present, subtype-selective agonists for the muscarinic receptors are not clinically available. Direct-acting nicotinic agonists may be classified on the basis of whether ganglionic (N_N) or neuromuscular (N_M) stimulation predominates, but agonist selectivity is very limited. Several molecular mechanisms for receptor signaling have been identified for muscarinic receptors (Table 5–1). In general, these receptors modulate the formation of second messengers or the activity of ion channels. In contrast, all nicotinic receptors cause the opening of a channel selective for sodium and potassium that results in cellular depolarization. This signaling mechanism occurs in the autonomic ganglia and at the neuromuscular junction.

Direct-acting cholinoceptor agonists are classified pharmacologically by the type of receptor—muscarinic or nicotinic—that is activated (Figure 5–1). Direct-acting agonists' physiologic effects are the result of their interaction with either the muscarinic or nicotinic receptors. Indirect-acting agonists are classified as such because they inhibit the hydrolysis and inactivation of endogenous acetylcholine (Figure 5–1). This increases the concentration of acetylcholine in the synapse and augments acetylcholine binding to receptors. Indirect-acting agonists are less specific in their stimulation of muscarinic compared to nicotinic receptors. The spectrum of action of direct- and indirect-acting cholinomimetic drugs and a summary of their pharmacokinetics are outlined in Table 5–2.

Direct-Acting Cholinergic Agonists

Direct-acting agonists are divided into two groups based on chemical structure. The first group consists of choline esters, typified by **acetylcholine, carbachol,** and **bethanechol.** The second

54

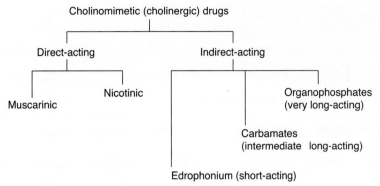

Figure 5–1. Algorithm of cholinomimetic drugs. Some drugs are direct-acting agonists that stimulate the muscarinic or nicotinic receptors. Alternatively, the drugs may be indirect-acting in that they inhibit the enzyme acetylcholinesterase that is responsible for terminating the action of acetylcholine.

group includes naturally occurring alkaloids such as **nicotine, muscarine,** and **pilocarpine.** Further classification is based on whether muscarinic or nicotinic receptor activation dominates.

Physiologic Effects

In general, direct-acting muscarinic agonists are parasympathomimetics in that they mimic stimulation of the parasympathetic system (Table 5–3). One exception is that these agents will also stimulate muscarinic receptors located on eccrine sweat glands which are responsible for thermoregulation and are under

sympathetic, not parasympathetic, nerve control. Additionally, vasodilation is observed with clinical use of these drugs; however, this is not a parasympathetic response. The vasodilation is the result of the release of endothelium-derived relaxing factor (EDRF) from uninnervated muscarinic receptors on endothelial cells lining the vascular walls. This vasodilation may result in a decrease in blood pressure.

The physiologic response for nicotinic receptor stimulation is dependent upon whether N_M or N_N receptors are activated. The tissue and organ level effects of N_N receptor stimulation in the ganglia

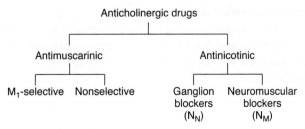

Figure 5–2. Grouping of cholinoreceptor direct-acting antagonists based on their inhibition of either muscarinic (M) or nicotinic (N) receptors. Further subdivisions for the muscarinic receptors include drugs that are specific antagonists of M_1 receptors located on nerve endings or nonspecific muscarinic antagonists. Nicotinic antagonists are subdivided based on whether the drug inhibits postsynaptic receptors at the neuromuscular junction (N_M) or postsynaptic receptors in the parasympathetic and sympathetic ganglia (N_N).

Table 5–1.	Subtypes and characteristics of cholinoceptors	

Receptor Type	Location	Postreceptor Mechanism[1]
Muscarinic (M)		
M_1	Nerves	IP_3, DAG cascade
M_2	Heart, nerves, smooth muscle	Inhibition of cAMP production, activation of K^+ channels
M_3	Glands, smooth muscle, endothelium	IP_3, DAG cascade
M_4[2]	CNS[3]	Inhibition of cAMP production
M_5[2]	CNS[3]	IP_3, DAG cascade
Nicotinic (N)		
N_M	Skeletal muscle neuromuscular junction	Na^+, K^+ depolarizing ion channel
N_N	Postganglionic cell body, dendrites	Na^+, K^+ depolarizing ion channel

[1]Mechanisms of receptor signaling are formation of second messengers diacylglycerol (DAG) and inositol-1,4,5-trisphosphate (IP_3), inhibition of the formation of second messenger cyclic-adenosine-monophosphate (cAMP), and ion channel activation for sodium (Na^+) influx or potassium (K^+) efflux.

[2]Functional receptors have not been identified.

[3]Questions remain concerning presence in the central nervous system (CNS).

depends on the organ system involved. The blood vessels are dominated by sympathetic innervation; therefore, nicotinic receptor activation of postganglionic neurons results in vasoconstriction. In contrast, the gastrointestinal (GI) system is dominated by parasympathetic control. Here stimulation of postganglionic neurons results in an increased motility and secretion. Stimulation of N_M receptors at the neuromuscular junction when activated by direct-acting nicotinic agonists results in fasciculations and muscle spasms. Prolonged stimulation of N_M receptors results in desensitization of the receptors and muscle paralysis. The latter event is a hazard of pesticides containing nicotine.

Clinical Use

A summary of the clinical applications of direct-acting muscarinic and nicotinic agonists is presented in Table 5–4.

Muscarinic agonists find a wide clinical application. In glaucoma, these drugs decrease intraocular pressure. They also assist in micturition in the hypotonic bladder after surgery or neurologic damage. In contrast, nicotinic agonists find limited clinical application except in tobacco abstention. The use of succinylcholine to provide skeletal muscle paralysis as an adjuvant to general anesthesia is related to inhibition at the neuromuscular junction. This drug will be discussed with the nicotinic antagonists in the last section of this chapter.

Adverse Events

The adverse effects associated with stimulation of muscarinic or nicotinic receptors vary depending upon the organ system. For muscarinic agonists, these include both central nervous system (CNS) and peripheral tissue responses. The CNS effect may include generalized

Table 5–2.	Cholinomimetics: spectrum of action and pharmacokinetics	

Drug	Spectrum of Action	Pharmacokinetic Features
Direct-acting		
Acetylcholine	B	Rapidly hydrolyzed by ChE; duration of action 5–30 s; poor lipid solubility
Bethanechol	M	Resistant to ChE, orally active, poor lipid solubility; duration of action 30 min to 2 h
Carbachol	B	Like bethanechol
Pilocarpine	M	Not an ester, good lipid solubility; duration of action 30 min to 2 h
Nicotine	N	Like pilocarpine; duration of action 1–6 h; high lipid solubility
Indirect-acting		
Edrophonium	B	Alcohol, quaternary amine, poor lipid solubility, not orally active; 5–15 min duration of action
Neostigmine	B	Carbamate, quaternary amine, poor lipid solubility, orally active, duration of action 30 min to 2 h
Physostigmine	B	Carbamate, tertiary amine, lipid soluble; duration of action 30 min to 2 h
Pyridostigmine, ambenonium	B	Carbamates like neostigmine, but longer duration of action (4–8 h)
Echothiophate	B	Organophosphate, moderate lipid solubility; duration of action 2–7 days
Parathion	B	Organophosphate insecticide, high lipid solubility; duration of action 7–30 days

M = muscarinic; N = nicotinic; B = both muscarinic and nicotinic; ChE = cholinesterase.

stimulation resulting in hallucinations or seizures. In the eye, miosis and spasm of ocular accommodation may occur. At higher doses, the peripheral responses may be generalized to excessive parasympathomimetic stimulation with bronchoconstriction and excessive mucus production, gastrointestinal distress, hyperactivity of the detrusor muscle of the bladder with increased frequency of voiding, and hypotension. Bradycardia may occur, but the hypotension usually evokes a reflex tachycardia. Finally, stimulation of muscarinic receptors on the eccrine sweat glands, which are under sympathetic control, may result in sweating.

Nicotinic agonists acting within the CNS may initiate seizures, coma, and respiratory depression. In the peripheral tissues, stimulation of the autonomic N_N receptors results in either parasympathetic or sympathetic manifestations, depending upon the organ system, as previously discussed. Significant clinical manifestations may include hypertension and cardiac arrhythmias. Prolonged stimulation of the N_M receptors at the neuromuscular junction and subsequent

Table 5–3.   Effects of cholinoceptor stimulation[1]

Organ	Response
Central nervous system	Complex stimulatory effects: mild alerting reaction (nicotinic), tremor, emesis, excitation of respiratory centers, convulsions
Autonomic nervous system	Complex stimulatory effects: stimulation of autonomic ganglia results in either parasympathetic or sympathetic response depending on each organ system (nicotinic), stimulation of target organ see below (muscarinic)
Eye	
Sphincter muscle of iris	Contraction (miosis)
Ciliary muscle	Contraction for near vision (accommodation, cyclospasm)
Heart	
Sinoatrial node	Decrease in rate (negative chronotropy)
Atria	Decrease in contractile strength (negative inotropy); decrease in refractory period
Atrioventricular node	Decrease in conduction velocity (negative dromotropy); decrease in refractory period
Ventricles	Small decrease in contractile strength
Blood vessels	Dilation (via EDRF[2])
Bronchi	Contraction (bronchoconstriction)
Gastrointestinal tract	
Motility	Increase
Sphincters	Relaxation (via enteric nervous system)
Secretion	Stimulation
Urinary bladder	
Detrusor	Contraction
Trigone and sphincter	Relaxation
Glands	Increased secretion: thermoregulatory sweat, lacrimal, salivary, bronchial, gastric, intestinal glands
Skeletal muscle	Activation of neuromuscular end plates; contraction of muscle

[1]Only the direct effects are indicated; homeostatic responses to these direct actions may be important.
[2]EDRF is the abbreviation for endothelium-derived relaxing factor. Evidence suggests EDRF is nitric oxide (NO).

muscle paralysis leads to decreased respiratory muscle function and hypoventilation. The chronic exposure to nicotine associated with tobacco use may result in additional pathophysiologic manifestations. Nicotine has a strong addictive potential. Chronic use of nicotine has an association with cancer, increased gastrointestinal ulcers, and increased risk of vascular disease and sudden coronary death.

Indirect-Acting Cholinergic Agonists

Indirect-acting cholinergic agonists fall into three major classes based on chemical structure and duration

Table 5–4.	Clinical applications of some cholinomimetics	
Clinical Applications	**Drug**	**Action**
Direct-Acting Agonists		
Postoperative and neurogenic ileus and urinary retention	Bethanechol	Activates bowel and bladder smooth muscle
Glaucoma	Carbachol	Activates pupillary sphincter and ciliary muscles of eye
Glaucoma, Sjögren's syndrome	Pilocarpine	Activates pupillary sphincter and ciliary muscle of eye; stimulates salivation
Smoking deterrence (patch, chewing gum)	Nicotine	Replaces rapid-onset actions (cigarette) with slower action
Indirect-Acting Agonists		
Postoperative and neurogenic ileus and urinary retention	Neostigmine	Amplifies endogenous ACh
Myasthenia gravis, reversal of neuromuscular blockade	Neostigmine, pyridostigmine, edrophonium	Amplifies endogenous ACh
Glaucoma	Physostigmine, echothiophate	Amplifies effects of ACh
Alzheimer dementia	Tacrine, donepezil, galantamine, rivastigmine	Amplifies effects of ACh in the CNS

ACH = acetylcholine; CNS = central nervous system.

of effect (Figure 5–1). These classes are alcohols (e.g., **edrophonium**), carbamates (e.g., **neostigmine**) and organophosphates (e.g., **echothiophate**). Both the carbamate and organophosphate classes bind to acetylcholinesterase and undergo hydrolysis. Following this enzymatic activity, the metabolite is released slowly, preventing the binding and inactivation of acetylcholine. The carbamates are released over a period of hours, whereas the organophosphates require days to weeks to be released by the acetylcholinesterase. The alcohol class (edrophonium) binds to the active site electrostatically and by hydrogen bonds. The binding is short lived—on the order of minutes. Based on the

binding, all three classes may be considered pseudoirreversible antagonists of acetylcholinesterase. Finally, some drugs in this class also have some direct-acting agonist activity. For example, neostigmine both inhibits acetylcholinesterase and directly activates the postsynaptic N_M receptor at the neuromuscular junction.

Physiologic Effects

By inhibiting acetylcholinesterase, indirect-acting cholinergic agonists amplify the actions of endogenous acetylcholine at both muscarinic and nicotinic synapses. Thus, these drugs may augment sympathetic or parasympathetic functions in the peripheral tissues. The response varies based on the organ system. In the GI tract, bladder, and lungs, parasympathetic activity predominates. At the neuromuscular junction, these drugs increase the force of muscle contractions, followed by fasciculations at higher concentrations, and ending ultimately with paralysis. Finally, cholinergic activity in the CNS parallels what was previously described for the direct-acting cholinergic agonists (Table 5–3). The one exception to this parallelism is that the indirectly acting drugs do not normally cause vasodilation because endothelial cells are not innervated, and do not release EDRF when these drugs are administered.

Clinical Use

The clinical use of indirect-acting agonists differs somewhat from the direct-acting muscarinic and nicotinic agonists. The carbamates receive wider clinical use compared to the organophosphates. The clinical use of the alcohol edrophonium is limited because of the short action of the drug (5–15 minutes). Unique to these indirect-acting agonists is their use in the treatment of myasthenia gravis and dementia (Table 5–4). Direct-acting muscarinic or nicotinic agonists are not currently in clinical use for either of these conditions.

Adverse Events

The clinical hazards of indirect-acting agonists parallel those of the direct-acting agonists with the following exceptions. First, vasodilation is late and uncommon, and bradycardia is more common than reflex tachycardia. The CNS manifestations are common following organophosphate overdose, with convulsions followed by respiratory and cardiovascular depression. A mnemonic for remembering the spectrum of adverse effects is DUMBBELSS (diarrhea, urination, miosis, bronchoconstriction, bradycardia, excitation of skeletal muscle and the CNS, lacrimation, salivation, and sweating). As with nicotinic agonists, prolonged stimulation of the N_M receptors at the neuromuscular junction results in muscle paralysis, and is a hazard of pesticides containing these indirect-acting agonists.

■ ANTICHOLINERGIC DRUGS

Direct-acting cholinoreceptor antagonists are classified based on their blockade of muscarinic or nicotinic receptors (Figure 5–2). Further subdivisions for the muscarinic receptors include drugs that are selective antagonists of M_1 receptors located on nerve endings as well as nonselective muscarinic antagonists. All antimuscarinic drugs currently available in the United States are nonselective antagonists.

Nicotinic antagonists are subdivided based on whether the drug inhibits postsynaptic N_M receptors at the neuromuscular junction or postsynaptic N_N receptors at the parasympathetic and sympathetic ganglia (Figure 5–3). The former have clinical application as general anesthesia adjuvants by inducing skeletal muscle paralysis. The latter drugs have limited clinical applications and will be discussed briefly.

Muscarinic Antagonists

Muscarinic antagonists may be further subdivided based on their clinical application and target organ system. Drugs used for either CNS or ophthalmic applications must be sufficiently lipid soluble to cross hydrophobic barriers such as the blood-brain barrier in the CNS. A major determinant for the

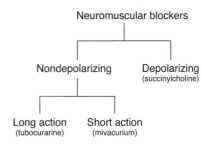

Figure 5–3. Neuromuscular blockers are clinically used to provide skeletal muscle paralysis at the neuromuscular junction (N_M) during general anesthesia. These drugs may be divided based on their mechanism of action as nondepolarizing and depolarizing drugs. Succinylcholine is the only clinically relevant drug in the latter class. Although the drug is an agonist to the N_M receptor, the subsequent muscle paralysis in the drug's physiologic response results in its clinical application as a skeletal muscle relaxant.

Table 5–5.	Effects of muscarinic blocking drugs	
Organ	**Effect**	**Mechanism**
Central nervous system	Sedation, antimotion-sickness action, antiparkinson action, amnesia, delirium	Block of muscarinic receptors, unknown subtypes
Eye	Cycloplegia, mydriasis	Block of M_3 receptors
Bronchi	Bronchodilation, especially if constricted	Block of M_3 receptors
Gastrointestinal tract	Relaxation, slowed peristalsis	Block of M_1, M_3 receptors
Genitourinary tract	Relaxation of bladder wall, increased bladder capacity	Block of M_3 receptors
Heart	Initial bradycardia, especially at low doses; then tachycardia	Tachycardia from block of M_2 receptors in the heart
Blood vessels	Block of muscarinic vasodilation; not manifest unless a muscarinic agonist is present	Block of M_3 receptors on endothelium of vessels
Glands	Marked reduction of salivation; moderate reduction of lacrimation, sweating; gastric secretion inhibited less effectively	Block of M_1, M_3 receptors
Skeletal muscle	None	

pharmacokinetics is the presence or absence of a permanently charged quaternary amine group on these drugs. The presence of this charged group diminishes the penetration across these hydrophobic barriers and, to some extent, the uptake by the GI system. **Atropine** is a plant alkaloid and a nonselective muscarinic antagonist. The drug is the prototypical nonselective muscarinic antagonist and is lipid soluble.

Physiologic Effects

The physiologic effects of muscarinic receptor inhibition are presented in Table 5–5. The peripheral actions of muscarinic blockers are mostly predicted by considering the removal of parasympathetic function on various organ systems. At therapeutic doses, cardiovascular effects include an initial bradycardia, possibly as a result of the blockade of postganglionic-presynaptic muscarinic receptors. The bradycardia is followed by tachycardia and increased atrioventricular conduction rate that would be predicted from the blockade of parasympathetic activity in the heart. In the respiratory system, bronchodilation and reduced secretion occurs. Inhibition of parasympathetic activity

in the GI system results in decreased motility, relaxation, and reduction in gastric secretions. In the genitourinary system there is a decrease in detrusor muscle tone and increased bladder capacity. Lacrimation, salivation, and sweating are also reduced. The reader should remember that lacrimation and salivation are under parasympathetic cholinergic activity; however, the eccrine sweat glands are under sympathetic cholinergic control. The CNS effects are less predictable. Most common are sedation, decreased motion sickness, and improved motor function in patients with Parkinson's disease.

Clinical Use

The clinical applications of muscarinic antagonists are presented in Table 5–6. Significant and clinically useful applications of these drugs include treatment of Parkinson's disease and reversal of bronchospasm. These two clinical applications of muscarinic antagonists will be discussed in Chapters 17 and 35, respectively. Direct ocular application of these drugs inhibits accommodation in the eye and causes dilation of the pupils. This application preceded that of the modern

Table 5–6.	Some clinical applications of antimuscarinic drugs	
Organ System	**Drugs[1]**	**Application**
CNS	Benztropine, trihexyphenidyl, biperiden	To treat the manifestations of Parkinson's disease
	Scopolamine	To prevent or reduce motion sickness
Eye	Atropine, homatropine, cyclopentolate, tropicamide	To produce mydriasis and cycloplegia
Bronchi	Ipratropium	To reverse bronchospasm in asthma and chronic obstructive pulmonary disease
Gastrointestinal tract	Glycopyrrolate, dicyclomine, methscopolamine	To reduce transient hypermotility
Genitourinary tract	Oxybutynin, glycopyrrolate, dicyclomine, tolterodine	To treat transient cystitis, postoperative bladder spasms, or incontinence

CNS = central nervous system.
[1]Only a few of many drugs are listed.

drug atropine. Extract of belladonna, the source of atropine, was used as a cosmetic to dilate the pupil centuries ago. **Scopolamine** decreases motion sickness and can be applied as a passive transdermal patch. This drug class also decreases hypertonicity of the bladder that results from neural damage above the micturition reflex arc, and can be used to decrease urgency and relieve stress incontinence. **Oxybutynin** is clinically used in this application, and may be applied as a passive transdermal patch. Rarely these drugs are also used clinically in cardiovascular or GI dysfunction, having been replaced by other drug classes with fewer adverse effects.

Adverse Effects

The traditional mnemonic for antimuscarinic toxicity may be "Dry as a bone, red as a beet, and mad as a hatter." This description reflects both the predictable antimuscarinic effects and some unpredictable actions. The "dry as a bone" response is the result of the inhibition of sweating, salivation, and lacrimation. Patients medicated with these drugs and involved in aerobic activities may experience hyperthermia. This effect results from these drugs' antagonism of the

thermoregulatory eccrine sweat glands. Moderate tachycardia is also common, with arrhythmias a much less common but life-threatening event. Dilation of cutaneous blood vessels occurs with toxic doses, and accounts for the "red as a beet" description. Finally, in the geriatric population, these drugs may exacerbate acute angle-closure glaucoma and urinary retention, especially in men with prostate hyperplasia. In the CNS, sedation, amnesia, and delirium with hallucinations contribute to the "mad as a hatter" description.

Nicotinic (N_M) Antagonists

Skeletal muscle contraction is evoked by postsynaptic N_M receptor-mediated signaling at the motor end plate. Activation of the N_M receptor results in channel opening, with subsequent influx of Na^+ and efflux of K^+ (motor end plate potential). This motor end plate potential, when large enough, results in adjacent muscle depolarization and propagation along the entire muscle fiber. Drugs that block the neuromuscular junction at the postsynaptic N_M receptor are clinically useful in producing muscle relaxation as an adjunct to major surgery. Neuromuscular blocking drugs are

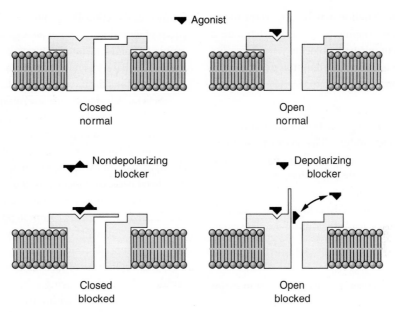

Figure 5–4. Schematic diagram of the interactions of drugs with the postsynaptic cholinergic (N_M) receptor on an end plate channel. **Top**: The action of the normal agonist, acetylcholine, in opening the channel. **Bottom**: **Left**, A nondepolarizing blocker is shown as preventing the opening of the channel when it binds to the receptor. **Right**, a depolarizing blocker, e.g., succinylcholine, both occupies the receptor and blocks the channel. Normal closure of the channel gate is prevented and the blocker may move rapidly in and out of the pore. Depolarizing blockers may desensitize the end plate by occupying the receptor and causing persistent depolarization. An additional effect of drugs on the end plate may occur through changes in the lipid environment surrounding the channel (not shown).

hydrophilic quaternary amines related to acetylcholine. As such, these drugs must be administered parenterally, and do not cross the blood-brain barrier into the central nervous system.

Most neuromuscular blocking drugs are direct-acting N_M receptor antagonists that are nondepolarizing. The prototypical drug is **tubocurarine** (Figure 5–3). These drugs all produce a reversible blockade of the postsynaptic N_M receptor (Figure 5–4). In general, they are metabolized and eliminated by either the kidney or the liver.

One neuromuscular blocking drug, **succinylcholine,** is defined as a depolarizing neuromuscular blocking drug (Figure 5–3). Succinylcholine is a direct-acting *agonist* that binds to the postsynaptic N_M receptor. The binding of succinylcholine to the N_M receptor

results in the opening of channels at the motor end plate and an initial depolarization—like that produced by acetylcholine—but greatly prolonged (Figure 5–4). This depolarization spreads to adjacent membranes causing contractions of surrounding muscle fibers. Visually this presents as twitching and fasciculation of the skeletal muscle. Because the muscle is unable to maintain tension without periodic depolarization and repolarization at the neuromuscular junction, the depolarized muscle undergoes relaxation and paralysis denoted "phase I blockade." With continued exposure to the drug, the motor end plate depolarization ceases, and repolarization occurs. Even with this repolarization, the motor end plate cannot undergo depolarization because it is desensitized. The mechanism for this desensitization is uncertain; however, blockade of the channel by succinylcholine may be important to the "phase II blockade" (Figure 5–4). Succinylcholine is included with neuromuscular blocking drugs because the final physiologic effect is inhibition of the neuromuscular junction.

Physiologic Effects

Both the nondepolarizing and depolarizing drugs produce flaccid muscle paralysis. The order of sensitivity of muscles to the nondepolarizing drugs proceeds from the smaller muscles (the first to undergo paralysis, and the last to recover) to larger ones, with the diaphragm being the most resistant. For succinylcholine, paralysis appears initially in the legs and arms followed by paralysis of the axial musculature.

Clinical Use

Nondepolarizing blockers are used frequently in major surgery to provide relaxation throughout the procedure. They are occasionally used in the intensive care unit to prevent respiratory complications when patients are on ventilators. The time of onset and duration of action varies with each drug. Succinylcholine is the only clinically relevant depolarizing neuromuscular blockade drug. It is used almost exclusively to provide brief relaxation during intubation (placing an endotracheal tube) when patients are being prepared for artificial ventilation.

Adverse Effects

Several of the nondepolarizing blockers can have cardiovascular effects (Table 5–7). Hypotension as a result of generalized histamine release occurs with older agents.

Cardiac dysfunction is also possible as a result of the effects of these drugs on autonomic ganglia, cardiac muscarinic receptors, or interaction with the general anesthetic. Respiratory paralysis occurs as a direct result of the inhibition of the intercostal muscles and diaphragm.

Several adverse events are unique to succinylcholine. Some inhaled anesthetics, such as isoflurane, strongly enhance and prolong the effects of this drug at the neuromuscular junction. Hyperkalemia may occur in patients with burns or spinal cord injury, peripheral nerve dysfunction, or muscular dysfunction. Emesis may occur as a result of increased intragastric pressure. Muscle pain is a common postoperative complaint, and muscle damage may occur. Finally, malignant hyperthermia is a rare autosomal dominant genetic disorder of skeletal muscle that occurs in certain individuals receiving general anesthetics with succinylcholine. The pathophysiologic mechanism appears to be an increase in intracellular free calcium from the sarcoplasmic reticulum. The syndrome has a rapid onset with tachycardia and hypertension. Severe muscle rigidity and hyperthermia are hallmark features. Hyperkalemia and eventual acidosis may also occur. Treatment is with **dantrolene**, a drug that inhibits intracellular calcium release, and measures that control body temperature and blood pressure.

Nicotinic (N_N) Antagonists

Postsynaptic N_N receptors are located in both parasympathetic and sympathetic ganglia. Similar to the N_M

Table 5–7.	Autonomic effects of some neuromuscular blocking drugs		
Drug	**Effect on Autonomic Ganglia**	**Effect on Cardiac Muscarinic Receptors**	**Ability to Release Histamine**
Nondepolarizing			
Atracurium	None	None	Slight
Mivacurium	None	None	Slight
Pancuronium	None	Blocks moderately	None
Tubocurarine	Blocks	None	Moderate
Vecuronium	None	None	None
Depolarizing			
Succinylcholine	Stimulates	Stimulates	Slight

Table 5–8.	Effects of ganglion-blocking drugs
Organ	**Effects**
Central nervous system	Antinicotinic actions may include reduction of nicotine craving and amelioration of Tourette's syndrome (mecamylamine only)
Eye	Moderate mydriasis and cycloplegia
Bronchi	Little effect; asthmatics may note bronchodilation
Gastrointestinal tract	Markedly reduced motility; constipation may be severe
Genitourinary tract	Reduced contractility of the bladder; impairment of erection and ejaculation
Heart	Moderate tachycardia in young adults; reduction in force of contraction and cardiac output
Blood vessels	Reduction in arteriolar tone, marked reduction in venous tone; blood pressure decrease and orthostatic hypotension may be severe
Glands	Reductions in salivation, lacrimation, sweating, and gastric secretion
Skeletal muscle	No significant effect

receptors, N_N receptors are susceptible to both nondepolarizing and depolarizing inhibition. The ganglion-blocking drugs used clinically are all nondepolarizing direct-acting competitive antagonists (**hexamethonium, mecamylamine, trimethaphan**); however, there is evidence that these drugs may also block the nicotinic ion channel.

Physiologic Effect

The physiologic effects of these drugs are presented in Table 5–8. Owing to the inhibition of sympathetic control of venous tone, these drugs cause venous pooling and orthostatic hypotension. Moderate tachycardia and decreased cardiac output due to reduced venous return and a negative inotropic effect may also occur.

Clinical Use

Owing to the fact that the adverse effects of these drugs are so severe, patients are able to tolerate these drugs for only a limited period. Additionally, some drugs demonstrate short half-lives or are orally inactive, reducing their clinical value. At present, two drugs are used clinically. Mecamylamine, a lipophilic synthetic amine that crosses into the CNS, is being studied to decrease nicotine addiction and to treat Tourette's syndrome. Trimethaphan is clinically used during a hypertensive crisis, and to produce controlled hypotension in some surgical scenarios.

Adverse Events

As a result of the inhibition of the autonomic nervous system by the ganglion-blocking drugs, patients tolerate them for only acute situations.

■ REHABILITATION FOCUS

Patients in rehabilitation may be prescribed either direct-acting or indirect-acting cholinomimetics. Physical therapists may have to adjust their patients' activities to account for the effects of these medications. Indications for these drugs include glaucoma, hypotonic bladder function, myasthenia gravis, and dementia. Many of these patients will be involved in rehabilitation and exertional activities as part of the therapy, and some myasthenia gravis patients benefit clinically from such activities. Cholinomimetics have the potential to significantly enhance or inhibit the rehabilitation process. Indirect-acting cholinomimetics are prescribed for patients with myasthenia gravis or Alzheimer's disease. In these situations, scheduling treatment periods when these drugs are at their maximal plasma level will enhance functional or cognitive activities and assist the therapist in providing a positive outcome.

Patients may also be medicated with either muscarinic or nicotinic antagonists. Muscarinic antagonists may be prescribed for patients with spastic bladder and incontinence, Parkinson's disease, or pulmonary dysfunction. In patients with spastic bladder and incontinence, the therapist may reduce inadvertent voiding by scheduling treatment periods at peak plasma levels of the drug. The clinical applications of antimuscarinics in the treatment of Parkinson's disease and pulmonary dysfunction are discussed in Chapters 17 and 35, respectively. The therapist should also remember that if treatment is undertaken at peak plasma levels of these drugs, and the activity involves sustained periods of exertion, hyperthermia may occur in the patient owing to inhibition of eccrine sweat glands by the antimuscarinic agent. Nicotinic skeletal muscle antagonists are commonly used in patients undergoing major surgery requiring mechanical ventilation. In these patients, optimal musculoskeletal function will return following elimination of the nicotinic antagonist. When possible, the therapist may consider establishing and reviewing treatment plans with the patients on the day prior to the surgery when cognitive and musculoskeletal function will be higher than immediately following the surgery.

Finally, patients may be self-medicating with nicotine via inhalation or buccal absorption; that is, smoking or dipping. These patients may experience various adverse sympathetic or parasympathetic responses based on other comorbidities. The physical therapist should advise these patients to abstain from these activities prior to treatment, or permanently if possible.

CLINICAL RELEVANCE FOR REHABILITATION

Adverse Drug Reactions
Direct- and indirect-acting parasympathomimetics
- Shortness of breath and altered heart rate may both occur with muscarinic agonists.

- Nicotine may increase blood pressure and possibly result in cardiac arrhythmias.
- Muscarinic agonists can increase frequency of urination and thus disrupt rehabilitation treatments.
- Muscarinic agonists can decrease visual acuity by preventing pupillary dilation in response to decreased light.

Anticholinergics
- Antimuscarinic drugs can prevent perspiration and lead to hyperthermia.
- Antimuscarinic drugs can increase heart rate and possibly predispose patients to arrhythmias.
- Antimuscarinic drugs can cause photosensitivity by decreasing pupillary constriction in response to bright light.
- Antimuscarinics can cause sedation and decrease cognitive function. High doses can cause hallucinations, especially in the elderly.

Effects Interfering with Rehabilitation
- Bronchoconstriction may decrease patients' ability to participate in aerobic activities.
- Hyperthermia, increased blood pressure and heart rate can also decrease patient participation in aerobic activities. These effects should be taken into account when developing a treatment plan.
- Sedation and decreased cognitive function can decrease patients' understanding of instructions for home treatment programs.
- Changes in light levels in the room in conjunction with sedation may increase the chance of falls.

Possible Therapy Solutions
- To avoid dyspnea and cardiac dysfunction, aerobic treatment prescriptions should be designed to allow the patient more time to achieve their aerobic goal.
- If sedation or decreased cognitive function is a problem, consider therapy at the end of a dosage period when the drug's plasma levels will be at their lowest.

Potentiation of Functional Outcomes Secondary to Drug Therapy
- Muscarinic antagonists used in the treatment of hypertonic bladder function can reduce incontinence during rehabilitation activities.

PROBLEM-ORIENTED PATIENT STUDY

Brief History: The patient is a 25-year-old male who was involved in a motor vehicle–motorcycle accident 4 weeks ago. The patient was transferred to rehabilitation yesterday. The patient is scheduled for evaluation for wheelchair mobility and transfer training today at 8:15 in the general gym in the rehabilitation department, immediately after breakfast.

Current Medical Status and Drug Therapy: As a result of the accident, the patient is a low spinal cord level paraplegic in stable condition. The patient has no cardiovascular dysfunction, but is currently on drugs to reduce spasticity, including oxybutynin to reduce spastic bladder activity.

Rehabilitation Setting: The patient appears eager to begin. The therapist and patient begin the evaluation by starting with a sliding board transfer from the wheelchair to the plinth. The patient becomes incontinent during his initial attempt with the sliding board activities, and voids involuntarily. The patient becomes embarrassed, and complains that this has happened previously when he attempted to sit up and reposition himself with his hands. The patient requests that rehabilitation activities for the day be terminated and he be returned to his room. In the afternoon, the patient does not want to come to the gym setting as he states that he is afraid that the same problem will arise again.

Problem/Clinical Options: Contraction of abdominal musculature in conjunction with a Valsalva maneuver during the initial sliding board transfer increased pressure on the spastic bladder resulting in incontinence during the sliding board transfer. The oxybutynin to assist in decreasing spasticity is normally prescribed three times a day. The first dosage for the day is usually taken at breakfast just prior to the rehabilitation activities in the gym. The onset of activity for oxybutynin is approximately 30 to 60 minutes following an oral dose, peak activity 3 to 6 hours later, and the duration of effect 6 to 10 hours. The patient receives the last dose of the day in the evening. Insufficient time had elapsed for the initial oxybutynin dose of the day to reach peak plasma levels prior to rehabilitation activity. The rehabilitation activity should be rescheduled in the morning for approximately 2 to 3 hours after the first dose of the day to maximize pharmacologic effect and minimize the patient's incontinence.

PREPARATIONS AVAILABLE

Direct-Acting Cholinomimetics

Acetylcholine (Miochol-E)
Ophthalmic: 1:100 (10-mg/mL) intraocular solution

Bethanechol (generic, Urecholine)
Oral: 5-, 10-, 25-, 50-mg tablets
Parenteral: 5 mg/mL for SC injection

Carbachol
Ophthalmic (topical, Isopto Carbachol, Carboptic): 0.75, 1.5, 2.25, 3% drops
Ophthalmic (intraocular, Miostat, Carbastat): 0.01% solution

Cevimeline (Evoxac)
Oral: 30-mg capsules

Pilocarpine (generic, Isopto Carpine)
Ophthalmic (topical): 0.25, 0.5, 1, 2, 3, 4, 6, 8, 10% solutions, 4% gel
Ophthalmic sustained-release inserts (Ocusert Pilo-20, Ocusert Pilo-40): release 20 and 40 mcg pilocarpine per hour for 1 week, respectively
Oral (Salagen): 5-mg tablets

Cholinesterase Inhibitors

Ambenonium (Mytelase)
Oral: 10-mg tablets

Demecarium (Humorsol)
Ophthalmic: 0.125, 0.25% drops

Donepezil (Aricept)
Oral: 5-, 10-mg tablets

Echothiophate (Phospholine)
Ophthalmic: Powder to reconstitute for 0.03, 0.06, 0.125, 0.25% drops

Edrophonium (generic, Tensilon)
Parenteral: 10 mg/mL for IM or IV injection

Galantamine (Reminyl)
Oral: 4-, 8-, 12-mg capsules; 4 mg/mL solution

Neostigmine (generic, Prostigmin)
Oral: 15-mg tablets
Parenteral: 1:1000 in 10 mL; 1:2000, 1:4000 in 1 mL

Physostigmine, eserine (generic)
Parenteral: 1 mg/mL for IM or slow IV injection

Pyridostigmine (Mestinon, Regonol)
Oral: 60-mg tablets; 180-mg sustained-release tablets; 15 mg/mL syrup
Parenteral: 5 mg/mL for IM or slow IV injection

Rivastigmine (Exelon)
Oral: 1.5-, 3-, 4.5-, 6-mg tablets; 2 mg/mL solution

Tacrine (Cognex)
Oral: 10-, 20-, 30-, 40-mg tablets

Antimuscarinic Anticholinergic Drugs[*,†]

Atropine (generic)
Oral: 0.4-mg tablets
Parenteral: 0.05, 0.1, 0.3, 0.4, 0.5, 0.8, 1 mg/mL for injection

Ophthalmic (generic, Isopto Atropine): 0.5, 1, 2% drops; 1% ointments

Belladonna alkaloids, extract or tincture (generic)
Oral: 0.27–0.33 mg/mL liquid

Clidinium (Quarzan)
Oral: 2.5-, 5-mg capsules

Cyclopentolate (generic, Cyclogyl, others)
Ophthalmic: 0.5, 1, 2% drops

Dicyclomine (generic, Bentyl, others)
Oral: 10-, 20-mg capsules; 20-mg tablets; 10 mg/5 mL syrup
Parenteral: 10 mg/mL for injection

Flavoxate (Urispas)
Oral: 100-mg tablets

Glycopyrrolate (generic, Robinul)
Oral: 1-, 2-mg tablets
Parenteral: 0.2 mg/mL for injection

Homatropine (generic, Isopto Homatropine)
Ophthalmic: 2, 5% drops

l-Hyoscyamine (Anaspaz, Cystospaz-M, Levsinex)
Oral: 0.125-, 0.15-mg tablets; 0.375-mg timed-release capsules; 0.125 mg/5 mL oral elixir and solution
Parenteral: 0.5 mg/mL for injection

Mepenzolate (Cantil)
Oral: 25-mg tablets

Methantheline (Banthine)
Oral: 50-mg tablets

Methscopolamine (Pamine)
Oral: 2.5-mg tablets

Oxybutynin (generic, Ditropan)
Oral: 5-mg tablets; 5-, 10-, 15-mg extended-release tablets; 5 mg/5 mL syrup

Propantheline (generic, Pro-Banthine)
Oral: 7.5-, 15-mg tablets

Scopolamine (generic)
Oral: 0.4-mg tablets
Parenteral: 0.3, 0.4, 0.65, 0.86, 1 mg/mL for injection
Ophthalmic (Isopto Hyoscine): 0.25% solution

Transdermal (Transderm Scop): 1.5-mg (delivers 0.5 mg) patch

Tolterodine (Detrol)
Oral: 1-, 2-mg tablets; 2-, 4-mg extended-release capsules

Tridihexethyl (Pathilon)
Oral: 25-mg tablets

Tropicamide (generic, Mydriacyl Ophthalmic, others)
Ophthalmic: 0.5, 1% drops

Ganglion Blockers

Mecamylamine (Inversine)
Oral: 2.5-mg tablets

Trimethaphan (Arfonad)
Parenteral: 50-mg/mL

Neuromuscular Blocking Drugs

Atracurium (Tracrium)
Parenteral: 10 mg/mL for injection

Cisatracurium (Nimbex)
Parenteral: 2, 10 mg/mL for IV injection

Doxacurium (Nuromax)
Parenteral: 1 mg/mL for IV injection

Metocurine (generic, Metubine Iodide)
Parenteral: 2 mg/mL for injection

Mivacurium (Mivacron)
Parenteral: 0.5, 2 mg/mL for injection

Pancuronium (generic, Pavulon)
Parenteral: 1, 2 mg/mL for injection

Pipecuronium (Arduan)
Parenteral: 1 mg/mL for IV injection

Rocuronium (Zemuron)
Parenteral: 10 mg/mL for IV injection

Succinylcholine (generic, Anectine)
Parenteral: 20, 50, 100 mg/mL for injection; 100, 500-mg per vial powders to reconstitute for injection

Tubocurarine (generic)
Parenteral: 3 mg (20 units)/mL for injection

Vecuronium (generic, Norcuron)
Parenteral: 10, 20 mg powder to reconstitute for injection

*Antimuscarinic drugs used in Parkinson's disease are listed in Chapter 17.

†Antimuscarinic drugs used in respiratory dysfunction are listed in Chapter 35.

REFERENCES

Direct Acting and Cholinesterase Inhibitors

Benowitz NL: Pharmacology of nicotine: Addiction and therapeutics. *Annu Rev Pharmacol Toxicol* 1996;36:597.

Brodde O-E, et al: Presence, distribution, and physiologic function of adrenergic and muscarinic receptor subtypes in the human heart. *Basic Res Cardiol* 2001;96:528.

Ehlert FJ: Contractile role of M2 and M3 muscarinic receptors in gastrointestinal, airway, and urinary bladder smooth muscle. *Life Sci* 2003;74:355.

Fox RI, Konttinen Y, Fisher A: Use of muscarinic agonists in the treatment of Sjögren's syndrome. *Clin Immunol* 2001;101:249.

Lucas RJ, et al: International Union of Pharmacology. XX. Current status of the nomenclature for nicotinic acetylcholine receptors and their subunits. *Pharmacol Rev* 1999;51:397.

Okamoto H, et al: Muscarinic agonist potencies at three different effector systems linked to the M(2) or M(3) receptor in longitudinal smooth muscle of guinea-pig small intestine. *Br J Pharmacol* 2002;135:1765.

Rand MJ: Neuropharmacological effects of nicotine in relation to cholinergic mechanisms. *Prog Brain Res* 1989;79:3.

Smoking and cardiovascular disease. *MMWR Morb Mortal Wkly Rep* 1984;32:677.

The Surgeon General: Smoking and Health. Washington, DC: US Department of Health and Human Services, 1964.

Vincent A, Drachman DB: Myasthenia gravis. *Adv Neurol* 2002;88:159.

Antimuscarinic Drugs

Andersson KE: Antimuscarinics for treatment of overactive bladder. *Lancet Neurol* 2004;3:46.

Andersson KE, Hedlund P: Pharmacologic perspective on the pathophysiology of the lower urinary tract. *Urology* 2002;60(5 Suppl 1):13.

Campbell SC: Clinical aspects of inhaled anticholinergic therapy. *Respir Care* 2001;46:275.

Chapple CR, Yamanishi T, Chess-Williams R: Muscarinic receptor types and management of the overactive bladder. *Urology* 2002;60(5 Suppl 1):82.

Kranke P, et al: The efficacy and safety of transdermal scopolamine for the prevention of postoperative nausea and vomiting: a quantitative systematic review. *Anesth Analg* 2002;95:133.

Lee AM, Jacoby DB, Fryer AD: Selective muscarinic receptor antagonists for airway diseases. *Curr Opin Pharmacol* 2001;1:223.

Olson K: Mushrooms. In *Poisoning & Drug Overdose,* 3rd ed. Olson K, ed. New York: McGraw-Hill, 1998.

Rascol O, et al: Antivertigo medications and drug-induced vertigo: A pharmacological review. *Drugs* 1995;50:777.

Shuessler B, et al: Pharmacologic treatment of stress urinary incontinence: Expectations for outcome. *Urology* 2003;62(4 Suppl 1):31.

Smellie JM, et al: Nocturnal enuresis: A placebo-controlled trial of two antidepressant drugs. *Arch Dis Child* 1996;75:62.

Watson NM: Use of the Agency for Health Care Policy and Research Urinary Incontinence Guideline in nursing homes. *J Am Geriatr Soc* 2003;51:1779.

Wellstein A, Pitschner HF: Complex dose-response curves of atropine in man explained by different functions of M_1- and M_2-cholinoceptors. *Naunyn Schmiedebergs Arch Pharmacol* 1988;338:19.

Young JM, et al: Mecamylamine: new therapeutic uses and toxicity/risk profile. *Clin Ther* 2001;23:532.

Neuromuscular Blockers

Atherton DP, Hunter JM: Clinical pharmacokinetics of the newer neuromuscular blocking drugs. *Clin Pharmacokinet* 1999;36:169.

Ericksson LI: Residual neuromuscular blockade. Incidence and relevance. *Anaesthetist* 2000;49(Suppl 1):S18.

Meakin GH: Recent advances in myorelaxant therapy. *Paediatr Anaesth* 2001;11:523.

Moore EW, Hunter JM: The new neuromuscular blocking agents: Do they offer any advantages? *Br J Anaesth* 2001;87:912.

Savarese JJ, et al: Pharmacology of muscle relaxants and their antagonists. In *Anesthesia,* 5th ed. Miller RD, ed. Churchill Livingstone, 2000.

White PF: *Perioperative Drug Manual,* 2nd ed. Philadelphia: Elsevier, 2005.

Rehabilitation

Blass JP, Cyrus PA, Bieber F, Gulanski B: Randomized, double-blind, placebo-controlled, multicenter study to evaluate the safety and tolerability of metrifonate in patients with probable Alzheimer disease. The Metrifonate Study Group. *Alzheimer Dis Assoc Disord* 2000;14:39.

Lohi EL, Lindberg C, Andersen O: Physical training effects in myasthenia gravis. *Arch Phys Med Rehabil* 1993;74:1178.

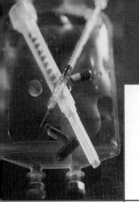

6

SYMPATHOMIMETICS AND SYMPATHOLYTICS

Receptors of the sympathetic system may be divided into alpha (α), beta (β), and dopamine (D) receptors. Drugs that bind to these receptors and modulate or mimic the function of the sympathetic nervous system may be divided into those which augment the system (*sympathomimetics*) and those which antagonize the system (*sympatholytics*). The sympathomimetics constitute a very important group of agonists used for cardiovascular, respiratory, and other conditions. They are readily divided into subgroups on the basis of their spectrum of affinity for α, β, or D receptors. Alternatively, sympathomimetics may be divided into subgroups based on whether their mode of action is direct or indirect. Sympatholytics are an important group of antagonists used in cardiovascular and other conditions. These drugs are divided into primary subgroups on the basis of their receptor (α and β) selectivity.

▉ SYMPATHOMIMETIC DRUGS

Mode of Action

Sympathomimetics (also called *adrenomimetics*) may directly activate their adrenoceptors, or they may act indirectly to increase the concentration of catecholamine transmitter in the synapse (Figure 6–1). Amphetamine derivatives and tyramine cause the release of stored catecholamines; these sympathomimetics are, therefore, mainly indirect in their mode of action. Another form of indirect action is seen with cocaine and the tricyclic antidepressants; these drugs inhibit reuptake of catecholamines by presynaptic nerve terminals that release them (Figure 4–3), and thus increase the synaptic activity of released transmitter.

Blockade of metabolism (i.e., block of catechol-*O*-methyltransferase [COMT] and-monoamine oxidase [MAO]) has little direct effect on autonomic activity, but MAO inhibition increases the stores of catecholamines in adrenergic synaptic vesicles and thus may potentiate the action of other indirect-acting sympathomimetics subsequently discussed.

Spectrum of Action

Both α and β receptors are further subdivided into subgroups. The distribution of these receptors is set forth in Table 4–3. Epinephrine may be considered a single prototype with effects at all receptor types (α_1, α_2, β_1, β_2, and β_3). In addition, separate prototypes—**phenylephrine** for α receptors and **isoproterenol** for β receptors—have been characterized. Dopamine receptors constitute a third class of adrenoceptors. The just-mentioned drugs have relatively little effect on dopamine receptors, but dopamine itself is a potent dopamine receptor agonist and when

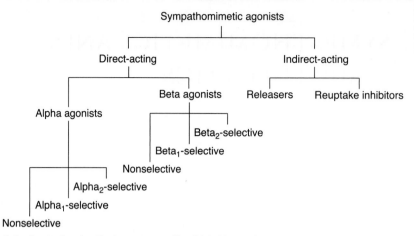

Figure 6–1. Sympathomimetic drugs are readily divided into subgroups on the basis of which receptors they activate: alpha, beta, or dopamine (not shown). Alternatively, these drugs are divided into subgroups on the basis of whether their mode of action is direct (at postsynaptic receptors) or indirect (other than at post-synaptic receptors).

given as a drug can also activate β receptors (intermediate doses) and α receptors (large doses). The relative affinities of these representative drugs are presented in Table 6–1.

Chemistry and Pharmacokinetics

The endogenous adrenoceptor agonists (**epinephrine, norepinephrine,** and **dopamine**) are catecholamines and are rapidly metabolized by COMT and MAO. As

Table 6–1.	**Relative selectivity of adrenoceptor agonists**
Drug	**Relative Receptor Affinities**
Alpha agonists	
Phenylephrine	$\alpha_1 > \alpha_2 >>>>> \beta$
Clonidine	$\alpha_2 > \alpha_1 >>>>> \beta$
Mixed α and β agonists	
Norepinephrine	$\alpha_2 = \alpha_1; \beta_1 >> \beta_2$
Epinephrine	$\alpha_2 = \alpha_1; \beta_1 = \beta_2$
Beta agonists	
Dobutamine[1]	$\beta_1 > \beta_2 >>>> \alpha$
Isoproterenol	$\beta_1 = \beta_2 >>>> \alpha$
Terbutaline, metaproterenol, albuterol	$\beta_2 >> \beta_1 >>>> \alpha$
Dopamine agonists	
Dopamine	$D_1 = D_2 >> \beta >> \alpha$
Fenoldopam	$D_1 >> D_2$

α = alpha; β = beta; D = dopamine.
[1]Dobutamine is a relatively β_1-selective synthetic catecholamine.

a result, these adrenoceptor agonists are almost inactive when given by the oral route (Table 6–2).

When released from presynaptic nerve terminals, norepinephrine, epinephrine, and dopamine are subsequently taken up into these same presynaptic nerve terminals and into perisynaptic cells; this uptake may also occur when they are given as drugs. These agonists have a short duration of action. When given parenterally, they do not enter the central nervous system (CNS) in significant amounts. Isoproterenol, a synthetic catecholamine, is similar to the endogenous transmitters but is not readily taken up into the presynaptic nerve terminals. Phenylisopropylamines, for example, amphetamines, are resistant to MAO; most of them are not catecholamines and are, therefore, also resistant to COMT. These agents are orally active; they enter the CNS; and their effects last much longer than those of catecholamines. Tyramine, which is not a phenylisopropylamine, is rapidly metabolized by MAO except in patients who are taking an MAO inhibitor drug. MAO inhibitors are sometimes used in the treatment of depression (Chapter 19).

Mechanisms of Action

Alpha Receptor Effects

Alpha$_1$ receptor effects are mediated primarily by the trimeric coupling protein G$_q$. When G$_q$ is activated, the alpha moiety of this protein activates the phosphoinositide cascade and causes the release of inositol-1,4,5-trisphosphate (IP$_3$) and diacylglycerol (DAG)

Table 6–2. Pharmacokinetics and clinical applications of some sympathomimetics

Drug	Oral Activity	Duration of Action	Clinical Applications
Catecholamines			
Epinephrine	No	Minutes	For anaphylaxis, glaucoma, and to cause vasoconstriction
Norepinephrine	No	Minutes	To cause vasoconstriction in hypotension
Isoproterenol	Poor	Minutes	For asthma, atrioventricular block (rare)
Dopamine	No	Minutes	For shock, heart failure
Dobutamine	No	Minutes	For shock, heart failure
Other sympathomimetics			
Amphetamines, phenmetrazine, others	Yes	Hours	For narcolepsy, obesity, attention deficit disorder
Ephedrine	Yes	Hours	For urinary incontinence, and to cause vasoconstriction in hypotension
Phenylephrine	Poor	Hours	To cause mydriasis, vasoconstriction, decongestion
Albuterol, metaproterenol, terbutaline	Moderate	Hours	For asthma
Oxymetazoline, xylometazoline	Yes	Hours	To cause nasal decongestion (long acting)
Cocaine	Poor	Minutes to hours	To cause vasoconstriction and local anesthesia

from membrane lipids (Figure 6–2). Calcium is subsequently released from stores in smooth muscle cells. Direct gating of calcium channels may also play a role in increasing intracellular calcium concentration. In smooth muscle cells, the cellular response to this elevated intracellular calcium is increased contraction. In contrast, α_2 receptor activation results in inhibition of adenylyl cyclase via the coupling protein G_i, and subsequent decrease of the second messenger cyclic adenosine monophosphate (cAMP) (Figure 6–3).

Beta Receptor Effects

Beta receptors (β_1, β_2, and β_3) stimulate adenylyl cyclase via the coupling protein G_s, which leads to an increase in cAMP concentration in the cell. cAMP acts as a second messenger mediating the cellular response to β receptor stimulation (Figure 6–3).

Dopamine Receptor Effects

D_1 receptors activate adenylyl cyclase in neurons and vascular smooth muscle. D_2 receptors are more important in the brain but probably also play a significant role as presynaptic receptors on peripheral nerves. These receptors inhibit adenylyl cyclase activity, open potassium channels, and decrease calcium influx.

Physiologic Effects

CNS

Catecholamines do not enter the CNS effectively. Sympathomimetics that can enter the CNS (e.g.,

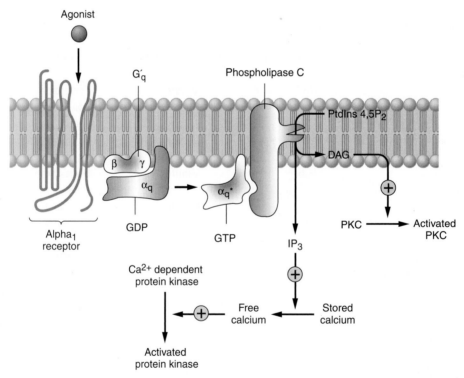

Figure 6–2. Activation of α_1 responses. Stimulation of α_1 receptors by catecholamines leads to the activation of a G_q coupling protein. The activated α subunit (α_q^*) of this G protein activates the effector, phospholipase C, which leads to the release of IP_3 (inositol 1,4,5-trisphosphate) and DAG (diacylglycerol) from phosphatidylinositol 4,5-bisphosphate (PtdIns 4,5-P_2). IP_3 stimulates the release of sequestered stores of calcium, leading to an increased concentration of cytoplasmic Ca^{2+}. The Ca^{2+} may then activate Ca^{2+}-dependent protein kinases, which in turn phosphorylate their substrates. DAG activates protein kinase C (PKC). See text for additional effects of α_1 receptor activation.

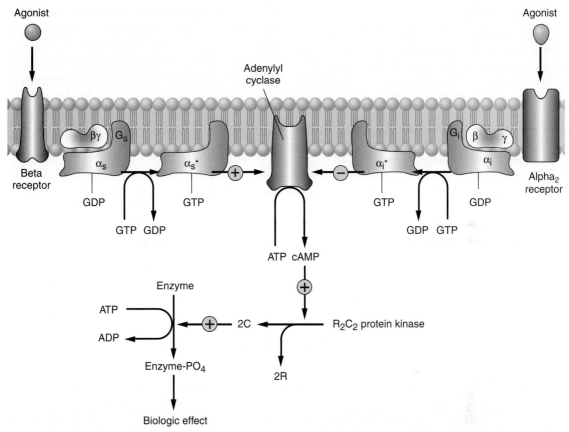

Figure 6–3. Activation and inhibition of adenylyl cyclase by agonists that bind to catecholamine receptors. Binding to β adreno-ceptors stimulates adenylyl cyclase by activating the stimulatory G protein (G_s) which leads to the dissociation of its α subunit charged with guanosine triphospate (GTP). This α_s subunit directly activates adenylyl cyclase, resulting in an increased rate of synthesis of cyclic adenosine monophosphate (cAMP). Alpha$_2$ adrenoceptor ligands inhibit adenylyl cyclase by causing dissoci-ation of the inhibitory G protein (G_i) into its subunits; i.e., an α_i subunit charged with GTP and a β-γ unit. The mechanism by which these subunits inhibit adenylyl cyclase is uncertain. cAMP binds to the regulatory subunit (R) of cAMP-dependent protein kinase, leading to the liberation of active catalytic subunits (C) that phosphorylate specific protein substrates and modify their activity. These catalytic units also phosphorylate the cAMP response element binding protein that modifies gene expression (not shown). See text for other actions of β and α_2 adrenoceptors.

amphetamines) have a spectrum of stimulant effects, beginning with mild alerting or reduction of fatigue and progressing to anorexia, euphoria, and insomnia. Some of these central effects probably reflect the release of dopamine in certain dopaminergic tracts. Very high doses lead to marked anxiety or aggressiveness, paranoia, and, rarely, convulsions. Direct-acting α_2 agonists such as clonidine are quite different in that they decrease sym-pathetic neuronal outflow and have sedative effects.

Eye

The smooth muscle of the pupillary dilator responds to topical phenylephrine and similar α agonists with mydriasis. Accommodation is not significantly affected. Outflow of aqueous humor may be facilitated by non-selective α agonists, with a subsequent reduction of intraocular pressure. Alpha$_2$-selective agonists also reduce intraocular pressure, apparently by reducing synthesis of aqueous humor.

Gastrointestinal Tract

The gastrointestinal tract is well endowed with both α and β receptors that are located on both smooth muscle and on neurons of the enteric nervous system. Activation of either α or β receptors leads to relaxation of the smooth muscle. Alpha$_2$ agonists may decrease salt and water secretion into the intestine.

Genitourinary Tract

The genitourinary tract contains α receptors in the bladder trigone and sphincter area; these receptors mediate contraction of the sphincter. Sympathomimetics are sometimes used to increase sphincter tone. Beta$_2$ agonists may cause significant uterine relaxation in pregnant women near term, but the doses required also cause significant tachycardia.

Vascular System

Different vascular beds respond differently depending on their dominant receptor type. Alpha, β, and D receptors all have effects on the vasculature. Alpha$_1$ agonists (e.g., phenylephrine) constrict skin and splanchnic blood vessels and increase peripheral vascular resistance and venous pressure. Because these drugs increase blood pressure, they often evoke a compensatory reflex bradycardia. Alpha$_2$ agonists (e.g., clonidine) cause vasoconstriction when administered intravenously or topically (e.g., as a nasal spray), but when given orally they accumulate in the CNS and reduce sympathetic outflow and blood pressure as described in Chapter 7. Beta$_2$ agonists (e.g., terbutaline) cause significant reduction in arteriolar tone in the skeletal muscle vascular bed and can reduce peripheral vascular resistance and arterial blood pressure.

Beta$_1$ agonists have relatively little effect on blood vessels. Dopamine causes vasodilation in the splanchnic and renal vascular beds by activating D$_1$ receptors. This effect has been used in the treatment of renal failure associated with shock. At higher doses, dopamine activates β receptors in the heart and elsewhere; at still higher doses, α receptors are activated.

Heart

The heart is well supplied with β$_1$ and β$_2$ receptors. The β$_1$ receptors predominate in some parts of the heart. Activation of both of these receptors results in increased normal and abnormal pacemaker activity (chronotropic), contractility, (inotropic), and conduction (dromotropic) responses.

Summary of Cardiovascular Actions

Sympathomimetics with both α and β$_1$ effects (e.g., norepinephrine) cause an increase in blood pressure and evoke increased baroreceptor activation (*baroreceptor reflex*). The increased afferent baroreceptor activity ultimately results in increased efferent vagal activity. This reflex vagal effect often dominates any direct β effects on the heart rate, so that a slow infusion of norepinephrine typically causes increased blood pressure and bradycardia (Table 6–3). The feedback regulation of blood pressure is further discussed in Chapter 4 (Figure 4–5). A pure α agonist (e.g., phenylephrine) will routinely slow the heart rate via the baroreceptor reflex, whereas a pure β agonist (e.g., isoproterenol) almost always increases the heart rate. The diastolic blood pressure is affected mainly by peripheral vascular resistance and the heart rate. The adrenoceptors with the greatest effects on vascular resistance

Table 6–3.	Effects of prototypical sympathomimetics on vascular resistance, blood pressure, and heart rate				
Drug	**Effect on**				
	Skin, Splanchnic Vessel Resistance	Skeletal Muscle Vessel Resistance	Renal Vessel Resistance	Mean Blood Pressure	Heart Rate
Phenylephrine	↑↑↑	—	↑	↑↑	↓
Isoproterenol	—	↓↓	—	↓↓	↑↑
Norepinephrine	↑↑↑↑	↑	↑	↑↑↑	↓

are α and β_2 receptors. The systolic blood pressure is the sum of the diastolic and pulse pressures. The pulse pressure is determined mainly by the stroke volume (a function of force of cardiac contraction), which is influenced by β_1 receptors.

Bronchi

The smooth muscle of the bronchi relaxes markedly in response to β_2 agonists. These agents are the most efficacious and reliable drugs available for reversing bronchospasm in asthma. See Chapter 35 for additional information.

Metabolic and Hormonal Effects

Beta$_1$ agonists increase renal renin secretion. Beta$_2$ agonists increase insulin secretion by the pancreas. Both increase glycogenolysis in the liver and release of glucose into the blood. The resulting hyperglycemia is countered by the increased insulin levels. Transport of glucose out of the liver is associated initially with hyperkalemia; transport into peripheral organs (especially skeletal muscle) is accompanied by movement of potassium into these cells, resulting in a later hypokalemia. All β agonists appear to stimulate lipolysis.

Clinical Uses

Clinical applications of selected sympathomimetics are shown in Table 6–2.

Anaphylaxis

Epinephrine is the drug of choice for the immediate treatment of anaphylactic shock. The catecholamine is sometimes supplemented with antihistamines and corticosteroids, but these agents are not as efficacious as epinephrine nor as rapidly acting.

CNS

The phenylisopropylamines, such as **amphetamine,** are widely used and abused for their CNS effects. Legitimate indications include narcolepsy, attention deficit disorder, and, with appropriate controls, weight reduction. The anorexiant effect may be helpful in initiating weight loss but is insufficient to maintain the loss unless patients also receive intensive dietary and psychologic counseling and support. The drugs are abused or misused for the purpose of deferring sleep and for

their mood-elevating, euphoria-producing action (Chapter 21).

Eye

Alpha agonists, especially phenylephrine, are often used topically to produce mydriasis and to reduce the conjunctival itching and congestion caused by irritation or allergy. These drugs do not cause cycloplegia. Epinephrine and a prodrug, **dipivefrin,** have been used topically in the treatment of glaucoma. Phenylephrine has also been used for glaucoma, mainly outside the United States. Newer α_2 agonists introduced for use in glaucoma include **apraclonidine** and **brimonidine.** As noted, the α_2-selective agonists appear to reduce aqueous synthesis.

Cardiovascular Applications

The cardiovascular applications of these drugs may be divided into clinical conditions in which the goal is increased blood flow, decreased blood flow, or increased blood pressure. Clinical conditions in which an increased blood flow is desired include acute heart failure and some types of shock. An increase in cardiac output and blood flow to the tissues is needed in these clinical situations. Beta$_1$ agonists may be useful in this situation because they increase cardiac contractility and reduce (to some degree) afterload by decreasing the impedance to ventricular ejection through a small β_2 effect. In contrast, clinical conditions in which a decrease in blood flow or increase in blood pressure is desired require vasoconstriction. Alpha$_1$ agonists are useful in situations where vasoconstriction is appropriate. These include local hemostatic and decongestant effects as well as spinal shock. In the latter, alpha agonists may temporarily maintain blood pressure and perfusion of the brain, heart, and kidneys. Shock due to septicemia or myocardial infarction, on the other hand, is usually made worse by vasoconstrictors because sympathetic discharge is usually already increased. Alpha agonists are often mixed with local anesthetics to reduce the loss of anesthetic from the area of injection into the circulation and improve hemostasis. Chronic orthostatic hypotension due to inadequate sympathetic tone can be treated with ephedrine or a newer orally active α_1 agonist, **midodrine.**

Upper and Lower Respiratory System

Owing to the previously discussed vasoconstrictive effects of α_1 agonists, these drugs are used to vasoconstrict the nasal vasculature and decrease sinus congestion. Both short- and long-acting β_2-selective agonists are drugs of choice in the treatment of asthma. The short-acting β_2-selective agonists are not recommended for prophylaxis, but they are safe and effective and may be lifesaving in the treatment of acute asthmatic bronchoconstriction. The long-acting β_2-selective agonists are recommended for prophylaxis. See Chapter 35 for additional information.

Genitourinary Tract

Beta$_2$ agonists (**ritodrine, terbutaline**) are used to suppress premature labor, but the cardiac stimulant effect may be hazardous to both mother and fetus. Nonsteroidal anti-inflammatory drugs, calcium channel blockers, and magnesium are also used for this indication. Long-acting oral sympathomimetics such as **ephedrine** are sometimes used to improve urinary continence in children with enuresis and in the elderly. This action is mediated by α receptors in the trigone of the bladder and, in men, the smooth muscle of the prostate.

Adverse Effects

Catecholamines

Because of their limited penetration into the brain, these drugs have little CNS toxicity when given systemically. In the periphery, their adverse effects are extensions of their pharmacologic α or β actions: excessive vasoconstriction, cardiac arrhythmias, myocardial infarction, and pulmonary edema or hemorrhage.

Other Sympathomimetics

The phenylisopropylamines may produce mild to severe CNS toxicity depending on dosage. In small doses, they induce nervousness, anorexia, and insomnia; in higher doses, they may cause anxiety, aggressiveness, or paranoid behavior. Convulsions may occur. Peripherally acting agents have toxicities that are predictable on the basis of the receptors they activate. Thus, α_1 agonists cause hypertension and β_1 agonists cause sinus tachycardia and serious arrhythmias. Beta$_2$ agonists cause skeletal muscle tremor, and at higher doses cardiac dysrhythmias. Both β_1 and β_2 receptor

stimulation may increase blood glucose levels. Note that none of these drugs is purely selective; at high doses, β_1-selective agents have β_2 actions and vice versa. Cocaine is of special importance as a drug of abuse (Chapter 21): its major toxicities include cardiac arrhythmias or infarction and convulsions. A fatal outcome is more common with acute cocaine overdose than with any other sympathomimetic.

■ SYMPATHOLYTIC DRUGS

Alpha- and β-receptor antagonists are divided into primary subgroups on the basis of their receptor selectivity (Figure 6–4). Because α- and β-blockers differ markedly in their effects and clinical applications these drugs are considered separately in the following discussion. The relative receptor selectivity of these drugs for either α or β receptors are listed in Table 6–4.

Alpha-Blocking Drugs

Subdivisions of the α-receptor antagonists are based on selective affinity for α_1 versus α_2 receptors. Other features used to classify these drugs are their reversibility and duration of action. **Phenoxybenzamine** is an irreversible, long-acting, prototypical blocking agent, and is only slightly α_1 selective. In contrast, **phentolamine** is a competitive, reversible, nonselective alpha blocking agent. **Prazosin** is an α_1 selective, reversible blocking agent. **Doxazosin, terazosin,** and **tamsulosin** are similar drugs. Unlike phenoxybenzamine, the other antagonists effects are competitive; that is, they may be surmounted

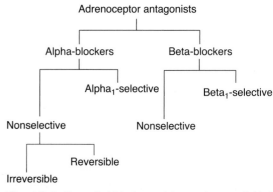

Figure 6–4. Drugs that block α and β receptors are divided into primary subgroups on the basis of their receptor selectivity. All of these agents are pharmacologic antagonists.

Table 6–4. **Relative selectivity of antagonists for adrenoceptors**

Drug	Receptor Affinity
α Antagonists	
Prazosin, terazosin, doxazosin	$\alpha_1 >>>> \alpha_2$
Phenoxybenzamine	$\alpha_1 > \alpha_2$
Phentolamine	$\alpha_1 = \alpha_2$
Mixed antagonists	
Labetalol, carvedilol	$\beta_1 = \beta_2 \geq \alpha_1 > \alpha_2$
β Antagonists	
Metoprolol, acebutolol, alprenolol, atenolol, betaxolol, celiprolol, esmolol	$\beta_1 >>> \beta_2$
Propranolol, carteolol, penbutolol, pindolol, timolol	$\beta_1 = \beta_2$

by increased concentrations of agonist for the α receptor. The advantage of α_1 selectivity is discussed later.

These drugs are all active by the oral and parenteral routes, although phentolamine is rarely given orally. Phenoxybenzamine has a short elimination half-life but a long duration of action of about 48 hours because it binds covalently to its receptor. Phentolamine has a duration of action of about 2 to 4 hours when used orally, and 20 to 40 minutes when given parenterally. Prazosin and the other α_1-selective receptor antagonists act for 8 to 24 hours.

Physiologic Effects

Nonselective antagonists, such as phenoxybenzamine, cause a predictable blockade of α-mediated responses to sympathetic nervous system discharge and exogenous sympathomimetics as presented in Table 4-3. The most important effects of nonselective α-receptor antagonists are those on the cardiovascular system. The reduction in vascular tone results in decreases in both arterial and venous pressures. There are no significant direct cardiac effects. However, the nonselective α-receptor antagonists do cause baroreceptor reflex-mediated tachycardia as a result of the drop in mean arterial pressure (Figure 4–5). This tachycardia may be exaggerated because the α_2 autoreceptors on the presynaptic side of the adrenergic synapse in the heart, which normally reduce the net release of norepinephrine, are also blocked (Figure 4–3). Phentolamine also has some non–alpha-mediated vasodilating effects. Because prazosin and the other selective receptor antagonists block vascular α_1

receptors much more effectively than the α_2-autoreceptors associated with cardiac sympathetic nerve terminals, these drugs cause much less tachycardia than the nonselective α-blocking agents when reducing blood pressure.

Clinical Uses

Nonselective α-blockers have limited clinical applications. The best-documented application is in the presurgical management of pheochromocytoma. Such patients may have severe hypertension and reduced blood volume, which should be corrected before subjecting the patient to the stress of surgery. Phenoxybenzamine is usually used during this preparatory phase; phentolamine is sometimes used during surgery. Nonselective α-blocking agents, such as phenoxybenzamine and phentolamine, may also be used in the treatment of Raynaud phenomenon, which sometimes responds to α-receptor blockade; however, calcium channel blockers (Chapter 7) may be preferable for many patients. Phenoxybenzamine also has serotonin receptor-blocking effects, which justify its occasional use in carcinoid tumor; and H_1 antihistamine effects, which leads to its use in mastocytosis. Accidental local infiltration of potent α agonists such as norepinephrine may lead to tissue ischemia and necrosis if not promptly reversed; infiltration of the ischemic area with phentolamine is sometimes used to prevent tissue damage. Overdose with drugs of abuse such as amphetamine, cocaine, or phenylpropanolamine may lead to severe hypertension because of their indirect sympathomimetic actions. This hypertension will usually respond well to α receptor antagonists. Sudden cessation of clonidine therapy leads to rebound hypertension; this phenomenon is also often treated with phentolamine.

The selective α-blockers (prazosin, **doxazosin,** and **terazosin**) are used in hypertension (Chapter 7) and in the management of urinary hesitancy and prevention of urinary retention in men with benign prostatic hyperplasia. A newer drug, **tamsulosin,** is currently replacing many of the previously used α_1-blocking agents in the treatment of benign prostatic hyperplasia. The efficacy of tamsulosin is based upon its specificity for inhibiting the α_{1A} receptor-mediated contraction of prostate smooth muscle, and minimal orthostatic hypotension effects.

Adverse Effects

The most important toxicities of the α-blockers are simple extensions of their α-blocking effects. The main manifestations are orthostatic hypotension and, in the case of the nonselective agents, marked reflex tachycardia. Tachycardia is less common and less severe with α_1-selective receptor antagonists. In patients with coronary disease, angina may be precipitated by the tachycardia. Oral administration of any of these drugs can cause nausea and vomiting. The α_1-selective agents are associated with an exaggerated orthostatic hypotensive response to the first dose in some patients. Therefore, the first dose is usually small and taken just before going to bed.

Beta-Blocking Drugs

All of the clinically used β-receptor antagonists are competitive inhibitors. **Propranolol** is the prototype. Drugs in this group are usually classified into subgroups on the basis of β_1 selectivity, partial agonist activity, local anesthetic action, and lipid solubility (Table 6–5). **Labetalol** and **carvedilol** have combined β- and α-blocking actions. **Nadolol,** propranolol, and timolol are typical nonselective β-receptor antagonists. These full antagonists may cause severe bronchospasm in patients with obstructive lung disease. Drugs such as **acebutolol, atenolol, esmolol, metoprolol,** and several other β-receptor antagonists demonstrate a greater selectivity for β_1 receptors compared to β_2 receptors. This property may be advantageous when treating patients with obstructive lung disease, minimizing inhibition of β_2 receptor–mediated bronchodilation. **Pindolol** and acebutolol have partial β_1 and β_2 agonist activity. Similarly, this intrinsic sympathomimetic activity may be an advantage in treating patients with obstructive lung disease. Theoretically, even at maximum dosage, these drugs cause less bronchoconstriction than full antagonists such as propranolol. Beta-blocking drugs have been developed for chronic oral use. The pharmacokinetics document that bioavailability and duration of action for these drugs

Table 6–5.	Properties of several β-receptor antagonists				
Drug	Selectivity	Partial Agonist Activity	Local Anesthetic Action	Lipid Solubility	Elimination Half-Life
Acebutolol	β_1	Yes	Yes	Low	3–4 h
Atenolol	β_1	No	No	Low	6–9 h
Esmolol	β_1	No	No	Low	10 min
Carvedilol[1]	None	No	No	No data	7–10 h
Labetalol[1]	None	Yes[2]	Yes	Moderate	5 h
Metoprolol	β_1	No	Yes	Moderate	3–4 h
Nadolol	None	No	No	Low	14–24 h
Pindolol	None	Yes[2]	Yes	Moderate	3–4 h
Propranolol	None	No	Yes	High	3.5–6 h
Timolol	None	No	No	Moderate	4–5 h

[1]Also cause α_1 receptor blockade.
[2]Partial agonist effects at β_2 receptors.

vary widely (Table 6–5). Nadolol is the longest acting β-receptor antagonist. Acebutolol, atenolol, and nadolol are less lipid-soluble than other β-receptor antagonists and probably enter the CNS to a lesser extent.

Physiologic Effects

Most of the organ-level effects of these drugs are predictable from blockade of the β receptor–mediated effects of sympathetic discharge and exogenous sympathomimetics as presented in Table 4–3. Mechanisms of blood pressure reduction include an initial reduction in cardiac output, but after a few days their action may include a decrease in vascular resistance as a contributing effect. The latter physiologic response may be accounted for by reduced angiotensin levels resulting from decreased β receptor–mediated renin release from the kidney.

Clinical Use

The clinical applications of β blockade are remarkably broad (Table 6–6). The cardiovascular clinical applications are discussed in Chapters 7 to 10. Pheochromocytoma is sometimes treated with a drug such as labetalol which combines both α and β blockade, especially if the tumor is producing large amounts of epinephrine as well as norepinephrine. Finally, the treatment of open-angle glaucoma involves the use of β-blocking drugs as well as other agents.

Adverse Effects

Cardiovascular adverse effects are extensions of the β blockade induced by these agents, and include bradycardia, atrioventricular blockade, and heart failure. Patients with obstructive lung disease may suffer severe bronchospasm. Beta-receptor antagonists have been shown experimentally to reduce insulin secretion, but

Table 6–6. Clinical applications of β-receptor antagonists

Application	Drugs	Effect
Hypertension	Atenolol, propranolol, metoprolol, timolol, others	Reduced cardiac output, reduced renin secretion
Angina pectoris	Propranolol, nadolol, others	Reduced cardiac rate and force
Arrhythmia prophylaxis after myocardial infarction	Propranolol, metoprolol, timolol	Reduced automaticity of all cardiac pacemakers
Supraventricular tachycardias	Propranolol, esmolol, acebutolol	Slowed AV conduction velocity
Heart failure	Carvedilol, labetalol, metoprolol	Decreased mortality, mechanism not understood
Hypertrophic cardiomyopathy	Propranolol	Slowed rate of cardiac contraction
Migraine	Propranolol	Prophylactic, mechanism uncertain
Familial tremor, other types of tremor, "stage fright"	Propranolol	Reduced β$_2$ effects on neuromuscular transmission; possible CNS effects
Thyroid storm, thyrotoxicosis	Propranolol	Reduced cardiac rate and arrhythmogenesis; other mechanisms may be involved
Glaucoma	Timolol, others	Reduced secretion of aqueous humor

AV = atrioventricular; CNS = central nervous system.

this does not appear to be a clinically important effect. Conversely, initial symptoms of hypoglycemia from insulin or oral hypoglycemic overdosing may be masked by β-receptor antagonists. These manifestations include tachycardia, tremors, and anxiety and provide the patient with useful warning signs. Additionally, mobilization of glucose from the liver may be impaired. Central nervous system adverse effects of β-receptor antagonists include sedation, fatigue, and sleep alterations. Atenolol, nadolol, and several other less lipid-soluble β-receptor antagonists are claimed to have less marked CNS action because they do not enter the CNS as readily as other members of this group. Beta-blockade therapy is also associated with slightly elevated low-density lipoprotein and triglyceride concentrations, and diminished high-density lipoprotein levels in the blood.

Chronic use of these drugs may result in up-regulation of β receptors on the myocardium. Abrupt discontinuation of these drugs following chronic use may result in these patients being at risk of adverse cardiovascular events, such as rebound tachycardia. This is especially true of shorter acting drugs such as propranolol and metoprolol. Prudence dictates that patients should be warned not to terminate these medications abruptly.

■ REHABILITATION FOCUS

Drugs with sympathomimetic and sympatholytic properties are used in a broad spectrum of pathophysiologic conditions that mirror the role of the autonomic nervous system in the body and catecholamine neurotransmitters in the CNS. Drugs with sympathomimetic or sympatholytic properties are found in many other drug groups and are discussed in various chapters in this book. Sympathomimetic drugs are prescribed in the treatment of upper and lower respiratory dysfunctions (Chapter 35), whereas sympatholytic drugs are prescribed in the treatment of various cardiovascular disorders (Chapters 7 to 10). Less obvious drugs with sympathomimetic clinical uses or adverse effects include tricyclic antidepressants and MAO$_A$ inhibitors used to treat depression (Chapter 19), and MAO$_B$ and COMT inhibitors used to treat Parkinson's disease (Chapter 17).

■ CLINICAL RELEVANCE FOR REHABILITATION

Adverse Drug Reactions
- Central nervous system stimulation with sympathomimetics may lead to restlessness and insomnia.
- Alpha$_1$ agonists may increase blood pressure and precipitate angina pectoris in patients during aerobic rehabilitation activities.
- Beta$_2$ agonists may increase heart rate and precipitate angina pectoris or cardiac dysrhythmias.
- Orthostatic hypotension is a problem with many of the sympatholytic drugs.
- Bronchoconstriction is a problem with the β-receptor antagonists.

Effects Interfering with Rehabilitation
- Orthostatic hypotension may cause patients to faint when transferring from sitting or supine positions to standing, exiting from a warm aquatherapy area, or if aerobic exercise is terminated without an appropriate cool-down period.
- Dyspnea may decrease the aerobic capacity of patients.
- Heart rate cannot be used as a marker of exertion for patients taking β-receptor antagonists.

Possible Therapy Solutions
- To prevent fainting associated with orthostatic hypotension, assist patients with positional changes and when exiting a warm pool. Always provide a cool-down period following a period of exercise.
- Allow increased time to complete aerobic tasks to prevent dyspnea and account for depressed cardiac activity.
- Check blood pressure and heart rate prior to and following aerobic activities. Monitor heart rate during aerobic activities.

Potentiation of Functional Outcomes Secondary to Drug Therapy
- Many of the sympatholytic drugs allow patients to participate in aerobic activities while minimizing increases in blood pressure, angina, or cardiac dysrhythmias.
- Patients with asthma or other respiratory dysfunction may benefit from the use of β$_2$ agonists prior to aerobic activities.

PROBLEM-ORIENTED PATIENT STUDY

Brief History: Your physical therapy practice is associated with a wellness center where the practice provides consulting advice on aerobic and resistive exercise training. All of the physical therapists in the practice have both physical therapy degrees and athletic training certifications. The patient is a 47-year-old male who works as an accountant for a local business. He has elected to join the wellness center to improve his general fitness status. According to the patient, at his last medical evaluation, the family physician suggested that he had prehypertension and that his "bad" cholesterol was high. The physician suggested that the patient begin a regular exercise program to lower his weight, blood pressure, and cholesterol levels.

Current Medical Status and Drug Therapy: At his initial evaluation, the following were recorded: body mass index 29, blood pressure 135/84 mm Hg, and heart rate 84 beats per minute. There has been no change in any of these parameters during the past month. The patient is currently taking no prescription drugs.

Rehabilitation Setting: At the initial evaluation and training session, an aerobics program with upper extremity resistive training was developed. The patient conducted the defined program at the initial session and in subsequent sessions, three times a week during the past month, without incident. The patient has no prescribed medications. The patient arrived today (Monday) to participate in his program. He stated that he missed Friday because of a cold which persisted through the weekend. He stated that during the weekend he began taking various over-the-counter cold preparations to relieve his cold symptoms. These preparations included the topical decongestant Afrin (oxymetazoline) to relieve the nasal congestion and Advil Cold and Sinus (ibuprofen and pseudoephedrine) taken orally. During the conversation with the patient the therapist notices that the patient is moving his left arm in a circular motion and rubbing his left shoulder. When questioned, the patient states that for the past couple of days his left shoulder has been hurting intermittently, as it was doing just now.

Problem/Clinical Options: The therapist recognizes that the locker room for the men is one flight of stairs down from the main workout area. The patient just ascended that flight of stairs and is complaining of left shoulder pain. Measurement of the patient's blood pressure and heart rate were 145/92 mm Hg and 108 beats per minute, respectively. The therapist realizes that the patient is presenting with the manifestations of angina pectoris due to insufficient blood flow in the coronary arteries, also known as exertional angina pectoris. This is a result of the elevated blood pressure due to the cold medications which contain the α_1 agonist pseudoephedrine. The elevated blood pressure increased cardiac workload. The exertion of climbing the flight of stairs in combination with the drug-induced cardiac changes resulted in the expression of the angina pectoris. The therapist recommends that the patient terminate his exercise program and return to his physician for further evaluation. For additional information on angina pectoris, see Chapter 8, and for nasal decongestants, see Chapter 35.

PREPARATIONS AVAILABLE[1]

Sympathomimetics

Amphetamine, racemic mixture (generic)
Oral: 5-, 10-mg tablets
Oral (Adderall): 1:1:1:1 mixtures of amphetamine sulfate, amphetamine aspartate, dextroamphetamine sulfate, and dextroamphetamine saccharate, formulated to contain a total of 5, 7.5, 10, 12.5, 15, 20, or 30 mg in tablets; or 10, 20, or 30 mg in capsules

Apraclonidine (Iopidine)
Topical: 0.5, 1% solutions

Brimonidine (Alphagan)
Topical: 0.15, 0.2% solution

Dexmedetomidine (Precedex)
Parenteral: 100 mcg/mL

Dexmethylphenidate (Focalin)
Oral: 2.5-, 5-, 10-mg tablets

Dextroamphetamine (generic, Dexedrine)
Oral: 5-, 10-mg tablets
Oral sustained-release: 5-, 10-, 15-mg capsules
Oral mixtures with amphetamine: see Amphetamine (Adderall)

Dipivefrin (generic, Propine)
Topical: 0.1% ophthalmic solution

Dobutamine (generic, Dobutrex)
Parenteral: 12.5 mg/mL in 20 mL vials for injection

Dopamine (generic, Intropin)
Parenteral: 40, 80, 160 mg/mL for injection; 80, 160, 320 mg/100 mL in 5% D/W for injection

Ephedrine (generic)
Oral: 25-mg capsules
Parenteral: 50 mg/mL for injection
Nasal: 0.25% spray

Epinephrine (generic, Adrenalin Chloride, others)
Parenteral: 1:1000 (1 mg/mL), 1:2000 (0.5 mg/mL), 1:10,000 (0.1 mg/mL), 1:100,000 (0.01 mg/mL) for injection
Parenteral autoinjector (Epipen): 1:2000 (0.5 mg/mL)
Ophthalmic: 0.1, 0.5, 1, 2% drops
Nasal: 0.1% drops and spray
Aerosol for bronchospasm (Primatene Mist, Bronkaid Mist): 0.16, 0.2 mg/spray
Solution for aerosol: 1:100

Fenoldopam (Corlopam)
Parenteral: 10 mg/mL for IV infusion

Hydroxyamphetamine (Paredrine)
Ophthalmic: 1% drops

Isoproterenol (generic, Isuprel)
Parenteral: 1:5000 (0.2 mg/mL), 1:50,000 (0.02 mg/mL) for injection

Mephentermine (Wyamine Sulfate)
Parenteral: 15, 30 mg/mL for injection

Metaraminol (Aramine)
Parenteral: 10 mg/mL for injection

Methamphetamine (Desoxyn)
Oral: 5-mg tablets

Methoxamine (Vasoxyl)
Parenteral: 20 mg/mL for injection

Methylphenidate (generic, Ritalin, Ritalin-SR)
Oral: 5-, 10-, 20-mg tablets
Oral sustained-release: 10-, 18-, 20-, 27-, 36-, 54-mg tablets; 20-, 30-, 40-mg capsules

Midodrine (ProAmatine)
Oral: 2.5-, 5-mg tablets

Modafinil (Provigil)
Oral: 100-, 200-mg tablets

---

[1]α_2-Agonists used in hypertension are listed in Chapter 7.
β_2-Agonists used in asthma are listed in Chapter 35.

Naphazoline (Privine)
Nasal: 0.05% drops and spray
Ophthalmic: 0.012, 0.02, 0.03% drops

Norepinephrine (generic, Levophed)
Parenteral: 1 mg/mL for injection

Oxymetazoline (generic, Afrin, Neo-Synephrine 12-Hour, others)
Nasal: 0.025, 0.05% sprays
Ophthalmic: 0.025% drops

Pemoline (generic, Cylert)
Oral: 18.75-, 37.5-, 75-mg tables; 37.5-mg chewable tablets

Phendimetrazine (generic)
Oral: 35-mg tablets, capsules; 105-mg sustained-release capsules

Phenylephrine (generic, Neo-Synephrine)
Oral: 10 mg chewable tablets
Parenteral: 10 mg/mL for injection
Nasal: 0.125, 0.16, 0.25, 0.5, 1% drops and spray; 0.5% jelly

Pseudoephedrine (generic, Sudafed, others)
Oral: 30-, 60-mg tablets; 60-mg capsules; 15-, 30-mg/5-mL syrups; 7.5-mg/0.8-mL drops
Oral extended-release: 120-, 240-mg tablets, capsules

Tetrahydrozoline (generic, Tyzine)
Nasal: 0.05, 0.1% drops
Ophthalmic: 0.05% drops

Xylometazoline (generic, Otrivin, Neo-Synephrine Long-Acting, Chlorohist LA)
Nasal: 0.05 drops, 0.1% drops and spray

Sympatholytics

Alpha Receptor Antagonists

Doxazosin (generic, Cardura)
Oral: 1-, 2-, 4-, 8-mg tablets

Phenoxybenzamine (Dibenzyline)
Oral: 10-mg capsules

Phentolamine (generic, Regitine)
Parenteral: 5 mg/vial for injection

Prazosin (generic, Minipress)
Oral: 1-, 2-, 5-mg capsules

Tamsulosin (Flomax)
Oral: 0.4-mg capsule

Terazosin (generic, Hytrin)
Oral: 1-, 2-, 5-, 10-mg tablets, capsules

Tolazoline (Priscoline)
Parenteral: 25 mg/mL for injection

Beta Receptor Antagonists

Acebutolol (generic, Sectral)
Oral: 200-, 400-mg capsules

Atenolol (generic, Tenormin)
Oral: 25-, 50-, 100-mg tablets
Parenteral: 0.5 mg/mL for IV injection

Betaxolol
Oral: 10-, 20-mg tablets (Kerlone)
Ophthalmic: 0.25%, 0.5% drops (generic, Betoptic)

Bisoprolol (Zebeta)
Oral: 5-, 10-mg tablets

Carteolol
Oral: 2.5-, 5-mg tablets (Cartrol)
Ophthalmic: 1% drops (generic, Ocupress)

Carvedilol (Coreg)
Oral: 3.125-, 6.25-, 12.5-, 25-mg tablets

Esmolol (Brevibloc)
Parenteral: 10 mg/mL for IV injection; 250 mg/mL for IV infusion

Labetalol (generic, Normodyne, Trandate)
Oral: 100-, 200-, 300-mg tablets
Parenteral: 5 mg/mL for injection

Levobunolol (Betagan Liquifilm, others)
Ophthalmic: 0.25, 0.5% drops

Metipranolol (Optipranolol)
Ophthalmic: 0.3% drops

Metoprolol (generic, Lopressor, Toprol)
Oral: 50-, 100-mg tablets
Oral sustained-release: 25-, 50-, 100-, 200-mg tablets
Parenteral: 1 mg/mL for injection

Nadolol (generic, Corgard)
Oral: 20-, 40-, 80-, 120-, 160-mg tablets

Penbutolol (Levatol)
Oral: 20-mg tablets

Pindolol (generic, Visken)
Oral: 5-, 10-mg tablets

Propranolol (generic, Inderal)
Oral: 10-, 20-, 40-, 60-, 80-, 90-mg tablets; 4-, 8-, 80-mg/mL solutions
Oral sustained release: 60-, 80-, 120-, 160-mg capsules
Parenteral: 1 mg/mL for injection

Sotalol (generic, Betapace)
Oral: 80-, 120-, 160-, 240-mg tablets

Timolol
Oral: 5-, 10-, 20-mg tablets (generic, Blocadren)
Ophthalmic: 0.25, 0.5% drops, gel (generic, Timoptic)

Synthesis Inhibitor

Metyrosine (Demser)
Oral: 250-mg capsules

REFERENCES

Sympathomimetics

Bray GA: Use and abuse of appetite-suppressant drugs in the treatment of obesity. *Ann Intern Med* 1993;119 (7 Part 2):707.

Brodde O-E, et al: Presence, distribution and physiological function of adrenergic and muscarinic receptor subtypes in the human heart. *Basic Res Cardiol* 2001;96:528.

Evans WE, McLeod HL: Pharmacogenomics—drug disposition, drug targets, and side effects. *N Engl J Med* 2003;348:538.

Ewan PW: Anaphylaxis. *BMJ* 1998;316:1442.

Goldenberg RL, Rouse DJ: Prevention of premature birth. *N Engl J Med* 1998;339:313.

Graham RM, et al: Alpha$_1$-adrenergic receptor subtypes. Molecular structure, function, and signaling. *Circ Res* 1996;78:737.

Jordan J: New trends in the treatment of orthostatic hypotension. *Curr Hypertens Rep* 2001;3:216.

Koshimizu T, et al: Recent progress in alpha$_1$-adrenoceptor pharmacology. *Biol Pharm Bull* 2002;25:401.

McCabe BJ: Dietary tyramine and other pressor amines in MAOI regimens: A review. *J Am Diet Assoc* 1986; 86:1059.

McClellan KJ, Wiseman LR, Wilde MI: Midodrine. A review of its therapeutic use in the management of orthostatic hypotension. *Drugs Aging* 1998;12:7.

Pierce KL, Lefkowitz RJ: Classical and new roles of beta-arrestins in the regulation of G-protein-coupled receptors. *Nat Rev Neurosci* 2001;2:727.

Post SR, Hammond HK, Insel PA: Beta-adrenergic receptors and receptor signaling in heart failure. *Annu Rev Pharmacol Toxicol* 1999;39:343.

Rockman HA, Koch WJ, Lefkowitz RJ: Seven-transmembrane-spanning receptors and heart function. *Nature* 2002; 415:206.

Small KM, McGraw DW, Liggett SB: Pharmacology and physiology of human adrenergic receptor polymorphisms. *Ann Rev Pharmacol Toxicol* 2003;43:381.

Soltau JB, Zimmerman TJ: Changing paradigms in the medical treatment of glaucoma. *Surv Ophthalmol* 2002;47(Suppl 1):S2.

Treatment of preterm labor with the beta-adrenergic agonist ritodrine. The Canada Preterm Labor Investigators Group. *N Engl J Med* 1992;327:308.

Tsao P, von Zastrow M: Downregulation of G protein–coupled receptors. *Curr Opin Neurobiol* 2000; 10:365.

Weyer C, Gautier JF, Danforth E Jr: Development of β_3-adrenoceptor agonists for the treatment of obesity and diabetes—an update. *Diabetes Metab* 1999;25:11.

Zhong H, Minneman KP: Alpha$_1$-adrenoceptor subtypes. *Eur J Pharmacol* 1999;375:26.

Sympatholytics

Alward WLM: Medical management of glaucoma. *N Engl J Med* 1998;339:1298.

Blaufarb I, Pfeifer TM, Frishman WH: Beta-blockers: Drug interactions of clinical significance. *Drug Saf* 1995; 13:359.

Bristow M: Antiadrenergic therapy of chronic heart failure: Surprises and new opportunities. *Circulation* 2003; 107:1100.

Cleland JG: Beta-blockers for heart failure: why, which, when, and where. *Med Clin North Am* 2003;87:339.

Cooper KL, McKiernan JM, Kaplan SA: Alpha-adrenoceptor antagonists in the treatment of benign prostatic hyperplasia. *Drugs* 1999;57:9.

Frishman WH: Carvedilol. *N Engl J Med* 1998;339:1759.

Lepor H, et al: The efficacy of terazosin, finasteride, or both in benign prostate hyperplasia. *N Engl J Med* 1996;335:533.

Teerlink JR, Massie BM: Beta-adrenergic blocker mortality trials in congestive heart failure. *Am J Cardiol* 1999;84(Suppl 9A):94R.

Wilt TJ, MacDonald R, Rutks I: Tamsulosin for benign prostatic hyperplasia. *Cochrane Database Syst Rev* 2003;(1):CD002081.

Wuttke H, et al: Increased frequency of cytochrome P450 2D6 poor metabolizers among patients with metoprolol-associated adverse effects. *Clin Pharmacol Ther* 2002;72:429.

Rehabilitation

Ades PA: Cardiac effects of beta-adrenoceptor blockade with intrinsic sympathomimetic activity during submaximal exercise. *Br J Clin Pharmacol* 1987;24(Suppl 1):29S.

Ades PA, et al: Exercise haemodynamic effects of beta-blockade and intrinsic sympathomimetic activity. *Eur J Clin Pharmacol* 1989;36:5.

Anderson SD, Brannan JD: Long-acting beta$_2$-adrenoceptor agonists and exercise-induced asthma: Lessons to guide us in the future. *Paediatr Drugs* 2004;6:161.

Gordon NF, Scott CB: Exercise and mild essential hypertension. *Prim Care* 1991;18:683.

Horan MJ, Roccella EJ: Nonpharmacologic treatment of hypertension: Does it work? *Eur Heart J* 1987;8 (Suppl B):77.

Petrella RJ: How effective is exercise training for the treatment of hypertension? *Clin J Sport Med* 1998; 8:224.

7

ANTIHYPERTENSIVE DRUGS

Hypertension is the most common cardiovascular disease and a precursor to other cardiovascular dysfunctions. The prevalence of hypertension increases with age and varies based on race and coexisting morbidities. Sustained arterial hypertension damages blood vessels and such changes in the kidney, heart, and brain lead to an increased incidence of renal failure, coronary disease, cardiac failure, and stroke.

◼ REGULATION OF BLOOD PRESSURE

The autonomic nervous system, especially the sympathetic branch, plays a significant role in the regulation of blood pressure. A general discussion of autonomic responses was presented in Chapter 4, specifically Table 4–3 and Figure 4–5. According to the hydraulic equation, arterial blood pressure (BP) is directly proportional to the product of the blood flow and the resistance to passage of blood through the vessels. The estimate for blood flow is cardiac output (CO), and the determinant for resistance is peripheral vascular resistance (PVR). The hydraulic equation is:

$$BP = CO \times PVR$$

In both normal and hypertensive individuals, blood pressure is maintained by moment-to-moment regulation of cardiac output and peripheral vascular resistance exerted at three anatomic sites (Figure 7–1). The primary locations are the precapillary arterioles, postcapillary venules, and the heart. A fourth anatomic control site, the kidney, contributes to maintenance of blood pressure by regulating the volume of intravascular fluid volume, a slower, longer-lasting control mechanism.

Baroreflexes, mediated by autonomic nerves, act in combination with humoral mechanisms, including the renal-mediated renin-angiotensin-aldosterone system, to coordinate function at these four control sites and to maintain normal blood pressure. Local release of vasoactive substances may also be involved in the regulation of vascular resistance. For example, nitric oxide (NO) and some prostaglandins dilate blood vessels. Other local agents constrict vessels.

Baroreflexes are responsible for rapid moment to moment adjustments in blood pressure, such as in transition from a reclining to an upright posture (Figure 7–2). Carotid baroreceptors are stimulated by the stretch of the vessel walls brought about by the internal blood pressure (Figure 7–2[1]). Baroreceptor activation inhibits discharge (Figure 7–2[2]) of tonically active sympathetic neurons (Figure 7–2[3]) in the vasomotor center of the medulla. Conversely, reduction in stretch results in a reduction in baroreceptor activity. Thus, in the case of a transition to

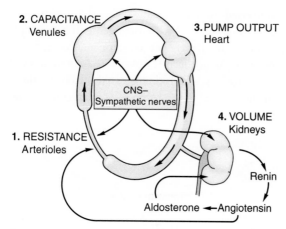

Figure 7–1. Anatomic sites of blood pressure control. These sites include vascular tone in venules and arterioles, the heart, and the kidney (by regulation of intravascular fluid volume).

upright posture, baroreceptors sense the reduced wall stretch that results from pooling of blood in the veins below the level of the heart as reduction in arterial pressure, and sympathetic discharge is increased. The increase in sympathetic outflow acts through nerve endings to constrict the arterioles, which increase peripheral vascular resistance. The sympathetic outflow also increases cardiac output, both directly through stimulation of the heart and through constriction of capacitance vessels that increases venous return to the heart. Both of these sympathetic responses restore normal blood pressure. This system requires two peripheral neurons, a preganglionic neuron and a postganglionic neuron, and two synapses to transmit from the central nervous system to the target tissue. The first synapse is within the autonomic ganglion (Figure 7–2[4]), between the preganglionic and post-ganglionic neurons. The second synapse is between the postganglionic neuron and the effector tissue (Figure 7–2[5]). The postganglionic neuron usually releases norepinephrine and activates α or β receptors (Figure 7–2[6]). The same baroreflex acts in response to any event that lowers arterial pressure, including a primary reduction in peripheral vascular resistance or a reduction in intravascular volume. A reduction in peripheral vascular resistance is an effect of vasodilators. A reduction in intravascular volume is an effect of diuretics, which increase loss of salt and water via the kidney.

By controlling blood volume, the kidney is primarily responsible for long-term blood pressure control. A reduction in renal perfusion pressure causes

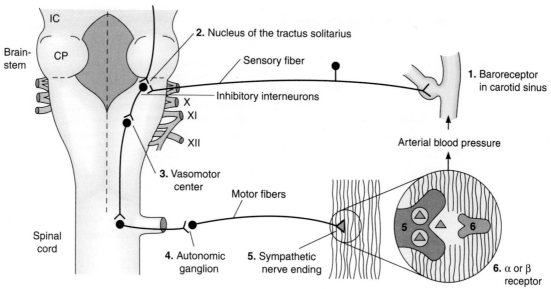

Figure 7–2. Baroreceptor reflex arc. For individual items 1 through 6, see section "Regulation of Blood Pressure" in text.

intrarenal redistribution of blood flow and increased reabsorption of salt and water. In addition, decreased pressure in renal arterioles and sympathetic neural activity (via β adrenoceptors) stimulate production of renin. Renin mediates conversion of angiotensinogen to angiotensin I (Figure 7–3). Angiotensin I is converted to angiotensin II by the angiotensin-converting enzyme (ACE). Angiotensin II has multiple physiologic effects that assist in increasing blood pressure. Angiotensin II causes direct constriction of resistance vessels and stimulates aldosterone synthesis in the adrenal cortex. Aldosterone is the hormonal

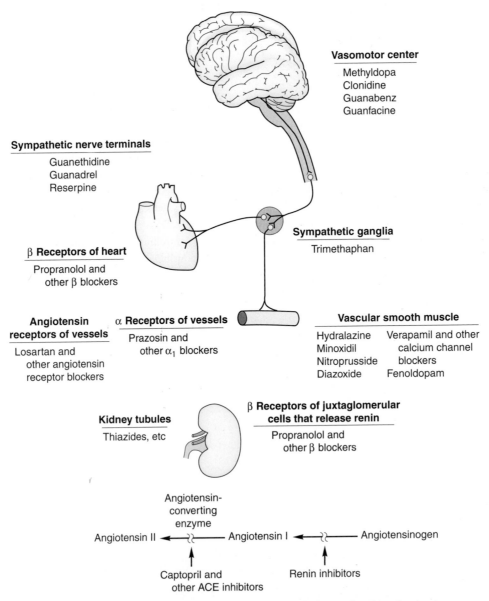

Figure 7–3. Sites of blood pressure control and actions of the major classes of antihypertensive drugs.

regulator for the sodium/potassium/proton exchange process in the distal convoluted tubules and collecting ducts of the kidney. Aldosterone stimulates renal sodium absorption with a resulting increase in intravascular blood volume. Finally, vasopressin (antidiuretic hormone, ADH) released from the posterior pituitary gland also plays a role in maintenance of blood pressure through its ability to regulate water reabsorption by the kidney.

HIGH BLOOD PRESSURE

A specific cause of hypertension can be established in only 10 to 15% of patients. In patients with no identified cause of hypertension, the high blood pressure is said to be "essential hypertension." In most cases, elevated blood pressure is associated with an overall increase in resistance to flow of blood through arterioles, whereas cardiac output is usually normal. No primary single abnormality has been identified as the cause of increased peripheral vascular resistance in essential hypertension. Elevated blood pressure is usually caused by a combination of several (multifactorial) abnormalities. Epidemiologic evidence points to genetic inheritance and environmental and dietary factors, such as increased salt and decreased potassium or calcium intake, as perhaps contributing to the development of hypertension. Increase in blood pressure with aging does not occur in populations with low daily sodium intake. Patients with labile hypertension appear more likely than normal controls to have blood pressure elevations after salt loading. The heritability of essential hypertension is estimated to be about 30%. Mutations in several genes have been linked to various rare causes of hypertension. Functional variations of the genes for angiotensinogen, ACE, and the β_2 adrenoceptor appear to contribute to some cases of essential hypertension.

THERAPEUTIC STRATEGIES

Blood pressure in a hypertensive patient is controlled by the same mechanisms that are operative in normotensive subjects. Regulation of blood pressure in hypertensive patients differs from healthy patients in that the baroreceptors and the renal blood volume–pressure control systems appear to be "set" at a higher level of blood pressure. All antihypertensive drugs act by interfering with these normal mechanisms. Effective lowering of pressure has been shown to prevent damage to blood vessels and to reduce morbidity and mortality rates substantially. The strategies for treating high blood pressure are based on these determinants of arterial pressure. These strategies include inhibition of sympathetic tone (sympatholytics), inhibition of vascular smooth muscle contraction (vasodilators), inhibition of angiotensin II formation (renin inhibitors and ACE inhibitors) and receptor activation (angiotensin receptor antagonists), and reduction of blood volume (diuretics). Thus, antihypertensive drugs are organized around a clinical indication, the need to treat a disease, rather than a single receptor type. A graphic overview of the sites of action of the antihypertensive drug classes with specific drug examples is presented in Figure 7–3, and an outline of the various classes of antihypertensive drugs is presented in Figure 7–4.

Sympatholytics

Sympatholytic antihypertensive drugs may be further divided into those that are antagonists at adrenoceptors, act within the central nervous system (CNS) to decrease sympathetic outflow, inhibit sympathetic activity at the autonomic ganglia, or modulate postganglionic neuronal function in the target tissue (Figure 7–3).

Adrenoceptor Antagonists
The α_1, α_2, and β_1 receptors all play a modulatory role in controlling blood pressure. The mechanisms of action and the physiologic effects of inhibiting these receptors were discussed in Chapter 6.

ALPHA ADRENOCEPTOR ANTAGONISTS

Clinical Use. The α_1-selective receptor antagonists such as **prazosin, doxazosin,** and **terazosin** are used for chronic treatment of hypertension as well as benign prostatic hyperplasia. These drugs decrease blood pressure by dilation of the arterial and, to a lesser extent, venous vasculature.

Adverse Effects. Orthostatic hypotension and reflex tachycardia both occur, although reflex tachycardia is less common with the α_1-selective blocking drugs.

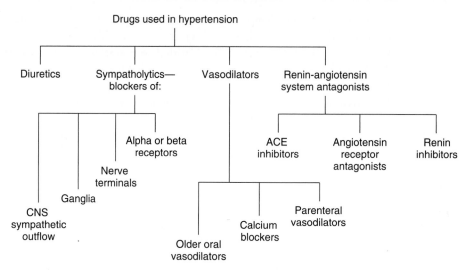

Figure 7–4. Various classes of drugs used in the treatment of hypertension. The general pharmacologic mechanisms include decreasing blood volume (diuretics), decreasing sympathetic tone (sympatholytics), direct relaxation of vascular smooth muscle (vasodilators), and inhibition of the effects of renin-angiotensin-aldosterone system (renin-angiotensin system antagonists).

BETA ADRENOCEPTOR ANTAGONISTS

Clinical Use. Cardiovascular applications include hypertension, angina, and cardiac arrhythmias. Treatment of chronic heart failure is a newer application for these drugs. Several large clinical trials have shown that certain β blockers (**labetalol, carvedilol,** and **metoprolol**) reduce morbidity and mortality when used properly in heart failure (Chapter 9).

Adverse Effects. Beta blockade of the heart may result in bradycardia, atrioventricular blockade, and acute heart failure. Additional care should be taken to watch for brochoconstriction in patients with asthma or chronic obstructive lung disease, and rhythm disturbances in patients with abrupt medication termination.

CNS-Acting Drugs

Alpha$_2$-selective agonists such as **clonidine, guanfacine,** and **methyldopa** cause a decrease in sympathetic outflow by a mechanism that involves activation of α_2 receptors in the CNS (Figure 7–3). These drugs readily enter the CNS when given orally. Methyldopa is a prodrug and is converted to methylnorepinephrine in the brain. Clonidine, guanfacine, and methyldopa reduce blood pressure by reducing cardiac output, vascular resistance, or both.

Adverse Effects. The major compensatory response is salt retention. Sudden discontinuation of clonidine may cause rebound hypertension, which may be quite severe. This rebound increase in blood pressure can be controlled by reinstitution of clonidine therapy. Clonidine also increases the risk of mental depression and should be used with caution in patients at risk. Methyldopa occasionally causes hematologic immunotoxicity, detected initially by test tube agglutination of red blood cells (positive Coombs test) and, in some patients, progresses to hemolytic anemia. All these drugs may cause sedation and dry mouth; methyldopa more so.

Ganglion-Blocking Drugs

Drugs that inhibit the nicotinic N$_N$ receptors in the ganglia are very efficacious, but because their adverse effects are severe, they are considered obsolete. **Hexamethonium** and **trimethaphan** are prototypical and are extremely powerful blood pressure–lowering drugs. The major compensatory response is salt retention. Toxicities reflect parasympathetic blockade (blurred vision, constipation, urinary hesitancy, sexual dysfunction) and sympathetic blockade (sexual dysfunction and orthostatic hypotension).

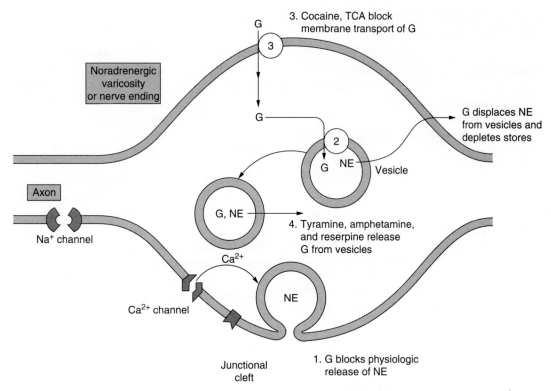

Figure 7–5. Pharmacodynamic mechanisms of drugs that act at the postganglionic sympathetic synapses to deplete or block the release of norepinephrine (NE). Reserpine blocks the uptake of NE into the vesicle (2). Guanethidine (G) both depletes NE in the vesicle (2) and prevents the release of NE into the synapse (1). Cocaine, tricyclic antidepressants (TCAs), tyramine, amphetamines, and reserpine may decrease the effectiveness of G (2, 3, and 4). Decreased effectiveness may occur by inhibiting uptake of G into the presynaptic terminal or the vesicle, or inappropriate release of G from the vesicle.

Postganglionic Sympathetic Blocking Drugs

Drugs that deplete the adrenergic nerve terminal of its norepinephrine stores or that deplete and block release of these stores can lower blood pressure (Figure 7–5). **Reserpine** is a prototypical drug that acts by the depletion mechanism; **guanethidine** acts by both depleting and blocking release. The major compensatory response is salt retention. In high dosages, both reserpine and guanethidine are very efficacious but produce a high incidence of adverse effects. Reserpine is still occasionally used in low doses as an adjunct to other agents. Guanethidine is rarely used. Reserpine readily enters the CNS; guanethidine does not. Both have long durations of action in the order of days to weeks. The most serious toxicities associated with reserpine are behavioral depression and pseudoparkinsonism,

which may require discontinuation of the drug. The major toxicities of guanethidine are orthostatic hypotension and sexual dysfunction. Guanethidine requires the catecholamine reuptake pump to reach its intracellular site of action in the postganglionic nerve terminal. Therefore, drugs that inhibit uptake of guanethidine into the adrenergic terminal or the vesicle (cocaine, tricyclic antidepressants, amphetamines) will interfere with the antihypertensive action of guanethidine.

Vasodilators

Drugs that dilate blood vessels by acting directly on smooth muscle cells through nonautonomic mechanisms are useful in treating some hypertensive patients. The four major mechanisms utilized by vasodilators

Table 7–1.	Mechanisms of action of vasodilators

Mechanism	Examples
Release of nitric oxide from drug or endothelium	Nitroprusside, hydralazine
Hyperpolarization of vascular smooth muscle through opening of potassium channels	Minoxidil sulfate, diazoxide
Reduction of calcium influx	Verapamil, diltiazem, nifedipine
Activation of dopamine type 1 receptors	Fenoldopam

are set forth in Table 7–1. Compensatory responses are marked for some vasodilators, especially hydralazine and minoxidil, and include salt retention and reflex tachycardia.

Vasodilators That Cause Release of Nitric Oxide

Hydralazine is an older vasodilator that has more effect on arterioles than on veins, is orally active, and is suitable for chronic therapy. Hydralazine apparently acts through the release of nitric oxide from endothelial cells. However, the drug is rarely used at high dosages because of its toxicity; therefore, its efficacy is limited. Toxicities of the drug include tachycardia, salt and water retention, and drug-induced lupus erythematosus. However, the latter effect is uncommon at dosages below 200 mg/day and is reversible upon stopping the drug. **Nitroprusside** is a short-acting agent (duration of action is a few minutes) that must be infused continuously and is used in hypertensive emergencies. The drug's mechanism of action involves the release of nitric oxide from the drug molecule itself. The released nitric oxide stimulates guanylyl cyclase and increases cyclic guanosine monophosphate (cGMP) concentration in smooth muscle, resulting in smooth muscle relaxation and vasodilation. The toxicity of nitroprusside includes excessive hypotension, tachycardia, and, if infusion is continued over several days, accumulation of cyanide or thiocyanate in the blood.

Vasodilators That Cause Cell Hyperpolarization

Minoxidil is another older vasodilator that has more effect on arterioles than on veins and is orally active. Minoxidil is a prodrug; its metabolite, minoxidil sulfate, hyperpolarizes and relaxes vascular smooth muscle by opening potassium channels. Minoxidil is

reserved for severe hypertension owing to its multiple side effects. Clinical use of minoxidil generally requires coadministration of a diuretic and β-receptor antagonist to minimize compensatory responses. The toxicity of minoxidil consists of severe compensatory responses, hirsutism, and pericardial abnormalities. **Diazoxide** is given as intravenous boluses or as an infusion and has a duration of action of several hours. Like minoxidil sulfate, diazoxide opens potassium channels, hyperpolarizing and relaxing smooth muscle cells. This parenteral vasodilator is used in hypertensive emergencies. The drug also reduces insulin release and can be used to treat hypoglycemia caused by insulin-producing tumors. The toxicity of diazoxide includes hypotension, hyperglycemia, and salt and water retention.

Vasodilators That Block Calcium Channels

Calcium channel blockers include **nifedipine, verapamil,** and **diltiazem;** they are effective vasodilators. Because they are orally active, these drugs are suitable for chronic use in hypertension of any severity. Many analogs of nifedipine are also available. Because they produce fewer compensatory responses, the calcium channel blockers are usually preferred to hydralazine and minoxidil. Their mechanism of action and toxicities are discussed in greater detail in Chapter 8.

Vasodilator That Activates Dopamine (D_1) Receptor

Dopamine D_1 receptor activation by **fenoldopam** causes prompt, marked, arteriolar vasodilation. This drug is given by intravenous infusion. The drug has a short duration of action of 10 minutes and is used for hypertensive emergencies.

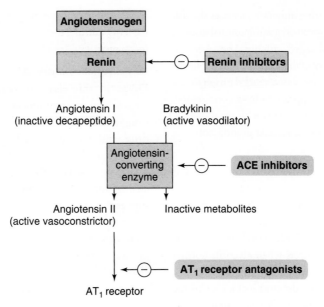

Figure 7–6. The action of renin inhibitors, angiotensin-converting enzyme inhibitors (ACE inhibitors), and angiotensin receptor (AT$_1$) antagonists. Renin converts angiotensinogen to angiotensin I. ACE is responsible for converting angiotensin I into the vasoconstrictor angiotensin II and for inactivating bradykinin. Bradykinin is a vasodilator normally present in very low concentrations. Blockade of ACE decreases the vasoconstrictor angiotensin II and increases the vasodilator bradykinin. The renin inhibitors and AT$_1$ receptor antagonists lack the effect on bradykinin levels, which may explain the lower incidence of cough observed with these drug classes.

Renin-Angiotensin-Aldosterone System

The sequence of angiotensin II formation is presented in Figure 7–6. Renin enzymatically converts angiotensinogen into angiotensin I (inactive peptide), which is subsequently converted into angiotensin II (active) by ACE. The three primary drug classes that alter the physiologic actions of this system are the renin inhibitors, ACE inhibitors, and the angiotensin II receptor (AT$_1$) antagonists. Of these drug classes, the most extensively used are the drugs that inhibit the enzyme variously known as ACE, kininase II, or peptidyl dipeptidase. Angiotensin II is a major stimulant of aldosterone release. The renin inhibitors, ACE inhibitors, and angiotensin receptor antagonists all reduce aldosterone levels.

Blockade of aldosterone release and its effects may lead to hyperkalemia. This potassium accumulation may be marked, especially if the patient has renal impairment, is consuming a high-potassium diet, or is taking potassium-sparing diuretics. Under these

circumstances, potassium concentrations may reach toxic levels. For additional information, see the section on Diuretic Medications below.

Renin Inhibitors

Inhibition of renin prevents the initiation of the renin-angiotensin-aldosterone cascade (Figure 7–6). Previous renin inhibitors were peptides and demonstrated low potency and bioavailability. **Aliskiren** represents a new class of low molecular weight, orally active renin inhibitors. Bioavailability of aliskiren is low at 2 to 3%, yet this drug produces a dose-dependent decrease in angiotensins I and II and aldosterone. Clinically, aliskiren produces a dose-dependent reduction in blood pressure in patients with essential hypertension. The most important adverse effect associated with aliskiren is decreased glomerular filtration. When aliskiren is used alone, hyperkalemia is minimal in patients with normal renal function. Concomitant use of aliskiren with either of the drug classes that inhibit the renin-angiotensin-aldosterone system, or potassium-sparing diuretics, increases the risk of hyperkalemia. Hyperuricemia, gastrointestinal distress, and skin rash are also associated with use. The exception to the generally high safety of this class of drugs applies to pregnancy because they may cause renal damage in the fetus. This class of drugs appears to have considerable promise in the treatment of patients with renal disease, hypertension, and other cardiovascular dysfunctions.

ACE Inhibitors

The prototypical drug for this class is **captopril**. ACE inhibition results in a reduction in blood levels of angiotensin II and aldosterone and probably an increase in endogenous vasodilators of the kinin family such as bradykinin (Figure 7–6). ACE inhibitors have a low incidence of serious adverse effects when given in normal dosage, and produce minimal compensatory responses. The adverse effects of ACE inhibitors include a chronic cough in up to 30% of patients. Decreases in glomerular filtration rate may occur in patients with preexisting renal vascular disease, although these drugs are protective in diabetic nephropathy. Hyperkalemia may occur in up to 11% of patients taking these drugs, and increases further when combined with potassium-sparing diuretics, renin inhibitors, or the subsequently discussed angiotensin receptor antagonists. As with the renin inhibitors, these drugs may cause renal damage in the fetus, and are, therefore, absolutely contraindicated in pregnancy.

AT₁ Receptor Antagonists

Drugs in this class are commonly referred to as **angiotensin receptor blockers** (ARBs). The protypical drug in this class is the orally active agent **losartan**; this drug and its many analogs competitively inhibit angiotensin II at its AT_1 receptor site (Figure 7–6). Losartan, **valsartan, irbesartan, candesartan,** and other analogs appear to be as effective in lowering blood pressure as the ACE inhibitors. The adverse effects of these drugs are similar to those of the ACE inhibitors; however, there is a lower incidence of chronic cough. They do cause fetal renal toxicity like that of the other drug classes inhibiting the renin-angiotensin-aldosterone system, and are thus contraindicated in pregnancy.

Diuretics

The tubular transport systems of the nephron regulate the solute, electrolyte, and water loss from the tubule. Each tubular segment has a unique major transport system. These transporters are found on the luminal (urinary) side of the epithelium. Diuretics are divided into several subgroups (Figure 7–7) based on their

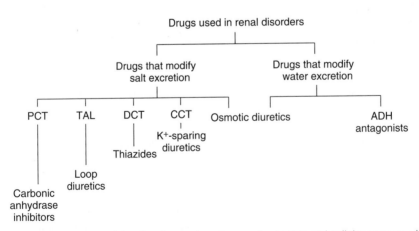

Figure 7–7. The subgroups of the diuretics are based on anatomic sites and cellular processes in the nephron. The effects of the diuretic agents are predictable from a knowledge of the function of the segment of the nephron in which they act. Each segment of the nephron has a different mechanism for reabsorbing sodium and other ions. Abbreviations for the different segments of the nephron are as follows: proximal convoluted tubule (PCT), thick ascending limb of the loop of Henle (TAL), distal convoluted tubule (DCT), and cortical collecting tubule (CCT).

Table 7–2. Electrolyte and systemic pH changes produced by the various diuretic subgroups

Group	Amount in Urine			Body pH
	NaCl	NaHCO$_3$	K$^+$	
Carbonic anhydrase inhibitors	↑	↑↑↑	↑	Acidosis
Loop diuretics	↑↑↑↑	–	↑	Alkalosis
Thiazides	↑↑	↑, –	↑	Alkalosis
K$^+$-sparing diuretics	↑	–	↓	Acidosis

inhibition of these different tubular transporters. Because the mechanisms for these diuretic subgroups differ, their adverse effects also differ. Table 7–2 highlights the electrolyte and systemic pH changes that result from the clinical use of these subgroups.

A summary of the passage of fluid through the nephron and tubular transport systems is provided in Figure 7–8. At the glomerulus, fluid is freely filtered through the glomerular membrane and into Bowman's space. Because the total plasma volume (about 4 L) is filtered many times daily (total filtrate about 180 L/day), the major function of the remainder of the nephron is to reabsorb essential substances. The proximal convoluted tubule carries out isosmotic reabsorption of amino acids, glucose, and numerous ions. This is also the major site for sodium chloride and sodium bicarbonate reabsorption. Bicarbonate itself is poorly reabsorbed through the luminal membrane, but conversion of bicarbonate to carbon dioxide via carbonic acid permits rapid reabsorption of the carbon dioxide. Bicarbonate can then be regenerated from carbon dioxide within the tubular cell and transported into the interstitium and back into the blood. Carbonic anhydrase is required for the bicarbonate reabsorption process and resides on the brush border and in the cytoplasm. This enzyme is the target of carbonic anhydrase inhibitor diuretic drugs. Sodium is separately reabsorbed from the lumen in exchange for hydrogen ions at the luminal surface of the cells and then transported into the interstitial space by the sodium pump at the basolateral surface. The proximal tubule is responsible for 60 to 70% of the total reabsorption of sodium and water. Active secretion and

reabsorption of weak acids and bases also occurs in the proximal tubule. Uric acid transport is especially important and is targeted by some of the drugs used in treating gout (Chapter 34).

The thick ascending limb of the loop of Henle reabsorbs sodium, potassium, and two chloride molecules out of the urine into the interstitium of the kidney (Figure 7–9). The segment is also a major site of calcium and magnesium reabsorption. Reabsorption of sodium, potassium, and chloride are all accomplished by a single carrier, which is the target of the loop diuretics. This cotransporter provides the concentration gradient for the countercurrent-concentrating mechanism in the kidney and is responsible for the reabsorption of 20 to 30% of the sodium filtered at the glomerulus. Because potassium is pumped into the cell from both the luminal and basal sides, an escape route must be provided; this occurs via a potassium-selective channel into the lumen. Because the potassium diffusing through these channels is not accompanied by an anion, a net positive charge is set up in the lumen. This positive potential drives the reabsorption of calcium and magnesium.

The distal convoluted tubule actively pumps sodium and chloride out of the lumen of the nephron via an electrically neutral cotransporter (Figure 7–10). This cotransporter is the target of the thiazide diuretics. The distal convoluted tubule is responsible for approximately 5 to 8% of sodium reabsorption. Calcium is also reabsorbed in this segment under the control of **parathyroid hormone** (PTH), and its role in osteoporosis is discussed in Chapter 25. Reabsorption of calcium from the tubule requires the Na$^+$-Ca^{2+}

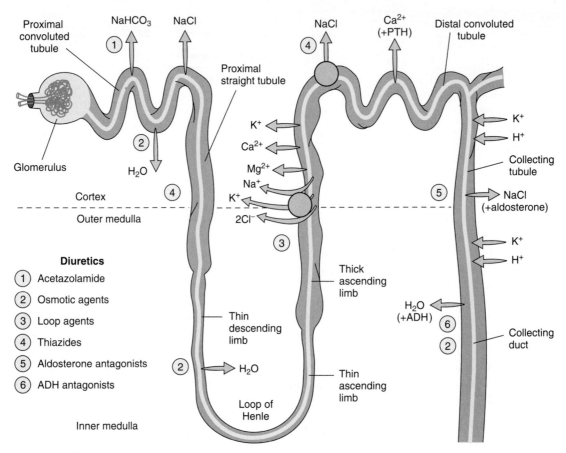

Figure 7–8. Overview of the tubule transport systems and sites of action of diuretics.

exchanger discussed in more detail in Chapter 9. Facilitation of this exchange and Ca^{2+} reabsorption is the reason these medications are occasionally used in the treatment of chronic renal stone formation.

The cortical collecting tubule is the last tubular site of sodium reabsorption and the final site of K^+ excretion. Sodium reabsorption in this segment is controlled by aldosterone (Figure 7–11). This segment is responsible for reabsorbing 2 to 5% of the total filtered sodium. The reabsorption of sodium occurs via channels and is accompanied by an equivalent loss of potassium or hydrogen ions. The collecting tubule is thus the primary site of potassium excretion and of urine acidification. The aldosterone receptor and the

sodium channels are sites of action of the potassium-sparing diuretics. Reabsorption of water occurs in the medullary collecting tubule under the control of ADH (Figure 7–11).

Six subgroups of diuretic classes have been characterized based on their pharmacodynamic mechanisms. These subgroups are osmotic, carbonic anhydrase inhibitors, loop, thiazide, potassium-sparing diuretics, and ADH antagonists (Figure 7–7). These drugs reduce vascular volume by either modifying salt excretion, water excretion, or both (Figure 7–8). Currently, only loop, thiazide, and potassium-sparing diuretics are commonly used to decrease vascular volume in the treatment of hypertension. Carbonic anhydrase inhibitors

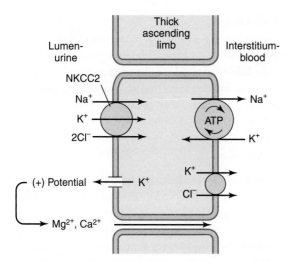

Figure 7–9. Ion transport pathways across the luminal and basolateral membranes of the thick ascending limb cell. The lumen-positive electrical potential created by K⁺ back diffusion drives divalent (and monovalent) cation reabsorption via the paracellular pathway. The major transport system is a Na⁺/K⁺/2Cl⁻ (NKCC2) cotransporter located in the luminal membrane.

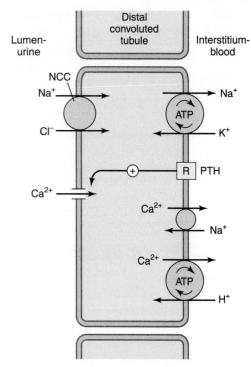

Figure 7–10. Ion transport pathways across the luminal and basolateral membranes of the distal convoluted tubule cell. As in all tubular cells, Na⁺/K⁺ ATPase is present in the basolateral membrane. The primary Na⁺ and Cl⁻ cotransporter (NCC) is electrically neutral and located in the luminal membrane. "R" represents the parathyroid hormone receptor.

such as **acetazolamide** are used to reduce intraocular pressure in glaucoma, to treat acute high-altitude sickness, and for edematous conditions associated with metabolic alkalosis. ADH antagonists such as **demeclocycline** and the newer "vaptans" are used in the treatment of the syndrome of inappropriate ADH secretion (SIADH). SIADH is associated with some neoplasms, with neurologic and pulmonary disorders, and as an adverse effect of some drugs. Finally, most diuretics act from the luminal side of the membrane and must be present in the urine. They are filtered at the glomerulus and some are also secreted by the weak acid-secretory carrier in the proximal tubule. Aldosterone receptor antagonists, such as spironolactone and eplerenone, are exceptions in that they enter the collecting tubule cell from the basolateral side and bind to the cytoplasmic aldosterone receptor.

Osmotic Diuretics

Mannitol, the prototypical osmotic diuretic, is given intravenously. Other drugs often classified with mannitol (but rarely used) include glycerin, isosorbide, and

urea. Because mannitol is freely filtered at the glomerulus but poorly reabsorbed from the tubule, mannitol remains in the lumen and "holds" water by virtue of its osmotic effect. The major location for this action is the proximal convoluted tubule, where the bulk of isosmotic reabsorption normally occurs. Reabsorption of water is also reduced in the descending limb of the loop of Henle and the collecting tubule.

Physiologic Effects. The volume of urine is increased. Most filtered solutes will be excreted in larger amounts unless they are actively reabsorbed. Sodium excretion is usually increased because the rate of urine flow through the tubule is greatly accelerated and sodium transporters cannot handle the volume rapidly enough. Mannitol can also reduce brain volume

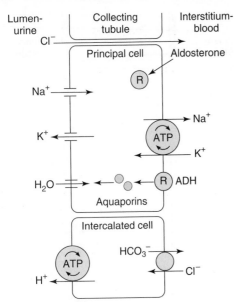

Figure 7–11. Ion transport pathways across the luminal and basolateral membranes of collecting tubule and collecting duct cells. Inward diffusion of Na^+ leaves a lumen-negative potential, which drives reabsorption of Cl^- and efflux of K^+. The Na^+-K^+ exchange function is regulated by aldosterone, which binds to an intracellular receptor (R). ADH acts on a receptor to facilitate insertion of aquaporins (water channels) into the luminal surface and reabsorption of water from the tubule. Hydrogen ion (H^+) secretion into the tubule with bicarbonate (HCO_3^-) reabsorption is also regulated here.

and intracranial pressure by osmotically extracting water from the tissue into the blood. A similar effect occurs in the eye.

Clinical Use. These drugs were formerly used to maintain high urine flow when renal blood flow is reduced or in conditions of solute overload from severe hemolysis or rhabdomyolysis, but are currently not used for these conditions. Mannitol and several other osmotic agents are useful in reducing intraocular pressure in acute glaucoma and intracranial pressure in neurologic conditions.

Adverse Effects. Removal of water from the intracellular compartment may cause hyponatremia and pulmonary edema. As the water is excreted, hypernatremia may follow. Headache, nausea, and vomiting are common.

Loop Diuretics

Furosemide is the prototypical loop agent. Furosemide, **bumetanide**, and **torsemide** are sulfonamide derivatives. **Ethacrynic acid** is a phenoxyacetic acid derivative but acts by the same mechanism. Loop diuretics inhibit the cotransport of sodium, potassium, and chloride (Figure 7–9). The loop diuretics are relatively short-acting. Diuresis usually occurs over a 4-hour period following a dose.

Physiologic Effects. The loop of Henle is responsible for a significant fraction of total renal sodium chloride reabsorption; therefore, a full dose of a loop diuretic produces a massive sodium chloride diuresis. If tissue perfusion is adequate, edema fluid is rapidly excreted and blood volume may be significantly reduced. The diluting ability of the nephron is reduced because the loop of Henle is the site of significant dilution of urine. Inhibition of the $Na^+/K^+/2Cl^-$ transporter also results in loss of the lumen-positive potential, which reduces reabsorption of divalent cations as well. As a result, calcium excretion is significantly increased. Ethacrynic acid is a moderately effective uricosuric drug if blood volume is maintained.

The presentation of large amounts of sodium to the collecting tubule as a function of loop diuresis may result in significant potassium wasting and excretion of protons; hypokalemic alkalosis may occur. The loop diuretics may also have pulmonary vasodilating effects; the mechanism is not known. Finally, prostaglandins are important in maintaining glomerular filtration. The efficacy of diuretics, especially loop diuretics, decreases when synthesis of prostaglandins is inhibited, as with nonsteroidal anti-inflammatory drugs (Chapter 34).

Clinical Use. The major application of loop diuretics is in the treatment of edematous states including heart failure and ascites. They are particularly valuable in acute pulmonary edema, in which the pulmonary vasodilating action plays a useful role. They are used in hypertension if response to thiazides is inadequate, but the short duration of the action of loop diuretics is a disadvantage in this condition. A less common but important application is in the treatment of severe hypercalcemia, which may occur in malignancy.

Adverse Effects. Loop diuretics cause potassium wasting, ultimately resulting in hypokalemia (Table 7–2). Large amounts of sodium are presented to the collecting tubules. The potassium is excreted by the latter segment in an effort to conserve sodium. The potassium wasting may be severe, and metabolic alkalosis may also occur. Because they are so efficacious, the loop diuretics can cause hypovolemia and associated orthostatic hypotension and reflex tachycardia. Ototoxicity is also an important toxic effect of the loop agents. The sulfonamides in this group may cause a typical sulfonamide allergy.

Thiazide Diuretics

Hydrochlorothiazide, the prototypical agent, and all the other members of this group are sulfonamide derivatives. Thiazides are active by the oral route and have a duration of action of 6 to 12 hours, which is considerably longer than the loop diuretics. The major action of thiazides is to inhibit sodium chloride transport in the early segment of the distal convoluted tubule (Figure 7–10).

Physiologic Effects. In full doses, thiazides produce moderate but sustained sodium and chloride diuresis. Hypokalemic metabolic alkalosis may occur (Table 7–2). Reduction in the transport of sodium into the tubular cell reduces intracellular sodium and promotes sodium-calcium exchange. As a result, reabsorption of calcium from the urine is increased and urine calcium content is decreased—the opposite of the effect of loop diuretics. Because they act in a diluting segment of the nephron, thiazides may interfere with excretion of water and cause dilutional hyponatremia. Thiazides also reduce blood pressure, and the maximal pressure-lowering effect occurs at doses lower than the maximal diuretic doses. When a thiazide is used with a loop diuretic, a synergistic effect occurs with marked diuresis.

Clinical Use. The major application of thiazides is in hypertension, for which their long duration and moderate intensity of action are particularly useful. Chronic therapy of edematous conditions such as mild heart failure is another important application, although loop diuretics are preferred. Chronic renal calcium stone formation can sometimes be controlled with thiazides because of their ability to reduce urine calcium concentration.

Adverse Effects. Massive sodium diuresis with hyponatremia is an uncommon but dangerous early effect of thiazides. As with loop diuretics, chronic therapy is often associated with potassium wasting potentially resulting in hypokalemia. Diabetic patients may have significant hyperglycemia. Serum uric acid and lipid levels are also increased in some individuals. Thiazides are sulfonamides and share sulfonamide allergenic potential.

Potassium-Sparing Diuretics

Spironolactone and **eplerenone** are steroid derivatives that act as pharmacologic antagonists of aldosterone in the collecting tubules (Figure 7–11). By combining with and blocking the intracellular aldosterone receptor, these drugs reduce the expression of genes controlling synthesis of epithelial sodium ion channels and Na^+/K^+ ATPase. **Amiloride** and **triamterene** act by blocking the sodium channels in the same portion of the nephron. Spironolactone and eplerenone have slow onsets and offsets of action of 24 to 72 hours. Amiloride and triamterene have duration of action of 12 to 24 hours.

Physiologic Effects. All drugs in this class cause an increase in sodium clearance and a decrease in potassium and hydrogen ion excretion and therefore qualify as potassium-sparing diuretics. They may also cause hyperkalemic metabolic acidosis (Table 7–2).

Clinical Use. Potassium wasting caused by chronic therapy with loop or thiazide diuretics, if not controlled by dietary potassium supplements, may be minimized by these drugs. The most common use is in the form of products that combine a thiazide with a potassium-sparing agent in a single pill. The aldosterone receptor antagonists of this group are also used to treat aldosteronism. Aldosteronism (elevated serum aldosterone levels) occurs in hepatic cirrhosis and heart failure. Spironolactone and eplerenone have been shown to have significant long-term benefits in heart failure (Chapter 9). Some of this effect may occur in the heart, an action that is not yet understood. Finally, spironolactone may also cause endocrine abnormalities, including gynecomastia and antiandrogenic effects. Eplerenone has fewer antiandrogenic effects.

Adverse Effects. The most important toxic effect is hyperkalemia. These drugs should never be given with potassium supplements or potassium-containing salt substitutes. Other aldosterone antagonists such as renin inhibitors, ACE inhibitors and angiotensin receptor antagonists, if used at all, should be used with great caution.

SUMMARY OF COMPENSATORY RESPONSES AND ADVERSE EFFECTS OF ANTIHYPERTENSIVE THERAPY

Physiologic compensatory responses to, and adverse effects from, antihypertensive therapy may affect rehabilitation therapy of patients in multiple clinical settings. Drug-mediated decreases in systemic pressure result in the activation of baroreflex and the renin-angiotensin system in an attempt to return to premedication pressures. The physiologic compensatory responses and adverse effects to the different antihypertensive drug classes are summarized in Table 7–3. Tachycardia is one compensatory response, and salt and water retention is another. Orthostatic hypotension is an adverse effect of several antihypertensive drug classes. Several of the compensatory responses to decreased pressure may be minimized with other antihypertensive medications (Figure 7–12). Thus, tachycardia may be counteracted with β-receptor antagonists or reserpine, and salt and water retention may be minimized with diuretics or drug classes that interfere with the angiotensin-aldosterone system.

REHABILITATION FOCUS

Clinical research has consistently documented that aerobic activity is one of the nonpharmacologic mechanisms for controlling hypertension and its sequelae.

Other nonpharmacologic therapies include low-sodium and low-fat diets, weight reduction, cessation of smoking, and moderate alcohol intake. Exercise may also assist in weight reduction. Antihypertensive drugs are commonly used by patients being treated in all rehabilitation settings.

Aerobic capacity may improve as a result of taking antihypertensive drugs. However, adverse events are also common when aerobic activities associated with rehabilitation are combined with antihypertensive drugs. Hypotension is a common potential hazard of antihypertensive drugs. Thus, care should be taken by the physical therapist in situations that may result in peripheral vasodilation. These include hydrotherapy in a warm environment or whirlpool of an entire lower extremity and absence of a cool-down period following a period of aerobic activity. In the former, the patient should be encouraged to exit the pool slowly or stand with support; in the latter, a cool-down period of moderate stretching may be required to avoid syncope. The therapist should also recognize that cardiac responses to exercise such as heart rate may be blunted by pharmacologic classes such as β-receptor antagonists and calcium channel blockers. β-receptor antagonists may also blunt bronchodilation and respiratory capacity in response to exercise. In contrast, some antihypertensive drugs such as direct-acting vasodilators and α_1 receptor antagonists may initiate reflex tachycardia that may be exacerbated by exercise. Blood electrolyte changes are a significant problem with several of the diuretic classes. These electrolyte changes may predispose some patients to arrhythmias, either directly or as a result of other drug interactions, and exercise may precipitate the arrhythmia.

Hypertension is known as the "silent killer" because clinical manifestations do not occur until the later stages of the disease. Furthermore, adverse effects resulting from clinical use of many antihypertensive drugs may be bothersome to the patient. Thus, patient compliance with regular drug use may be poor. The therapist must recognize that such noncompliance can predispose the patient to adverse effects during the rehabilitation treatment, especially if increased sympathetic activity is a result of the treatment process.

Table 7–3. Compensatory responses to and adverse effects of antihypertensive drugs

Class and Drug	Compensatory Responses	Adverse Effects
Diuretics		
Hydrochlorothiazide	Minimal	Hypokalemia, slight hyperlipidemia, hyperuricemia, hyperglycemia, lassitude, weakness, impotence
Sympatholytics		
Clonidine	Salt and water retention	Dry mouth, severe rebound hypertension if drug is suddenly stopped
Methyldopa	Salt and water retention	Sedation, positive Coombs test, hemolytic anemia
Trimethaphan	Salt and water retention	Severe orthostatic hypotension, constipation, blurred vision, sexual dysfunction
Reserpine (low dose)	Minimal	Diarrhea, nasal stuffiness, sedation, depression
Alpha$_1$-Selective Antagonists		
Prazosin	Salt and water retention, slight tachycardia	Orthostatic hypotension (limited to first few doses)
Beta-Selective Antagonists		
Propranolol	Minimal	Sleep disturbances, sedation, impotence, cardiac disturbances, bronchoconstriction
Vasodilators		
Hydralazine	Salt and water retention, marked tachycardia	Lupus-like syndrome (but lacking renal effects)
Minoxidil	Marked salt and water retention, very marked tachycardia	Hirsutism, pericardial effusion, orthostatic hypotension
Nitroprusside	Salt and water retention	Cyanide toxicity (CN$^-$ released)
Calcium Channel Blockers		
Nifedipine	Minor salt and water retention	Constipation, cardiac disturbances, flushing
ACE Inhibitors		
Captopril	Minimal	Cough, decreases glomerular filtration rate and exacerbates preexisting renal disease, nephrotoxic in the fetus
Angiotensin II Receptor Antagonists		
Losartan	Minimal	Decreases glomerular filtration rate and exacerbates preexisting renal disease, nephrotoxic in the fetus
Renin Inhibitor		
Aliskiren	Minimal	Decreases glomerular filtration rate, nephrotoxic in the fetus, hyperuricemia

ACE = angiotensin-converting enzyme.

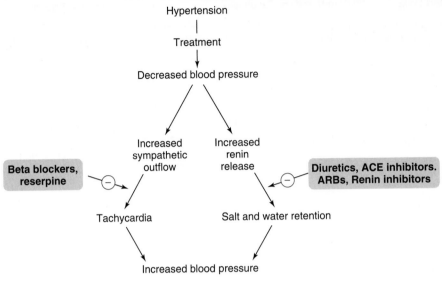

Figure 7–12. Compensatory responses to decreased blood pressure when treating hypertension. Arrows with minus signs indicate medication classes used to minimize the compensatory response. ARB = angiotensin receptor blocker.

Sympathetic activity increases as result of exercise, orthopedic strengthening, functional return to work rehabilitation, or even painful wound healing procedures. Beta-receptor antagonists such as propranolol, when taken chronically, may result in arrhythmias if abruptly stopped; and α_2 receptor agonists, such as clonidine, may result in rebound hypertension if abruptly stopped.

CLINICAL RELEVANCE FOR REHABILITATION

Adverse Drug Reactions
- Orthostatic hypotension is a common problem with some classes of antihypertensive drugs.
- Bronchoconstriction is a problem with β-receptor antagonists.
- Beta-receptor antagonists blunt the early manifestations of hypoglycemia.
- Several antihypertensive drug classes depress heart rate and contractility.

- Loop and thiazide diuretics can cause hypokalemia.
- Potassium-sparing diuretics can cause hyperkalemia.
- When taken with potassium-sparing diuretics, drugs inhibiting the renin-angiotensin-aldosterone system increase the risk of hyperkalemia.

Effects Interfering with Rehabilitation
- Orthostatic hypotension may cause patients to faint when transferring from a sitting or supine position to standing, exiting from a warm aquatherapy area, or if aerobic exercise is terminated without an appropriate cool-down period.
- Dyspnea may decrease aerobic capacity.
- Manifestations of hypoglycemia occurring during aerobic activities may be delayed.
- Heart rate cannot be used as a marker of exertion for patients taking β-receptor antagonists.
- Cardiac output may be depressed during aerobic activities by several drug groups.
- Altered plasma potassium levels can cause paresthesias, decrease skeletal muscle function, increase cramps, and increase the risk of cardiac dysfunction.

Possible Therapy Solutions

- Check blood pressure and heart rate prior to and following aerobic activities.
- Monitor heart rate during aerobic activities.
- To prevent fainting associated with orthostatic hypotension, assist patients with positional changes and when exiting a warm pool. Always provide a cool-down period following exercise.
- Allow increased time to complete aerobic tasks to prevent dyspnea and account for depressed cardiac activity.
- Use perceived exertion (Borg Rating of Perceived Exertion Scale) when determining aerobic activity in patients being treated with β-receptor antagonists.
- Have patients check glucose levels prior to aerobic activities if the patients are taking hypoglycemic drugs.
- Review the clinical manifestations of altered plasma potassium levels and determine if patients are taking medications that may alter these levels.

Potentiation of Functional Outcomes Secondary to Drug Therapy

- These drugs allow patients to participate in aerobic activities while minimizing increases in blood pressure.

PROBLEM-ORIENTED PATIENT STUDY

Brief History: The patient is a 46-year-old male who attended college on a 4-year baseball pitching scholarship. The patient was right-handed and pitched 3 years, being sidelined as a result of overuse injury toward the end of the fourth season. The patient is now employed as a trader on the floor of a major commodities exchange. The employment is stressful and requires constant standing and elevation of his right arm throughout the day while making bids in the commodities pits. Outside of this activity, the patient lives a sedentary lifestyle with no additional aerobic recreational activities except for walking between the commodities exchange and the train station and other community ambulation. During the years following college, the patient occasionally sought medical care for complaints of right shoulder pain. The patient has a 5-year history of essential hypertension that is stable on current drugs; otherwise, there are no other morbidities noted in the medical history.

Current Medical Status and Drug Therapy: One week previous the patient elected to have arthroscopic surgery for right shoulder girdle repair. The patient spent one night in the acute care facility prior to discharge and was referred to the outpatient rehabilitation clinic for assistance in return to functional activity. The patient has a body mass index of 27, and vital signs are 130/80 mm Hg for blood pressure and 66 bpm for the heart rate at rest. Current drugs are hydrochlorothiazide and propranolol in a single formulation (Inderide). The patient is also provided with an opiate analgesic to reduce postsurgical pain.

Rehabilitation Setting: The patient arrives for the first evaluation and treatment at 6:00 p.m. following work. Passive range of motion in gravity-eliminated position and in the pain-free range is examined for the right upper extremity. The patient's active range of motion in gravity eliminated and gravity resisted is limited by both pain and the physician's guidelines. The patient expresses urgency in regaining right arm function in order to return to work. The physical therapist has worked closely with the referring physician on other patients following arthroscopic surgical repair of the shoulder girdle, and has an established and agreed-upon general treatment

(continued)

PROBLEM-ORIENTED PATIENT STUDY (*Continued*)

guideline. This involves having the patients in a therapool up to neck level. Initial treatments allow buoyancy of the shoulder for pain-free function, and at 35°C the temperature allows muscular relaxation. The patient enters the pool up to his neck and under the guidance of the therapist begins the rehabilitation activities. After about 15 minutes into the session, the patient begins to complain of shortness of breath, and starts up the pool stairs with the assistance of the therapist. At the top of the stairs, the patient complains of being "lightheaded," and is assisted to a chair where he faints for several seconds prior to returning to consciousness. Blood pressure is 90/50 mm Hg and heart rate is 74 bpm. The patient is coherent and returns to standing after several minutes.

Problem/Clinical Options: The referring physician should be contacted by the physical therapist to document the incident and determine whether additional referral back to the physician is required prior to additional rehabilitation activities. The initial difficulty in breathing was a combination of the presence of the β-receptor antagonist (which diminished bronchodilation during the exertional activities), and hydrostatic pressure on the chest (from immersion up to the neck in the therapool). The subsequent hypotension upon leaving the therapool was the result of peripheral pooling of the blood while in the therapool, and partial inhibition of the homeostatic baroreflexes by the β-receptor antagonist and thiazide diuretic. This baroreflex should have increased return blood flow to the heart and cardiac output, preventing the syncope. Finally, the opiate analgesic may have diminished respiratory drive. See Chapter 20 for additional information on these drugs.

PREPARATIONS AVAILABLE

Alpha Adrenoceptor Antagonists

Doxazosin (generic, Cardura)
Oral: 1-, 2-, 4-, 8-mg tablets

Phenoxybenzamine (Dibenzyline)
Oral: 10-mg capsules

Phentolamine (generic, Regitine)
Parenteral: 5 mg/vial for injection

Prazosin (generic, Minipress)
Oral: 1-, 2-, 5-mg capsules

Terazosin (generic, Hytrin)
Oral: 1-, 2-, 5-, 10-mg tablets, capsules

Tolazoline (Priscoline)
Parenteral: 25 mg/mL for injection

CNS-Acting Sympatholytics

Clonidine (generic, Catapres)
Oral: 0.1-, 0.2-, 0.3-mg tablets
Transdermal (Catapres-TTS): patches that release 0.1, 0.2, 0.3 mg/24 h

Guanfacine (Tenex)
Oral: 1-, 2-mg tablets

Methyldopa (generic)
Oral: 250-, 500-mg tablets
Parenteral: 50 mg/mL for injection

Beta Receptor Antagonists

Acebutolol (generic, Sectral)
Oral: 200-, 400-mg capsules

Atenolol (generic, Tenormin)
Oral: 25-, 50-, 100-mg tablets
Parenteral: 0.5 mg/mL for IV injection

Betaxolol
Oral: 10-, 20-mg tablets (Kerlone)
Ophthalmic: 0.25%, 0.5% drops (generic, Betoptic)

Bisoprolol (Zebeta)
Oral: 5-, 10-mg tablets

Carteolol
Oral: 2.5-, 5-mg tablets (Cartrol)
Ophthalmic: 1% drops (generic, Ocupress)

Carvedilol (Coreg)
Oral: 3.125-, 6.25-, 12.5-, 25-mg tablets

Esmolol (Brevibloc)
Parenteral: 10 mg/mL for IV injection; 250 mg/mL for IV infusion

Labetalol (generic, Normodyne, Trandate)
Oral: 100-, 200-, 300-mg tablets
Parenteral: 5 mg/mL for injection

Levobunolol (Betagan Liquifilm, etc)
Ophthalmic: 0.25, 0.5% drops

Metipranolol (Optipranolol)
Ophthalmic: 0.3% drops

Metoprolol (generic, Lopressor, Toprol)
Oral: 50-, 100-mg tablets
Oral sustained release: 25-, 50-, 100-, 200-mg tablets
Parenteral: 1 mg/mL for injection

Nadolol (generic, Corgard)
Oral: 20-, 40-, 80-, 120-, 160-mg tablets

Penbutolol (Levatol)
Oral: 20-mg tablets

Pindolol (generic, Visken)
Oral: 5-, 10-mg tablets

Propranolol (generic, Inderal)
Oral: 10-, 20-, 40-, 60-, 80-, 90-mg tablets; 4, 8, 80 mg/mL solutions
Oral sustained release: 60-, 80-, 120-, 160-mg capsules
Parenteral: 1 mg/mL for injection

Sotalol (generic, Betapace)
Oral: 80-, 120-, 160-, 240-mg tablets

Timolol
Oral: 5-, 10-, 20-mg tablets (generic, Blocadren)

Ganglion-Blocking Agents

Mecamylamine (Inversine)
Oral: 2.5-mg tablets

Postganglionic Sympathetic Blocking Medications

Guanadrel (Hylorel)
Oral: 10-, 25-mg tablets

Guanethidine (Ismelin)
Oral: 10-, 25-mg tablets

Reserpine (generic)
Oral: 0.1-, 0.25-mg tablets

Vasodilators

Diazoxide (Hyperstat IV)
Parenteral: 15 mg/mL ampule
Oral (Proglycem): 50-mg capsule; 50 mg/mL oral suspension

Fenoldopam (Corlopam)
Parenteral: 10 mg/mL for IV infusion

Hydralazine (generic, Apresoline)
Oral: 10-, 25-, 50-, 100-mg tablets
Parenteral: 20 mg/mL for injection

Minoxidil (generic, Loniten) Clinical
Oral: 2.5-, 10-mg tablets
Topical (Rogaine, etc): 2% lotion

Nitroprusside (generic, Nitropress)
Parenteral: 50-mg/vial

Calcium Channel Blockers

Amlodipine (Norvasc)
Oral: 2.5-, 5-, 10-mg tablets

Bepridil (Vascor)
Oral: 200-, 300-mg tablets

Diltiazem (generic, Cardizem)
Oral: 30-, 60-, 90-, 120-mg tablets (unlabeled in hypertension)
Oral sustained release (Cardizem CD, Cardizem SR, Dilacor XL): 60-, 90-, 120-, 180-, 240-, 300-, 360-, 420-mg capsules
Parenteral: 5 mg/mL for injection

Felodipine (Plendil)
Oral extended release: 2.5-, 5-, 10-mg tablets

Isradipine (DynaCirc)
Oral: 2.5-, 5-mg capsules; 5-, 10-mg controlled-release tablets

Nicardipine (generic, Cardene)
Oral: 20-, 30-mg capsules
Oral sustained release (Cardene SR): 30-, 45-, 60-mg capsules
Parenteral (Cardene I.V.): 2.5 mg/mL for injection

Nisoldipine (Sular)
Oral: 10-, 20-, 30-, 40-mg extended release tablets

Nifedipine (generic, Adalat, Procardia)
Oral: 10-, 20-mg capsules (unlabeled in hypertension)
Oral extended release (Adalat CC, Procardia-XL): 30-, 60-, 90-mg tablets

Verapamil (generic, Calan, Isoptin)
Oral: 40-, 80-, 120-mg tablets
Oral sustained release (generic, Calan SR, Verelan): 120-, 180-, 240-mg tablets; 100-, 120-, 180-, 200-, 240-, 300-mg capsules
Parenteral: 2.5 mg/mL for injection

Renin Inhibitors

Aliskiren (Tektruna)
Oral: 150-, 300-mg tablets

ACE Antagonists

Benazepril (Lotensin)
Oral: 5-, 10-, 20-, 40-mg tablets

Captopril (generic, Capoten)
Oral: 12.5-, 25-, 50-, 100-mg tablets

Enalapril (Vasotec)
Oral: 2.5-, 5-, 10-, 20-mg tablets
Parenteral (Enalaprilat): 1.25 mg/mL for injection

Fosinopril (Monopril)
Oral: 10-, 20-, 40-mg tablets

Lisinopril (Prinivil, Zestril)
Oral: 2.5-, 5-, 10-, 20-, 40-mg tablets

Moexipril (Univasc)
Oral: 7.5-, 15-mg tablets

Perindopril (Aceon)
Oral: 2-, 4-, 8-mg tablets

Quinapril (Accupril)
Oral: 5-, 10-, 20-, 40-mg tablets

Ramipril (Altace)
Oral: 1.25-, 2.5-, 5-, 10-mg capsules

Trandolapril (Mavik)
Oral: 1-, 2-, 4-mg tablets

AT$_1$ Receptor Antagonists

Candesartan (Atacand)
Oral: 4-, 8-, 16-, 32-mg tablets

Eprosartan (Teveten)
Oral: 400-, 600-mg tablets

Irbesartan (Avapro)
Oral: 75-, 150-, 300-mg tablets

Losartan (Cozaar)
Oral: 25-, 50-, 100-mg tablets

Olmisartan (Benicar)
Oral: 5-, 20-, 40-mg tablets

Telmisartan (Micardis)
Oral: 20-, 40-, 80-mg tablets

Valsartan (Diovan)
Oral: 40-, 80-, 160-, 320-mg tablet

Diuretics

Acetazolamide (generic, Diamox)
Oral: 125-, 250-mg tablets
Oral sustained release: 500-mg capsules
Parenteral: 500-mg powder for injection

Amiloride (generic, Midamor, combination drugs)
Oral: 5-mg tablets

Bendroflumethiazide (Naturetin)
Oral: 5-, 10-mg tablets

Benzthiazide (Exna, combination drugs)
Oral: 50-mg tablets

Brinzolamide (Azopt)
Ophthalmic: 1% suspension

Bumetanide (generic, Bumex)
Oral: 0.5-, 1-, 2-mg tablets
Parenteral: 0.5 mg/2 mL ampule for IV or IM injection

Chlorothiazide (generic, Diuril, etc)
Oral: 250-, 500-mg tablets; 250 mg/5 mL oral suspension
Parenteral: 500-mg for injection

Chlorthalidone (generic, Thalitone, combination drugs)
Oral: 15-, 25-, 50-, 100-mg tablets

Demeclocycline (Declomycin)
Oral: 150-mg tablets and capsules; 300-mg tablets

Dichlorphenamide (Daranide)
Oral: 50-mg tablets

Dorzolamide (Trusopt)
Ophthalmic: 2% solution

Eplerenone (Inspra)
Oral: 25-, 50-, 100-mg tablets

Ethacrynic acid (Edecrin)
Oral: 25-, 50-mg tablets
Parenteral: 50-mg IV injection

Furosemide (generic, Lasix, etc)
Oral: 20-, 40-, 80-mg tablets; 8 mg/mL solutions
Parenteral: 10 mg/mL for IM or IV injection

Hydrochlorothiazide (generic, Microzide, Hydro-DIURIL, combination drugs)
Oral: 12.5-mg capsules; 25-, 50-, 100-mg tablets; 10 mg/mL solution

Hydroflumethiazide (generic, Diucardin)
Oral: 50-mg tablets

Indapamide (generic, Lozol)
Oral: 1.25-, 2.5-mg tablets

Mannitol (generic, Osmitrol)
Parenteral: 5, 10, 15, 20, 25% for injection

Methazolamide (generic, Neptazane)
Oral: 25-, 50-mg tablets

Methyclothiazide (generic, Aquatensen)
Oral: 2.5-, 5-mg tablets

Metolazone (Mykrox, Zaroxolyn) (Note: Bio-availability of Mykrox is greater than that of Zaroxolyn.)
Oral: 0.5 (Mykrox); 2.5-, 5-, 10-mg (Zaroxolyn) tablets

Polythiazide (Renese)
Oral: 1-, 2-, 4-mg tablets

Quinethazone (Hydromox)
Oral: 50-mg tablets

Spironolactone (generic, Aldactone)
Oral: 25-, 50-, 100-mg tablets

Torsemide (Demadex)
Oral: 5-, 10-, 20-, 100-mg tablets
Parenteral: 10 mg/mL for injection

Triamterene (Dyrenium)
Oral: 50-, 100-mg capsules

Trichlormethiazide (generic, Diurese, etc)
Oral: 2-, 4-mg tablets

REFERENCES

Antihypertensive Medications
ALLHAT Officers and Coordinators for the ALLHAT Collaborative Research Group: Major cardiovascular events in hypertensive patients randomized to doxazosin vs chlorthalidone: The antihypertensive and lipid-lowering treatment to prevent heart attack trial. *JAMA* 2000;283:1967.

ALLHAT Officers and Coordinators for the ALLHAT Collaborative Research Group: Major outcomes of high-risk hypertensive patients randomized to angiotensin-converting enzyme inhibitor or calcium channel blockers vs diuretic: The antihypertensive and lipid-lowering treatment to prevent heart attack trial. *JAMA* 2002;288:2981.

August P: Initial treatment of hypertension. *N Engl J Med* 2003;348:610.

Burnier M: Cardiovascular drugs: Angiotensin II type 1 receptor blockers. *Circulation* 2001;103:904.

Cooper H, et al: Diuretics and risk of arrhythmic death in patients with left ventricular dysfunction. *Circulation* 1999;100:1311.

Cooper ME, Johnston CI: Optimizing treatment of hypertension in patients with diabetes. *JAMA* 2000;283:3177.

Garg J, Messerli AW, Bakris GL: Evaluation and treatment of patients with systemic hypertension. *Circulation* 2002;105:2458.

He J, Ogden L, Vupputuri S: Dietary sodium intake and subsequent risk of cardiovascular disease in overweight adults. *JAMA* 1999;282:2027.

Hyman DJ, Pavlik VN: Characteristics of patients with uncontrolled hypertension in the United States. *N Engl J Med* 2001;345:479.

Kaplan NM: Management of hypertension in patients with type 2 diabetes mellitus: Guidelines based on current evidence. *Ann Intern Med* 2001;135:1079.

Palmer BF: Renal dysfunction complicating the treatment of hypertension. *N Engl J Med* 2002;347:1256.

Remuzzi G, Ruggenenti P, Perico N: Chronic renal diseases: Renoprotective benefits of renin-angiotensin-system inhibition. *Ann Intern Med* 2002;136:604.

Sixth report of the Joint National Committee on prevention, detection, evaluation, and treatment of high blood pressure. *Arch Intern Med* 1997;157:2413.

Stevens VJ, et al: Long-term weight loss and changes in blood pressure: Results of the trials of hypertension prevention, phase II. *Ann Intern Med* 2001;134:1.

Vollmer WM, et al: Effects of diet and sodium intake on blood pressure: Subgroup analysis of the DASH-Sodium trial. *Ann Intern Med* 2001;135:1019.

Diuretics

ALLHAT Officers and Coordinators for the ALLHAT Collaborative Research Group: Major outcomes in high-risk hypertensive patients randomized to angiotensin-converting enzyme inhibitor or calcium channel blocker vs diuretic: The antihypertensive and lipid-lowering treatment to prevent heart attack trial (ALLHAT). *JAMA* 2002;288:2981.

Brater DC: Pharmacology of diuretics. *Am J Med Sci* 2000;319:38.

Brenner BM (ed): *The Kidney,* 65th ed. Philadelphia: Saunders, 2001.

Ellison DH: Diuretic drugs and the treatment of edema: From clinic to bench and back again. *Am J Kidney Dis* 1994;23:623.

Forns X, et al: Management of ascites and renal failure in cirrhosis. *Semin Liver Dis* 1994;14:82.

Giebisch G, et al: Renal and extrarenal sites of action of diuretics. *Cardiovasc Drugs Ther* 1993;7:11.

Greenberg A: Diuretic complications. *Am J Med Sci* 2000;319:10.

Greger R: Physiology of renal sodium transport. *Am J Med Sci* 2000;319:51.

Hackett PH, Roach RC: High-altitude illness. *N Engl J Med* 2001;345:107.

Puschett JB: Pharmacological classification and renal actions of diuretics. *Cardiology* 1994;84(Suppl 2):4.

Schrot RJ, Muizelaar JP: Mannitol in acute traumatic brain injury. *Lancet* 2002;359:1633.

Sorrentino MJ: Drug therapy for congestive heart failure. *Postgrad Med* 1997;101:83.

Renin Inhibitors

Azizi M: Renin inhibition. *Curr Opin Nephrol Hypertens* 2006;15:505.

Cheng H, Harris RC: Potential side effects of renin inhibitors—mechanisms based on comparison with other renin-angiotensin blockers. *Expert Opin Drug Saf* 2006;5:631.

Danser AH, Deinum J: Renin, prorenin and the putative (pro)renin receptor. *Hypertension* 2005;46:1069.

Kelly DJ, Wilkinson-Berka JL, Gilbert RE: Renin inhibition: New potential for an old therapeutic target. *Hypertension* 2005;46:471.

O'Brien E: Aliskiren: A renin inhibitor offering a new approach for the treatment of hypertension. *Expert Opin Investig Drugs* 2006;15:1269.

Rehabilitation

Basu SK, Kinsey CD, Miller AJ, Lahiri A: Improved efficacy and safety of controlled-release diltiazem compared to nifedipine may be related to its negative chronotropic effect. *Am J Ther* 2000;7:17.

Davis MM, Jones DW: The role of lifestyle management in the overall treatment plan for prevention and management of hypertension. *Semin Nephrol* 2002;22:35.

Di Somma S, et al: Treatment of hypertension associated with stable angina pectoris: favourable interaction between new metoprolol formulation (OROS) and nifedipine. *Cardiologia* 1996;41:635.

Eagles CJ, Kendall MJ: The effects of combined treatment with beta₁-selective receptor antagonists and lipid-lowering drugs on fat metabolism and measures of fatigue during moderate intensity exercise:

A placebo-controlled study in healthy subjects. *Br J Clin Pharmacol* 1997;43:291.

Gordon NF, Scott CB: Exercise and mild essential hypertension. *Prim Care* 1991;18:683.

Horan MJ, Roccella EJ: Nonpharmacologic treatment of hypertension: Does it work? *Eur Heart* J 1987;8(Suppl B):77.

Johnston DL, Manyari DE, Kostuk WJ: The clinical and hemodynamic effects of propranolol, pindolol and verapamil in the treatment of exertional angina pectoris. *Can Med Assoc* J 1984;130:1449.

Miller BW, et al: Exercise during hemodialysis decreases the use of antihypertensive medications. *Am J Kidney Dis* 2002;39:828.

Petrella RJ: How effective is exercise training for the treatment of hypertension? *Clin J Sport Med* 1998;8:224.

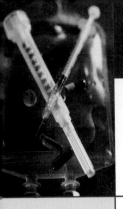

8

DRUGS USED IN THE TREATMENT OF ANGINA PECTORIS

The name *angina pectoris* refers to a strangling or pressure-like pain caused by cardiac ischemia. Angina is the most common condition involving tissue ischemia in which vasodilator drugs or cardiac depressants are used. The pain may be located substernally, radiating to the neck, in the left upper extremity, occasionally in the right upper extremity, or in the epigastrium. However, not all cardiac ischemia is associated with pain. Clinical conditions exist, such as silent myocardial infarction, in which myocardial ischemia or necrosis may occur without pain. Anginal pain is often atypical in women.

This chapter reviews the pathophysiology of angina and the therapeutic strategies for its treatment. Pharmacologic treatments are divided into vasodilators and cardiac depressants (Figure 8–1). In addition to the drugs discussed in this chapter, patients with angina are often treated with lipid-lowering drugs to minimize additional lipid plaque formation and antithrombotics or anticoagulants to control thrombosis at the site of these plaques. These drugs are discussed in Chapters 11 and 26.

■ DETERMINANTS OF CARDIAC OXYGEN DEMAND

The pharmacologic treatment of coronary insufficiency is based on physiologic factors that control the myocardial oxygen requirement. A major determinant of oxygen requirement is myocardial fiber tension. The higher the tension, the greater the oxygen requirement. Several variables contribute to fiber tension (Figure 8–2).

Among the diastolic factors, venous tone determines the capacity of the venous circulation and controls the amount of blood sequestered there versus the amount returned to the heart. Venous tone is maintained by sympathetic activity and increases when sympathetic activity increases. Venous tone and blood volume together determine preload, and preload is the major diastolic determinant of myocardial oxygen requirement.

The systolic factors include afterload, heart rate, contractility, and ejection time. Afterload is the pressure that the ventricle must overcome to eject blood into the arterial system. Afterload is determined by arterial blood pressure and large artery stiffness. Heart rate contributes to time-integrated fiber tension because at fast heart rates, fibers spend more time contracted at systolic tension levels. Because coronary perfusion is maximal during diastole, faster heart rates lead to decreased myocardial perfusion; that is, faster rates abbreviate the time spent in diastole and decrease myocardial perfusion. Systolic blood pressure and heart rate may be multiplied to yield the *double product*, a measure of cardiac work and, therefore, of oxygen requirement.

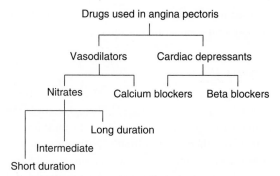

Figure 8–1. Pharmacologic classes used in the treatment of angina pectoris.

In patients with atherosclerotic angina, effective drugs reduce the double product. Force of cardiac contraction is another systolic factor controlled mainly by sympathetic activity to the heart. Finally, ejection time for ventricular contraction is inversely related to force of contraction but is also influenced by impedance to outflow. Increased ejection time increases oxygen requirement.

PATHOPHYSIOLOGY OF ANGINA PECTORIS

Atherosclerotic angina is also known as exertional angina or classic angina. This type of angina is associated with atheromatous plaques that partially occlude one or more coronary arteries. When cardiac work increases, for example, during exercise, the obstruction to flow results in the accumulation of acidic metabolites

and ischemic changes that stimulate myocardial pain fibers. Rest usually leads to relief of the pain within 5 to 15 minutes. Atherosclerotic angina constitutes about 90% of angina cases.

Vasospastic angina is also known as rest angina, variant angina, or Prinzmetal's angina and accounts for less than 10% of cases. Vasospastic angina involves reversible spasm of large coronary arteries, usually at the site of an atherosclerotic plaque. Spasm may occur at any time, even during sleep. Vasospastic angina superimposed on atherosclerotic angina may deteriorate into **unstable angina,** also known as crescendo angina or acute coronary syndrome. This form of angina is characterized by increased frequency and severity of attacks that result from a combination of atherosclerotic plaques, platelet aggregation at fractured plaques, and vasospasm. Unstable angina is thought to be the immediate precursor of a myocardial infarction and is treated as a medical emergency.

THERAPEUTIC STRATEGIES

The defect that causes anginal pain is inadequate coronary oxygen delivery relative to the myocardial oxygen requirement. At present, this defect is corrected by either increasing oxygen delivery or by reducing the oxygen requirement (Figure 8–3).

Currently popular pharmacologic therapies include the nitrates, the calcium channel blockers, and the β-receptor antagonists. These drug classes all reduce the oxygen requirement in atherosclerotic angina.

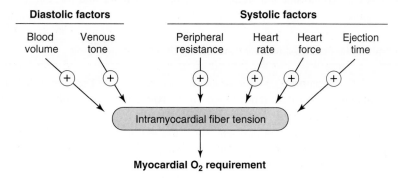

Figure 8–2. Determinants of the volume of oxygen required by the heart. Both diastolic and systolic factors contribute to the oxygen requirement; most of these factors are directly influenced by sympathetic discharge.

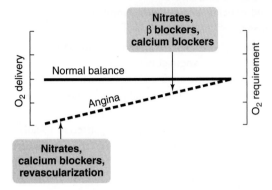

Figure 8–3. Strategies for the treatment of angina pectoris. Angina is characterized by reduced coronary oxygen delivery versus oxygen requirement. In some cases, this can be corrected by increasing oxygen delivery (**box on left:** revascularization or, in the case of reversible vasospasm, nitrates and calcium channel blockers). More often, drugs are used to reduce oxygen requirement (**box on right:** nitrates, β-receptor antagonists, and calcium channel blockers).

Nitrates and calcium channel blockers, but not β-receptor antagonists, can also increase oxygen delivery by reducing vasospasm, a useful effect only in vasospastic angina. Myocardial revascularization corrects coronary obstruction either by bypass grafting or by angioplasty (enlargement of the coronary lumen by means of a special catheter).

The therapy for unstable angina differs from that of exertional or vasospastic angina. Urgent angioplasty is the treatment of choice in most patients with unstable angina, and platelet clotting is the major target of drug therapy. The antithrombotics, **eptifibatide** and **tirofiban**, are used in this condition (Chapter 11). Intravenous nitroglycerin is sometimes of value.

Nitrates

The drugs of this pharmacologic class are sometimes referred to as "*organic nitrates.*" **Nitroglycerin** is the prototypical agent of this class and is the most important of the therapeutic nitrates. Nitroglycerin, also known as glyceryl trinitrate, is available in several forms (Table 8–1). Because treatment of acute attacks and prevention of attacks are both important aspects of therapy, the pharmacokinetics of these different dosage forms are clinically significant.

Glyceryl trinitrate is rapidly denitrated in the liver and in smooth muscle, first to glyceryl dinitrate and more slowly to glyceryl mononitrate. The dinitrate retains a significant vasodilating effect; the mononitrate is much less active. Because of the high enzyme activity in the liver, the first-pass effect for nitroglycerin is large—about 90%. The efficacy of swallowed nitroglycerin probably results from the high levels of glyceryl dinitrate in the blood. The effects of sublingual nitroglycerin are mainly the result of the unchanged drug because this route avoids the first-pass effect (Chapter 3). Other nitrates are similar to nitroglycerin in their pharmacokinetics and pharmacodynamics. **Isosorbide dinitrate** is another commonly used nitrate, and is available in sublingual and oral forms. Isosorbide dinitrate is rapidly denitrated in the liver and smooth muscle to isosorbide mononitrate, which is also active. **Isosorbide mononitrate** is available as a separate drug for oral use. Several other nitrates are

Table 8–1.	Pharmacokinetically distinct forms of nitrate drugs used in angina	
Category	**Example**	**Duration of Action**
Short	Sublingual nitroglycerin or isosorbide dinitrate	10–30 min (isosorbide dinitrate has a somewhat longer half-life than nitroglycerin)
Intermediate	Oral regular or sustained-release nitroglycerin or isosorbide dinitrate or mononitrate	4–8 h (much of the effect is due to active metabolites)
Long	Transdermal nitroglycerin patch	8–10 h (blood levels may persist for 24 h, but tolerance limits the duration of action)

available for oral use and, like the oral nitroglycerin preparation, have an intermediate duration of action of 4 to 6 hours. Parenteral passive transdermal delivery is also available. Patches or ointment containing nitroglycerin provide maintenance therapy by providing consistent blood levels for hours at a time.

Denitration of the nitrates within smooth muscle cells releases *nitric oxide* (NO), which stimulates guanylyl cyclase. Increased guanylyl cyclase activity increases the second messenger cyclic guanosine monophosphate (cGMP) and leads to smooth muscle relaxation by dephosphorylation of myosin light chain phosphate (Figure 8–4). This mechanism is identical to that of the direct-acting vasodilator nitroprusside (Chapter 7).

Physiologic Effect. The main beneficial effects of these drugs in the treatment of angina are on the cardiovascular system (Table 8–2); however, additional effects in other tissues are also observed. In the cardiovascular system, smooth muscle relaxation leads to peripheral venodilation, which results in reduced cardiac size and cardiac output through reduced preload. Reduced afterload, from arteriolar dilation, may contribute to an increase in ejection volume and a further decrease in cardiac size. The veins are the most sensitive to the action of nitrates, arteries less so, and arterioles are least sensitive. Venodilation leads to a decrease in venous return to the heart (preload) and subsequent reduction of intracardiac volume during diastole. The decrease in diastolic dilation reduces myocardial fiber tension. This

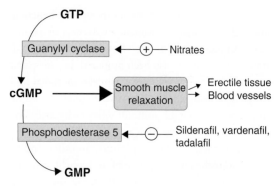

Figure 8–4. Mechanism of vasodilation by nitrates and drugs used in erectile dysfunction. Nitrate-stimulated guanylyl cyclase activity increases cyclic guanosine monophosphate (cGMP) resulting in smooth muscle relaxation and vasodilation. Sildenafil and similar drugs used in erectile dysfunction inhibit a phosphodiesterase isoform (PDE-5) that metabolizes cGMP in smooth muscle of the corpora cavernosa. The increased cGMP relaxes the erectile smooth muscle, allowing for greater inflow of blood and a more effective and prolonged erection. This effect also occurs to a lesser extent in the smooth muscle of other tissues, especially the vessels. Because nitrates and PDE-5 inhibitors both increase cGMP by complementary mechanisms, they can have a synergistic effect on decreasing blood pressure.

decrease in fiber tension reduces myocardial oxygen demand. Arteriolar dilation leads to reduced peripheral resistance and blood pressure. These changes contribute to an overall reduction in myocardial fiber tension, oxygen consumption, and the double product.

Table 8–2.	Beneficial and deleterious cardiovascular effects of nitrates in the treatment of angina

Effect	Result
Potential Beneficial Effects	
Decreased ventricular volume	Decreased myocardial oxygen requirement
Decreased arterial pressure	
Decreased ejection time	
Vasodilation of epicardial coronary arteries	Relief of coronary artery spasm
Increased collateral flow	Improved perfusion to ischemic myocardium
Decreased left ventricular diastolic pressure	Improved subendocardial perfusion
Potential Deleterious Effects	
Reflex tachycardia	Increased myocardial oxygen requirement
Reflex increase in contractility	
Decreased diastolic perfusion time due to tachycardia	Decreased myocardial perfusion

Thus, the primary mechanism for therapeutic benefit in atherosclerotic angina is reduction of the oxygen requirement. An increase in coronary flow via collateral vessels in ischemic areas has also been proposed. In vasospastic angina, a reversal of coronary spasm and increased flow can be demonstrated. Nitrates have no direct effects on cardiac muscle, but a significant reflex tachycardia and increased force of contraction are predictable when nitroglycerin reduces the blood pressure. In other organs, nitrates relax the smooth muscle of the bronchi, gastrointestinal tract, and genitourinary tract, but these effects are too small to be clinically useful. Intravenous nitroglycerin is sometimes used in unstable angina and has been demonstrated to reduce platelet aggregation. There are no significant effects on other tissues.

As previously stated, vasodilators used in hypertension such as **nitroprusside** and nitrates used in angina act by releasing nitric oxide. Nitroprusside and other drugs in this class are strong arteriolar vasodilators, in contrast to nitrates, which are relatively less effective dilators of arterioles. The more limited arteriolar vasodilation caused by nitrates ensures that excessive dilation will not occur in normal vessels to the detriment of flow through partially obstructed ones. Drugs such as nitroprusside would vasodilate both partially obstructed and normal coronary arterioles, and more so in the latter. Blood flow in the unobstructed arteriole then would increase disproportionately compared to the partially obstructed coronary arteriole, ultimately decreasing blood flow through the partially obstructed coronary arteriole and potentially exacerbating the tissue ischemia *(coronary steal)*. For this reason, drugs such as nitrates that act primarily on veins are very useful in angina because they demonstrate minimal coronary steal.

Clinical Uses. As previously noted, nitroglycerin is available in several formulations (Table 8–1). The standard form for treatment of acute exertional anginal pain is the sublingual tablet, which has a duration of action of 10 to 20 minutes. Isosorbide dinitrate is similar or slightly longer in duration of action. Swallowed normal-release nitroglycerin has a duration of action of 4 to 6 hours. Sustained-release oral forms have a somewhat longer duration of action. Transdermal formulations, in ointment or patch, can maintain blood levels for up to 24 hours. Tolerance develops after 8 to 10 hours, however, with rapidly diminishing effectiveness thereafter. Therefore, conventional medical practice is to recommend that nitroglycerin patches be removed after 10 to 12 hours to allow recovery of sensitivity to the drug.

Adverse Effects. The most common adverse effects of nitrates are the responses evoked by vasodilation (Table 8–2). These include tachycardia from the baroreceptor reflex, orthostatic hypotension as a direct extension of the venodilator effect, and throbbing headache from meningeal artery vasodilation. Nitrates interact with sildenafil and similar drugs promoted for erectile dysfunction. Both classes of drugs increase cGMP in vascular smooth muscle causing a synergistic relaxation of vascular smooth muscle with potentially dangerous hypotension and hypoperfusion of critical organs (Figure 8–4).

β-Receptor Antagonists

These drugs are described in detail in Chapter 6. All β-receptor antagonists are effective in the prophylaxis of atherosclerotic angina attacks.

Physiologic Effects. Beneficial effects include decreases in heart rate, cardiac contractility, and blood pressure. Like the nitrates and calcium channel blockers, the β-receptor antagonists reduce the double product.

Clinical Use. β-receptor antagonists are used only for prophylactic therapy of angina, but are extremely important in this application. They are of no value in an acute attack. These drugs are effective in preventing exertional angina, but are ineffective against the vasospastic form. The combination of β-receptor antagonists with nitrates is useful in the treatment of angina because the adverse compensatory effects discussed below are minimized.

Adverse Effects. Adverse cardiac effects caused by β-receptor antagonists include increased end diastolic pressure and increased ejection time. For additional adverse effects, see Chapter 6.

Calcium Channel Blockers

These drugs were discussed in the treatment of hypertension (Chapter 7). Several of the calcium channel blockers are approved for use in angina (Table 8–3). These drugs may be divided into two main classes: dihydropyridines and miscellaneous agents. **Nifedipine** is the prototypical dihydropyridine, whereas **diltiazem** and **verapamil** are familiar examples of the miscellaneous class. Although calcium channel blockers differ markedly in structure, all are orally active and most have half-lives of 3 to 6 hours.

These drugs block voltage-gated L-type calcium channels, which are the calcium channels most important in cardiac and smooth muscle. These agents decrease calcium influx during action potentials in a frequency- and voltage-dependent manner. As a result of the reduced intracellular calcium, cardiac and vascular smooth muscle contractility is decreased. None of these L-type channel blockers interfere with calcium-dependent neurotransmission or hormone release because those processes do not utilize L-type channels.

Physiologic Effects. Calcium channel blockers decrease cardiac contractility, relax blood vessels, and, to a lesser extent, relax the uterus, bronchi, and gut. The physiologic response to these drugs varies with the specific agent (Table 8–3). Diltiazem and verapamil have a greater inhibitory effect on cardiac rate and contraction compared to their vasodilatory effect. Because they block calcium-dependent conduction in the atrioventricular (AV) node, verapamil and diltiazem may be used to treat AV nodal arrhythmias (Chapter 10). Nifedipine and other dihydropyridines evoke greater vasodilation, and the resulting sympathetic reflex prevents bradycardia and may actually increase the heart rate. All the calcium channel blockers reduce blood pressure and reduce the double product in patients with angina.

Clinical Use. Calcium channel blockers are effective as prophylactic therapy in both exertional and vasospastic angina. Nifedipine has also been used to abort acute anginal attacks. In atherosclerotic angina, these drugs are particularly valuable when combined with nitrates. In addition to well-established uses in angina, hypertension, and supraventricular tachycardia, some of these agents are used in the treatment of migraine headaches, preterm labor, and Raynaud's phenomenon

Table 8–3.	Clinical indications and toxicities of some calcium channel blocking drugs	
Drug	**Indications**	**Adverse Effects**
Dihydropyridines		
Amlodipine	Angina, hypertension	Headache, peripheral edema
Felodipine	Hypertension, Raynaud's phenomenon, congestive heart failure	Dizziness, headache
Isradipine	Hypertension	Headache, fatigue
Nicardipine	Angina, hypertension, congestive heart failure	Peripheral edema, dizziness, headache, flushing
Nifedipine	Angina, hypertension, migraine, cardiomyopathy, Raynaud's phenomenon	Hypotension, dizziness, flushing, nausea, constipation, dependent edema
Nimodipine	Subarachnoid hemorrhage, migraine	Headache
Nisoldipine	Hypertension	Probably similar to nifedipine
Nitrendipine	Investigational for angina, hypertension	Probably similar to nifedipine
Miscellaneous		
Diltiazem	Angina, hypertension, Raynaud's phenomenon	Hypotension, dizziness, flushing, bradycardia
Verapamil	Angina, hypertension, arrhythmias, migraine, cardiomyopathy	Hypotension, myocardial depression, constipation, dependent edema

(Table 8–3). Finally, **nimodipine,** another dihydropyridine, is approved only for the management of stroke associated with subarachnoid hemorrhage.

Adverse Events. A summary of the adverse events related to calcium channel blockers when used alone is presented in Table 8–3. These drugs cause constipation, pretibial edema, nausea, flushing, and dizziness. More serious adverse effects include heart failure, atrioventricular blockade, and sinoatrial node depression; these are more common with verapamil than with the dihydropyridines.

COMBINING ANTIANGINAL AGENTS

A summary of the beneficial effects compared to the adverse effects of nitrates, calcium channel blockers, or β-receptor antagonists used alone, or in combination with each other, is presented in Table 8–4. Each drug class used alone has some undesirable effects. These adverse effects are mitigated when used in combination. Thus, the combined use of nitrates with calcium channel blockers or β-receptor antagonists enhances their clinical benefits by decreasing net myocardial oxygen requirement, and minimizes adverse events.

NONPHARMACOLOGIC THERAPY

Myocardial revascularization can be achieved by *coronary artery bypass grafting* (CABG) or *percutaneous*
coronary intervention (PCI). The latter procedure includes both *percutaneous transluminal coronary angioplasty* (PTCA) to dilate the vessel and the placement of an intraluminal stent to maintain the patency. These procedures are extremely important in the treatment of severe angina. They are the only methods capable of consistently increasing coronary flow in atherosclerotic angina and increasing the double product.

REHABILITATION FOCUS

Exercise is a well-recognized component of cardiac rehabilitation following a myocardial infarction. Such exercise programs yield physical, psychological, and financial benefits to the patient. Additionally, a regular moderate exercise program also appears to reduce the potential for subsequent myocardial infarction, and may do so at a reduced financial cost to the patient and the health-care system. Such exercise programs are not limited to use of the treadmill, but may also utilize upper body activities or functional activities related to returning to work in order to achieve the same goal. These programs are currently being safely supervised by physical therapists. Therefore, therapists require an understanding of the potential benefits and liabilities of antianginal drug effects

Table 8–4.	Effects of nitrates alone and with β blockers or calcium channel blockers in angina pectoris		
	Nitrates Alone	**β Blockers or Calcium Blockers Alone**	**Combined Nitrate and β Blocker or Calcium Blocker**
Heart rate	*Reflex increase*	**Decrease**	**Decrease**
Arterial pressure	Decrease	**Decrease**	**Decrease**
End-diastolic pressure	**Decrease**	*Increase*	**Decrease**
Contractility	*Reflex increase*	**Decrease**	No effect or **decrease**
Ejection time	Reflex decrease	*Increase*	No effect
Net myocardial oxygen requirement	**Decrease**	**Decrease**	**Decrease**

Undesirable effects that increase myocardial oxygen requirement are shown in *italics;* major therapeutic effects are shown in **bold and underlined**.

during periods of increased functional activity or exercise.

Patients may experience angina as the sole manifestation or as a component of a larger cardiovascular pathophysiologic presentation. To prevent or reduce angina, antianginal drugs are prescribed. Physical therapists must take into account the antianginal drugs being taken by patients during assessments and treatments. The therapist must know whether the drug is being taken prophylactically or on an as-needed basis by the patient. In the former case, the therapist must affirm that the patient has taken the drug regularly prior to participating in the rehabilitation activity. In the latter case, the therapist must affirm that the patient has the drug at hand during the assessment or treatment time because it may be needed. Many activities in rehabilitation can increase sympathetic stimulation of the heart, resulting in an anginal attack. Therapists recognize that exercise or functional and strength conditioning can increase the incidence of anginal attacks; in addition, activities such as painful wound treatment or apprehension at ambulation following a stroke or orthopedic surgery can also induce such an attack.

Finally, the therapist should remember that not all antianginal drugs enhance exercise tolerance in patients. Passive nitroglycerin may benefit the patient during functional activity. In contrast, β-receptor antagonists may reduce bronchodilation or cause bronchoconstriction and adversely affect cardiac responses to exercise. Calcium channel blockers and nitrates may induce orthostatic hypotension.

◼ CLINICAL RELEVANCE FOR REHABILITATION

Adverse Drug Reactions

Many of the drugs clinically used for angina pectoris are also used in the treatment of hypertension and the adverse effects are similar to those discussed in Chapter 7.

- Orthostatic hypotension is a common problem with several classes of antianginal drugs.
- Bronchoconstriction is a problem with the β-receptor antagonists.

- Beta-receptor antagonists blunt the early manifestations of hypoglycemia.
- Several antianginal drugs depress cardiac rate.
- Several antianginal drugs depress cardiac contractility.
- Nitrates cause reflex tachycardia.

Effects Interfering with Rehabilitation

- Orthostatic hypotension may cause patients to faint when transferring from a sitting or supine position to standing, exiting from a warm aquatherapy area, or if aerobic exercise is terminated without an appropriate cool-down period.
- Dyspnea may limit the aerobic capacity of patients.
- Cardiac output may be depressed by these drugs, further limiting aerobic activities.
- Manifestations of hypoglycemia occurring during aerobic activities may be diminished in patients taking β-receptor antagonists.
- Heart rate cannot be used as a marker of exertion for patients taking β-receptor antagonists.

Possible Therapy Solutions

- Check blood pressure and heart rate prior to and following aerobic activities.
- Monitor heart rate during aerobic activities.
- Have patients check glucose levels prior to aerobic activities if the patients are taking hypoglycemic drugs.
- To prevent fainting associated with orthostatic hypotension, assist patients with positional changes and when exiting a warm pool. Always provide a cool-down period following a period of exercise.
- Allow increased time to complete aerobic tasks to prevent dyspnea.
- Use perceived exertion (Borg Rating of Perceived Exertion Scale) when determining aerobic activity in patients being treated with β-receptor antagonists.

Potentiation of Functional Outcomes Secondary to Drug Therapy

- Patients with exertional angina may experience chest pain prior to aerobic activities or painful treatments such as wound debridement. Administration of drugs such as nitrates prior to the activity can help prevent chest pain.

PROBLEM-ORIENTED PATIENT STUDY

Brief History: The patient is a 52-year-old male with a 14-year history of hypertension and coronary artery disease, and is a union pipe fitter employed at a private shipyard. Job description includes climbing on scaffolding for activities performed in the process of ship construction. Three days ago, while at his job, the patient fell 8 feet off a platform, striking a raised object with the right leg in the area of the thigh. The impact resulted in a compound fracture to the right femur. Other relevant history includes moderate alcohol intake, 25 plus year history of smoking one-half pack of cigarettes a day, and a body mass index of 28.

Current Medical Status and Drug Therapy: The compound fracture of the femur was reduced with internal fixation by means of a medullary rod during orthopedic surgery 2 days ago. The patient was listed as stable following surgery. The chart states initial evaluation of upper body strength and trunk control unremarkable and patient is independent in transfer from bed to chair. Evaluation of patient was carried out in his room during the previous day prior to scheduling for rehabilitation in the acute care facilities gym today. Patient is scheduled today for ambulation assessment in parallel bars prior to determination and training for the type of ambulation assistive device required. The most recent blood pressure listed in the chart was 135/88 mm Hg, and heart rate was 60 bpm at rest. The current drugs include metoprolol, hydrochlorothiazide, and quinapril for chronic treatment of hypertension and additional drugs for pain control. The patient is also prescribed sublingual nitroglycerin as needed.

Rehabilitation Setting: The patient arrives in rehabilitation at 11:00 in a wheelchair. The patient expresses apprehension about standing and attempting to walk due to fear of excessive pain. The physical therapist convinces the patient to attempt standing in the parallel bars with use of a gait belt and two assistants. The patient stands with both hands on the parallel bars for assistance in rising. Prior to taking his first step, the patient begins to complain of chest pain on the left side and radiating down the left arm. The patient is quickly seated again, and the following vital signs recorded: blood pressure is 145/92 mm Hg, heart rate is 78 bpm and regular, and diaphoresis and paleness were also noted. A decision is made to return the patient to his room, and to inform the nursing staff of the changes in his status. The patient declines an afternoon session when contacted on the same day.

Problem/Clinical Options: Upon rising, the patient probably experienced pain due to the right femur injury. This resulted in increased sympathetic discharge to the heart. The combined increase in pain-associated sympathetic discharge and exertional activity of rising from the chair resulted in increased cardiac oxygen demand and ischemia. This increased oxygen demand clinically manifested as exertional angina. To minimize a recurrence of this exertional angina at the next scheduled session, the therapist should recommend to the nursing staff that sublingual nitroglycerin be given to the patient to carry with him to the session. The patient could then take the drug 5 to 10 minutes prior to beginning the exertion. The therapist should remember that a maximum of three nitroglycerin tablets may be taken at no longer than 5-minute intervals if pain occurs. If three tablets do not relieve the pain, medical evaluation for possible myocardial infarction is advisable.

PREPARATIONS AVAILABLE

Nitrates and Nitrites

Isosorbide dinitrate (generic, Isordil, Sorbitrate)
Oral: 5-, 10-, 20-, 30-, 40-mg tablets; 5-, 10-mg chewable tablets
Oral sustained-release (generic, Sorbitrate SA, Iso-Bid): 40-mg tablets and capsules
Sublingual: 2.5-, 5-, 10-mg sublingual tablets

Isosorbide mononitrate (Ismo, others)
Oral: 10-, 20-mg tablets; extended-release 30-, 60-, 120-mg tablets

Nitroglycerin
Sublingual: 0.3-, 0.4-, 0.6-mg tablets; 0.4 mg/metered dose aerosol
Oral sustained-release (generic, Nitrong): 2.6-, 6.5-, 9-mg tablets; 2.5-, 6.5-, 9-, 13-mg capsules

Buccal (Nitrogard): 2-, 3-mg buccal tablets
Parenteral (Nitro-Bid IV, Tridil, generic): 0.5, 5 mg/mL for IV administration
Transdermal patches (Minitran, Nitro-Dur, Transderm-Nitro): to release at rates of 0.1, 0.2, 0.3, 0.4, 0.6, or 0.8 mg/h.
Topical ointment (generic, Nitrol): 20 mg/mL ointment (1 inch, or 25 mm, of ointment contains about 15 mg nitroglycerin)

Calcium Channels Blockers

See Chapter 7.

Beta Receptor Antagonists

See Chapter 6.

REFERENCES

Braunwald E, et al: ACC/AHA Guidelines for the management of patients with unstable angina and non-ST-segment elevation myocardial infarction: Executive summary and recommendations. A Report of the American College of Cardiology/American Heart Association Task Force on Practice Guidelines (Committee on the Management of Patients with Unstable Angina). *Circulation* 2000;102:1193.

Braunwald E, et al: ACC/AHA Guideline update for the management of patients with unstable angina and non-ST-segment elevation myocardial infarction—2002. *Circulation* 2002;106:1893.

Gibbons RJ, et al: ACC/AHA/ACP-ASIM guidelines for the management of patients with chronic stable angina: Executive summary and recommendations. A Report of the American College of Cardiology/American Heart Association Task Force on Practice Guidelines (Committee on Management of Patients with Chronic Stable Angina). *J Am Coll Cardiol* 1999;33:2829.

Gibbons RJ, et al: ACC/AHA 2002 guideline update for the management of patients with chronic stable angina—summary article. *J Am Coll Cardiol* 2003;41:159.

Kawanishi DT, et al: Response of angina and ischemia to long-term treatment in patients with chronic stable angina: A double blind randomized individualized dosing trial of nifedipine, propranolol, and their combination. *J Am Coll Cardiol* 1992;19:409.

Yusuf S, et al: Effects of an angiotensin-converting enzyme inhibitor, ramipril, on cardiovascular events in high-risk patients. The Heart Outcomes Prevention Evaluation Study Investigators. *N Engl J Med* 2000;342:145.

Rehabilitation

Abete P, et al: High level of physical activity preserves the cardioprotective effect of preinfarction angina in elderly patients. *J Am Coll Cardiol* 2001;38:1357.

Acker J Jr, Martin D: Angina and ST-segment depression during treadmill and arm ergometer testing in patients with coronary artery disease. *Phys Ther* 1988;68:195.

Basu SK, Kinsey CD, Miller AJ, Lahiri A: Improved efficacy and safety of controlled-release diltiazem compared to nifedipine may be related to its negative chronotropic effect. *Am J Ther* 2000;7:17.

Ehsani AA: Cardiac rehabilitation. *Cardiol Clin* 1984;2:63.

Hambrecht R, et al: Percutaneous coronary angioplasty compared with exercise training in patients with stable coronary artery disease: a randomized trial. *Circulation* 2004;109:1371.

Mahmarian JJ, et al: Transdermal nitroglycerin patch therapy reduces the extent of exercise-induced myocardial ischemia: Results of a double-blind, placebo-controlled trial using quantitative thallium-201 tomography. *J Am Coll Cardiol* 1994;24:25.

Rigotti NA, Thomas GS, Leaf A: Exercise and coronary heart disease. *Annu Rev Med* 1983;34:391.

Vongvanich P, Paul-Labrador MJ, Merz CN: Safety of medically supervised exercise in a cardiac rehabilitation center. *Am J Cardiol* 1996;77:1383.

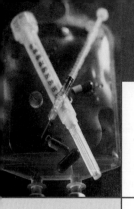

9

DRUGS USED IN HEART FAILURE

Heart failure occurs when the cardiac output is inadequate to provide the oxygen needed by the body. Heart failure is a highly lethal condition, with a 5-year mortality rate conventionally said to be about 50%. In systolic failure, cardiac contractility and the ejection fraction of the heart are reduced. In diastolic failure, stiffening and loss of adequate relaxation plays a major role in reducing cardiac output, although the ejection fraction may be normal. Because other cardiovascular conditions such as myocardial infarction are now being treated more effectively, more patients are surviving long enough to develop heart failure. Thus, heart failure is increasing in prevalence. Although research suggests that the primary defect in early heart failure resides in the excitation-contraction coupling machinery of the heart, the clinical condition also involves many other processes and organs, including the baroreceptor reflex, the sympathetic nervous system, the kidneys, angiotensin II and other peptides, and death of cardiac cells. The most common cause of heart failure in the United States is coronary artery disease.

This chapter reviews normal cardiac contractility and the pathophysiology and major clinical manifestations of heart failure. Drugs used to treat heart failure include positive inotropic agents, vasodilators, diuretics, and several miscellaneous drug classes (Figure 9–1). The positive inotropic agents increase the contractility of the heart, whereas the vasodilators and miscellaneous drugs have effects at both cardiac and noncardiac sites. Several drugs acting at noncardiac sites, such as the vasculature, kidneys, and central nervous system, have been discussed in Chapters 6 through 8.

CONTROL OF NORMAL CARDIAC CONTRACTILITY

The force of contraction of heart muscle is determined by several processes that lead to the movement of actin and myosin filaments in the cardiac sarcomere (Figure 9–2). During systole, contraction results from the interaction of calcium with the actin-troponin-tropomyosin system, thereby releasing the actin-myosin interaction from inhibition. The calcium involved in this interaction is released from the *sarcoplasmic reticulum* (SR). The amount released depends on the amount stored in the SR and on the amount of trigger calcium that enters the cell during the action potential.

Several factors related to intracellular calcium physiology have been proposed as key components for cardiac contractility and potential sites for pharmacologic manipulation. The first factor is sensitivity of the contractile proteins to calcium (Figure 9–2, Site 6). Increased sensitivity of these proteins to calcium improves cardiac contractility; however, the determinants of calcium sensitivity—the curve relating the shortening of cardiac myofibrils to the cytoplasmic

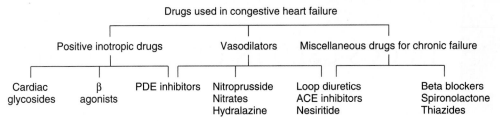

Figure 9–1. Drugs used in the treatment of heart failure. Several pharmacologic classes have a combination of physiologic effects and do not fall into a single category. ACE = angiotensin-converting enzyme inhibitors; PDE = phosphodiesterase. Spironolactone is a potassium-sparing diuretic that inhibits the aldosterone receptor in the collecting tubules of the kidney and nonrenal tissue sites.

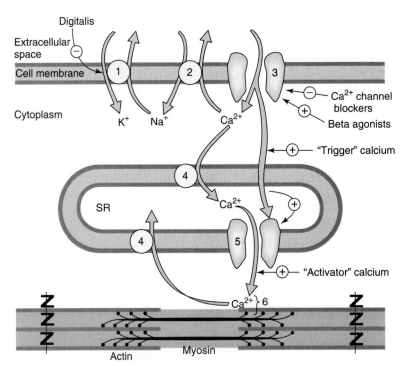

Figure 9–2. Schematic diagram of a cardiac muscle sarcomere, with the sites of action of several drug classes that alter contractility (numbered structures). Site 1 is Na+/K+–ATPase, the sodium pump. Site 2 is the Na-Ca2+ exchanger. Site 3 is the voltage-gated calcium channel. Site 4 is a calcium transporter that pumps calcium into the sarcoplasmic reticulum (SR). Site 5 is a calcium channel in the membrane of the SR that is activated to release stored calcium by an influx of calcium that enters the cell through calcium channels; i.e., "trigger" calcium. Site 6 is the actin-troponin-tropomyosin complex at which "activator" calcium released from the sarcoplasmic reticulum brings about contractile interaction of actin and myosin.

calcium concentration—are incompletely understood. Next, increasing the amount of calcium stored and released from the SR improves cardiac contractility. The SR membrane contains a very efficient calcium uptake transporter (Figure 9–2, Site 4), which maintains free cytoplasmic calcium at very low levels during diastole by pumping calcium into the SR. The amount of calcium sequestered in the SR is determined in part by the amount available for transport into the SR. This in turn is dependent on the balance of calcium influx (Figure 9–2, Site 3), primarily through the voltage-gated membrane calcium channels, and calcium efflux, the amount removed from the cell primarily via the sodium-calcium exchanger (Figure 9–2, Site 2). The amount of calcium released from the sarcoplasmic reticulum (Figure 9–2, Site 5) is regulated in part by the calcium influx through the cell membrane at Site 3 in Figure 9–2. A small rise in free cytoplasmic calcium, brought about by calcium influx during the action potential, triggers the opening of calcium channels in the membrane of the SR, and results in the rapid release of a large amount of the ion into the cytoplasm in the vicinity of the actin-troponin-tropomyosin complex. The amount of calcium that enters the cell depends on the availability of L-type calcium channels and the duration of their opening. As described in Chapter 4, sympathetic stimulation of the heart increases calcium influx through an action on these L-type calcium channels.

The sodium-calcium exchanger uses the influx of extracellular sodium to move calcium against its concentration gradient from the cytoplasm to the extracellular space (Figure 9–2, Site 2). Under physiologic conditions, extracellular concentrations of these ions are much less labile than intracellular concentrations. The ability of the sodium-calcium exchanger to carry out this transport is thus strongly dependent on the intracellular concentrations of both calcium and sodium, especially sodium. By removing intracellular sodium, the Na^+/K^+ adenosine triphosphatase (ATPase) (Figure 9–2, Site 1) is the major determinant of sodium concentration in the cell. The sodium influx through voltage-gated channels, which occurs as a normal part of almost all cardiac action potentials, is another determinant. As described below, Na^+/K^+ ATPase appears to be the primary target of cardiac glycosides.

PATHOPHYSIOLOGY

The fundamental physiologic defect in heart failure is a decrease in cardiac contractility. Decreased contractility results in cardiac output that is inadequate to maintain homeostasis. This is best shown by the ventricular function curve, also known as the Frank-Starling curve (Figure 9–3). The ventricular function curve reflects some compensatory responses of the body and may also be used to demonstrate the response to drugs. As ventricular ejection decreases, the end-diastolic fiber length increases as shown by

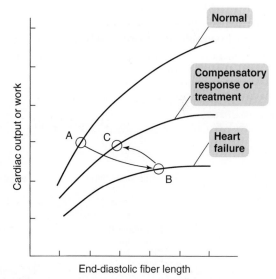

Figure 9–3. Ventricular function (Frank-Starling) curves. The abscissa can be any measure of preload-fiber length, filling pressure, or pulmonary capillary wedge pressure. The ordinate is a measure of useful external cardiac work, stroke volume, or cardiac output. In heart failure, output is reduced at all fiber lengths and the heart dilates because ejection fraction is decreased. As a result, the heart moves from point A to point B. Compensatory sympathetic discharge or effective clinical treatment allows the heart to eject more blood, and the heart moves to point C on the middle curve.

the shift from point A to point B in Figure 9–3. Operation at point B is intrinsically less efficient than operation at shorter fiber lengths because of the increase in myocardial oxygen requirement associated with increased fiber stretch (Figure 8–2).

The compensatory responses of the body to depressed cardiac output are extremely important and are mediated mainly by the sympathetic nervous system and the renin-angiotensin-aldosterone system. They are summarized in Figure 9–4. The major responses include tachycardia, increased preload and afterload, and cardiomegaly. Tachycardia is an early manifestation of heart failure and is the result of increased sympathetic tone. Increased peripheral vascular tone results in increased preload and afterload, and is another early response of heart failure mediated by increased sympathetic activity. The activation of the renin-angiotensin-aldosterone system results in retention of salt and water by the kidney. This is also an early compensatory response and is facilitated by increased sympathetic activity. Finally, cardiomegaly, enlargement of the heart, is a slower compensatory response and is mediated at least in part by sympathetic

activity. Angiotensin II also plays an important role in cardiomegaly, and may be directly responsible for these cardiac changes. Although these compensatory responses temporarily improve cardiac output, they also increase cardiac workload. Eventually, the increased load contributes to further long-term decline in cardiac function.

Heart failure presents with multiple clinical signs and symptoms. Patients may manifest varying degrees of impaired cardiac reserve and exercise tolerance. Tachycardia is usually present along with the potential for cardiac arrhythmias. Increased salt and water retention results in weight gain, edema in the lower extremities when in an upright position, and pulmonary congestion. The lower extremity edema manifests as pitting edema and patients' complaints of heavy feet. Pulmonary congestion results in exertional dyspnea, positional orthopnea, and paroxysmal nocturnal dyspnea. When these clinical signs of congestion are present, the pathophysiology is described as congestive heart failure.

Clinically, heart failure may be divided into chronic "compensated" heart failure and acute "decompensated" heart failure. Chronic heart failure is further subdivided

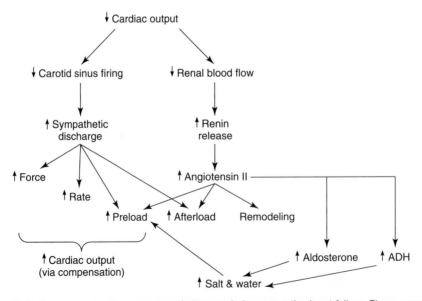

Figure 9–4. Some compensatory responses that occur during congestive heart failure. These responses play an important role in the progression of the disease. Responses include increased sympathetic activity and increases in renin-angiotensin-aldosterone and antidiuretic hormone (ADH).

into four classes according to a scale suggested by the New York Heart Association. Class I failure is associated with no limitations on ordinary activities and symptoms that occur only with greater than ordinary exercise. Class II is characterized by some limitation of ordinary activities, which results in fatigue and palpitations. Class III presents with no symptoms at rest, but fatigue and other clinical manifestations appear with less than ordinary physical activity. Class IV is associated with symptoms even when the patient is at rest. In contrast, acute heart failure manifests as the fairly rapid (hours to days) development of worsening peripheral edema, respiratory distress with exertion and later at rest, and diaphoresis and cyanosis; acute failure requires urgent medical intervention.

■ THERAPEUTIC STRATEGIES

Figure 9–1 presents the pharmacologic classes used in the treatment of acute and chronic heart failure. These drug classes include positive inotropic agents (cardiac glycosides, beta (β) agonists, and phosphodiesterase inhibitors), and vasodilators (nitrates and other direct vasodilators). Recent approval of nesiritide, a recombinant

Table 9–1.	Steps in the treatment of chronic heart failure

1. Reduce workload of the heart
   a. Limit activity level
   b. Reduce weight
   c. Control hypertension
2. Restrict sodium
3. Restrict water (rarely required)
4. Give diuretics
5. Give ACE inhibitors or angiotensin receptor antagonists
6. Give digitalis if systolic dysfunction with third heart sound or atrial fibrillation present
7. Give β-receptor antagonists to patients with stable class 2 to 4 heart failure
8. Give vasodilators

ACE = angiotensin-converting enzyme.

form of brain natriuretic peptide, has increased interest in the use of vasodilating and natriuretic peptides in heart failure. The miscellaneous drug category includes aldosterone receptor antagonists, angiotensin inhibitors, loop and thiazide diuretics, and β-receptor antagonists.

Diuretics have long been considered first-line therapy for heart failure. Cardiac glycosides (digitalis) were also part of the traditional regimen, but careful studies indicate that digitalis has been greatly overused. Clinical results have shown that angiotensin-converting enzyme inhibitors, β-receptor antagonists, and aldosterone receptor antagonists are the only agents in current use that actually prolong life in patients with chronic heart failure. A summary of the treatment algorithm used in the treatment of heart failure is presented in Table 9–1.

Pharmacologic therapies for heart failure include the removal of retained salt and water with diuretics, direct treatment of the depressed heart with positive inotropic drugs such as cardiac glycosides, reduction of preload and afterload with vasodilators, and reduction of afterload and retained salt and water by angiotensin inhibitors. In addition, considerable evidence suggests that angiotensin inhibitors diminish pathologic structural cardiac changes that often follow myocardial infarction and lead to failure. Current clinical evidence suggests that acute heart failure should be treated with a loop diuretic, a prompt-acting positive inotropic agent such as a β agonist or phosphodiesterase inhibitor, and vasodilators as required to optimize filling pressures and blood pressure. In contrast, evidence suggests that therapy directed at noncardiac targets may be more valuable in chronic heart failure than traditional drugs such as digitalis that focus on improving cardiac contractility. Thus, chronic failure is best treated with diuretics plus an angiotensin-converting enzyme (ACE) inhibitor and, if tolerated, a β-receptor antagonist. Positive inotropic drugs such as cardiac glycosides reduce symptoms in chronic failure if systolic dysfunction is prominent.

Positive Inotropic Agents

Cardiac Glycosides

The cardiac glycosides are often called "digitalis" because several come from the digitalis (foxglove) plant. **Digoxin** is the prototypic agent and the only one commonly used in the United States. A very similar molecule, digitoxin, which also comes from the foxglove, is no longer available in the United States. Inhibition of Na^+/K^+–ATPase of the cell membrane by digitalis is well documented and is considered to be the primary biochemical mechanism of action of digitalis (Figure 9–2, Site 1). Translation of this effect into an increase in cardiac contractility involves the Na^+/Ca^{2+} exchange mechanism (Figure 9–2, Site 2). Inhibition of Na^+/K^+–ATPase results in a small increase in intracellular sodium. The increased sodium alters the driving force for sodium-calcium exchange so that less calcium is removed from the cell. The increased intracellular calcium is stored in the sarcoplasmic reticulum (Figure 9–2, Site 4) and, upon release, (Figure 9–2, Site 5) increases contractile force (Figure 9–2, Site 6). Other mechanisms of action for digitalis have been proposed but these are probably not as important as the inhibition of ATPase. The consequences of Na^+/K^+–ATPase inhibition are seen in both the mechanical and the electrical

function of the heart. Digitalis also has a cardioselective parasympathomimetic effect. This action involves sensitization and increased firing of the baroreceptors resulting in decreased efferent sympathetic activity and increased vagal stimulation. Muscarinic transmission in atrial and atrioventricular (AV) nodal cells is also facilitated.

Physiologic Response. The cardiovascular response to digitalis is mediated by both the direct effect on cardiac cells and the indirect effect mediated through the parasympathetic system (Table 9–2). These effects are divided into mechanical and electrical effects. The mechanical effects include an increase in contractility resulting in increased ventricular ejection, decreased end-systolic and end-diastolic dilation, increased cardiac output, and increased renal perfusion. These beneficial effects permit a decrease in the compensatory sympathetic and renal responses previously described. The decrease in sympathetic tone is especially beneficial: reduced heart rate, preload, and afterload permit the heart to function more efficiently (Figure 9–3, point C).

Table 9–2.	Major actions of cardiac glycosides on cardiac electrical functions		
	Tissue		
Variable	**Atrial Muscle**	**AV Node**	**Purkinje System Ventricles**
Effective refractory period	↓ (PANS)[1]	↑ (PANS)	↓ (Direct) [2]
Conduction velocity	↑ (PANS)	↓ (PANS)	Negligible
Automaticity	↑ (Direct)	↑ (Direct)	↑ (Direct)
Electrocardiogram before arrhythmias	Negligible	↑ PR interval	↓ QT interval; T-wave inversion; ST-segment depression
Arrhythmias[3]	Atrial tachycardia; fibrillation	AV nodal tachycardia; AV blockade	Premature ventricular contractions; bigeminy, ventricular tachycardia, ventricular fibrillation

AV = atrioventricular.
[1]PANS = parasympathomimetic actions.
[2]Direct = direct membrane actions.
[3]Digitalis-induced arrhythmias are more likely in the presence of hypokalemia, hypomagnesemia, or hypercalcemia.

The electrical effects include early cardiac parasympathomimetic responses and later detrimental arrhythmogenic responses. An increased PR interval, caused by the decrease in AV conduction velocity, and flattening of the T wave are often seen. The effects on the atria and AV node are largely parasympathetic in origin. The increase in the AV nodal refractory period is particularly important when atrial flutter or fibrillation is present because the refractoriness of the AV node determines the ventricular rate in these arrhythmias. The effect of digitalis is to slow the ventricular rate. Shortened QT, inversion of the T, and ST depression may occur later.

Clinical Uses. Digitalis is the traditional positive inotropic agent used in the treatment of chronic heart failure. However, careful clinical studies indicate that while digitalis improves functional status by reducing symptoms, it does not prolong life. As discussed later, other agents such as diuretics, ACE inhibitors, and vasodilators may be equally effective and less toxic in some patients, and some of these alternative therapies do prolong life. In atrial flutter and fibrillation, reduction of the conduction velocity, or increasing the refractory period of the atrioventricular node, is desirable so that the ventricular rate is controlled at a level compatible with efficient filling and ejection. The parasympathomimetic action of digitalis often accomplishes this therapeutic objective, although high doses may be required. Alternative drugs for rate control include β-receptor antagonists and calcium channel blockers, but these drugs have negative inotropic effects. Because the half-lives of cardiac glycosides are long, the drugs accumulate significantly in the body, and dosing regimens must be carefully designed and monitored. The therapeutic and toxic concentrations are presented in Table 9–3.

Adverse Effects. Increased automaticity, caused by intracellular calcium overload, is the most important manifestation of toxicity. This increase in calcium results in delayed after-depolarizations, which may evoke extrasystoles, tachycardia, or fibrillation in any part of the heart. In the ventricles, the extrasystoles are recognized as *premature ventricular contractions* (PVCs). When PVCs are coupled to normal beats in a 1:1 fashion, the rhythm is called bigeminy. Cardiac glycosides also have significant drug interactions

Table 9–3.	Clinical use of digoxin
Digoxin Concentration	**Value[1]**
Therapeutic plasma concentration	0.5–1.5 ng/mL
Toxic plasma concentration	>2 ng/mL

[1]These values are appropriate for adults with normal renal and hepatic function.

which, when combined with its narrow therapeutic window, often result in adverse events. Quinidine causes a well-documented reduction in digoxin clearance and can increase the serum digoxin level if digoxin dosage is not adjusted. Digitalis effects are inhibited by extracellular potassium and magnesium and facilitated by extracellular calcium. Loop diuretics and thiazides, often used in treating heart failure, may induce hypokalemia and hypomagnesemia, and thus precipitate digitalis toxicity. Digitalis-induced vomiting may induce hypomagnesemia and similarly facilitate toxicity. These ion interactions are important in treating digitalis toxicity. The major signs of digitalis toxicity are arrhythmias, nausea, vomiting, and diarrhea. Rarely, confusion or hallucinations and visual aberrations may occur. The treatment of digitalis arrhythmias is important because this manifestation of digitalis toxicity is common and dangerous. Chronic intoxication is characterized by increased automaticity and the arrhythmias noted in Table 9–2. Acute severe intoxication is caused by suicidal or accidental extreme overdose and results in cardiac depression leading to cardiac arrest rather than tachycardia or fibrillation.

β Agonists

Dobutamine and **dopamine** are useful in many cases of acute failure in which systolic function is markedly depressed. These agents stimulate cardiac β_1 adrenoreceptors and enhance calcium influx (Figure 9–2, Site 3). The increased calcium influx increases cardiac contractility with, in heart failure, minimal increase in heart rate. However, they are not appropriate for chronic failure because of tolerance and lack of oral efficacy. Manifestations of toxicity include significant arrhythmogenic effects and angina.

Phosphodiesterase Inhibitors

Inamrinone and **milrinone** are the major representatives of this infrequently used group. These drugs increase cyclic adenosine monophosphate (cAMP) by inhibiting its breakdown by phosphodiesterase, and cause an increase in cardiac intracellular calcium similar to that produced by β_1 adrenoceptor agonists (Figure 9–2, Site 3). Again, the increase in contractility occurs with, in heart failure, a minimal increase in heart rate. Phosphodiesterase inhibitors also cause vasodilation, which may be responsible for a major part of their beneficial effect. At sufficiently high concentrations, these agents may also increase the sensitivity of the contractile protein system to calcium (Figure 9–2, Site 6). These agents are used in the treatment of acute heart failure, and should not be used in chronic failure because they have been shown to increase morbidity and mortality. Manifestations of toxicity include nausea, vomiting, thrombocytopenia, hepatic and bone marrow toxicities, and arrhythmias.

Vasodilators

Vasodilators, including nitrate and other direct-acting drugs, were previously discussed in Chapters 7 and 8. Vasodilator therapy with **nitroprusside** or **nitroglycerin** is often used for acute severe heart failure with congestion. The use of these vasodilator drugs is based on the reduction in cardiac size and improved efficiency that can be realized with proper adjustment of venous return and reduction of resistance to ventricular ejection. Vasodilator therapy can be dramatically effective, especially in cases in which increased afterload is a major factor in causing the failure, such as in continuing hypertension in an individual who has just had a myocardial infarct. Chronic heart failure sometimes responds favorably to oral vasodilators such as **hydralazine** or **isosorbide dinitrate**, especially in African Americans.

Natriuretic Peptides

The atria and other tissues of mammals contain a family of peptides consisting of *atrial natriuretic peptide* (ANP), *brain natriuretic peptide* (BNP), and *C-type natriuretic peptide* (CNP). The release of both ANP

and BNP appears to be related to blood volume. ANP and BNP exhibit similar natriuretic, diuretic, and hypotensive activities. CNP has less natriuretic and diuretic activity than ANP and BNP, but is a potent vasodilator. The physiologic role of CNP is unclear. Several factors increase the release of ANP from the heart. These include atrial stretch, volume expansion, changing from the standing to the supine position, and exercise. In each case, the increase in ANP release is probably due to increased atrial stretch. Increased sympathetic stimulation (of α_{1A} adrenoceptors) and release of glucocorticoids and vasopressin also stimulate ANP release. Plasma ANP concentration increases in various pathologic states including heart failure, primary aldosteronism, chronic renal failure, and a syndrome of inappropriate antidiuretic hormone (SIADH) release. Natriuretic peptides participate in the physiologic regulation of sodium excretion and blood pressure. Administration of ANP to normal subjects produces prompt and marked increases in sodium excretion and urine flow. Secretion of renin, aldosterone, and vasopressin is inhibited by ANP. These changes may also increase sodium and water excretion. ANP decreases arterial blood pressure. This hypotensive action is due to vasodilation, resulting from relaxation of vascular smooth muscle via guanylyl cyclase activity. ANP also reduces sympathetic tone to the peripheral vasculature and antagonizes the vasoconstrictor action of angiotensin II and other vasoconstrictors. These actions may contribute to the hypotensive action of the peptide. Patients with heart failure have high plasma levels of ANP and BNP, which have emerged as diagnostic and prognostic markers in this condition. Plasma BNP concentration has been shown to be closely correlated with the New York Heart Association functional class of symptomatic heart failure. The clinical benefits of the recombinant BNP (**nesiritide**) appear mainly to be due to vasodilation, although its natriuretic effects may also contribute. Nesiritide is given by IV bolus or infusion for acute failure only. Excessive hypotension is the most common adverse effect, and renal damage is also of serious concern.

Miscellaneous Category

Loop, thiazide, and aldosterone antagonist diuretics, angiotensin inhibitors, and β-receptor antagonists have been discussed in Chapter 6 and 7. This discussion will focus on the clinical benefit of these medications in the treatment of heart failure. Diuretics are usually used in heart failure treatment before any other drugs are considered. **Furosemide,** a loop diuretic, is a very useful agent for immediate reduction of the pulmonary congestion and severe edema associated with acute heart failure or severe chronic failure. Thiazides, such as **hydrochlorothiazide,** are sometimes sufficient for mild chronic failure. Clinical studies suggest that **spironolactone** and **eplerenone,** which are both aldosterone antagonist diuretics, have significant long-term benefits in chronic failure. ACE inhibitors, such as **captopril,** have been shown to reduce morbidity and mortality in chronic heart failure. Although they have no direct positive inotropic action, these agents reduce aldosterone secretion, salt and water retention, and vascular resistance. They are now considered, along with diuretics, among the first-line drugs for chronic heart failure. The angiotensin receptor antagonists such as **losartan** appear to have the same benefits as ACE inhibitors, although experience with these newer drugs is not as extensive as with ACE inhibitors. Finally, certain β-receptor antagonists (**carvedilol, labetalol,** and **metoprolol**) have been shown in long-term studies to reduce progression of chronic heart failure. The benefit of these agents had long been recognized in patients with hypertrophic cardiomyopathy, but has now been shown to occur also in patients without cardiomyopathy. The β-receptor antagonists are not of value in acute failure and may be detrimental if systolic dysfunction is marked.

■ REHABILITATION FOCUS

Exercise programs for patients with congestive heart failure result in improved exertion tolerance, endurance, and improved quality of life. Effective formats for these programs may include hydrotherapy, aerobic activities, strengthening, or a combination of both strengthening and aerobic activities. Many exercise programs involving physical therapists are hospital based, although non-hospital-based programs are also safe and effective. The therapist should be aware of the interactions between the drugs, patients, and their exercise programs.

Drugs used to improve cardiac performance or decrease cardiac workload improve patient participation in these programs. However, prescription drug effects may result in adverse events previously discussed. Additional care should also be taken by therapists when aerobic activities such as hydrotherapy are combined with drugs that produce orthostatic hypotension. Finally, appropriate cool-down periods are required following aerobic activities in patients taking these drugs to prevent syncope due to peripheral distribution of blood.

■ CLINICAL RELEVANCE FOR REHABILITATION

Adverse Drug Reactions
- Cardiac glycosides can cause arrhythmias.
- Thiazide and loop diuretics can cause hypokalemia.
- Hypokalemia can exacerbate the toxic effects of cardiac glycosides.
- Drugs that cause hyperkalemia inhibit the effects of cardiac glycosides.
- Drugs that inhibit the renin-angiotensin-aldosterone system including aldosterone receptor antagonists can cause hyperkalemia.
- Bronchoconstriction is a problem with the β-receptor antagonists, especially in asthmatics.
- Beta-receptor antagonists blunt the early manifestations of hypoglycemia in diabetics.
- Beta-receptor antagonists can depress cardiac contractility.
- Beta-receptor antagonists can depress cardiac rate.
- Vasodilators and loop diuertics can cause orthostatic hypotension.
- Vasodilators can cause reflex tachycardia.

Effects Interfering with Rehabilitation
- Orthostatic hypotension may cause patients to faint when transferring from a sitting or supine position to standing, exiting from warm aquatherapy area, or if aerobic exercise is terminated without an appropriate cool-down period.
- Dyspnea may decrease the aerobic capacity of patients.
- Heart rate should not be used as a marker of exertion for patients taking β-receptor antagonists.

- Cardiac output may be depressed during aerobic activities.
- Manifestations of hypoglycemia occurring during aerobic activities may be delayed.
- Altered plasma potassium levels can cause paresthesia, decrease skeletal muscle function, and increase cramps.
- Aerobic activities may initiate cardiac arrhythmias.

Possible Therapy Solutions
- Check blood pressure and heart rate prior to and following aerobic activities.
- Monitor heart rate during aerobic activities.
- To prevent fainting associated with orthostatic hypotension, assist patients with positional changes and when exiting a warm pool. Always provide a cool-down period following a period of exercise.

- To prevent dyspnea and to account for depressed cardiac activity, allow increased time to complete aerobic tasks.
- Use perceived exertion (Borg Rating of Perceived Exertion Scale) when determining aerobic activity in patients being treated with β-receptor antagonists.
- Have patients check glucose levels prior to aerobic activities if the patients are taking hypoglycemic drugs.
- Note clinical manifestations of altered plasma potassium levels and determine if patients are prescribed medications which may alter these levels.

Potentiation of Functional Outcomes Secondary to Drug Therapy
- Effective therapy improves cardiac function and reserve in many patients with heart failure, allowing them to participate in aerobic activities associated with rehabilitation.

PROBLEM-ORIENTED PATIENT STUDY

Brief History: The patient is a 65-year-old male with a history of congestive heart failure resulting from long-standing cardiomyopathy. The patient has a history of coronary artery disease including a triple coronary artery bypass graft 5 years ago. The patient has a body mass index of 30 and a 40-year plus history of smoking cigarettes. The patient quit smoking 10 years ago.

Current Medical Status and Drug Therapy: The patient was hospitalized recently for orthopedic surgery involving a right total knee replacement. The patient spent 3 days in acute care followed by a transfer to a rehabilitation facility where he spent 5 days. The patient was discharged from the rehabilitation setting with minimal assistance and household ambulation in a quad-walker. Current drugs include nadolol, benazepril, furosemide, and spironolactone. Opiate analgesic medication is provided for as-needed pain relief.

Rehabilitation Setting: The patient was referred to the outpatient clinic to continue ambulation training and endurance and for re-evaluation of assistive devices. The patient was initially evaluated 2 days ago at the clinic. At that time, his vital signs were blood pressure 120/70 mm Hg and heart rate 68 beats per minute (bpm). The patient arrives today at 10:30 for his second appointment, ambulating with a quad-walker approximately 15 feet from the car into the general treatment area. The patient appears pale while seated prior to beginning ambulation training, but states that he has consistently been taking all drugs on a regular basis on the preceding days. His vital signs are 145/90 mm Hg and heart rate is 70 bpm. The physical therapist is concerned. Prior to beginning the ambulation training with a cane, while attaching the gait belt, the physical therapist notices 3+/5 pitting edema at the ankles. During this process that patient talks about the new barbecue

PROBLEM-ORIENTED PATIENT STUDY (*Continued*)

restaurant that recently opened, and that he had a barbecue platter with French fries and ice tea for dinner there last night. The patient is assisted to standing and begins ambulation with the cane for approximately 35 feet. The patient becomes extremely dyspneic with labored breathing and wheezing, lips appear cyanotic, and diaphoresis is noted about the head, neck, and hands. A chair is immediately brought, and the patient is assisted into seating. His vital signs are now 160/94 mm Hg for blood pressure and 86 bpm.

Problem/Clinical Options: The physical therapist should immediately contact the referring physician's office to determine whether the patient should be transferred to emergency facilities or to the office of the referring physician. This patient's medical history and current medical problems are extensive. Progression through prior ambulation

training was probably delayed because of the high body mass index, age, and congestive heart failure. The current adverse event at this rehabilitation treatment session was probably precipitated by the previous evening's activities. The dinner the previous evening included a significant amount of sodium and water, exceeding the diuretic's action, resulting in both systemic and pulmonary edema. Nadolol, a nonselective β-receptor antagonist, may have exacerbated the dyspnea by preventing bronchodilation. Although not documented, the patient probably suffers from chronic obstructive pulmonary disease due to the 40-year plus history of cigarette smoking. This comorbidity also exacerbated the dyspnea. Finally, the opiate drug for pain may have decreased respiratory drive. See Chapter 20 for additional information on these drugs.

PREPARATIONS AVAILABLE

Digitalis

Digoxin* (generic, Lanoxicaps, Lanoxin)
Oral: 0.125-, 0.25-mg tablets; 0.05-, 0.1-, 0.2-mg capsules*; 0.05 mg/mL elixir
Parenteral: 0.1, 0.25 mg/mL for injection

*Digoxin capsules (Lanoxicaps) have greater bioavailability than digoxin tablets.

Sympathomimetics Most Commonly Used in Congestive Heart Failure

Dobutamine (generic, Dobutrex)
Parenteral: 12.5 mg/mL for IV infusion

Dopamine (generic, Intropin)
Parenteral: 40, 80, 160 mg/mL for IV injection; 80, 160, 320 mg/dL in 5% dextrose for IV infusion

Angiotensin-Converting Enzyme Inhibitors Labeled for Use in Congestive Heart Failure

Captopril (generic, Capoten)
Oral: 12.5-, 25-, 50-, 100-mg tablets

Enalapril (Vasotec, Vasotec I.V.)
Oral: 2.5-, 5-, 10-, 20-mg tablets
Parenteral: 1.25 mg enalaprilat/mL

Fosinopril (Monopril)
Oral: 10-, 20-, 40-mg tablets

Lisinopril (Prinivil, Zestril)
Oral: 2.5-, 5-, 10-, 20-, 40-mg tablets

Quinapril (Accupril)
Oral: 5-, 10-, 20-, 40-mg tablets

Ramipril (Altace)
Oral: 1.25-, 2.5-, 5-, 10-mg capsules

Trandolapril (Mavik)
Oral: 1-, 2-, 5-mg tablets

Angiotensin Receptor Blockers

Candesartan (Atacand)
Oral: 4-, 8-, 16-, 32-mg tablets

Eprosartan (Teveten)
Oral: 400-, 800-mg tablets

Irbesartan (Avapro)
Oral: 75-, 150-, 300-mg tablets

Losartan (Cozaar)
Oral: 25-, 50-, 100-mg tablets

Olmesartan (Benicar)
Oral: 5-, 20-, 40-mg tablets

Telmisartan (Micardis)
Oral: 20-, 40-, 80-mg tablets

Valsartan (Diovan)
Oral: 40-, 80-, 160-, 320-mg tablets

β Blockers that Have Reduced Mortality in Heart Failure

Bisoprolol (Zebeta, unlabeled use)
Oral: 5-, 10-mg tablets

Carvedilol (Coreg)
Oral: 3.125-, 6.25-, 12.5-, 25-mg tablets

Metoprolol (Lopressor, Toprol XL)
Oral: 50-, 100-mg tablets; 25-, 50-, 100-, 200-mg extended-release tablets
Parenteral: 1 mg/mL for IV injection

Phosphodiesterase Inhibitors

Inamrinone (generic)
Parenteral: 5 mg/mL for IV injection

Milrinone (generic, Primacor)
Parenteral: 1 mg/mL for IV injection; 200 mcg/mL premixed for IV infusion

Natriuretic Peptide

Nesiritide (Natrecor)
Parenteral: 1.5 mg lyophilized reconstituted for IV bolus or infusion

Diuretics

See Chapter 7.

REFERENCES

Basic Pharmacology

Kelly RA, Smith TW: Recognition and management of digitalis toxicity. *Am J Cardiol* 1992;69:108G.

Post SR, Hammond HK, Insel PA: β-Adrenergic receptors and receptor signaling in heart failure. *Annu Rev Pharmacol Toxicol* 1999;39:343.

Zipes, D, et al (eds): *Braunwald's Heart Disease. A Textbook of Cardiovascular Medicine,* 7th ed. Philadelphia: Elsevier Saunders, 2005.

Pathophysiology of Heart Failure

McPhee SJ, Ganong WF: *Pathophysiology of disease. An Introduction to Clinical Medicine,* 5th ed. New York: McGraw-Hill, 2006.

Schrier RW, Abraham WT: Hormones and hemodynamics in heart failure. *N Engl J Med* 1999;341:577.

Acute Myocardial Infarction

Hennekens CH, et al: Adjunctive drug therapy of acute myocardial infarction: Evidence from clinical trials. *N Engl J Med* 1996;335:1660.

Ryan TJ, et al: 1999 Update ACC/AHA Guidelines for the management of acute myocardial infarction. *Circulation* 1999;100:1016.

Chronic Heart Failure

Cohn J, et al: A randomized trial of the angiotensin receptor blocker valsartan in heart failure. *N Engl J Med* 2002;345:1667.

CONSENSUS Trial Study Group: Effects of enalapril on mortality in severe congestive heart failure. *N Engl J Med* 1987;316:1429.

Digitalis Investigation Group: The effect of digoxin on mortality and morbidity in patients with heart failure. *N Engl J Med* 1997;336:525.

Foody JM, Farrell MH, Krumholtz H: Beta blocker therapy in heart failure. *JAMA* 2002;287:883.

Goodley E: Newer drug therapy for congestive heart failure. *Arch Intern Med* 1999;159:1177.

Klein L, et al: Pharmacologic therapy for patients with chronic heart failure and reduced systolic function: Review of trials and practical considerations. *Am J Cardiol* 2003;91(Suppl 9A):18F.

Mann DL, et al: New therapeutics for chronic heart failure. *Annu Rev Med* 2002;53:59.

Packer M, et al: The effect of carvedilol on morbidity and mortality in patients with chronic heart failure. *N Engl J Med* 1996; 334:334.

Pitt B, et al: The effect of spironolactone on morbidity and mortality in patients with severe heart failure. *N Engl J Med* 1999;341:709.

Natriuretic Peptides

Boomsma F, van den Meiracker AH: Plasma A- and B-type natriuretic peptides: Physiology, methodology and clinical use. *Cardiovasc Res* 2001;51:442.

Melo LG, Pang SC, Ackermann U: Atrial natriuretic peptide: Regulator of chronic arterial blood pressure. *News Physiol Sci* 2000;15:143.

Vesely DL: Atrial natriuretic peptides in pathophysiological diseases. *Cardiovasc Res* 2001;51:647.

Rehabilitation

Cider A, Schaufelberger M, Sunnerhagen KS, Andersson B: Hydrotherapy—a new approach to improve function in the older patient with chronic heart failure. *Eur J Heart Fail* 2003;5:527.

Coats AJ, et al: Effects of physical training in chronic heart failure. *Lancet* 1990;335:63.

Corvera-Tindel T, et al: Effects of a home walking exercise program on functional status and symptoms in heart failure. *Am Heart J* 2004;147:339.

DiBianco R, et al: Doxazosin for the treatment of chronic congestive heart failure: Results of a randomized double-blind and placebo-controlled study. *Am Heart J* 1991;121:372.

Oka RK, et al: Impact of a home-based walking and resistance training program on quality of life in patients with heart failure. *Am J Cardiol* 2000;85:365.

Pflugfelder PW, et al: Clinical consequences of angiotensin-converting enzyme inhibitor withdrawal in chronic heart failure: A double-blind, placebo-controlled study of quinapril. The Quinapril Heart Failure Trial Investigators. *J Am Coll Cardiol* 1993;22:1557.

Smart N, Marwick TH: Exercise training for patients with heart failure: A systematic review of factors that improve mortality and morbidity. *Am J Med* 2004;116:693.

Udelson JE, et al: Effects of amlodipine on exercise tolerance, quality of life, and left ventricular function in patients with heart failure from left ventricular systolic dysfunction. *Am Heart J* 2000; 139:503.

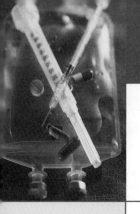

10

ANTIARRHYTHMIC DRUGS

Cardiac arrhythmias reduce cardiac output and commonly occur in the presence of pre-existing heart disease. They are the most common cause of death in patients who have had a myocardial infarction, and over 80% of patients with an acute myocardial infarction have arrhythmias. Cardiac arrhythmias also occur in up to 25% of patients treated with digitalis and in 50% of anesthetized patients. Patients with electrolyte imbalances also demonstrate arrhythmias, and diuretics are significant sources of such imbalances. Arrhythmias may require treatment because of rhythms that are too rapid, too slow, or asynchronous. Some arrhythmias may precipitate more serious or even lethal rhythm disturbances. For example, *premature ventricular contractions* (PVCs) can precipitate ventricular fibrillation, which is fatal unless corrected promptly. In such patients, antiarrhythmic drugs may be lifesaving. In contrast, pharmacologic treatment of asymptomatic or minimally symptomatic arrhythmias is avoided until clinically necessary because of the ability of many of these drugs themselves to induce lethal arrhythmias. In this chapter, we will review the conduction sequence and electrophysiology of normal cardiac rhythm, highlight the mechanisms of arrhythmias, and discuss the antiarrhythmic drugs used in their treatment.

The most widely used classification of antiarrhythmic drugs recognizes four classes (Figure 10–1) and is based on their mechanisms of action. These mechanisms are blockade of sodium channels (class I), blockade of cardiac β receptors (class II), blockade of potassium channels (class III), and blockade of calcium channels (class IV). A fifth group of miscellaneous antiarrhythmic drugs with no single mechanism of action is also recognized.

ELECTROPHYSIOLOGY OF NORMAL CARDIAC RHYTHM

Cardiac Electrical Conduction Pathway

The electrical impulse that triggers a normal cardiac contraction originates at regular intervals in the *sinoatrial* (SA) pacemaker node (Figure 10–2), usually at a frequency of 60 to 100 beats per minute. This impulse spreads rapidly through the atria and enters the *atrioventricular node* (AV), which is normally the only conduction pathway between the atria and ventricles. Conduction through the AV node is slow, requiring about 0.15 second. This delay provides time for atrial contraction to propel blood into the ventricles. The impulse then propagates over the His-Purkinje system and invades all parts of the ventricles. Ventricular activation is complete in less than 0.1 second; therefore, contraction of all of the ventricular muscle is synchronous and hemodynamically effective. A comparison of this cardiac electrical activity to the electrocardiogram is

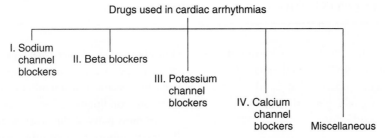

Figure 10–1. Classes of drugs used in the treatment of cardiac arrhythmias. They comprise four major classes and an additional miscellaneous group.

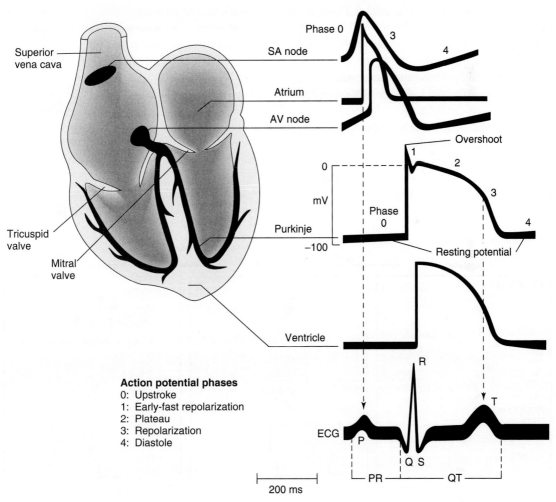

Action potential phases
0: Upstroke
1: Early-fast repolarization
2: Plateau
3: Repolarization
4: Diastole

Figure 10–2. Schematic representation of the heart and normal cardiac electrical activity (intracellular recordings from areas indicated and ECG). Sinoatrial node (SA), atrioventricular (AV) node, and Purkinje cells all display pacemaker activity (phase 4 depolarization). The ECG is the body surface manifestation of the depolarization and repolarization waves of the heart. The P wave is generated by atrial depolarization, the QRS by ventricular muscle depolarization, and the T wave by ventricular repolarization. Thus, the PR interval is a measure of conduction time from atrium to ventricle, and the QRS duration indicates the time required for all of the ventricular cells to be activated (i.e., the intraventricular conduction time). The QT interval reflects the duration of the ventricular action potential.

137

presented in Figure 10–2. Arrhythmias consist of cardiac depolarizations that deviate from the above description in one or more aspects; that is, there is an abnormality in the site of origin of the impulse, its rate or regularity, or its conduction.

Action Potentials in the Cardiac Cell

The transmembrane potential of cardiac cells is determined by the concentrations of *sodium* (Na^+), *potassium* (K^+), *calcium* (Ca^{2+}), and *chloride* (Cl^-) on either side of the membrane and the permeability of the membrane to each ion. These water-soluble ions are unable to diffuse freely across the lipid cell membrane in response to their electrical and concentration gradients; they require aqueous ion channels for such diffusion. Thus, ions move across cell membranes in response to their gradients only at specific times during the cardiac cycle when these ion channels are open. The movements of these ions produce currents that form the basis of the cardiac action potential. Individual channels are relatively ion selective, and the flux of ions through them is controlled by "gates" composed

of flexible peptide chains. Each type of ion channel has its own type of gate, and each type of gate is modulated by specific transmembrane voltage, ionic, or metabolic conditions.

In most parts of the heart, sodium channels are the most important determinant of conduction of the action potential (AP) and have been extensively characterized. From a functional point of view, it is convenient to describe the behavior of the sodium channel in terms of three functional states (Figure 10–3). The channel contains two gates, an *activation* (*m*) and inactivation (*h*) gate. At rest, the activation gate is closed, and the inactivation gate is open (Figure 10–3a). *Depolarization* to the threshold voltage results in opening of the activation gate (Figure 10–3b). The sodium influx is brief because the opening of the activation gate is soon followed by the closing of the inactivation gate (Figure 10–3c). Upon repolarization, recovery from inactivation (Figure 10–3c) takes place, making the sodium channels again available for excitation (Figure 10–3a). Most calcium channels are activated and inactivated in what

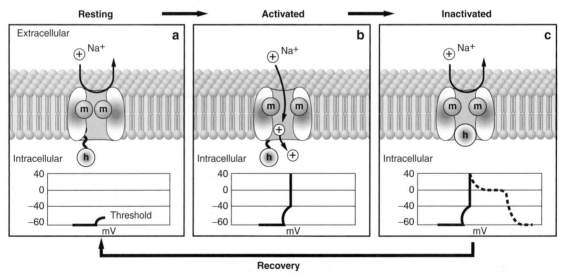

Figure 10–3. A schematic representation of Na^+ channels cycling through different conformational states during the cardiac action potential. Transitions between resting (a), activated (b), and inactivated (c) states are dependent on membrane potential and time. The activation gate is shown as (m) and the inactivation gate as (h). Potentials typical for each state are shown under each channel schematic as a function of time. The dashed line indicates that part of the action potential during which most Na^+ channels are completely or partially inactivated and unavailable for reactivation.

appears to be the same way as sodium channels, but in cardiac L-type calcium channels, the transitions occur more slowly and at more positive potentials than in sodium channels.

At rest, most cardiac cells are not significantly permeable to sodium, but at the start of each action potential, they become quite permeable. The cellular action potentials shown in Figure 10–2 are the result of ion fluxes through voltage-gated channels and carrier mechanisms. These processes are further diagrammed in Figure 10–4. In normal atrial, Purkinje, and ventricular cells, the action potential upstroke (phase 0) is dependent on sodium current (I_{Na}). After a very brief activation

of the *m* gate, the channel enters a more prolonged period of inactivation on account of the *h* gate closing. At the AV node, calcium current (I_{Ca}) dominates the phase 0 upstroke. The plateau of the AP (phases 1 and 2) is dominated by calcium current (I_{Ca}) and a potassium repolarizing current (I_K). At the end of the plateau, I_K causes rapid repolarization (phase 3). During the plateau of the action potential, most sodium channels are inactivated. The time between phase 0 and sufficient recovery of sodium channels in phase 3 to permit a new propagated response to external stimulus is the refractory period. Thus, the *effective refractory period* (ERP) of the cardiac cell is a function of how rapidly

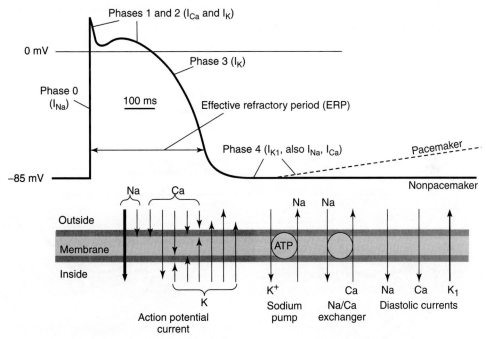

Figure 10–4. Components of the membrane action potential (AP) in a typical Purkinje or ventricular cardiac cell. The deflections of the AP, designated as phases 0 to 3, are generated by several ionic currents. The actions of the sodium pump and sodium–calcium exchanger are mainly involved in maintaining ionic steady state during repetitive activity. Note that small but significant currents occur during diastole (phase 4) in addition to the pump and exchanger activity. In nonpacemaker cells, the outward potassium current during phase 4 is sufficient to maintain a stable negative resting potential as shown by the solid line at the right end of the tracing. In pacemaker cells, however, the potassium current is smaller and the depolarizing currents (sodium, calcium, or both) during phase 4 are large enough to gradually depolarize the cell during diastole (*dashed line*). The phase 4 slope is increased by sympathetic stimulation and results in a positive chronotropic effect. With parasympathetic stimulation, the reverse effect occurs, resulting in a decrease in phase 4 slope and a negative chronotropic effect.

sodium channels recover from inactivation. The prolongation of this recovery time results in an increase in the ERP and is dependent upon the membrane potential, which varies with repolarization time and extracellular potassium concentration. A more positive resting membrane potential results in fewer sodium channels opening and a depressed sodium current. The carrier processes, such as the Na^+/K^+–ATPase pump and the sodium–calcium exchanger, contribute little to the shape of the AP; however, these membrane transporters are critical for the maintenance of the ion gradients on which the sodium, calcium, and potassium currents depend. Antiarrhythmic medications act on I_{Na}, I_{Ca}, or I_K, individually or in combination, or on the second-messenger systems that modulate these currents.

ARRHYTHMOGENIC MECHANISMS

Factors precipitating arrhythmias include ischemia, hypoxia, acidosis or alkalosis, electrolyte abnormalities, excessive catecholamine exposure, autonomic influences, toxicity due to digitalis or antiarrhythmic drugs, overstretching of cardiac fibers, and the presence of scarred or otherwise diseased cardiac tissue. All arrhythmias result from disturbances in impulse formation, disturbances in impulse conduction, or both.

Impulse formation in the SA pacemaker node can be accelerated by increasing phase 4 depolarization. This increase is caused by stimulation of cardiac β_1 receptors, positive *chronotropic* drugs, fiber stretch, acidosis, and partial depolarization by currents of injury. Vagal discharge and β-receptor antagonists slow the SA pacemaker node by decreasing the phase 4 depolarization. Latent pacemaker cells and normally quiescent atrial and ventricular cells can also demonstrate abnormal pacemaker activity under some pathophysiologic conditions such as ischemia, hypoxia, or hypokalemia.

Disturbances in conduction are the second major cause of cardiac arrhythmias. Severely depressed conduction may result in a simple block such as at the AV node. AV blockade is particularly significant because the AV node is normally the only conduction pathway between the atria and ventricles.

Another common abnormality of conduction is *reentry*, also known as circus movement (Figure 10–5). Here a single impulse reenters in a retrograde direction

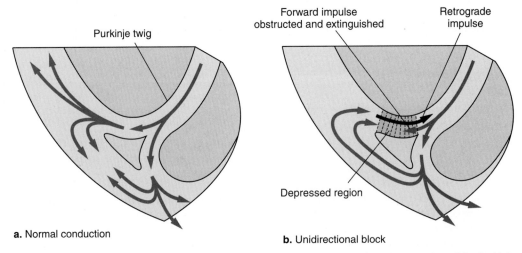

a. Normal conduction

b. Unidirectional block

Figure 10-5. Schematic diagram of a reentry circuit that might occur in small bifurcating branches of the Purkinje system where they enter the ventricular wall. (a) Normally, electrical excitation branches around the circuit are transmitted to the ventricular branches and become extinguished at the other end of the circuit due to collision of impulses. (b) An area of unidirectional block develops in one of the branches, preventing antegrade impulse transmission at the site of block, but the retrograde impulse may be propagated through the site of block if the impulse finds excitable tissue; that is, the refractory period is shorter than the conduction time. This impulse will then re-excite tissue it had previously passed through, and a reentry arrhythmia will be established.

and excites areas of the heart more than once. The path of the reentering impulse may be confined to very small areas. Alternatively, multiple reentry circuits, determined by the properties of the cardiac tissue, may meander through the heart in apparently random paths. Furthermore, the circulating impulse gives off "daughter impulses" that can spread to the rest of the heart. Depending on how many round trips through the pathway the impulse makes before dying out, the arrhythmia may be manifested as one or a few extra beats or as a sustained tachycardia. In order for reentry to occur, three conditions must coexist. First, there must be an anatomic or physiologic obstacle to conduction, thus establishing a circuit around which the reentrant wavefront can propagate. Second, there must be unidirectional block at some point in the circuit; that is, conduction must die out in one direction but continue in the opposite direction. Third, the conduction time around the circuit must be long enough so that the retrograde impulse does not enter the refractory tissue as it travels around the obstacle, that is, the conduction time must exceed the effective refractory period for the tissue. Under such conditions, as shown in Figure 10–5b, the normal impulse gradually decreases as it invades progressively more depolarized tissue and finally stops. Altering the refractory period, either by lengthening or shortening, may make reentry less likely. The longer the refractory period in tissues near the site of the block, the greater the chance that the tissues will still be refractory when reentry is attempted. Alternatively, the shorter the refractory period in the depressed region, the less likely it is that unidirectional block will occur. Several classes of antiarrhythmic drugs suppress arrhythmias by altering the refractory period in cardiac tissues where reentry occurs.

A few of the clinically important arrhythmias are *atrial flutter*, *atrial fibrillation* (AF), *AV nodal reentry* (a common type of *supraventricular tachycardia* [SVT]), *premature ventricular contractions* (PVCs), *ventricular tachycardia* (VT), and *ventricular fibrillation* (VF). Examples of electrocardiographic recordings of normal sinus rhythm and some of these common arrhythmias are shown in Figure 10–6. *Torsade de pointes* is a ventricular arrhythmia of great pharmacologic importance because it is often induced by antiarrhythmic drugs and

other drugs that prolong the QT interval. The electrocardiographic morphology is that of a polymorphic ventricular tachycardia, often displaying waxing and waning QRS amplitude. Torsade is also associated with long QT syndrome, a heritable abnormal prolongation of the QT interval caused by mutations in the I_K or I_{Na} channel molecules.

THERAPEUTIC STRATEGIES

Arrhythmias are caused by abnormal pacemaker activity or abnormal impulse propagation. Thus, the aim of therapy for arrhythmias is to reduce ectopic pacemaker activity and modify conduction or refractoriness in reentry circuits to disable circus movement. As previously stated, the major mechanisms are blockade of sodium channels (class I), blockade of cardiac β receptors (class II), blockade of potassium channels (class III), and blockade of calcium channels (class IV).

Antiarrhythmic drugs decrease the automaticity of ectopic pacemakers more than that of the SA node. They also reduce conduction and excitability and increase the refractory period to a greater extent in depolarized tissue than in normally polarized tissue. This is accomplished chiefly by selectively blocking the sodium or calcium channels of depolarized cells. Therapeutically useful channel-blocking agents have a high affinity for activated channels during phase 0, or inactivated channels during phases 2 and 3, but very low affinity for resting channels during phase 4. Therefore, these drugs block electrical activity when there is a fast tachycardia, where many channel activations and inactivations per unit time occur. These drugs also block electrical activity when there is significant loss of resting potential; many channels are inactivated during rest at less negative potentials. Thus, channels used frequently or those in an inactivated state are more susceptible to blockade than channels at rest at more negative potentials.

In cells with abnormal automaticity, most of these drugs reduce the phase 4 slope by blocking either sodium or calcium channels and thereby reducing the ratio of influx of positive ions compared to efflux of positive ions. This results in a slower phase 4 depolarization in susceptible cells. In addition, some agents may increase the threshold; that is, make it more positive.

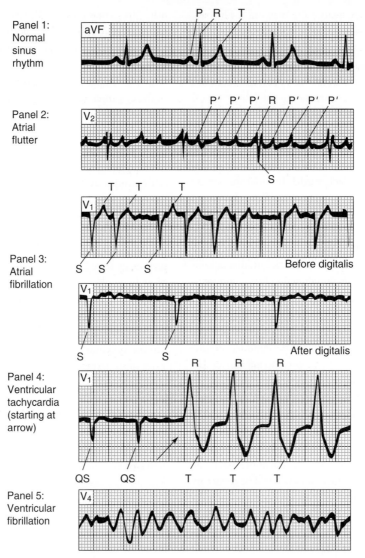

Figure 10-6. Typical ECGs of normal sinus rhythm and some common arrhythmias. Major waves (P, Q, R, S, and T) are labeled in each electrocardiographic record except in panel 5, in which electrical activity is completely disorganized and none of these deflections is recognizable.

In reentry arrhythmias, which depend on critically depressed antegrade conduction, most antiarrhythmic agents slow conduction further by one or both of two mechanisms. These agents may decrease the steady-state number of available unblocked channels, which reduces the excitatory currents to a level below that required for propagation. Alternatively, these drugs may prolong the recovery time of the channels still able to reach the rested and available state, which increases the ERP. As a result, early extrasystoles are unable to propagate at all; later impulses propagate more slowly and are subject to bidirectional conduction block.

By these mechanisms, antiarrhythmic drugs can suppress ectopic automaticity and abnormal conduction occurring in depolarized cells, rendering them electrically silent, while minimally affecting the electrical activity in normal repolarized parts of the heart. However, as dosage is increased, most of these agents also depress conduction in normal tissue, eventually resulting in drug-induced arrhythmias. Furthermore, a drug concentration that is antiarrhythmic under the initial circumstances of treatment may promote arrhythmias during tachycardia, acidosis, hyperkalemia, or ischemia.

Class I Antiarrhythmics (Local Anesthetics, [I_{NA}] Channel Blockers)

The class I drugs are further subdivided on the basis of their effects on action potential duration. Class IA

agents, such as **procainamide**, prolong the AP. Class IB drugs, such as **lidocaine**, shorten the AP in some cardiac tissues. Class IC drugs, such as **flecainide**, have no effect on AP duration. General pharmacokinetics for this class are presented in Table 10–1, and the pharmacodynamic effects on the cardiac action potential are presented in Figure 10–7.

Physiologic Effects

As local anesthetics, all class I drugs slow or block conduction, especially in depolarized cells, and slow or abolish abnormal pacemakers wherever these processes depend on sodium channels. Useful sodium channel-blocking drugs bind to their receptors much more readily when the channel is open or inactivated than when it is fully repolarized and recovered from its previous activity. Ion channels in arrhythmic tissue spend more time in

Table 10–1.	Properties of the prototype antiarrhythmic drugs					
Drug	Class	Half-life	Route	PR Interval	QRS Duration	QT Interval
Disopyramide	IA	6–8 h	Oral	↓ or ↑[1]	↑↑	↑↑
Procainamide	IA	3–4 h	Oral, IV	↓ or ↑[1]	↑↑	↑↑
Quinidine	IA	6 h	Oral, IV	↓ or ↑[1]	↑↑	↑↑↑
Lidocaine	IB	1–2 h	IV	—	—[2]	—
Mexiletine	IB	12 h	Oral	—	—[2]	—
Tocainide	IB	12 h	Oral	—	—[2]	—
Flecainide	IC	20 h	Oral	↑ (slight)	↑↑	—
Esmolol	II	10 min	IV	↑↑	—	—
Propranolol	II	8 h	Oral, IV	↑↑	—	—
Amiodarone	IA, III	1–10 weeks	Oral, IV	↑	↑↑	↑↑↑↑
Ibutilide	III	6 h	Oral	↑	—	↑↑↑
Sotalol	III, II	7 h	Oral	↑	—	↑↑↑
Verapamil	IV	7 h	Oral, IV	↑↑	—	—
Diltiazem	IV	4–8 h	Oral, IV	↑	—	—
Adenosine	Misc	3 s	IV	↑↑↑	—	—

[1]PR may decrease through antimuscarinic action or increase through channel-blocking action.
[2]Lidocaine, mexiletine, and tocainide slow conduction velocity in ischemic, depolarized ventricular cells but not in normal tissue.

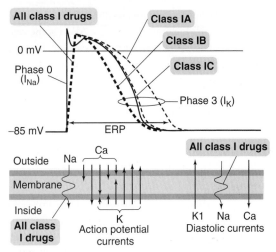

Figure 10–7. Schematic diagram of the effects of class I agents. Note that all class I drugs reduce both phase 0 and phase 4 sodium currents (*wavy lines*) in susceptible cells. Class IA drugs also reduce potassium current (I_K) and prolong the AP duration. This results in significant prolongation of the effective refractory period. Class IB and class IC drugs have different (or no) effects on potassium current and thus shorten or have no effect on the AP duration.

the open or inactivated states than do channels in normal tissue. Therefore, these antiarrhythmic drugs block channels in abnormal tissue more effectively than channels in normal tissue. As a result, antiarrhythmic sodium channel blockers selectively depress tissue that is frequently depolarizing or is relatively depolarized during rest. Such conditions occur during a fast tachycardia for the former and in hypoxic tissue in the latter.

CLASS IA: **Procainamide** is a class IA prototype. Other drugs with class IA actions include **quinidine** and **disopyramide. Amiodarone,** often classified as class III, also has typical class IA actions. These drugs affect both atrial and ventricular arrhythmias. They block I_{Na} and, therefore, slow conduction velocity in the atria, Purkinje fibers, and ventricular cells. At high doses, they also slow AV conduction. The reduction in ventricular conduction results in increased QRS duration in the electrocardiogram (ECG) (Table 10–1). In addition, class IA drugs block I_K. Therefore, they increase AP duration and the ERP, in addition to slowing conduction velocity and ectopic pacemakers. The increase in AP duration

generates an increase in QT interval. Amiodarone has similar effects on sodium current and has the greatest AP-prolonging effect.

CLASS IB: **Lidocaine** is the prototype IB drug. **Mexiletine** and **tocainide** are other class IB agents. Lidocaine selectively affects ischemic or depolarized Purkinje and ventricular tissue and has little effect on atrial tissue. The drug reduces AP duration, but because it slows recovery of sodium channels from inactivation, it does not shorten and may even prolong the ERP. Mexiletine and tocainide have similar effects. Because these agents have little effect on normal cardiac cells, they have little effect on the ECG (Table 10–1). **Phenytoin,** an anticonvulsant and not a true local anesthetic, is sometimes classified with the class IB antiarrhythmic agents because it can be used to reverse digitalis-induced arrhythmias. Phenytoin resembles lidocaine in lacking significant effect on the normal ECG.

CLASS IC: **Flecainide** is the prototype drug with class IC actions. **Encainide, moricizine,** and **propafenone** are rarely used members of this class. These drugs have no effect on ventricular AP duration or the QT interval. They are powerful depressants of sodium current, however, and can markedly slow conduction velocity in atrial and ventricular cells. They increase the QRS duration of the ECG.

Clinical Uses

CLASS IA: Procainamide can be used in all types of arrhythmias; both atrial and ventricular arrhythmias may be responsive. Quinidine and disopyramide have similar uses. Procainamide is also commonly used in arrhythmias during the acute phase of myocardial infarction.

CLASS IB: Lidocaine is useful in acute ventricular arrhythmias, especially those involving ischemia, such as following myocardial infarction. Atrial arrhythmias are not responsive unless caused by digitalis. Mexiletine and tocainide have similar actions and are given orally. Lidocaine is usually given intravenously, but intramuscular administration is also possible. Lidocaine is never given orally because it has a very high first-pass effect and its metabolites are potentially cardiotoxic.

CLASS IC: Flecainide is effective in both atrial and ventricular arrhythmias but is approved only for refractory ventricular tachycardias that tend to progress to VF at unpredictable times resulting in "sudden death," and for certain intractable supraventricular arrhythmias.

Adverse Effects

In the following discussion, the reader should note that hyperkalemia potentially exacerbates the cardiac toxicity of all class I drugs.

CLASS IA: Procainamide causes hypotension, especially when used parenterally, and a reversible syndrome similar to lupus erythematosus. Quinidine causes cinchonism, which may manifest as headache, vertigo, tinnitus, cardiac depression, gastrointestinal upset, and autoimmune reactions such as thrombocytopenic purpura. As noted in Chapter 9, quinidine reduces the clearance of digoxin and may increase the serum concentration of the glycoside significantly. Disopyramide has marked antimuscarinic effects and may precipitate heart failure. All class IA drugs may precipitate new arrhythmias. Torsade de pointes is particularly associated with quinidine and other drugs (except amiodarone) that prolong AP duration. The toxicities of amiodarone are discussed below.

CLASS IB: Lidocaine, mexiletine, and tocainide may cause typical local anesthetic toxicity. Such toxicity may result in central nervous system (CNS) stimulation, possibly including convulsions and cardiovascular depression. Allergies such as rashes are also a potential effect and may extend to anaphylaxis. Tocainide may cause agranulocytosis. These drugs may also precipitate arrhythmias, but this is less common than with class IA and IC drugs.

CLASS IC: Flecainide and its congeners are more likely than other antiarrhythmic agents to exacerbate or precipitate arrhythmias. Therefore, these drugs are said to have a proarrhythmic effect. For this reason, class IC drugs are now restricted to use in arrhythmias that fail to respond to other drugs. These drugs also cause local anesthetic-like CNS toxicity.

Class II Antiarrhythmics (β-Receptor Antagonists)

Beta blockers are discussed in more detail in Chapter 6. **Propranolol** and **esmolol** are the prototypic antiarrhythmic β-receptor antagonists. Their mechanism in arrhythmias is primarily cardiac β_1 receptor blockade and reduction in cyclic adenosine monophosphate (cAMP). This results in the reduction of both I_{Na} and I_{Ca} and the suppression of abnormal pacemakers. The AV node is particularly sensitive to β-receptor antagonists. The PR interval is usually prolonged by class II drugs (Table 10–1). Under some conditions, these drugs may have some direct local anesthetic effect in the heart, that is, sodium channel blockade, but this is probably rare at the concentrations achieved clinically.

Clinical Uses

Esmolol, a very short-acting β-receptor antagonist for intravenous administration, is used exclusively in acute arrhythmias. Propranolol, **metoprolol**, and **timolol** are commonly used as prophylactic drugs in patients who have had a myocardial infarction. Chronic therapy with these drugs provides a protective effect for 2 years or longer after the infarct.

Adverse Effects

The toxicities of β-receptor antagonists are the same in patients with arrhythmias as in patients with other conditions (Chapter 6). While patients with arrhythmias are often more prone to β-receptor antagonist-induced depression of cardiac output than are patients with normal hearts, judicious use of these drugs reduces progression of chronic heart failure (Chapter 9) and reduces the incidence of potentially fatal arrhythmias in heart failure.

Class III Antiarrhythmics (Potassium [I_K] Channel Blockers)

Sotalol and **ibutilide** are prototypic class III drugs. Sotalol has both effective β-receptor antagonist activity and an action potential prolonging antiarrhythmic action. **Dofetilide** is similar to ibutilide. **Amiodarone** is usually classified as a class III drug because it markedly prolongs AP duration by blocking potassium channels; in addition, it blocks sodium channels. **Bretylium** is an older agent that combines general sympatholytic actions and a potassium channel-blocking effect in ischemic tissue.

Physiologic Effects

The hallmark of class III drugs is prolongation of the AP duration (Figure 10–8). This AP prolongation is caused by blockade of I_K potassium channels that are

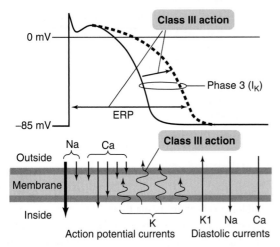

Figure 10–8. Schematic diagram of the effects of class III agents. All class III drugs prolong the AP duration in susceptible cardiac cells by reducing the outward phase 3 potassium current (I_K, *wavy lines*). The main effect is to prolong the effective refractory period. Note that the phase 4 diastolic potassium current (I_{K1}) is not affected by these drugs.

responsible for the repolarization of the AP. The AP prolongation results in an increase in ERP and reduces the ability of the heart to respond to rapid tachycardias. Sotalol, ibutilide, dofetilide, and amiodarone produce this effect on most cardiac cells. The action of these drugs is therefore apparent in the ECG as an increase in QT interval. N-acetylprocainamide, a metabolite of procainamide (class IA), also significantly prolongs the AP and the QT interval. Bretylium, on the other hand, produces AP prolongation mainly in ischemic cells and causes little change in the ECG.

Clinical Uses and Adverse Effects
Bretylium is rarely used clinically. Bretylium is now used only in the emergency treatment of refractory postmyocardial infarction arrhythmias, especially recurrent ventricular fibrillation, and only after lidocaine and cardioversion have failed. This drug may precipitate new arrhythmias or marked hypotension. Sotalol is much more commonly used and is available by the oral route (Table 10–1). Sotalol may precipitate torsade de pointes arrhythmia as well as signs of excessive β blockade such as sinus bradycardia or asthma. Ibutilide and dofetilide are recommended for atrial flutter and fibrillation. Their most important

toxicity is induction of torsade de pointes. The toxicities of class IA drugs, which share the I_K potassium channel-blocking action of class III agents, are discussed with the class IA drugs.

Amiodarone is a special case. Amiodarone is effective in most types of arrhythmias and is considered the most efficacious of all antiarrhythmic drugs. This may be because it has a broad spectrum of activity. Amiodarone blocks sodium, calcium, and potassium channels and β₁ receptors. Because of the toxicities of amiodarone, it is approved for use mainly in arrhythmias that are resistant to other drugs. Nevertheless, the drug is actually used extensively in a wide variety of arrhythmias. Amiodarone causes microcrystalline deposits in the cornea and skin, hyperthyroidism or hypothyroidism, paresthesias, tremor, and pulmonary fibrosis. Amiodarone rarely causes new arrhythmias, perhaps because of its broad spectrum of action.

Class IV Antiarrhythmics (Calcium Channel Blockers)

Verapamil is the prototypic class IV antiarrhythmic. **Diltiazem** is also an effective antiarrhythmic drug, although it is not Food and Drug Administration (FDA)—approved for this purpose. Nifedipine and the other dihydropyridines are not useful as antiarrhythmics, probably because they decrease arterial pressure sufficiently to evoke a compensatory sympathetic discharge to the heart. The latter effect facilitates rather than suppresses arrhythmias.

Physiologic Response
Verapamil and diltiazem are most effective in arrhythmias that must traverse the AV node, a calcium-dependent cardiac tissue. These agents cause a selective depression of calcium current in tissues that require the participation of L-type calcium channels (Figure 10–9). Conduction velocity is decreased, and effective refractory period is increased by these drugs. The PR interval is consistently increased (Table 10–1).

Clinical Use and Adverse Effects
Calcium channel blockers are effective for converting AV nodal reentry, also known as nodal tachycardia, to normal sinus rhythm. Their major use is in the prevention of these nodal arrhythmias in patients prone to recurrence.

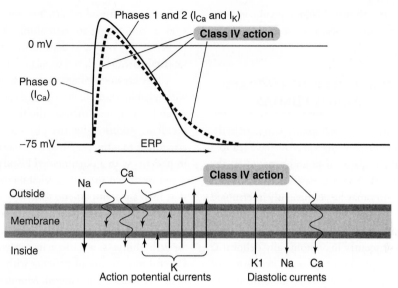

Figure 10–9. Schematic diagram of the effects of class IV drugs in a calcium-dependent cardiac cell in the AV node. At the AV node, the AP upstroke is mainly due to calcium current. Class IV drugs reduce inward calcium current during the AP and during phase 4 (*wavy lines*). As a result, conduction velocity is slowed in the AV node and refractoriness is prolonged. Pacemaker depolarization during phase 4 is slowed as well if caused by excessive calcium current.

These drugs are orally active, but are also available for parenteral use (Table 10–1). Diltiazem is clinically used for treatment of atrial flutter and fibrillation. The most important toxicity of verapamil is an excessive pharmacologic effect because cardiac contractility, AV conduction, and blood pressure can be significantly depressed. Diltiazem has a less depressant effect on blood pressure. See Chapter 8 for additional discussion of toxicity.

Miscellaneous Antiarrhythmic Drugs

Adenosine is a normal component of the body, but when given in high doses (6 to 12 mg) as an intravenous bolus the drug markedly slows or completely blocks conduction in the AV node (Table 10–1), probably by hyperpolarizing this tissue through increased I_K and reduced I_{Ca}. Adenosine is extremely effective in abolishing AV nodal arrhythmias, and because of very low toxicity, it has become the drug of choice for acute episodes of this type of arrhythmia. Adenosine has an extremely short duration of action of about 15 seconds. Toxicity includes flushing and hypotension, but because of their short duration, these effects do not limit the use of the drug. Chest pain and dyspnea can also occur.

The actions of **digitalis** are discussed in Chapter 9. The cardiac parasympathomimetic action of digoxin is sometimes exploited in the treatment of rapid atrial or AV nodal arrhythmias. In atrial flutter or fibrillation, digitalis slows AV conduction sufficiently to protect the ventricles from excessively high rates (Figure 10–6, panel 3). In AV nodal reentrant arrhythmias, digitalis may exert enough depressant effect to abolish the arrhythmia. The latter use of digitalis has become less common since the introduction of calcium channel blockers and adenosine as antiarrhythmic drugs.

Potassium depresses ectopic pacemakers, including those caused by digitalis toxicity. Hypokalemia is associated with an increased incidence of arrhythmias, especially in patients receiving digitalis. Conversely, excessive potassium levels depress conduction and can cause reentry arrhythmias. As both insufficient and excessive potassium may cause arrhythmias, potassium therapy in arrhythmias is directed toward normalizing this ion within the body.

Magnesium has not been as well studied as potassium but appears to have similar depressant effects on digitalis-induced arrhythmias. Magnesium also appears to be effective in some cases of torsade de pointes arrhythmia.

NONPHARMACOLOGIC THERAPY OF CARDIAC ARRHYTHMIAS

Antiarrhythmic drugs can precipitate lethal arrhythmias in some patients, and clinical trials have led to a reevaluation of their relative risks and benefits. At the start of the twentieth century, experimental research suggested that reentry may be permanently interrupted by transecting the reentry circuit. This concept has now been applied to treat clinical arrhythmias that occur as a result of reentry in anatomically delineated pathways. For example, interruption of accessory AV connections can permanently cure arrhythmias in patients with the Wolff-Parkinson-White syndrome. Such interruption was originally performed during open heart surgery but is now often accomplished by delivery of radio frequency energy through an appropriately positioned intracardiac catheter. Since the procedure causes minimal morbidity, it is being increasingly applied to other reentry arrhythmias with defined pathways, such as AV nodal reentry, atrial flutter, and some forms of atrial fibrillation and ventricular tachycardia. Other nonpharmacologic forms of therapy, such as external cardiac defibrillation, implanted cardiac defibrillators (ICDs), and implanted pacemakers, have become extremely important. The increasing use of nonpharmacologic antiarrhythmic therapies reflects both advances in the relevant technologies and an increasing appreciation of the dangers of long-term therapy with currently available drugs.

REHABILITATION FOCUS

Arrhythmias are manifestations of several cardiovascular disorders and effects of various drugs and electrolyte abnormalities. Both decreases and increases in arrhythmia incidence during rehabilitation have been reported in patients with a known history of arrhythmias. Therefore, careful monitoring is required in these patients during physical therapy. Prevention of arrhythmias with antiarrhythmic drugs in patients during rehabilitation has

demonstrated mixed results. Yet, rehabilitated patients who are also taking antiarrhythmic drugs demonstrate higher quality of life, as defined by emotional stability, satisfaction with work and social life, and return to work.

The cardiovascular stress of activities associated with rehabilitation, such as graded exercising in cardiac rehabilitation, may increase the risk of an arrhythmic incident. Additionally, the physical therapist should remember that the potential for increased arrhythmias in patients with a documented history of arrhythmias is not restricted to cardiac rehabilitation. Any activity that increases sympathetic tone may increase the risk of arrhythmias. The patient being rehabilitated in a work-hardening program may be just as likely to have an arrhythmia as a patient in cardiac rehabilitation. Careful monitoring of patients with a known history of arrhythmias is encouraged. Monitored ECG during ambulation and exercise training is the preferred method. If electrocardiographic monitoring is unavailable, determination of an abnormal pulse, dizziness, or nausea may also allow the clinician to detect arrhythmias during rehabilitation.

CLINICAL RELEVANCE FOR REHABILITATION

Adverse Drug Reactions

- Orthostatic hypotension is a problem with class II, IV, and some class III antiarrhythmic drugs.
- Bronchoconstriction is a problem with class II antiarrhythmic drugs.
- Class II antiarrhythmic drugs blunt the early manifestations of hypoglycemia.
- Several antiarrhythmic drug classes depress cardiac rate and contractility.
- All antiarrhythmic drug classes have some representatives that can induce cardiac arrhythmias.
- Potassium-sparing diuretics and drugs inhibiting the angiotensin-aldosterone system increase plasma potassium and exacerbate the reentry-causing effects of class I antiarrhythmics. Thiazide and loop diuretics decrease plasma potassium and increase spontaneous automaticity-induced arrhythmias.
- Amiodarone can cause hyperthyroidism or hypothyroidism.

Effects Interfering with Rehabilitation

- Orthostatic hypotension may cause patients to faint when transferring from a sitting or supine position to standing, exiting from warm aquatherapy area, or if aerobic exercise is terminated without an appropriate cool-down period.
- Dyspnea may decrease the aerobic capacity of patients.
- Heart rate cannot be used as a marker of exertion for patients taking class II antiarrhythmic drugs.
- Cardiac output may be diminished by these drugs during aerobic activities.
- Manifestations of hypoglycemia occurring during aerobic activities may be diminished in patients taking class II antiarrhythmic drugs.
- Ability to participate in aerobic activities may be decreased because of thyroid dysfunction in patients receiving amiodarone.

Possible Therapy Solutions

- Check blood pressure and heart rate prior to and following aerobic activities.
  - If the patient is not taking class II antiarrhythmic drugs, monitor heart rate during aerobic activities.

- If the patient is diabetic and medicated with class II antiarrhythmic drugs, have her or him check glucose levels prior to aerobic activities.
- To prevent fainting associated with orthostatic hypotension, assist patients with positional changes and when exiting a warm pool. Finally, always provide a cool-down period following a period of aerobic activity.
- Allow increased time to complete aerobic tasks to prevent dyspnea and account for depressed cardiac output.
- Use perceived exertion (Borg Rating of Perceived Exertion Scale) when determining aerobic activity in patients being treated with class II antiarrhythmic drugs.

Potentiation of Functional Outcomes Secondary to Drug Therapy

- Control of arrhythmias with these drugs allows patients improved aerobic tolerance during various rehabilitation activities. These include:
  Cardiac rehabilitation
  Return to work conditioning
  Musculoskeletal strengthening and endurance activities

PROBLEM-ORIENTED PATIENT STUDY

Brief History: The patient is a 42-year-old female with a history of paroxysmal atrial fibrillation and mitral valve prolapse since childhood. The patient is under the care of a cardiologist for this condition. The patient has a body mass index of 25 and no other documented morbidities. The patient is employed at a manufacturing plant making carbon fiber aerospace components. Her job description requires final examination of the component at the end of the manufacturing process and then repetitive motion involved in stacking objects weighing approximately 8 to 15 pounds during an 8-hour

shift. The bottom of the component stack starts at the knees and maximal stack height is at the shoulders. Owing to production requirements, if the components touch the floor, they must be retrieved and discarded. The examination of the components requires specific engineering skills and expertise. Fourteen days ago, the patient dropped one of the components and bent over to retrieve the item and felt a sudden pain on the right side in the lumbar area. The patient was taken to the emergency room in extreme pain and discharged with a prescription for a pain-relief drug. The patient was subsequently seen by

(continued)

PROBLEM-ORIENTED PATIENT STUDY (*Continued*)

the corporate physician 2 days later and referred to a physical therapy clinic for pain relief and a functional return to work program.

Current Medical Status and Drug Therapy: The patient states that she takes diltiazem regularly to prevent arrhythmias and is currently on no other drugs except analgesics.

Rehabilitation Setting: The patient is driven to the outpatient clinic by another person and she received assistance getting out of the vehicle. Except for clinic visits, the patient states that she has been involved in almost no physical activities, except basic physiologic needs, and has remained in bed or on the couch since the accident. The first three treatments at the clinic were to minimize pain and begin to return to functional mobility with minimal physical exertion. The patient states that she terminated the prescribed drug for the low back pain yesterday because of sedation and constipation and has attempted to control the pain with over-the-counter drugs. Today, the patient arrives to begin the functional return to work program. The rehabilitation session begins with determination of vital signs. The

heart rate is 78 bpm and regular, and blood pressure is 132/89 mm Hg at rest prior to beginning the program. The patient is 15 minutes into the functional return to work program when she complains of chest palpitations that she recognizes as an arrhythmia. Determinations of vital signs show a heart rate of 120 bpm and irregular and blood pressure of 159/98 mm Hg. After several minutes, the chest palpitations recede and heart rate becomes regular but still elevated at 100 bpm.

Problem/Clinical Options: The elevated blood pressure, tachycardia, and irregular rhythm during the functional return to work activity suggest that activity induced the arrhythmia. The situation may have been precipitated by the patient's period of inactivity since the accident which resulted in deconditioning. Additionally, the corporate referring physician may not have been aware of the patient's cardiac disease. The therapist should contact both the referring physician and the patient's cardiologist to determine if the patient should be transferred to another location for additional medical care and for approval of additional functional activities prior to the next scheduled appointment.

PREPARATIONS AVAILABLE

Sodium Channel Blockers (Class I)

Disopyramide (generic, Norpace)
Oral: 100-, 150-mg capsules
Oral controlled-release (generic, Norpace CR): 100-, 150-mg capsules

Flecainide (Tambocor)
Oral: 50-, 100-, 150-mg tablets

Lidocaine (generic, Xylocaine)
Parenteral: 100 mg/mL for IM injection; 10, 20 mg/mL for IV injection; 40, 100, 200 mg/mL

for IV admixtures; 2, 4, 8 mg/mL premixed IV (5% D/W) solution

Mexiletine (Mexitil)
Oral: 150-, 200-, 250-mg capsules

Moricizine (Ethmozine)
Oral: 200-, 250-, 300-mg tablets

Procainamide (generic, Pronestyl, others)
Oral: 250-, 375-, 500-mg tablets and capsules
Oral sustained release (generic, Procan-SR): 250-, 500-, 750-, 1000-mg tablets
Parenteral: 100, 500 mg/mL for injection

Propafenone (Rythmol)
Oral: 150-, 225-, 300-mg tablets

Quinidine sulfate (83% quinidine base) (generic)
Oral: 200-, 300-mg tablets
Oral sustained release (Quinidex Extentabs):
300-mg tablets

Quinidine gluconate (62% quinidine base) (generic)
Oral sustained release: 324-mg tablets
Parenteral: 80 mg/mL for injection

Quinidine polygalacturonate (60% quinidine base) (Cardioquin)
Oral: 275-mg tablets

β Receptor Antagonists Labeled for Use as Antiarrhythmics (Class II)

Acebutolol (generic, Sectral)
Oral: 200-, 400-mg capsules
Parenteral: 10 mg/mL, 250 mg/mL for IV injection

Propranolol (generic, Inderal)
Oral: 10-, 20-, 40-, 60-, 80-, 90-mg tablets
Oral sustained release: 60-, 80-, 120-, 160-mg capsules
Oral solution: 4, 8 mg/mL
Parenteral: 1 mg/mL for injection

Potassium Channel Blockers (Class III)

Amiodarone (Cordarone)
Oral: 200-, 400-mg tablets
Parenteral: 150 mg/3 mL for intravenous infusion

Bretylium (generic)
Parenteral: 2, 4, 50 mg/mL for injection

Dofetilide (Tikosyn)
Oral: 125-, 250-, 500-mcg capsules

Ibutilide (Corvert)
Parenteral: 0.1 g/mL solution for IV infusion

Sotalol (generic, Betapace)
Oral: 80-, 120-, 160-, 240-mg capsules

Calcium Channel Blockers (Class IV)

Diltiazem (generic, Cardizem, Dilacor)
Oral: 30-, 60-, 90-, 120-mg tablets; 60-, 90-, 120-, 180-, 240-, 300-, 340-, 420-mg extended- or sustained-release capsules (not labeled for use in arrhythmias)
Parenteral: 5 mg/mL for intravenous injection

Verapamil (generic, Calan, Isoptin)
Oral: 40-, 80-, 120-mg tablets;
Oral sustained release (Calan SR, Isoptin SR): 100-, 120-, 180-, 240-mg capsules
Parenteral: 5 mg/2 mL for injection

Miscellaneous

Adenosine (Adenocard)
Parenteral: 3 mg/mL for injection

Magnesium sulfate
Parenteral: 125, 500 mg/mL for intravenous infusion

REFERENCES

Antzelevitch C, Shimizu W: Cellular mechanisms underlying the long QT syndrome. *Curr Opin Cardiol* 2002;17:43.

Dumaine R, Antzelevitch C: Molecular mechanisms underlying the long QT syndrome. *Curr Opin Cardiol* 2002;17:36.

Gollob MH, Seger JJ: Current status of the implantable cardioverter-defibrillator. *Chest* 2001;119:1210.

Grant AO: Molecular biology of sodium channels and their role in cardiac arrhythmias. *Am J Med* 2001; 110:296.

Hondeghem LM: Classification of antiarrhythmic agents and the two laws of pharmacology. *Cardiovasc Res* 2000;45:57.

Morady F: Radio-frequency ablation as treatment for cardiac arrhythmias. *N Engl J Med* 1999;340:534.

Nattel S: New ideas about atrial fibrillation 50 years on. *Nature* 2002;415:219.

Roden DM: Pharmacogenetics and medication-induced arrhythmias. *Cardiovasc Res* 2001;50:224.

Srivatsa U, Wadhani N, Singh AB: Mechanisms of antiarrhythmic medication actions and their clinical relevance for controlling disorders of cardiac rhythm. *Curr Cardiol Rep* 2002;4:401.

Rehabilitation

Ali A, et al: Effects of aerobic exercise training on indices of ventricular repolarization in patients with chronic heart failure. *Chest* 1999;116:83.

Belardinelli R: Arrhythmias during acute and chronic exercise in chronic heart failure. *Int J Cardiol* 2003; 90:213.

Di Somma S, et al: Treatment of hypertensive patients with ventricular arrhythmias: comparison and combination of beta-blocker and anti-arrhythmic therapy. *J Int Med Res* 1989;17:113.

Dolatowski RP, et al: Dysrhythmia detection in myocardial revascularization surgery patients. *Med Sci Sports Exerc* 1983;15:281.

Falk RH: Flecainide-induced ventricular tachycardia and fibrillation in patients treated for atrial fibrillation. *Ann Intern Med* 1989;111:107.

Galante A, et al: Incidence and risk factors associated with cardiac arrhythmias during rehabilitation after coronary artery bypass surgery. *Arch Phys Med Rehabil* 2000; 81:947.

Hertzeanu HL, et al: Ventricular arrhythmias in rehabilitated and nonrehabilitated post-myocardial infarction patients with left ventricular dysfunction. *Am J Cardiol* 1993;71:24.

Koch G, Lindstrom B. Efficacy of oral mexiletine in the prevention of exercise-induced ventricular ectopic activity. *Eur J Clin Pharmacol* 1978;13:237.

Viitasalo MT, Kala R, Eisalo A, Halonen PI. Ventricular arrhythmias during exercise testing, jogging, and sedentary life: A comparative study of healthy physically active men, healthy sedentary men, and men with previous myocardial infarction. *Chest* 1979;76:21.

11

DRUGS AFFECTING THE BLOOD

D rug classes presented in this chapter include nutrients and growth factors affecting formation of blood cells and platelets (hematopoiesis) (Figure 11–1) and drugs used in the control of blood clotting (*hemostasis*) (Figure 11–2).

BLOOD CELL FORMATION

Hematopoiesis is the production of circulating erythrocytes (red blood cells, RBCs), platelets, and leukocytes from undifferentiated stem cells. This remarkable process produces over 200 billion new blood cells per day in the normal person and even greater numbers of cells in people with conditions that cause loss or destruction of blood cells. The hematopoietic machinery resides primarily in the bone marrow in adults and requires a constant supply of essential nutrients such as iron, vitamin B_{12}, and folic acid. Hematopoietic growth factors, proteins that regulate the proliferation and differentiation of hematopoietic cells, are also required. The circulating blood cells play essential roles in oxygenation of tissues, coagulation, protection against infectious agents, and tissue repair. Blood cell deficiency is a relatively common occurrence that can have profound effects on health. Inadequate supplies of either the growth factors or, much more commonly, the essential nutrients, result in deficiency of functional blood cells.

Anemia is a deficiency of oxygen-carrying erythrocytes. Regardless of the cause, anemia presents clinically with pallor, fatigue, dizziness, exertional dyspnea, and tachycardia. The most common causes of anemia are insufficient supply of iron, vitamin B_{12}, or folic acid. Treatment of these types of anemia involves replacement of the missing nutrient. Treatment of certain forms of anemia and treatment of deficiency of other types of blood cells requires transfusion of the appropriate cell type or administration of recombinant hematopoietic growth factors. These growth factors stimulate the production of various lineages of blood cells and regulate blood cell function. Almost a dozen glycoprotein growth factors regulate the differentiation and maturation of stem cells within the bone marrow. Several growth factors, produced by recombinant DNA technology, have Food and Drug Administration (FDA) approval for treatment of patients with blood cell deficiencies.

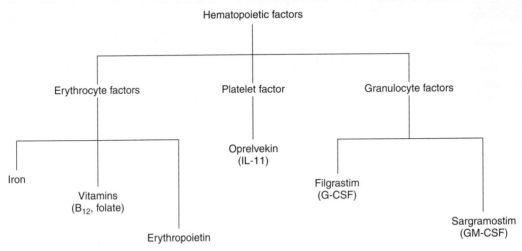

Figure 11–1. Drugs used in the treatment of anemia. The hematopoietic factors are initially classified based on the blood component stimulated. Erythrocyte factors are subsequently divided into nutrients such as iron or vitamins and erythropoietin, a growth factor that stimulates erythrocyte formation.

▪ NUTRIENTS TO PREVENT OR CORRECT RED BLOOD CELL DEFICIENCIES

Iron

Iron is the essential metallic component of heme, the molecule responsible for the bulk of oxygen transport in the blood. Iron is available in a wide variety of foods but is especially abundant in meat. Iron in the heme of hemoglobin and myoglobin in meat is efficiently absorbed intact without having to be broken down into elemental iron. Nonheme iron in the diet is absorbed less efficiently than heme iron (i.e., its bioavailability is lower). Iron in the body is present in myoglobin, hemoglobin, *transferrin*, and ferritin. Both myoglobin and hemoglobin are heme-based proteins; the former is found in muscle and the latter in red blood cells. Transferrin is a transport protein and ferritin is a storage protein. Deficiency of iron occurs most often in women because of menstrual blood loss and in vegetarians or malnourished individuals because of inadequate dietary iron intake. Children and pregnant women have increased requirements for iron.

Regulation of Iron Stores. The body has a complex system for regulating the uptake and storage of iron because adequate supplies are required for normal hematopoiesis, yet *excess* free iron is extremely toxic. Regulation of body iron content occurs through modulation of intestinal absorption. There is no mechanism for the efficient excretion of iron. As a result, abnormally increased gastrointestinal iron absorption can be a cause of organ damage because of excess iron stores (hemochromatosis). Free iron from iron supplements and iron stripped from complexes in food is absorbed as the ferrous ion (Fe^{2+}) and oxidized in the intestinal mucosal cell to the ferric ion (Fe^{3+}) form. Heme iron is absorbed as a complex and the heme component is degraded to release free iron. Iron is stored as Fe^{3+} in the intestinal mucosa (in ferritin, a complex of iron and the protein apoferritin) or carried elsewhere in the body (bound to transferrin). Excess iron is stored as ferritin in the reticuloendothelial system and, in cases of gross overload, in parenchymal cells of the skin, liver, heart, and other organs. An accumulation of stored iron occurs in hemolytic anemias due to the excess destruction of red blood cells and in hemochromatosis, an inherited abnormality of iron absorption. Minimal amounts of iron are eliminated from the body with sweat and saliva and in exfoliated skin and intestinal mucosal cells.

Clinical Use. The treatment or prevention of iron deficiency anemia is the only indication for iron administration. Iron deficiency can be diagnosed from red blood cell morphology (pale, microcytic cell size, diminished hemoglobin content) and from measurements of serum and bone marrow iron stores. The anemia is treated by oral ferrous iron supplementation and, in special cases, by parenteral administration of iron preparations. Iron is not given to patients with hemolytic anemia because their iron stores are elevated, not depressed.

Adverse Effects. Acute iron toxicity is most common in children and usually occurs as a result of accidental ingestion of iron supplement tablets. Depending on the dose, necrotizing gastroenteritis, shock, metabolic acidosis, coma, and death may result. Chronic toxicity occurs most often in individuals who receive frequent transfusions (e.g., patients with sickle cell anemia) and in those with hemochromatosis. Immediate treatment of acute iron intoxication is necessary and usually consists of removal of unabsorbed tablets from the gut, correction of acid-base and electrolyte abnormalities, and parenteral administration of **deferoxamine**, which chelates circulating iron, or **deferasirox**, an oral chelator. Chronic iron toxicity, such as in hemochromatosis, is usually treated by phlebotomy (therapeutic withdrawal of blood).

Vitamin B$_{12}$

Vitamin B$_{12}$ (cobalamin) is a cobalt-containing molecule that is produced by bacteria. This vitamin cannot be synthesized by multicellular organisms.

Pharmacokinetics and Pharmacodynamics. Vitamin B$_{12}$ contained in dietary meat (especially liver), eggs, and dairy products is absorbed from the gastrointestinal tract in the presence of *intrinsic factor*, a protein product of the parietal cells of the stomach. Defective secretion of intrinsic factor by gastric mucosal cells results in vitamin B$_{12}$ deficiency and pernicious anemia, which is particularly common in the elderly. Vitamin B$_{12}$ is stored in the liver in large amounts; a normal individual has enough to last 5 years. Nutritional deficiency is rare except in strict vegetarians after many years without meat, eggs, or dairy products. Plasma transport is accomplished by binding to transcobalamin II. When parenteral vitamin B$_{12}$ is given, any vitamin B$_{12}$ that exceeds the transport protein binding capacity is excreted.

Vitamin B$_{12}$ is essential in two reactions: conversion of methylmalonyl-coenzyme A (CoA) to succinyl-CoA and conversion of homocysteine to methionine. The second reaction is linked to folic acid metabolism and is required for the transfer of one-carbon units in DNA synthesis. Impairment of DNA synthesis affects all cells, but because red blood cells must be produced continuously, deficiency of either vitamin B$_{12}$ or folic acid usually manifests first as anemia. In addition, an important manifestation of vitamin B$_{12}$ deficiency is the development of neurologic defects, which may become irreversible if not treated promptly. The two available forms of vitamin B$_{12}$, cyanocobalamin and hydroxocobalamin, have equivalent effects. However, hydroxocobalamin has a longer circulating half-life because it is more firmly bound to plasma proteins.

Clinical Use and Toxicity. The major application of vitamin B$_{12}$ is in the treatment of pernicious anemia and anemia that results from a lack of intrinsic factor following gastric resection. Because vitamin B$_{12}$ deficiency anemia is almost always caused by inadequate absorption, therapy should be by parenteral administration of vitamin B$_{12}$. Neither form of vitamin B$_{12}$ (cyanocobalamin and hydroxocobalamin) has significant toxicity.

Folic Acid

The richest dietary sources of folic acid are yeast, liver, kidney, and green vegetables. Since 1998, all products made from enriched grains in the United States have been supplemented with folic acid in an effort to reduce the incidence of neural tube defects, which are birth defects associated with folic acid deficiency during pregnancy.

Pharmacokinetics and Pharmacodynamics. Folic acid is readily absorbed from the gastrointestinal tract. Only modest amounts are stored in the body, so a decrease in dietary intake is followed by anemia within a few months. Like vitamin B$_{12}$, folic acid is required for normal synthesis of amino acids, purines, and DNA.

Rapidly dividing cells, which require rapid DNA synthesis, are highly sensitive to folic acid deficiency. A deficiency in folic acid usually presents as megaloblastic anemia. In addition, deficiency of folic acid during pregnancy increases the risk of fetal neural tube defects such as spina bifida.

Clinical Use and Toxicity. Folic acid deficiency is most often caused by dietary insufficiency or malabsorption. Anemia resulting from folic acid deficiency is readily treated by oral folic acid supplementation. Folic acid supplementation can correct the anemia but not the neurologic deficits of vitamin B_{12} deficiency. Therefore, vitamin B_{12} deficiency must be ruled out before folic acid is used as the sole therapeutic agent in the treatment of a patient with megaloblastic anemia. Folic acid has no recognized toxicity.

HEMATOPOIETIC GROWTH FACTORS

Erythropoietin

Erythropoietin is an important protein hormone produced by the kidney that stimulates red blood cell production in the bone marrow; reduction in its synthesis is responsible for the anemia associated with renal failure. Through activation of specific receptors on erythroid progenitors in the bone marrow, erythropoietin both stimulates the production of mature erythrocytes and increases their release from the bone marrow. Erythropoietin is routinely used for anemia associated with renal failure and is sometimes effective for patients with other forms of anemia (e.g., primary bone marrow disorders or anemia secondary to cancer chemotherapy or HIV treatment, bone marrow transplantation, AIDS, or cancer). Erythropoietin is also one of the drugs banned by athletic organizations. The most serious adverse effects of erythropoietin therapy are cardiovascular and thrombotic events, and worsening hypertension. These can be minimized by avoiding a rapid rise in hematocrit and keeping serum hemoglobin at or below 12 g/dL. **Darbepoetin alpha**, a glycosylated form of erythropoietin with a much longer half-life, is often used to treat patients with anemia due to chronic renal failure.

Myeloid Growth Factors

Filgrastim (granulocyte colony-stimulating factor; G-CSF) and **sargramostim** (granulocyte-macrophage colony-stimulating factor; GM-CSF) stimulate the production and function of neutrophils. GM-CSF also stimulates the production of other myeloid and megakaryocyte progenitors. G-CSF and, to a lesser degree, GM-CSF mobilize hematopoietic stem cells (i.e., increase their concentration in peripheral blood).

Both growth factors are used to accelerate the recovery of neutrophils after cancer chemotherapy and to treat other forms of secondary and primary neutropenia (e.g., aplastic anemia, congenital neutropenia). When given to patients soon after autologous stem cell transplantation, G-CSF reduces the time to engraftment (the process by which newly transplanted stem cells start to produce new blood cells) and the duration of neutropenia. G-CSF is also used to mobilize peripheral blood stem cells in preparation for *autologous* and allogeneic stem cell transplantation. The toxicity of G-CSF is minimal, although the drug sometimes causes bone pain (ostealgia). GM-CSF can cause more severe effects, including fever, arthralgias, and capillary damage with edema. Allergic reactions are rare. **Pegfilgrastim**, a covalent conjugation product of filgrastim and a form of polyethylene glycol, has a much longer serum half-life than recombinant G-CSF.

Megakaryocyte Growth Factors

Both **thrombopoietin** and **oprelvekin** (recombinant interleukin-11 [IL-11]) stimulate the growth of megakaryocytic progenitors and increase the number of peripheral platelets (thrombocytes). IL-11 is used for the treatment of patients who have had a prior episode of thrombocytopenia after a cycle of cancer chemotherapy. In such patients, it reduces the need for platelet transfusions. The most common side effects of IL-11 are fatigue, headache, dizziness, and fluid retention. The fluid retention may also result in anemia, dyspnea, and transient atrial arrhythmias. Thrombopoietin, an investigational drug that is not yet approved by the FDA, is mainly produced by hepatocytes, and its pharmacodynamic effects appear to be similar to those of IL-11.

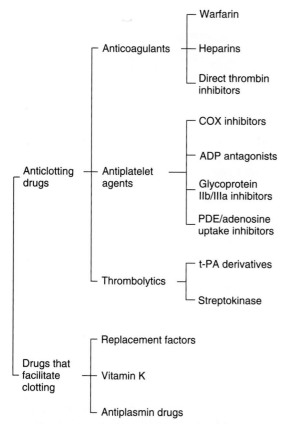

Figure 11–2. Drugs used in the treatment of altered hemostasis can be divided into those that inhibit thrombosis and those that facilitate clotting. Those used to prevent or dissolve blood clots are divided into three classes that describe their mechanisms of action: anticoagulants, antiplatelet agents, and thrombolytics. Drugs to prevent excessive bleeding are divided into three classes. These classes are replacement of clotting factors, vitamin K supplementation (required for manufacture of clotting factors), and drugs that inhibit plasmin (an enzyme that degrades blood clots).

■ DRUGS USED IN COAGULATION DISORDERS

Hemostasis is the spontaneous arrest of bleeding from a damaged blood vessel. Appropriate hemostasis requires normal function of both the coagulation cascade (Figure 11–3) and platelets. The coagulation cascade is a series of proteolytic reactions that produce active proteases and ultimately generate thrombin,

which converts fibrinogen to fibrin, a key structural component of a fibrous clot. The normal vascular endothelial cell is not thrombogenic, and circulating blood platelets and clotting factors do not normally adhere to it. However, when endothelial damage exposes the underlying tissue, platelets in the vicinity immediately undergo a reaction that causes them to stick to the exposed collagen (platelet adhesion) and to each other (platelet aggregation), and the coagulation cascade is activated. The platelet plug quickly arrests bleeding but must be reinforced by fibrin for long-term effectiveness. Disorders of hemostasis can be divided into excessive clotting (*thrombosis*) and excessive bleeding (bleeding diathesis).

The drugs used to treat disorders of hemostasis can similarly be divided into two primary groups (Figure 11–2): (1) anticlotting drugs used to decrease clotting in patients who either have evidence of a pathologic thrombus or are at risk for thrombotic vascular occlusion (anticoagulants, thrombolytics, and antiplatelet drugs); and (2) drugs used to restore clotting in patients with clotting deficiencies. The first group includes some of the most commonly used drugs in the United States. Anticlotting drugs are used in the prevention and treatment of myocardial infarction and other acute coronary syndromes, atrial fibrillation, ischemic stroke, and deep vein thrombosis (DVT). The anticoagulant and thrombolytic drugs are effective in treatment of both venous and arterial thrombosis, whereas antiplatelet drugs are used primarily for treatment or prevention of arterial thrombosis. Drugs in the second group are used to facilitate clotting in patients with excessive bleeding due to overanticoagulation or other causes (e.g., hemophilia).

Anticlotting Drugs

Anticoagulants

Anticoagulants inhibit the formation of fibrin clots. Three major types of anticoagulants are available: **heparin** and related products, which must be used parenterally; **direct thrombin inhibitors**, which also must be used parenterally; and the orally active coumarin derivatives (e.g., **warfarin**). The groups differ in chemistry, pharmacokinetics, and pharmacodynamics.

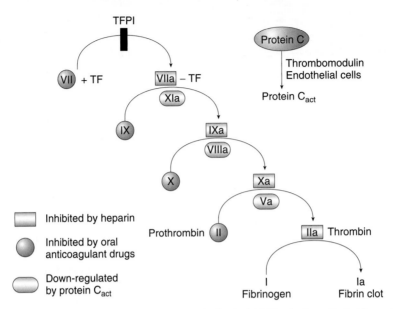

Figure 11–3. A model of the coagulation cascade, including its inhibition by the activated form of the protein C. Tissue factor (TF) is important in initiating the cascade. Tissue factor pathway inhibitor (TFPI) inhibits the action of the VIIA–TF complex.

Properties of the heparins and warfarin are compared in Table 11–1.

HEPARIN. Heparin is a large sulfated polysaccharide polymer obtained from animal sources. Each batch contains molecules of varying size, with an average molecular weight of 15,000 to 20,000. Heparin is highly acidic. In rare instances of dangerously elevated anticoagulation with excessive heparin, heparin can be rapidly neutralized by intravenous administration of the highly basic protein **protamine**. Heparin must be given parenterally (intravenously or subcutaneously). Intramuscular injection is avoided because of the risk of hematoma formation.

Low molecular weight (LMW) fractions of heparin have been developed. These have molecular weights of 2,000 to 6,000 (e.g., **enoxaparin**). LMW heparins have greater and more reliable bioavailability and longer durations of action than regular heparin; thus, doses can be given subcutaneously less frequently (e.g., once or twice a day). **Fondaparinux** is a small synthetic drug that contains a key pentasaccharide that also is present in pharmacologically active molecules of unfractionated and LMW heparins. Fondaparinux is administered subcutaneously once daily. **Danaparoid** (not available in the United States) is a LMW heparinoid, and is chemically distinct from heparin. This drug is given either intravenously or subcutaneously.

Mechanism and Effects. Unfractionated heparin binds to endogenous antithrombin III (ATIII), a powerful endogenous anticlotting protease. The heparin–ATIII complex combines with and irreversibly inactivates thrombin (activated factor II) and several other factors, particularly factor Xa (Figure 11–3). In the presence of heparin, ATIII destroys thrombin and factor Xa approximately 1000-fold faster than in its absence. Because it acts on existing blood components, heparin provides anticoagulation immediately after administration. The action of heparin is monitored with the activated partial thromboplastin time (aPTT) or partial thromboplastin time (PTT) laboratory tests (Table 11–1).

LMW heparins and fondaparinux bind ATIII, and these complexes have the same inhibitory effect on factor Xa as the regular heparin–ATIII complex.

Table 11–1. Properties of heparins and warfarin

Property	Heparins	Warfarin
Structure	Large polymers, acidic	Small lipid-soluble molecule
Route of administration	Parenteral	Oral
Site of action	Blood	Liver
Onset of action	Rapid (seconds)	Slow, limited by half-lives of factors being replaced
Mechanism of action	Activates antithrombin III, which inactivates factors including thrombin and factor Xa	Impairs posttranslational modification of factors II, VII, IX, X
Monitoring	aPTT[1] for unfractionated heparin but not LMW heparins[2]	PT[3]
Antidote	Protamine for unfractionated heparin but not LMW heparins	Vitamin K, plasma
Use	Mostly acute, over days	Chronic, over weeks to months
Use in pregnancy	Yes	No

[1]Heparin may be monitored by a protamine titration or anti-Xa assay, and therapeutic concentrations result in values of 0.2–0.4 units (protamine titration) or 0.3–0.7 units (anti-Xa assay). Activated partial thromboplastin time (aPTT) may also be used to monitor heparin. The units of the aPTT are seconds. Therapeutic concentrations of heparin result in aPTT of 2.0–2.5 that of control values; however, concerns exist as to whether this range for the aPTT may underanticoagulate patients.

[2]Low molecular weight (LMW) heparins are monitored by factor anti-Xa assay, and therapeutic concentrations are 0.5–0.1 U/mL.

[3]Prothrombin time (PT): The PT is calculated as a "normalized ratio." The clotting time for a patient taking warfarin is divided by the control time. This PT ratio is adjusted with a correction factor to yield the international normalized ratio (INR). Therapeutic concentrations of warfarin result in an INR of 2.0–3.5.

However, LMW heparin–ATIII and fondaparinux–ATIII complexes provide a more selective action because they fail to affect thrombin. The aPTT test does not reliably measure the anticoagulant effect of the LMW heparins and fondaparinux. Because the LMW heparins and fondaparinux have fairly reliable pharmacokinetic properties, their use usually precludes the need for laboratory monitoring of the coagulation effect. However, the lack of a readily available test for monitoring drug effect is a potential problem in special circumstances such as in patients with impaired renal function who may exhibit reduced drug clearance.

Clinical Use. Because of its rapid effect, heparin is used when anticoagulation is needed immediately (e.g., when starting anticoagulation therapy). Common uses include treatment of DVT, pulmonary embolism, and acute myocardial infarction. Heparin is used in combination with thrombolytics for revascularization and in combination with glycoprotein IIb/IIIa inhibitors during angioplasty and placement of coronary stents. Because heparin does not cross the placental barrier, it is the drug of choice when an anticoagulant must be used in pregnancy. LMW heparins and fondaparinux have similar clinical applications.

Adverse Effects. Increased bleeding is the most serious adverse effect of heparin and the related molecules; the bleeding may result in hemorrhagic stroke. If excessive unfractionated heparin has been given, protamine can be used as an antidote to lessen the risk of hemorrhage. Protamine only partially reverses the effects of LMW heparins and does not affect the action of fondaparinux. Regular heparin causes moderate transient thrombocytopenia in many patients and severe thrombocytopenia and paradoxic thrombosis in a small percentage of patients. The latter individuals produce an antibody that binds to a complex of heparin and platelet factor 4. LMW heparins, fondaparinux, and danaparoid are less likely to cause this immune-mediated thrombocytopenia. Prolonged use for 3 to 6 months or longer of full doses of regular heparin is associated with osteoporosis.

DIRECT THROMBIN INHIBITORS. Direct thrombin inhibitors are derived from proteins made by *Hirudo medicinalis*, the medicinal leech. **Lepirudin** is the recombinant form of the leech protein hirudin, and **bivalirudin** is a modified form of hirudin. **Argatroban** is a small, nonprotein molecule. All three drugs are administered parenterally. Lepirudin can accumulate in patients with renal failure, whereas argatroban can accumulate in patients with liver disease.

Mechanism and Effects. These drugs inhibit coagulation by binding directly to thrombin, thus avoiding the need for endogenous antithrombin III. Unlike the heparins, these drugs inhibit both soluble thrombin and the thrombin enmeshed within clots. Bivalirudin also inhibits platelet activation.

Clinical Use. Lepirudin and argatroban are used as alternatives to heparin in patients who require anticoagulation and who also have a history of heparin-induced thrombocytopenia. Bivalirudin is used in combination with aspirin during percutaneous transluminal coronary angioplasty. Like unfractionated heparin, the action of these drugs is monitored with the aPTT laboratory test.

Adverse Effects. Like other anticoagulants, the direct thrombin inhibitors can cause bleeding. No reversing agents are available. Prolonged infusion of lepirudin can induce formation of antibodies that form a complex with lepirudin and prolong its action.

COUMARIN ANTICOAGULANTS. The coumarin anticoagulants (e.g., **warfarin**) are small, lipid-soluble molecules that are readily absorbed after oral administration. Because they cross the placenta and have teratogenic effects, they are not used in pregnancy. Warfarin is highly bound to plasma proteins (>99%), and its elimination depends on metabolism by cytochrome P450 enzymes. Warfarin is the only member of the group used in the United States.

Mechanism and Effects. Warfarin and other coumarins interfere with the normal posttranslational modification of clotting factors in the liver, a process that requires vitamin K. The vitamin K–dependent factors include factors II (thrombin), VII, IX, and X (Figure 11–2). Because these factors have half-lives of 8 to 60 hours in the plasma, an anticoagulant effect is observed only after sufficient time has passed for the existing functional factors to be eliminated. The action of warfarin can be reversed with vitamin K, but recovery requires the synthesis of new functional clotting factors and is therefore slow, requiring 6 to 24 hours. More rapid reversal can be achieved by transfusion with fresh or frozen plasma that contains normal clotting factors. The effect of warfarin is monitored by the prothrombin time (PT) corrected by means of the International Normalization Ratio (INR) (Table 11–1).

Clinical Use and Adverse Effects. Warfarin is used for chronic anticoagulation in all of the clinical situations described previously for heparin except those that occur in pregnant women. Bleeding is the most important adverse effect of warfarin. Early in therapy, a period of hypercoagulability with subsequent dermal vascular necrosis can occur. This is most commonly due to reduced synthesis of protein C, an endogenous vitamin K–dependent anticoagulant with a relatively short half-life. Warfarin can cause bone defects and hemorrhage in the developing fetus and is contraindicated in pregnancy.

Because warfarin has a narrow therapeutic window, its involvement in drug interactions is of major concern. Cytochrome P450–inducing drugs (e.g., barbiturates, carbamazepine, phenytoin) increase clearance of warfarin and reduce the anticoagulant effect of a given dose. Cytochrome P450–inhibitors (e.g., amiodarone, selective serotonin reuptake inhibitors, cimetidine) reduce clearance of warfarin and increase its anticoagulant effects. Variations in dietary vitamin K can also alter the anticoagulant effects of warfarin. Increases in vitamin K in the diet decrease the anticoagulant effect of warfarin, and decreases in vitamin K have the opposite effect. A major source of vitamin K is leafy green vegetables.

Antiplatelet Drugs

Platelet aggregation plays a central role in the clotting process and is especially important in clots that form in the arterial circulation, including those responsible for coronary and cerebral artery occlusion. Platelet aggregation is facilitated by thromboxane, adenosine diphosphate (ADP), fibrin, serotonin, and other endogenous substances. Endogenous substances that increase the formation of cyclic adenosine monophosphate (cAMP) in platelets (e.g., prostacyclin) inhibit platelet aggregation.

Classification and Prototypes. Antiplatelet drugs include *aspirin*, antagonists of ADP receptors (clopidogrel and ticlopidine), glycoprotein IIb/IIIa receptor inhibitors (abciximab, tirofiban, and eptifibatide) and inhibitors of phosphodiesterase 3 (dipyridamole and cilostazol). The antiplatelet drugs increase bleeding time, which is the basis of a laboratory test that is sometimes used to monitor their effects.

Mechanisms of Action. **Aspirin** and other nonsteroidal anti-inflammatory drugs (NSAIDs) are discussed in Chapter 34. These drugs inhibit the formation of all prostaglandins, including thromboxane, by inhibiting the enzyme cyclooxygenase (COX). Although all NSAIDs impart an increased risk of bleeding, particularly in the gastrointestinal tract, only aspirin is used therapeutically as an antiplatelet drug. Aspirin is particularly effective because of its irreversible inhibition of COX. In blood vessels, there is a delicate balance between the inhibitory effect on platelet function of prostacyclin, which is produced by endothelial cells, and the platelet-activating effect of thromboxane, which is released by previously activated platelets. Platelets, which lack the machinery for synthesis of new proteins, are unable to escape the inhibitory effect of aspirin on thromboxane formation. In contrast, endothelial cells, which contain a nucleus and the capacity to synthesize proteins, continue to produce some COX and prostacyclin. Aspirin therapy, therefore, tips the prostacyclin/thromboxane balance toward prostacyclin and inhibition of platelet function. Since all of the other NSAIDs inhibit COX reversibly, they have a less selective antiplatelet effect. In fact, if other NSAIDs are administered concomitantly, they may decrease the antiplatelet effect of aspirin.

The mechanism of antiplatelet action of **ticlopidine** and **clopidogrel** involves irreversible inhibition of the ADP receptor, resulting in inhibition of ADP-mediated platelet aggregation. Because these drugs irreversibly modify the platelet ADP receptor, platelets are affected for the remainder of their lifespan, which is about 10 days (as is the case with aspirin).

Abciximab is a monoclonal antibody that reversibly inhibits the binding of fibrin and other ligands to the platelet *glycoprotein IIb/IIIa* receptor. **Eptifibatide** and **tirofiban** also reversibly block the glycoprotein IIb/IIIa receptor. Glycoprotein IIb/IIIa, a member of the integrin family of adhesion molecules, is the most abundant receptor on the surface of activated platelets. The binding of fibrinogen (the primary ligand) and other ligands (e.g., von Willebrand factor) to the glycoprotein IIb/IIIa receptor cross links platelets, resulting in platelet aggregation and formation of the platelet plug.

Dipyridamole and the newer drug **cilostazol** exert their antiplatelet activity by inhibiting *phosphodiesterase 3*, an enzyme that inactivates cAMP, and also by inhibiting the uptake of adenosine, which increases platelet cAMP through activation of *adenosine receptors*. These two molecular effects act in concert to boost the intracellular concentration of cAMP, an inhibitor of platelet activation. Activation of adenosine A_2 receptors acts through G_s to stimulate adenylyl cyclase. Blockade of adenosine uptake by dipyridamole or cilostazol increases the local concentration of adenosine and thereby increases the rate of production of cAMP in platelets. At the same time, the inhibition of the enzyme that inactivates intracellular cAMP prolongs the duration of action of this second messenger.

Clinical Use. Aspirin is used to prevent future infarcts in individuals who have had one or more myocardial infarcts. Aspirin may also reduce the incidence of first infarcts. The drug is used extensively to prevent transient ischemic attacks (TIAs), ischemic stroke, and other thrombotic events. Clopidogrel and ticlopidine are useful in preventing TIAs and ischemic stroke, especially in patients who cannot tolerate aspirin. Clopidogrel is also used to reduce thrombosis in patients who have recently received a coronary artery stent. The glycoprotein IIb/IIIa inhibitors (abciximab, eptifibatide, and tirofiban) prevent restenosis after coronary angioplasty and are used in acute coronary syndromes (e.g., unstable angina and non-Q-wave acute myocardial infarction). Dipyridamole and cilostazol are used to treat intermittent claudication (muscle pain on exercise), a manifestation of peripheral arterial disease.

Adverse Effects. Aspirin causes gastrointestinal, renal, and CNS effects, as discussed in more detail in Chapter 34. All antiplatelet drugs significantly enhance the effects of other anticlotting agents. However, their inhibitory effects on hemostasis cannot be monitored with the aPTT or PT anticoagulation tests. Ticlopidine causes bleeding in up to 5% of patients, severe neutropenia in about 1%, and very rarely thrombotic thrombocytopenic purpura, a serious condition characterized by hemolysis

and end-organ damage. Clopidogrel is less hematotoxic. The major toxicities of glycoprotein IIb/IIIa receptor-blocking drugs (abciximab, eptifibatide, and tirofiban) are bleeding and, with chronic use, thrombocytopenia. The most common adverse effects of dipyridamole and cilostazol are headaches and palpitations.

Thrombolytic Drugs

The thrombolytic drugs currently available are alteplase, tenecteplase, and reteplase (forms of tissue plasminogen activator [t-PA]), urokinase, and streptokinase (Table 11–2). All are given intravenously.

Mechanism of Action. Plasmin is an endogenous fibrinolytic enzyme. By splitting fibrin into fragments, plasmin promotes the breakdown and dissolution of clots (Figure 11–4). Thrombolytic enzymes catalyze the conversion of the inactive precursor, plasminogen, to plasmin.

TISSUE PLASMINOGEN ACTIVATOR (t-PA). t-PA is a large human protein that directly converts fibrin-bound plasminogen to plasmin (Figure 11–4). **Alteplase** is normal human plasminogen activator produced by recombinant DNA technology. **Reteplase** is a mutated

Table 11–2.	Properties of thrombolytic enzymes		
Agent	**Source**	**Duration of Action (min)**	**Comments**
Alteplase, reteplase, tenecteplase	Recombinant human proteins	2–10	Active tissue plasminogen activator, (t-PA); converts plasminogen to plasmin; intravenous infusion (alteplase) or bolus doses (reteplase, tenecteplase). Most expensive. Reteplase and tenecteplase are longer acting than alteplase.
Streptokinase	Bacterial product	20–25	Streptokinase combines with plasminogen; the combination converts plasminogen to plasmin; intravenous infusion required. Least expensive.
Urokinase	Human kidney cell culture	<20	Active plasminogen activator

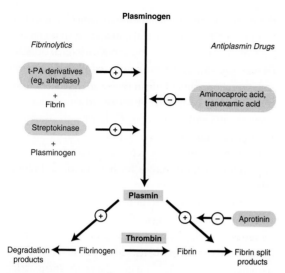

Figure 11–4. Diagram of the fibrinolytic system. The useful thrombolytic drugs are shown on the left. Aminocaproic acid and tranexamic acid inhibit plasmin formation, while aprotinin inhibits plasmin's enzymatic activity.

form of human t-PA with similar effects, but a slightly faster onset of action and longer duration of action. **Tenecteplase** is another mutated form of t-PA with a longer half-life.

UROKINASE. Urokinase is extracted from cultured human kidney cells. Like t-PA, this human enzyme directly converts plasminogen to plasmin.

STREPTOKINASE. Streptokinase is obtained from bacterial cultures. Although not itself an enzyme, streptokinase forms a complex with endogenous plasminogen. The complex catalyzes the rapid conversion of plasminogen to plasmin.

Clinical Use. The major application of the thrombolytic agents is in the emergency treatment of acute myocardial infarction when emergency coronary angioplasty is either not available or contraindicated. Under ideal conditions in which treatment is initiated within 12 hours of the thrombotic event, these agents can cause prompt recanalization (restoration of the lumen) of the occluded vessel.

Alteplase is also approved for the treatment of acute ischemic stroke with the caveats that drug therapy must be initiated within 3 hours of the onset of symptoms, and only after hemorrhagic stroke has been ruled out by an imaging procedure. The thrombolytic agents are also used in cases of pulmonary embolism with hemodynamic instability, severe DVTs, and ascending thrombophlebitis of the iliofemoral vein with severe lower extremity edema.

Adverse Effects. Bleeding is the most important hazard and occurs with approximately the same frequency with all of the thrombolytics. Cerebral hemorrhage is the most serious manifestation. Streptokinase, a bacterial protein, often evokes the production of antibodies and loses its effectiveness or induces severe allergic reactions on subsequent therapy. Patients who have had streptococcal infections may have preformed antibodies to the drug. Because they are human proteins, urokinase, t-PA, and variants of t-PA are not subject to this problem, but they are much more expensive than streptokinase and not much more effective.

DRUGS USED IN BLEEDING DISORDERS

Inadequate blood clotting may result from vitamin K deficiency, genetically determined errors of clotting factor synthesis (e.g., *hemophilia*), a variety of drug-induced conditions, or *thrombocytopenia*. Treatment, therefore, involves administration of preformed clotting factors, vitamin K, or antiplasmin drugs. Thrombocytopenia can be treated by administration of platelets.

Clotting Factors

The most important agents used to treat hemophilia are fresh plasma and human blood-clotting factors, especially factor VIII and factor IX, which are either purified from blood products or produced by recombinant DNA technology. Factor VIII is used to treat classic hemophilia (hemophilia A) and factor IX is used for Christmas disease (hemophilia B). Several other clotting factor preparations are available. These products are extremely expensive and factors purified from human blood carry a risk of infection and immunologic reactions. Contamination by blood-borne pathogens (e.g., human immunodeficiency virus [HIV] and hepatitis) are major concerns for factors purified from blood. Patients receiving clotting factors and undergoing rehabilitation should be closely monitored for undermedication, especially when resistive exercises or physical impact activities are involved in the process. Such activities may result in bleeding into muscle sheaths and joint spaces and manifest clinically as myalgia and arthralgia. Chronic complications of repeated hemarthrosis may result in ankylosis and functional loss of use of these joints.

Vitamin K

Deficiency of vitamin K, a group of chemically related fat-soluble vitamins, is particularly common in newborns and in older individuals with abnormalities of fat absorption. The deficiency is readily treated with oral or parenteral vitamin K supplements using **phytonadione (vitamin K$_1$)**, the member of the group that is available for therapeutic use. In the United states, all newborns receive an injection of vitamin K$_1$. Large doses of vitamin K$_1$ are also used to reverse the anticoagulant effect of excess warfarin.

Antiplasmin Agents

Antiplasmin agents are valuable for the management of acute bleeding episodes in hemophiliacs and others with bleeding disorders. **Aminocaproic acid** and (outside the United States) **tranexamic acid** are orally active agents that inhibit fibrinolysis by inhibiting plasminogen activation (Figure 11–4). Aprotinin is a serine protease inhibitor that inhibits fibrinolysis by both plasmin and plasmin-streptokinase complex. Aprotinin is approved for use in patients undergoing coronary artery bypass grafting who are at high risk of excessive blood loss. Its use is associated with increased risk of myocardial infarction, stroke, and renal damage.

▮ REHABILITATION FOCUS

The drug classes discussed in this chapter have significant impact on rehabilitation outcomes. Furthermore, a significant number of patients are treated with these drugs during rehabilitation. Anemia is a problem experienced by many patients, including those receiving cancer chemotherapy and those with renal or heart failure. Exercise programs combined with drug therapy improve quality of life in these patients and reduce morbidity and mortality. However, when patients are being treated with hematopoietic factors, the therapist should consider that the aerobic capacity or the immune response may be depressed. Additional review of patients' medical records for hematocrit and blood cell counts is warranted.

Patients in rehabilitation are often being treated with anticlotting drugs. This patient population includes neurologic, postsurgical, cardiac, and some general medicine patients. Medications for these patients may include anticoagulants or antiplatelet drugs. To prevent adverse events during rehabilitation, these patients require appropriate medication. Clinicians should carefully monitor laboratory coagulation test results, when these are available. Awareness of the values prior to beginning a treatment session is important, especially if treatment is aerobic-related rehabilitation or sharp debridement of wounds. This will assure that the treatment session is appropriately scaled to the patient's level of medication.

Adverse effects associated with overmedication may present as myalgia or arthralgia associated with bleeding into tissues. These symptoms may not occur until 1 or 2 days following a rehabilitation session involving impact-related physical activities. Similarly, patients with hemophilia-type bleeding disorders who are undermedicated may present with myalgia and arthralgia following impact-related physical activities.

▮ CLINICAL RELEVANCE FOR REHABILITATION

Adverse Drug Reactions

- Bleeding caused by anticoagulants and antithrombotics may cause myalgia and arthralgia.
- Patients with bleeding disorders who are undermedicated may also complain of myalgia and arthralgia.
- Hematopoietic growth factors may cause ostealgia.
- Anticoagulants, antithrombotics, and thrombolytics all inhibit clotting.

Effects Interfering with Rehabilitation

- Arthralgia, myalgia, or ostealgia may decrease the function of the patient due to pain and may adversely affect functional outcomes of treatment.
    - The clinician should differentiate pain associated with exercise from that associated with the adverse effects of these drugs.
- Increased bleeding (delayed clotting) may alter some wound care activities.
    - If excessive bleeding caused by anticoagulants, antithrombotics, or thrombolytics is a concern, alternatives to sharp debridement of necrotic tissue associated with the wound should be considered.

Possible Therapy Solutions

- If the patient presents with any manifestations of bleeding, contact the referring health-care provider.

Potentiation of Functional Outcomes Secondary to Drug Therapy

- Prevention of anemia by supplementation with iron, appropriate vitamins, or hematopoietic growth factors will improve cardiovascular function and exercise tolerance.
    - Careful monitoring of laboratory values related to complete blood count will assist in developing an appropriate rehabilitation protocol.

PROBLEM-ORIENTED PATIENT STUDY

Brief History: The patient is a 66-year-old retired male in a conditioning program at a wellness center. The program includes walking on a treadmill, upper extremity resistive exercise with light weights, and abdominal exercises. The patient started the program in May and has been participating for 2 months without incident. At this time of the year, the wellness center provides an area for the exchange by members of produce from their gardens.

Current Medical Status and Drug Therapy: He has angina pectoris and is currently taking warfarin in addition to antianginal drugs.

Rehabilitation Setting: The conditioning program is 5 days a week; however, the patient routinely participates an average of 4 days a week. The patient's current status and program modification are reviewed on an every other week basis by a physical therapist at the wellness center. Last week, the patient was absent. This week, the patient participated on Monday and Tuesday, and his progress was reviewed on Wednesday. During the initial discussion, the patient states he was out of town visiting his grandchildren and he kept up with all his medications but not his conditioning program. He also discussed the fact that he missed the fresh vegetables last week while away. Today, he complains of pain in his shoulders and in his knees. He figures it was the result of not keeping up with the conditioning program last week and getting started again. The therapist notices a circumferential bruise around the right wrist that appears several days old. When questioned, the patient states that must have been his grandchildren leading him by the wrist last week. The therapist tells the patient to contact the health-care provider who prescribed the warfarin to have his anticoagulation level determined.

Problem/Clinical Options: The pain in the shoulders and knees may be related to restarting the conditioning program following the 1-week abstinence. However, the circumferential bruise at the wrist, when combined with the other manifestations, suggests excessive anticoagulation with warfarin. Immediate referral to the prescribing health-care professional is recommended.

PREPARATIONS AVAILABLE

Hematopoietic Factors

Darbepoetin alfa (Aranesp)
Parenteral: 25, 40, 60, 100, 200, 300, 500 mcg/mL for IV or SC injection

Epoetin alfa (erythropoietin, EPO) (Epogen, Procrit)
Parenteral: 2000, 3000, 4000, 10000, 20000, 40000 IU/mL vials for IV or SC injection

Filgrastim (G-CSF) (Neupogen)
Parenteral: 300-mcg vials for IV or SC injection

Oprelvekin (interleukin-11) (Neumega)
Parenteral: 5-mg vials for SC injection

Pegfilgrastim (Neulasta)
Parenteral: 10 mg/mL solution in single-dose syringe

Sargramostim (GM-CSF) (Leukine)
Parenteral: 250-, 500-mcg vials for IV infusion

Drugs Used in Coagulation Disorders

Abciximab (ReoPro)
Parenteral: 2 mg/mL for IV injection

Alteplase recombinant (t-PA) (Activase*)
Parenteral: 50-, 100-mg lyophilized powder to reconstitute for IV injection

Aminocaproic acid (generic, Amicar)
Oral: 500-mg tablets; 250 mg/mL syrup
Parenteral: 250 mg/mL for IV injection

Antihemophilic factor (factor VIII, AHF) (Alphanate, Bioclate*, Helixate,* Hemofil M, Koate-HP, Kogenate,* Monoclate, Recombinate,* others)
Parenteral: in vials

Anti-inhibitor coagulant complex (Autoplex T, Feiba VH Immuno)
Parenteral: in vials

Antithrombin III (Thrombate III)
Parenteral: 500, 1000 IU powder to reconstitute for IV injection

Argatroban
Parenteral: 100 mg/mL in 2.5-mL vials

Bivalirudin (Angiomax)
Parenteral: 250 mg per vial

Cilostazol (Pletal)
Oral: 50-, 100-mg tablets

Clopidogrel (Plavix)
Oral: 75-mg tablets

Coagulation factor VIIa recombinant (NovoSeven*)
Parenteral: 1.2-, 4.8-mg powder/vial for IV injection

Dalteparin (Fragmin)
Parenteral: 2500, 5000, 10,000 antifactor Xa units/0.2 mL for SC injection only

Danaparoid (Orgaran)
Parenteral: 750 anti-Xa units/vial

Dipyridamole (Persantine)
Oral: 25-, 50-, 75-mg tablets
Oral combination product (Aggrenox): 200-mg extended-release dipyridamole plus 25-mg aspirin

Enoxaparin (low molecular weight heparin, Lovenox)
Parenteral: prefilled, multiple-dose syringes for SC injection only

Eptifibatide (Integrilin)
Parenteral: 0.75, 2 mg/mL for IV infusion

Factor VIIa: see Coagulation factor VIIa recombinant

Factor VIII: see Antihemophilic factor

Factor IX complex, human (AlphaNine SD, Bebulin-VH, BeneFix*, Konyne 80, Mononine, Profilnine SD, Proplex T, Proplex SX-T)
Parenteral: in vials

Fondaparinux (Arixtra)
Parenteral: 2.5 mg in 0.5 mL single-dose prefilled syringes

Heparin sodium (generic, Liquaemin)
Parenteral: 1000, 2000, 2500, 5000, 10,000, 20,000, 40,000 units/mL for injection

Lepirudin (Refludan*)
Parenteral: 50 mg powder for IV injection

Phytonadione (vitamin K₁) (generic, Mephyton, AquaMephyton)
Oral: 5-mg tablets
Parenteral: 2, 10 mg/mL aqueous colloidal solution or suspension for injection

Protamine (generic)
Parenteral: 10 mg/mL for injection

Reteplase (Retavase*)
Parenteral: 10.8 IU powder for injection

Streptokinase (Streptase)
Parenteral: 250,000, 750,000, 1,500,000 IU per vial powders to reconstitute for injection

Tenecteplase (TNKase)*
Parenteral: 50 mg powder for injection

Ticlopidine (Ticlid)
Oral: 250-mg tablets

Tirofiban (Aggrastat)
Parenteral: 50, 250 mcg/mL for IV infusion

Tranexamic acid (Cyklokapron)
Oral: 500-mg tablets
Parenteral: 100 mg/mL for IV infusion

Urokinase (Abbokinase)
Parenteral: 250,000 IU per vial for systemic use

Warfarin (generic, Coumadin)
Oral: 1-, 2-, 2.5-, 3-, 4-, 5-, 6-, 7.5-, 10-mg tablets

*Recombinant product.

REFERENCES

Anemia and Hematopoietic Factors

Cook JD: Diagnosis and management of iron-deficiency anaemia. *Best Pract Res Clin Haematol* 2005;18:309.

Fisher JW: Erythropoietin: physiology and pharmacology update. *Exp Biol Med* 2003;228:1.

Gazitt Y: Comparison between granulocyte colony-stimulating factor and granulocyte-macrophage colony stimulating factor in the mobilization of peripheral blood stem cells. *Curr Opin Hematol* 2002;9:190.

Linker CA: Blood. *Current Medical Diagnosis and Treatment.* New York: McGraw-Hill, 2004, Chapter 13.

Ozer H, et al: 2000 update of recommendations for the use of hematopoietic colony-stimulating factors: evidence-based, clinical practice guidelines. American Society of Clinical Oncology Growth Factors Expert Panel. *J Clin Oncol* 2001; 19:1583.

Anticlotting Drugs

Blood Coagulation

Dahlback B: Blood coagulation. *Lancet* 2000;355:1627.

Anticoagulant Drugs

Dalen JE, Hirsh J, Guyatt GH (eds): Sixth ACCP Consensus Conference on Antithrombotic Therapy. *Chest* 2001;119(Suppl):1.

Ridker PM, et al: Long-term, low-intensity warfarin therapy for the prevention of recurrent venous thromboembolism. *N Engl J Med* 2003;348:15.

Fibrinolytic Drugs

Davydov L, et al: Tenecteplase: A review. *Clin Ther* 2001; 23:982.

Thrombolytic therapy with streptokinase in acute ischemic stroke. The Multicenter Acute Stroke Trial–Europe Study Group. *N Engl J Med* 1996;335:145.

Antithrombotic Drugs

American Heart Association: Guidelines 2000 for cardiopulmonary resuscitation and emergency cardiovascular care. Part 7. *Circulation* 2000;102:I–172.

Hurlen M, et al: Warfarin, aspirin, or both after myocardial infarction. *N Engl J Med* 2002;347:969.

Rehabilitation

Burke DT: Prevention of deep venous thrombosis: overview of available therapy options for rehabilitation patients. *Am J Phys Med Rehabil* 2000;79:S3.

Deligiannis A: Exercise rehabilitation and skeletal muscle benefits in hemodialysis patients. *Clin Nephrol* 2004;61(Suppl 1):S460.

Gabrilove J: Anemia and the elderly: clinical considerations. *Best Pract Res Clin Haematol* 2005;18:417.

Ginzburg E, et al: Thromboprophylaxis in medical and surgical patients undergoing physical medicine and rehabilitation: consensus recommendations. *Am J Phys Med Rehabil* 2006;85:159.

Hebbeler SL, et al: Daily vs twice daily enoxaparin in the prevention of venous thromboembolic disorders during rehabilitation following acute spinal cord injury. *J Spinal Cord Med* 2004;27:236.

Johansen KL: Physical functioning and exercise capacity in patients on dialysis. *Adv Ren Replace Ther* 1999;6:141.

Lawrence DP, et al: Evidence report on the occurrence, assessment, and treatment of fatigue in cancer patients. *J Natl Cancer Inst Monogr* 2004;40.

Lindholm E, et al: Effects of recombinant erythropoietin in palliative treatment of unselected cancer patients. *Clin Cancer Res* 2004;10:6855.

Smith KJ, et al: The cardiovascular effects of erythropoietin. *Cardiovasc Res* 2003; 59:538.

Merli GJ: Treatment of deep venous thrombosis and pulmonary embolism with low molecular weight heparin in the geriatric patient population. *Clin Geriatr Med* 2001;17:93.

Nissenson AR: Recombinant human erythropoietin: Impact on brain and cognitive function, exercise tolerance, sexual potency, and quality of life. *Semin Nephrol* 1989;9:25.

Shioji K, et al: Heparin and exercise treatment in a patient with arteriosclerosis obliterans. *Jpn Circ J* 1997;61:715.

Zorowitz RD, et al: Antiplatelet and anticoagulant medication usage during stroke rehabilitation: the Post-Stroke Rehabilitation Outcomes Project (PSROP). *Top Stroke Rehabil* 2005;12:11.

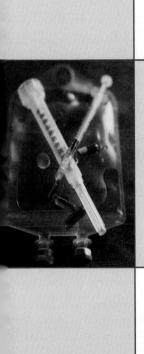

DRUGS AFFECTING THE CENTRAL NERVOUS SYSTEM

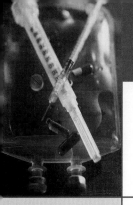

INTRODUCTION TO THE PHARMACOLOGY OF CENTRAL NERVOUS SYSTEM DRUGS

Drugs acting in the central nervous system (CNS) were among the first to be discovered by primitive humans and are still the most widely used group of pharmacologic agents. In addition to their use in therapy, many drugs acting on the CNS are used without prescription to increase one's sense of well-being.

The mechanisms by which various drugs act in the CNS have not always been clearly understood. Since the causes of many of the conditions for which these drugs are used (e.g., schizophrenia, anxiety) are themselves poorly understood, it is not surprising that in the past much of CNS pharmacology has been purely descriptive. However, dramatic advances in the methodology of CNS pharmacology now make it possible to study the action of a drug on individual cells and even on single ion channels within synapses. This information has provided the basis for several major developments in studies of the CNS.

First, it is clear that nearly all drugs with CNS effects act on specific receptors that modulate synaptic transmission, either directly by affecting the receptors themselves or indirectly through various second-messenger coupling systems, ion channels, or other mechanisms. Second, drugs are among the most important tools for studying all aspects of CNS physiology, from the mechanism of convulsions to the laying down of long-term memory. As will be described below, synthetic agonists that mimic natural transmitters (and in many cases are more selective than the endogenous substances) and antagonists are extremely useful in such studies. Third, unraveling the actions of drugs with known clinical efficacy has led to some of the most fruitful hypotheses regarding the mechanisms of disease. For example, information on the action of antipsychotic drugs on dopamine receptors has provided the basis for important hypotheses regarding the pathophysiology of schizophrenia. Studies of the effects of a variety of agonists and antagonists on gamma-aminobutyric acid (GABA) receptors have resulted in new concepts pertaining to the pathophysiology of several diseases, including anxiety and epilepsy.

This chapter provides an introduction to the functional organization of the CNS and its synaptic transmitters as a basis for understanding the actions of the drugs described in the following chapters.

ION CHANNELS AND NEUROTRANSMITTER RECEPTORS

Most drugs that act on the CNS appear to do so by changing ion flow through transmembrane channels of nerve cells. The membranes of nerve cells contain two types of ion channels defined

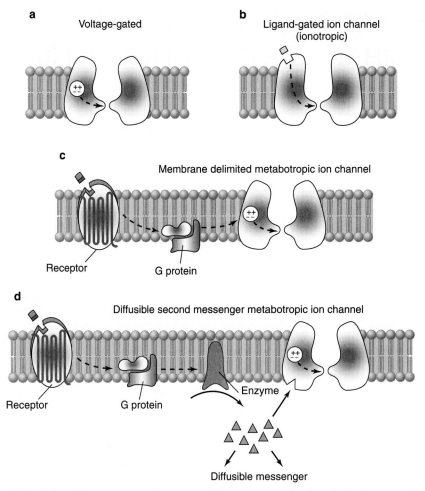

Figure 12–1. Types of ion channels and neurotransmitter receptors in the CNS. (a) A voltage-gated channel in which a voltage sensor controls the gating (broken arrow) of the channel. (b) A ligand-gated channel in which the binding of the neurotransmitter to the channel controls the gating (broken arrow) of the channel. (c) A G protein-coupled receptor, which when bound, activates a G protein which then interacts directly with an ion channel. (d) A G protein-coupled receptor, which when bound, activates a G protein which then activates an enzyme. The activated enzyme generates a diffusible second messenger that interacts with an ion channel.

on the basis of the mechanisms that control their gating (opening and closing) as *voltage-gated* and *ligand-gated channels* (Figure 12–1a and b). Voltage-gated channels respond to changes in the membrane potential of the cell. In nerve cells, voltage-gated sodium channels are concentrated near and on the axon and are responsible for the action potential which transmits the signal from cell body to nerve terminal.

There are also many types of voltage-sensitive calcium and potassium channels on the cell body, dendrites, and initial segment, which act on a slower time scale and modulate the rate at which the neuron discharges. Ligand-gated channels, also called *ionotropic receptors*, are opened by the binding of neurotransmitters to the channel. The channel is formed of subunits, and the receptor is an integral part of the channel complex.

These channels are insensitive or only weakly sensitive to membrane potential. Activation of these channels typically results in a brief (a few milliseconds to tens of milliseconds) opening of the channel. Ligand-gated channels are responsible for fast synaptic transmission typical of hierarchical pathways in the CNS (see below).

Research has now well established that the traditional view of completely separate voltage-gated and ligand-gated channels requires substantial modifications. Neurotransmitters also bind to G protein-coupled receptors (metabotropic receptors) that can modulate voltage-gated ion channels. Neurotransmitter-controlled ion channels are found on cell bodies and on both the presynaptic and postsynaptic sides of synapses. In neurotransmitter-controlled ion channels, coupling may occur by one of two mechanisms. First, control may occur through a receptor that is coupled to the ion channel through a portion of the G protein itself (Figure 12–1c). Two types of voltage-gated ion channels are involved in this type of signaling: calcium channels and potassium channels. When G proteins interact with calcium channels, they inhibit channel function. This mechanism accounts for the presynaptic inhibition that occurs when presynaptic metabotropic receptors are activated. In contrast, when these receptors are postsynaptic, they activate (cause the opening of) potassium channels, resulting in a slow postsynaptic inhibition. Second, control may be through a receptor coupled to a G protein that modulates the concentration of diffusible second messengers, such as cyclic adenosine monophosphate (cAMP), inositol trisphosphate (IP_3), and diacylglycerol (DAG), which secondarily modulate ion channels (Figure 12–1d).

An important consequence of the involvement of G proteins in receptor signaling is that, in contrast to the brief effect of transmitters on ionotropic receptors, the effects of metabotropic receptor activation can last tens of seconds to minutes. Metabotropic receptors predominate in the diffuse neuronal systems in the CNS.

THE SYNAPSE AND SYNAPTIC POTENTIALS

Communication between neurons in the CNS occurs through chemical synapses in the vast majority of cases. An action potential in the presynaptic fiber propagates into the synaptic terminal and opens voltage-sensitive calcium channels in the membrane of the terminal. Calcium flows into the terminal, and the increase in intraterminal calcium concentration promotes the fusion of synaptic vesicles with the presynaptic membrane. The transmitter contained in the vesicles is released into the synaptic cleft and diffuses to the receptors on the postsynaptic membrane. Binding of the transmitter to its receptor causes a brief change in membrane conductance (permeability to ions) of the postsynaptic cell.

The binding of the neurotransmitter to the postsynaptic membrane can result in two types of postsynaptic potentials; excitatory or inhibitory. Excitatory postsynaptic potentials (EPSPs) are usually generated by the opening of sodium or calcium channels. In some synapses, depolarizing potentials result from the *closing* of potassium channels. Inhibitory postsynaptic potentials (IPSPs) are usually generated by the opening of potassium or chloride channels. For example, activation of postsynaptic metabotropic receptors increases the efflux of potassium. *Presynaptic* inhibition can occur via a decrease in calcium influx elicited by activation of presynaptic metabotropic receptors.

SITES OF DRUG ACTION

Virtually all of the drugs that act in the CNS produce their effects by modifying some step in chemical synaptic transmission. Figure 12–2 illustrates some of the steps that can be altered. These transmitter-dependent actions can be divided into presynaptic and postsynaptic categories. Drugs acting on the synthesis, storage, metabolism, and release of neurotransmitters fall into the presynaptic category. Synaptic transmission can be depressed by blockade of transmitter synthesis or storage (Figure 12–2, Sites 2 and 3). For example, **reserpine** depletes the synapses of monoamines by interfering with intracellular storage. Blockade of transmitter catabolism (Figure 12–2, Site 4) can increase transmitter concentrations and has been reported to increase the amount of transmitter released per impulse. Drugs can also alter the release of transmitter (Figure 12–2, Site 5). For example, the

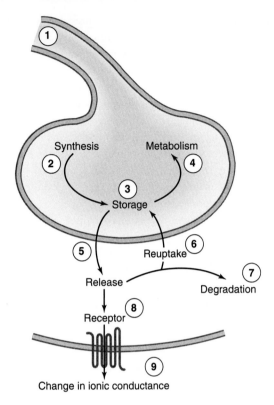

Figure 12–2. Sites of drug action. Schematic drawing of steps at which drugs can alter synaptic transmission. (1) Action potential in presynaptic fiber; (2) synthesis of transmitter; (3) storage; (4) metabolism; (5) release; (6) reuptake; (7) degradation; (8) receptor for the transmitter; (9) receptor-induced increase or decrease in ionic conductance.

stimulant **amphetamine** induces the release of catecholamines from adrenergic nerve endings and **botulinum** toxin blocks the release of acetylcholine. After a transmitter has been released into the synaptic cleft, its action is terminated either by uptake or degradation (Figure 12–2, Sites 6 and 7, respectively). For some neurotransmitters, there are uptake mechanisms into the synaptic terminal and also into surrounding neuroglia. **Cocaine**, for example, blocks the uptake of catecholamines at adrenergic synapses and thus potentiates the action of these amines. In contrast, no uptake mechanism has been found for any of the numerous CNS peptides, and it has yet to be demonstrated

whether specific enzymatic degradation terminates the action of peptide transmitters. The transmitter acetylcholine is inactivated within the synapse by enzymatic degradation. Anticholinesterase drugs block the degradation of acetylcholine and thereby prolong its action.

In the postsynaptic region, the transmitter receptor provides the primary site of drug action (Figure 12–2, Site 8). Drugs can act either as neurotransmitter agonists, such as the opioids, which mimic the action of endogenous peptides such as enkephalin, or as neurotransmitter antagonists, acting to block receptor function. Receptor antagonism is a common mechanism of action for CNS drugs. Drugs can also act directly on the ion channel of ionotropic receptors. For example, barbiturates can enter and block the channel of many excitatory ionotropic receptors. In the case of metabotropic receptors, drugs can act at any of the steps downstream of the receptor. Perhaps the best example is provided by the methylxanthines (such as **caffeine**), which can modify neurotransmitter responses mediated through the second-messenger cAMP. At high concentrations, the methylxanthines elevate the level of cAMP by blocking its metabolism and thereby prolong its action in the postsynaptic cell.

The selectivity of CNS drug action is based almost entirely on the fact that different transmitters are used by different groups of neurons. Furthermore, these transmitters are often segregated into neuronal systems that subserve different CNS functions. Without such segregation, it would be impossible to selectively modify CNS function even if one had a drug that operated on a single neurotransmitter system.

CELLULAR ORGANIZATION OF THE BRAIN

Most of the neuronal systems in the CNS can be divided into two broad categories: hierarchical systems and nonspecific (diffuse) neuronal systems.

Hierarchical Systems

These systems include all of the pathways directly involved in sensory perception and motor control. The pathways are generally clearly delineated anatomically

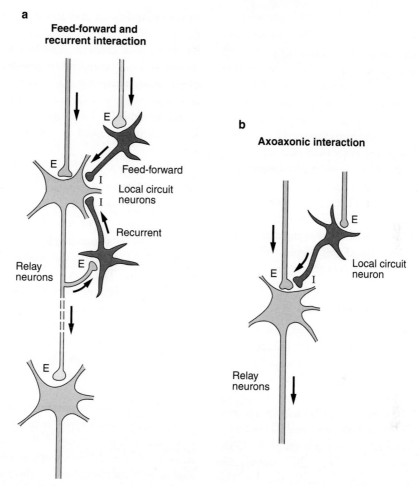

Figure 12–3. Pathways in the central nervous system. **(a)** Two relay neurons (light gray) and two types of inhibitory pathways, recurrent and feed-forward. The inhibitory feed-forward and recurrent neurons are shown in dark gray, and represent local circuit neurons. **(b)** The pathway responsible for presynaptic inhibition in which the axon of an inhibitory neuron (dark gray) synapses on the axon terminal of an excitatory fiber (light gray). E signifies an excitatory synapse; I, an inhibitory synapse.

and contain large myelinated, rapidly conducting fibers. The information is typically phasic (i.e., dependent on the frequency of action potential firing), and the information is processed sequentially at each successive relay nucleus on its way to its destination. A lesion at any link will incapacitate the system. Within each nucleus and in the cortex, there are two types of cells: relay or projection neurons and local circuit neurons (Figure 12–3a). Projection neurons form

interconnecting pathways transmitting signals over long distances. The cell bodies are relatively large and their axons are long. These neurons are excitatory, and their synaptic influences, which involve ionotropic receptors, are very short-lived. The excitatory transmitters released from these cells are glutamate and aspartate.

Local circuit neurons are typically smaller than projection neurons, and their axons arborize in the immediate vicinity of the cell body. The vast majority of these neurons are inhibitory, and they release either GABA or glycine. They synapse primarily on the cell body of the projection neurons but can also synapse on the dendrites of projection neurons as well as with each other. A special class of local circuit neurons in the spinal cord forms axoaxonic synapses on the terminals of sensory axons (Figure 12–3b). Two common types of pathways for these neurons include recurrent feedback pathways and feed-forward pathways (Figure 12–3a). Although there is a great variety of synaptic connections in these hierarchical systems, the fact that a limited number of transmitters are utilized by these neurons indicates that any major pharmacologic manipulation of this system will have a profound effect on the overall excitability of the CNS.

Nonspecific or Diffuse Neuronal Systems

Diffuse systems are broadly distributed, with neurons frequently sending processes to many different areas. These systems differ in fundamental ways from the hierarchical systems. The axons of these neurons are very fine and contain unmyelinated, slowly conducting fibers. The axons branch repeatedly and diverge into many areas. Branches from the same neuron can innervate several functionally different parts of the CNS. The axons commonly have periodic enlargements (varicosities) that contain transmitter vesicles. The transmitters in diffuse systems are often amines (norepinephrine, dopamine, 5-hydroxytryptamine [serotonin]) or peptides that exert actions on metabotropic receptors and, therefore, initiate long-lasting synaptic effects. Based on all of these observations, it is clear that the diffuse systems cannot convey specific topographic or highly transient types of information; rather large areas of the CNS must be affected at the same time and in a rather uniform way. These systems have been implicated in such global functions as sleeping and waking, attention, appetite, and emotional states.

▇ CENTRAL NEUROTRANSMITTERS

To be accepted as a neurotransmitter, a candidate chemical must (1) be present in higher concentration in the synaptic area than in other areas (i.e., must be localized in appropriate areas), (2) be released by electrical or chemical stimulation via a calcium-dependent mechanism, and (3) produce the same sort of postsynaptic response that is seen with physiologic activation of the synapse (i.e., must exhibit synaptic mimicry). Table 12–1 lists the most important chemicals currently accepted as neurotransmitters in the CNS.

Acetylcholine

Approximately 5% of brain neurons have receptors for acetylcholine (ACh). Most CNS responses to ACh are mediated by a large family of G protein-coupled muscarinic M_1 receptors that lead to slow excitation when activated. The ionic mechanism of slow excitation involves a decrease in membrane permeability to potassium. At a few sites, ACh causes slow inhibition of the neuron by activating the M_2 subtype of receptor, which opens potassium channels. Nicotinic receptors are present in the CNS but are less common than muscarinic receptors. A number of pathways contain acetylcholine, including neurons in the neostriatum, the medial septal nucleus, and the reticular formation. Cholinergic pathways appear to play an important role in cognitive functions, especially memory. Presenile dementia of the Alzheimer type is reportedly associated with a profound loss of cholinergic neurons. However, the specificity of this loss has been questioned since the levels of other putative transmitters, for example, somatostatin, are also decreased. Drugs affecting the activity of cholinergic systems in the brain include the acetylcholinesterase inhibitors used in Alzheimer's disease (e.g., **donepezil**, **rivastigmine**) and the muscarinic blocking agents used in parkinsonism (e.g., **benztropine**).

Dopamine

The major pathways containing dopamine are the projections linking the substantia nigra in the basal ganglia to the neostriatum; the ventral tegmental region to limbic structures, particularly the limbic cortex; the medullary-periventricular; the incertohypothalamic; and the tuberoinfundibular tracts. All dopamine

Table 12–1. Neurotransmitter pharmacology in the central nervous system

Transmitter	Anatomical Distribution	Major Receptor Subtypes	Receptor Mechanisms
Acetylcholine	Cell bodies at all levels, short and long axons	Muscarinic, M_1; blocked by pirenzepine and atropine	Excitatory; $\downarrow$ K^+ conductance; $\uparrow$ IP_3 and DAG
		Muscarinic, M_2; blocked by atropine	Inhibitory; $\uparrow$ K^+ conductance; $\downarrow$ cAMP
	Motoneuron–Renshaw cell synapse	Nicotinic, N	Excitatory; $\uparrow$ cation conductance
Dopamine	Cell bodies at all levels, short, medium, and long axons	D_1; blocked by phenothiazines	Inhibitory; $\uparrow$ cAMP
		D_2; blocked by phenothiazines and haloperidol	Inhibitory (presynaptic); $\downarrow$ Ca^{2+} conductance;
			Inhibitory (postsynaptic); $\uparrow$ K^+ conductance; $\downarrow$ cAMP
Norepinephrine	Cell bodies in pons and brain stem projecting to all levels	$Alpha_1$; blocked by prazosin	Excitatory; $\downarrow$ K^+ conductance; $\uparrow$ IP_3 and DAG
		$Alpha_2$; activated by clonidine	Inhibitory (presynaptic); $\downarrow$ Ca^{2+} conductance
			Inhibitory (postsynaptic); $\uparrow$ K^+ conductance; $\downarrow$ cAMP
		$Beta_1$; blocked by propranolol	Excitatory; $\downarrow$ K^+ conductance; $\uparrow$ cAMP
		$Beta_2$; blocked by propranolol	Inhibitory; may involve $\uparrow$ in electrogenic sodium pump
Serotonin (5-hydroxy-tryptamine)	Cell bodies in midbrain and pons projecting to all levels	$5\text{-}HT_{1A}$; buspirone is a partial agonist	Inhibitory; $\uparrow$ K^+ conductance
		$5\text{-}HT_{2A}$; blocked by clozapine, risperidone, and olanzapine	Excitatory; $\downarrow$ K^+ conductance; $\uparrow$ IP_3 and DAG
		$5\text{-}HT_3$; blocked by ondansetron	Excitatory; $\uparrow$ cation conductance
		$5\text{-}HT_4$	Excitatory; $\downarrow$ K^+ conductance; $\uparrow$ cAMP

(continued)

Table 12–1.	Neurotransmitter pharmacology in the central nervous system (*continued*)		
Transmitter	**Anatomical Distribution**	**Major Receptor Subtypes**	**Receptor Mechanisms**
GABA	Supraspinal interneurons; spinal interneurons involved in presynaptic inhibition	$GABA_A$; facilitated by benzodiazepines and zolpidem	Inhibitory; ↑ Cl⁻ conductance
		$GABA_B$; activated by baclofen	Inhibitory (presynaptic); ↓ Ca^{2+} conductance Inhibitory (postsynaptic); ↑ K^+ conductance
Glutamate, aspartate	Relay neurons on all levels	Four subtypes; NMDA subtype blocked by phencyclidine, ketamine and memantine	Excitatory; ↑ cation conductance
		Metabotropic subtypes	Inhibitory (presynaptic); ↓ Ca^{2+} conductance, ↓ cAMP Excitatory (postsynaptic); ↓ K^+ conductance; ↑ IP_3 and DAG
Glycine	Interneurons in spinal cord and brain stem	Single subtype; blocked by strychnine	Inhibitory; ↑ Cl⁻ conductance
Opioid peptides	Cell bodies at all levels	Three major subtypes: mu, delta, kappa	Inhibitory (presynaptic); ↓ Ca^{2+} conductance; ↓ cAMP Inhibitory (postsynaptic); ↑ K^+ conductance; ↓ cAMP

receptors are metabotropic. Dopamine exerts slow inhibitory actions at synapses in specific neuronal systems via G protein-coupled activation of potassium channels. The D_2 receptor is the main dopamine subtype in basal ganglia neurons, and it is widely distributed at the supraspinal level. In addition to the two receptors listed in Table 12–1, three other dopamine receptor subtypes have been identified (D_3, D_4, and D_5). Drugs affecting the activity of dopaminergic pathways include antipsychotics (e.g., **chlorpromazine**), CNS stimulants (e.g., **amphetamine**), and antiparkinsonism drugs (e.g., **levodopa**).

Norepinephrine

Noradrenergic neuron cell bodies are mainly located in the brain stem (locus ceruleus) and the lateral tegmental area of the pons (reticular formation). These neurons diverge to provide most regions of the CNS with diffuse noradrenergic input. All noradrenergic receptor subtypes are metabotropic. Inhibitory effects are caused by activation of α_2 receptors, which leads to an increase in potassium conductance. Excitatory effects are produced by both direct and indirect mechanisms. The direct mechanism involves the blockade of a potassium conductance that normally slows neuronal discharge. Depending on the type of neuron, this effect is mediated by either α_1 or β receptors. The indirect mechanism involves disinhibition; that is, inhibitory local circuit neurons are inhibited. Facilitation of excitatory synaptic transmission is in accordance with many of the behavioral processes thought to involve noradrenergic pathways (e.g., attention and arousal). CNS stimulants, monoamine oxidase inhibitors, and tricyclic antidepressants have important effects on the activity of noradrenergic pathways.

Serotonin

Most serotonin (5-hydroxytryptamine, 5-HT) pathways originate from cell bodies in the raphe or midline regions of the pons and upper brain stem; these pathways contain unmyelinated fibers that innervate most regions of the CNS. Multiple 5-HT receptor subtypes have been identified and, with the exception of the 5-HT_3 subtype, all are metabotropic. In most areas of the central nervous system, 5-HT has a strong inhibitory action. This action is mediated by 5-HT_{1A} receptors and is associated with membrane hyperpolarization caused by an increase in potassium conductance. In fact, 5-HT_{1A} receptors and $GABA_B$ receptors are both associated with the same family of potassium channels. The ionotropic 5-HT_3 receptor exerts a rapid excitatory action at a very limited number of sites in the CNS. Both excitatory and inhibitory actions can occur on the same neuron if appropriate receptors are present. Most of the agents used in the treatment of major depressive disorders affect serotonergic pathways (e.g., tricyclic antidepressants [TCAs], selective serotonin reuptake inhibitors [SSRIs]). The actions of some CNS stimulants and newer antipsychotic drugs may also be mediated via effects on serotonergic transmission. Reserpine, which may cause severe depression of mood, depletes vesicular stores of both serotonin and norepinephrine in CNS neurons. Other proposed regulatory functions of 5-HT–containing neurons include sleep, temperature, appetite, and neuroendocrine control.

Glutamic Acid (Glutamate)

Most neurons in the brain are excited by glutamic acid. This excitation is caused by the activation of both ionotropic and metabotropic receptors. The ionotropic receptors can be further divided into three subtypes on the basis of drugs that selectively activate them: kainate (KA), α-amino-3-hydroxy-5-methylisoxazole-4-propionate (AMPA), and N-methyl-D-aspartate (NMDA). The AMPA- and KA-activated channels are often referred to as non-NMDA channels and are permeable to sodium and potassium. The NMDA-activated channel is highly permeable to sodium, potassium, and calcium ions. NMDA receptors appear to play a role in synaptic plasticity related to learning and memory. **Memantine** is an NMDA antagonist used for treatment of Alzheimer's dementia. Excessive activation of NMDA receptors after neuronal injury may be responsible for cell death. Although clinical trials have been disappointing, the blockade of NMDA receptors has been shown to attenuate the neuronal damage caused by anoxia in experimental animals. Glutamate metabotropic receptor activation can result in G protein-coupled activation of phospholipase C or inhibition of adenylyl cyclase. Depending on the type of synapse, these receptors can initiate a slow postsynaptic excitation or a presynaptic inhibition.

GABA and Glycine

GABA is the primary neurotransmitter mediating IPSPs in neurons in the brain; it is also important in the spinal cord. The $GABA_A$ receptor is located on chloride ion channels and the binding of GABA opens the channel, hyperpolarizing the cell. $GABA_B$ receptors are coupled to G proteins that either activate potassium channels or inhibit calcium channels. Fast IPSPs are blocked by $GABA_A$ receptor antagonists, and slow IPSPs are blocked by $GABA_B$ receptor antagonists. A large majority of the local circuit neurons synthesize GABA, including neurons located in the dorsal horn of the spinal cord. Drugs that influence $GABA_A$ receptors include sedative-hypnotics (e.g., benzodiazepines, barbiturates) and some anticonvulsants (e.g., **gabapentin**, **vigabatrin**). $GABA_B$ receptors are activated by the drug **baclofen**, a very useful drug for the treatment of muscle spasticity (e.g., in cerebral palsy). Glycine receptors, which are more numerous in the gray matter of the spinal cord than in the brain, are blocked by **strychnine**, a spinal convulsant. Research evidence generally supports that glycine is released from spinal cord inhibitory local circuit neurons involved in postsynaptic inhibition.

Peptide Transmitters

Many peptides have been identified in the CNS, and some meet most or all of the criteria for acceptance as neurotransmitters. These peptides include opioid peptides (enkephalins, endorphins, dynorphins), neurotensin, substance P, somatostatin, cholecystokinin, vasoactive intestinal polypeptide, neuropeptide Y, and thyrotropin-releasing hormone. As in the peripheral autonomic nervous system, peptides often coexist with a conventional nonpeptide transmitter in the same neuron. The best defined peptide transmitters are the opioid peptides (beta-endorphin, met- and leu-enkephalin, and dynorphin), which are distributed at all levels of the neuraxis. The most important therapeutic actions of opioid analgesics (e.g., **morphine**) are mediated by receptors for these endogenous peptides. Substance P is a mediator of slow EPSPs in neurons involved in nociceptive sensory pathways in the spinal cord and brain stem. Peptide transmitters differ from nonpeptide transmitters in that (1) the peptides are synthesized in the cell body and transported to the nerve ending via axonal transport, and (2) no reuptake or specific enzyme mechanisms have been identified for terminating their actions.

Endocannabinoids

The primary psychoactive ingredient in marijuana or cannabis, Δ^9-tetrahydrocannabinol (Δ^9-THC), affects the brain mainly by activating a specific cannabinoid receptor, CB1. Several brain lipid derivatives (e.g., 2-arachidonyl-glycerol and anandamide) are the endogenous ligands for CB1 receptors. These ligands are not stored, as are classic neurotransmitters, but instead are rapidly synthesized in response to depolarization and consequent calcium influx. Endogenous cannabinoids are released postsynaptically after membrane depolarization but act presynaptically (retrograde transmission) to decrease transmitter release. Cannabinoids may affect memory, cognition, and pain perception by this mechanism.

Nitric Oxide

The gaseous substance nitric oxide (NO) is synthesized in many tissues in response to a variety of stimuli. The CNS contains a substantial amount of nitric oxide synthase (NOS) within certain classes of neurons. Neuronal NOS is an enzyme activated by calcium-calmodulin, and activation of NMDA receptors, which increases intracellular calcium, resulting in the generation of NO. While a physiologic role for nitric oxide has been clearly established for vascular and erectile smooth muscle, its role in synaptic transmission and synaptic plasticity remains controversial.

■ REHABILITATION FOCUS

Drugs acting in the CNS are the most widely used group of pharmacologic agents. These drugs can provide a wide range of therapeutic benefit, but, because of the organization of the CNS, they can also produce a wide range of adverse drug reactions. Drugs acting in the CNS can have effects (both positive and negative) at all three levels of the International Classification of Functioning, Disability and Health (ICF) Model of Disability: body function and structure, activity, and participation. For example, a benzodiazepine (e.g., **diazepam**), useful as a sleeping (hypnotic) agent and skeletal muscle relaxant, can impair motor function because of its GABAergic influence. This can have an effect on muscle activation, the ability to carry out basic motor functions, and the ability to participate in the responsibilities of life situations. On the other hand, a dopamine antagonist (e.g., **clozapine**) when used to treat schizophrenia, can have profound positive effects on an individual's ability to participate in his or her own responsibilities in life situations.

REFERENCES

Bettler B, et al: GABA$_B$ receptors: Drugs meet clones. *Curr Opin Neurobiol* 1998;8:345.

Conn PJ, Pin JP: Pharmacology and functions of metabotropic glutamate receptors. *Annu Rev Pharmacol Toxicol* 1997;37:205.

Costa E: From GABA$_A$ receptor diversity emerges a unified vision of GABAergic inhibition. *Annu Rev Pharmacol Toxicol* 1998;38:321.

Dingledine R, et al: The glutamate receptor ion channels. *Pharmacol Rev* 1999;51:7.

Hall ZW: *An Introduction to Molecular Neurobiology.* Sinauer, 1992.

Hokfelt T, et al: Neuropeptides—an overview. *Neuropharmacology* 2000;39:1337.

Laube B, et al: Modulation of glycine receptor function: A novel approach for therapeutic intervention at inhibitory synapses? *Trends Pharmacol Sci* 2002;23:519.

Martin GR, et al: The structure and signaling properties of 5-HT receptors: An endless diversity? *Trends Pharmacol Sci* 1998;19:2.

Miller RJ: Presynaptic receptors. *Annu Rev Pharmacol Toxicol* 1998;38:201.

Missale C, et al: Dopamine receptors: From structure to function. *Physiol Rev* 1998;78:189.

Nestler EJ, et al: *Molecular Neuropharmacology.* New York: McGraw-Hill, 2001.

Seal RP, Amara SG: Excitatory amino acid transporters: A family in flux. *Annu Rev Pharmacol Toxicol* 1999; 39:431.

Walmsley B, et al: Diversity of structure and function at mammalian central synapses. *Trends Neurosci* 1998; 21:81.

Wilson RI, Nicoll RA: Endocannabinoid signaling in the brain. *Science* 2002;296:678.

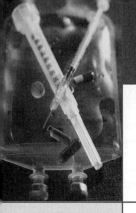

13

SEDATIVE-HYPNOTIC DRUGS

Assignment of a drug to the sedative-hypnotic class indicates that its major therapeutic use is to cause sedation (with concomitant relief of anxiety) or to encourage sleep. Because there is considerable chemical variation within this group, this drug classification is based on clinical uses rather than on similarities in chemical structure. Anxiety states and sleep disorders are common problems, and sedative-hypnotics are widely prescribed drugs worldwide. Drugs in this class include alcohols, benzodiazepines, barbiturates, carbamates, and several newer hypnotics, including eszopiclone, zaleplon, and zolpidem (Figure 13–1).

An effective sedative (anxiolytic) agent should reduce anxiety and exert a calming effect. The degree of central nervous system (CNS) depression caused by a sedative should be the minimum consistent with therapeutic efficacy. A hypnotic drug should produce drowsiness and encourage the onset and maintenance of a state of sleep. Hypnotic effects involve more pronounced depression of the CNS than sedation, and this is achieved with most drugs in this class simply by increasing the dose. Graded dose-dependent depression of CNS function is a characteristic of sedative-hypnotics. However, individual drugs differ in the relationship between the dose and the degree of CNS depression. Two examples of such dose-response relationships are shown in Figure 13–2. The linear slope for barbiturates means an increase in dose above that needed for hypnosis may lead to a state of general anesthesia. At still higher doses, these types of sedative-hypnotics may depress respiratory and vasomotor centers in the medulla, leading to coma and death. Deviation from a linear dose-response relationship, as shown for benzodiazepine drugs, will require much greater dosage increments in order to achieve CNS depression more profound than hypnosis. This greater margin of safety for benzodiazepines and the newer hypnotics (e.g., zolpidem) is an important reason for their widespread use to treat anxiety states and sleep disorders.

GENERAL PHARMACOKINETIC PROPERTIES

Lipid solubility plays a major role in determining the rate at which a particular sedative-hypnotic enters the CNS. Most of the sedative-hypnotic drugs are lipid soluble and are absorbed well from the gastrointestinal tract, with good distribution to the brain. This property is responsible for the rapid onset of CNS effects of triazolam, thiopental (Chapter 15), and the newer hypnotics. Oral absorption of **triazolam** and the newer hypnotics is extremely rapid, and that of **diazepam** and the active metabolite of clorazepate is more rapid than other commonly used

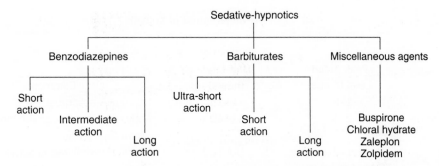

Figure 13–1. Drugs used as sedative-hypnotics. Benzodiazepine and barbiturate drug classes are further subdivided into short-, intermediate-, and long-acting groups depending on their respective half-lives.

benzodiazepines. **Clorazepate** is converted to its active form, **desmethyldiazepam** (nordiazepam), by acid hydrolysis in the stomach. Most of the barbiturates and other older sedative-hypnotics are absorbed rapidly into the blood following their oral administration.

All sedative-hypnotics cross the placental barrier during pregnancy. If sedative-hypnotics are given in the predelivery period, they may contribute to depression of neonatal vital functions. Sedative-hypnotics are also detectable in breast milk and may exert depressant effects in the nursing infant.

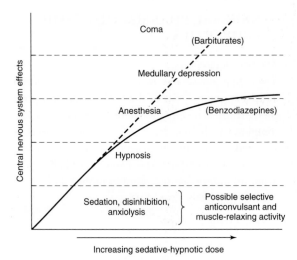

Figure 13–2. Dose-response curves demonstrating the relationships between dose of benzodiazepines and barbiturates and their CNS effects. Benzodiazepines have a higher therapeutic index than barbiturates.

Metabolic transformation to more water-soluble metabolites is necessary for clearance of sedative-hypnotics from the body. The microsomal drug-metabolizing enzyme systems of the liver are most important in this regard. Few sedative-hypnotics are excreted from the body in unchanged form, so elimination half-life depends mainly on the rate of metabolic transformation. Metabolic rates and pathways vary among different drugs. Many active benzodiazepines are converted initially to active metabolites with long half-lives. After several days of therapy with some drugs (e.g., diazepam, **flurazepam**), accumulation of active metabolites can lead to excessive sedation. Cumulative and residual effects appear to be less of a problem with **oxazepam** and **lorazepam**, which have shorter half-lives and are conjugated to form inactive metabolites. With the exception of **phenobarbital**, which is excreted partly unchanged in the urine (20 to 30% in humans), the barbiturates are also metabolized by hepatic enzymes. Zolpidem and zaleplon are rapidly metabolized to inactive metabolites by the liver and have very short elimination half-lives of 1.5 to 3.5 hours and 1 hour, respectively. Eszopiclone is metabolized more slowly and has a half-life of 6 hours. Dosage reductions of zolpidem and zaleplon are recommended in patients with hepatic dysfunction, in elderly patients, and in patients taking cimetidine. Drugs that induce hepatic cytochrome P450s may increase the clearance of eszopiclone, zaleplon, and zolpidem.

The duration of CNS actions of sedative-hypnotic drugs ranges from just a few hours (e.g., zaleplon < zolpidem = triazolam < **chloral hydrate**) to more than

Table 13–1.	Pharmacokinetic properties of benzodiazepines in humans		
Drug	Peak Blood Level (hours)	Elimination Half-Life[1] (hours)	Comments
Alprazolam	1–2	12–15	Rapid oral absorption
Chlordiazepoxide	2–4	15–40	Active metabolites; erratic bioavailability from IM injection
Clorazepate	1–2 (Nordiazepam)	50–100	Prodrug; hydrolyzed to active form (nordiazepam) in stomach
Diazepam	1–2	20–80	Active metabolites; erratic bioavailability from IM injection
Flurazepam	1–2	40–100	Active metabolites with long half-lives
Lorazepam	1–6	10–20	No active metabolites
Oxazepam	2–4	10–20	No active metabolites
Triazolam	1	2–3	Rapid onset; short duration of action

[1]Includes half-lives of major metabolites.

30 hours (e.g., **chlordiazepoxide**, clorazepate, diazepam, phenobarbital).

Some pharmacokinetic properties of selected benzodiazepines are listed in Table 13–1.

Factors Affecting Biodisposition

The biodisposition of sedative-hypnotics can be influenced by several factors, particularly alterations in hepatic function resulting from disease or drug-induced increases or decreases in microsomal enzyme activities (Chapter 3). In very old patients and in patients with severe liver disease, the elimination half-lives of these drugs are often increased significantly. In such cases, multiple normal doses of these sedative-hypnotics often result in excessive CNS effects.

The activity of hepatic microsomal drug-metabolizing enzymes may be increased in patients exposed to certain older sedative-hypnotics on a chronic basis (enzyme induction). Barbiturates (especially phenobarbital) are most likely to cause this effect, which may result in an increase in their hepatic metabolism as well as that of other drugs. Increased biotransformation of other pharmacologic agents as a result of enzyme induction by barbiturates is a potential mechanism

underlying drug interactions. In contrast, the benzodiazepines and the newer hypnotics do not change hepatic drug-metabolizing enzyme activity with continuous use.

GENERAL PHARMACODYNAMIC PROPERTIES

The benzodiazepines, the barbiturates, zolpidem and newer hypnotics, and many other drugs bind to molecular components of the GABA$_A$ receptor present in neuronal membranes in the CNS. This receptor complex, which functions as a chloride ion channel, is activated by the inhibitory neurotransmitter gamma-aminobutyric acid (GABA) (Chapter 12). GABA is the major inhibitory neurotransmitter in the CNS.

Major Drug Groups

Benzodiazepines
Benzodiazepines potentiate GABAergic inhibition at all level of the neuraxis, including the spinal cord, hypothalamus, hippocampus, substantia nigra, cerebellar cortex, and cerebral cortex. Receptors (or binding sites)

for benzodiazepines form part of the GABA$_A$ receptor-chloride ion channel molecular complex. The GABA$_A$ receptor exists in several different forms (isoforms), consisting of alpha, beta, and gamma subunits. Benzodiazepines bind to several of these GABA$_A$ receptor isoforms. Benzodiazepines appear to increase the efficiency of GABAergic synaptic inhibition. The benzodiazepines do not substitute for GABA but appear to enhance GABA's effects without directly activating GABA receptors or opening the associated chloride channels (Figure 13–3). The enhancement in chloride ion conductance induced by the interaction of benzodiazepines with GABA$_A$ receptors takes the form of an increase in the *frequency* of channel-opening events. This action of benzodiazepines can be antagonized by the drug flumazenil (discussed below).

Barbiturates

Barbiturates also facilitate the actions of GABA at multiple sites in the CNS, but, in contrast to benzodiazepines, they appear to increase the *duration* of the GABA-gated chloride channel openings. At high concentrations, the barbiturates may also be GABAmimetic, directly activating chloride channels. These effects involve a binding site or sites distinct from the benzodiazepine binding sites. The actions of barbiturates are not antagonized by flumazenil. Barbiturates are less selective in their actions than benzodiazepines, since they also depress the actions of excitatory neurotransmitters (e.g., glutamic acid) and exert nonsynaptic membrane effects in parallel with their effects on GABA neurotransmission. These multiple sites of action of barbiturates may be the basis for their ability to induce full surgical anesthesia (Chapter 15) and for their more pronounced central depressant effects (which result in their low margin of safety) compared to benzodiazepines.

Newer Hypnotic Drugs

The hypnotics **eszopiclone**, **zolpidem**, and **zaleplon** are not benzodiazepines (BZ) but appear to exert their CNS effects via interaction with certain benzodiazepine-binding sites, classified as BZ$_1$ subtypes. In contrast to benzodiazepines, zolpidem and other newer hypnotics bind more selectively because these drugs only interact

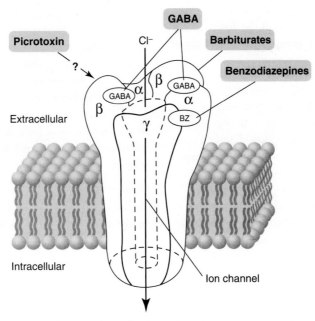

Figure 13–3. Mechanism of action of sedative-hypnotics. (Reproduced, with permission, from Zorumski CF, Isenburg KE: Insights into the structure and function of GABA-benzodiazepine receptors: Ion channels and psychiatry. Am J Psychiatry 1991;148:162.)

with $GABA_A$ receptor isoforms that contain α_1 subunits. Their CNS depressant effects are antagonized by flumazenil.

Receptor-Ligand Interactions

Two major types of therapeutic ligand-benzodiazepine binding site interactions have been reported: (1) *Agonists* facilitate GABA actions, and this occurs at multiple BZ-binding sites in the case of the benzodiazepines. The nonbenzodiazepines eszopiclone, zolpidem, and zaleplon are selective agonists at the BZ_1-binding site. (2) *Antagonists* are typified by the synthetic benzodiazepine derivative flumazenil, which blocks the actions of benzodiazepines but does not antagonize the actions of barbiturates or ethanol.

Benzodiazepine Agonists

Organ Level Effects

The CNS effects of most sedative-hypnotics depend on dose, as shown in Figure 13–2. These effects range from sedation and relief of anxiety (anxiolysis), through hypnosis (facilitation of sleep), to anesthesia and coma. Depressant effects are additive when two or more drugs are given together. The steepness of the dose-response curve varies among drug groups; those with flatter curves, such as benzodiazepines, are safer for clinical use.

Sedation

Benzodiazepines, barbiturates, and most older sedative-hypnotic drugs exert calming effects with concomitant reduction of anxiety at relatively low doses. In most cases, however, the anxiolytic actions of sedative-hypnotics are accompanied by some decremental effects on psychomotor and cognitive functions. In experimental animal models, sedative-hypnotic drugs are able to disinhibit punishment-suppressed behavior. This disinhibition has been equated with antianxiety effects of sedative-hypnotics, and it is not a characteristic of all drugs that have sedative effects (e.g., antidepressants). However, the disinhibition of previously suppressed behavior may be more related to behavioral disinhibitory effects of sedative-hypnotics, including euphoria, impaired judgment, and loss of self-control, which can occur at dosages in the range of those used for management of anxiety. The benzodiazepines also exert dose-dependent anterograde amnesic effects (inability to remember events occurring during the drug's duration of action).

Hypnosis

All sedative-hypnotics will induce sleep if high enough doses are given. The effects of sedative-hypnotics on the stages of sleep depend on several factors, including the specific drug, the dose, and the frequency of its administration. The effects of benzodiazepines and older sedative-hypnotics on patterns of normal sleep are as follows: (1) the latency of sleep onset (time to fall asleep) is decreased; (2) the duration of stage 2 nonrapid eye movement (NREM) sleep is increased; (3) the duration of rapid eye movement (REM) sleep is decreased; and (4) the duration of stage 4 NREM slow-wave sleep is decreased. Zolpidem also decreases REM sleep but has minimal effect on slow-wave sleep. Eszopiclone and zaleplon decrease the latency of sleep onset with little effect on NREM or REM sleep.

More rapid onset of sleep and prolongation of stage 2 are presumably clinically useful effects. However, the significance of sedative-hypnotic drug effects on REM and slow-wave sleep is not clear. Deliberate interruption of REM sleep may cause anxiety and irritability followed by a rebound increase in REM sleep in individuals taking sedative-hypnotics. A similar pattern of "REM rebound" can be detected following abrupt cessation of drug treatment with sedative-hypnotics, especially when drugs with short durations of action are used at high doses. The use of sedative-hypnotics for more than 1 to 2 weeks leads to some tolerance to their effects on sleep patterns.

Anesthesia

As shown in Figure 13–2, certain sedative-hypnotics in high doses will depress the CNS to the point known as stage III of general anesthesia (see Chapter 15). However, the suitability of a particular agent as an adjunct in anesthesia depends mainly on the physicochemical properties that determine its rapidity of onset and duration of effect. Among the barbiturates, thiopental and **methohexital** are very lipid soluble, penetrating brain tissue rapidly following intravenous administration, a characteristic favoring their use for induction of anesthesia. Rapid tissue redistribution accounts for the short duration of action of these drugs, a feature useful in recovery from anesthesia.

Benzodiazepines, including diazepam, lorazepam, and **midazolam**, are used intravenously in anesthesia (Chapter 15), often in combination with other agents. Not surprisingly, benzodiazepines given in large doses as adjuncts to general anesthetics may contribute to a persistent postanesthetic respiratory depression. This is probably related to their relatively long half-lives and the formation of active metabolites.

Anticonvulsant Effects

Most of the sedative-hypnotics are capable of inhibiting the development and spread of epileptic activity in the CNS. Some selectivity exists in that some members of the group can exert anticonvulsant effects without marked CNS depression (although psychomotor function may be impaired). Several benzodiazepines, including **clonazepam**, diazepam, and lorazepam, are sufficiently selective to be clinically useful in the management of seizure states (see Chapter 14). Of the barbiturates, phenobarbital and **metharbital** (converted to phenobarbital in the body) are effective in the treatment of generalized tonic-clonic seizures. The newer hypnotics eszopiclone, zaleplon, and zolpidem lack anticonvulsant activity.

Muscle Relaxation

Some sedative-hypnotics, particularly members of the carbamate and benzodiazepine groups, exert inhibitory effects on polysynaptic reflexes and internuncial transmission, and at high doses may also depress transmission at the skeletal neuromuscular junction. These somewhat selective actions have been used for relaxing voluntary muscle in joint disease or muscle spasm (see section on Clinical Uses below). None of the newer hypnotics has significant muscle-relaxing activity.

Effects on Respiration and Cardiovascular Function

At hypnotic doses in healthy patients, the effects of sedative-hypnotics on respiration are comparable to changes during natural sleep. However, even at therapeutic doses, sedative-hypnotics can produce significant respiratory depression in patients with pulmonary disease. Effects on respiration are dose related, and depression of the medullary respiratory center is the usual cause of death due to overdose of sedative-hypnotics.

At doses up to those causing hypnosis, no significant effects on the cardiovascular system are observed in healthy patients. However, in hypovolemic states, heart failure, and other diseases that impair cardiovascular function, normal doses of sedative-hypnotics may cause cardiovascular depression, probably as a result of actions on the medullary vasomotor centers. At toxic doses, myocardial contractility and vascular tone may both be depressed by central and peripheral effects, leading to circulatory collapse. Respiratory and cardiovascular effects are more marked when sedative-hypnotics are given intravenously.

Tolerance and Dependence

Tolerance (decreased responsiveness to a drug following repeated exposure) is a common feature of sedative-hypnotic use. Tolerence may result in an increase in the dose needed to maintain symptomatic improvement or to promote sleep. Partial cross-tolerance also occurs between the sedative-hypnotics described here and with **ethanol**—a feature of great clinical importance, as explained below. The mechanisms responsible for tolerance to sedative-hypnotics are not well understood. An increase in the rate of drug metabolism (metabolic tolerance) may be partly responsible in the case of chronic administration of barbiturates, but changes in responsiveness of the CNS (pharmacodynamic tolerance) are of greater importance for most sedative-hypnotics. In the case of benzodiazepines, the development of tolerance in animals is associated with down-regulation of brain benzodiazepine receptors. Tolerance has been reported to occur with the extended use of zolpidem. Minimal tolerance has been observed with the use of zaleplon or eszopiclone.

The perceived desirable properties of relief of anxiety, euphoria, disinhibition, and promotion of sleep have led to the compulsive misuse of virtually all sedative-hypnotics. For this reason, most sedative-hypnotic drugs are classified as Schedule III or Schedule IV drugs for prescribing purposes. The consequences of abuse of these agents can be defined in both psychologic and physiologic terms. The psychologic component may initially parallel simple neurotic behavior patterns difficult to differentiate from those of the inveterate coffee drinker or cigarette smoker. When the pattern of sedative-hypnotic use becomes compulsive, more serious complications develop, including physiologic dependence and tolerance.

Physiologic dependence can be described as an altered physiologic state that requires continuous drug administration to prevent the appearance of an **abstinence** or **withdrawal syndrome**. In the case of sedative-hypnotics, the withdrawal syndrome is characterized by states of increased anxiety, insomnia, and CNS excitability that may progress to convulsions. Most sedative-hypnotics, including benzodiazepines and ethanol, are capable of causing physiologic dependence when used on a chronic basis. However, the severity of withdrawal symptoms differs between individual drugs and depends also on the magnitude of the doses used immediately prior to cessation of use. When higher doses of sedative-hypnotics are used, abrupt withdrawal leads to more serious withdrawal signs. Differences in the severity of withdrawal symptoms between individual sedative-hypnotics relate in part to half-life, since drugs with long half-lives are eliminated slowly enough to accomplish gradual withdrawal with few physical symptoms. The

use of drugs with very short half-lives for hypnotic effects may lead to signs of withdrawal even between doses. For example, triazolam, a benzodiazepine with a half-life of about 4 hours, has been reported to cause daytime anxiety when used to treat sleep disorders. The abrupt cessation of zolpidem, zaleplon, or eszopiclone may also result in withdrawal symptoms though usually of lesser intensity than those seen with benzodiazepines.

Benzodiazepine Antagonists: Flumazenil

Flumazenil is a benzodiazepine derivative with high affinity for the benzodiazepine receptor that acts as a *competitive antagonist*. It is the only benzodiazepine receptor antagonist available for clinical use at present. It blocks many of the actions of benzodiazepines (and the newer hypnotics such as zolpidem) but does not antagonize the CNS effects of other sedative-hypnotics (barbiturates, alcohols), opioids, or general anesthetics. Flumazenil is approved for use in reversing the CNS depressant effects of benzodiazepine overdose and to hasten recovery following use of these drugs in anesthetic and diagnostic procedures. While the drug reverses the sedative effects of benzodiazepines, antagonism of benzodiazepine-induced respiratory depression is less predictable. When given

---

Box 13–1. Buspirone

Buspirone has selective anxiolytic effects, and its pharmacologic characteristics are quite different from those of drugs described in this chapter. Buspirone relieves anxiety without causing marked sedative or euphoric effects, and the drug has no hypnotic, anticonvulsant, or muscle relaxant properties. Buspirone may exert its anxiolytic effects by acting as a partial agonist at brain 5-HT$_{1A}$ receptors, but it also has affinity for brain dopamine D$_2$ receptors. Buspirone-treated patients show no rebound anxiety or withdrawal signs on abrupt discontinuance. Buspirone has minimal abuse liability. In marked contrast to the benzodiazepines, the anxiolytic effects of buspirone may take more than a week to become established, making the drug unsuitable for management of acute anxiety states.

The drug is used in generalized anxiety states but is not very effective in panic disorders.

Buspirone causes less psychomotor impairment than diazepam and does not affect driving skills. The drug does not potentiate the CNS depressant effects of conventional sedative-hypnotic drugs, ethanol, or antidepressants, and elderly patients do not appear to be more sensitive to its actions. Tachycardia, palpitations, nervousness, gastrointestinal distress, and paresthesias may occur more frequently than with benzodiazepines. Buspirone also causes a dose-dependent pupillary constriction. Blood pressure may be elevated in patients receiving monoamine oxidase (MAO) inhibitors.

Box 13–2. Hangover Syndrome and Chronic Use of Sedative Hypnotics

Although the benzodiazepines continue to be widely used in the treatment of anxiety states and for insomnia, their adverse effects include daytime sedation and drowsiness (hangover syndrome), synergistic depression of the CNS with other drugs (especially alcohol), and the possibility of psychologic and physiologic dependence with repeated use. Anxiolytic drugs that act through non-GABAergic systems might have a reduced propensity for such actions. Several non-benzodiazepines, including buspirone, have such characteristics. In addition, the newer hypnotics zolpidem and zaleplon are more selective in their central actions even though they appear to act through benzodiazepine receptors.

---

intravenously, flumazenil acts rapidly but has a short half-life (0.7 to 1.3 hours) owing to rapid hepatic clearance. Since all benzodiazepines have a longer duration of action than flumazenil, sedation commonly recurs, requiring repeated administration of the antagonist.

Adverse effects of flumazenil include agitation, confusion, dizziness, and nausea. Flumazenil may cause a severe precipitated abstinence syndrome in patients who have developed physiologic benzodiazepine dependence. Transient improvement in mental status has been reported with flumazenil when used in patients with hepatic encephalopathy.

CLINICAL USES

Treatment of Anxiety States

The psychologic, behavioral, and physiologic responses that characterize anxiety can take many forms. Typically, the awareness of anxiety is accompanied by enhanced vigilance, motor tension, and autonomic hyperactivity. In many cases, anxiety is secondary to organic disease states—for example, acute myocardial infarction, angina pectoris, or gastrointestinal ulcers—which themselves require specific therapy. Another class of secondary anxiety states (situational anxiety) results from circumstances that may have to be dealt with only once or a few times, including anticipation of frightening medical or dental procedures and family illness or tragedy. Even though situational anxiety tends to be self-limiting, the short-term use of sedative-hypnotics is often employed for the treatment of this and certain disease-associated anxiety states. Similarly, the use of a sedative-hypnotic as premedication prior to surgery or some unpleasant medical procedure is rational and proper (Table 13–2).

Table 13–2.	Clinical uses of sedative-hypnotics

For relief of anxiety
For insomnia
For sedation and amnesia before medical and surgical procedures
For treatment of epilepsy and seizure states
As a component of balanced anesthesia (intravenous administration)
For control of ethanol or other sedative-hypnotic withdrawal states
For muscle relaxation in specific neuromuscular disorders

The benzodiazepines continue to be widely used for the management of anxiety states. **Alprazolam** and clonazepam are thought to have greater efficacy than other benzodiazepines in panic and phobic disorders. The choice of benzodiazepines for anxiety is based on several sound pharmacologic principles: (1) a relatively high therapeutic index (Figure 13–2), plus availability of flumazenil for treatment of overdose; (2) a low risk of drug interactions based on liver enzyme induction; (3) slow elimination rates, which may favor persistence of useful CNS effects.

Disadvantages of the benzodiazepines include the risk of dependence, the formation of active metabolites, amnestic effects, and their high cost. In addition, the benzodiazepines exert additive CNS depression when administered with other drugs, including ethanol. Patients should be warned of this possibility to avoid impairment of performance of any task requiring mental alertness and motor coordination.

In the treatment of generalized anxiety disorders, panic disorders, and certain phobias, newer antidepressants such as **paroxetine** and **venlafaxine** are now considered by many authorities to be drugs of first choice (see Chapter 19). However, these agents have minimal effectiveness in acute anxiety states.

Sedative-hypnotics for the treatment of anxiety should be used with appropriate caution so as to minimize adverse effects. A prescribed dose should not impair mentation or motor functions during waking hours. Some patients may tolerate the drug better if most of the daily dose is given at bedtime, with smaller doses during the day. Typically, prescriptions are written for short periods, since there is little justification for long-term therapy. Health-care providers should make an effort to assess the efficacy of drug therapy from the patient's subjective responses. People taking sedatives should be cautioned about the consumption of alcohol and the concurrent use of over-the-counter medications containing antihistaminic or anticholinergic drugs or alcohol.

Alternatives to the previously mentioned anxiolytic drugs are buspirone (Box 13–1) and beta-blocking drugs. Beta-blocking drugs (e.g., propranolol) may be used as antianxiety agents in situations such as performance anxiety. The sympathetic nervous system overactivity associated with anxiety appears to be satisfactorily relieved by the β blockers, and a slight improvement in the nonsomatic components of anxiety may also occur. Adverse CNS effects of propranolol include lethargy, vivid dreams, and a decreased cardiac response to exercise.

Treatment of Sleep Problems

Nonpharmacologic therapies that are useful for sleep problems include proper diet and exercise, avoiding stimulants before retiring, ensuring a comfortable sleeping environment, and retiring at a regular time each night. In some cases, however, the patient will need and should be given a sedative-hypnotic for a limited period. It should be noted that the abrupt discontinuance of most drugs in this class can lead to rebound insomnia.

Benzodiazepines are useful in primary insomnia and for the management of certain other sleep disorders. The drug selected should be one that provides sleep of fairly rapid onset (decreased sleep latency) and sufficient duration, with minimal "hangover" effects (Box 13–2) such as drowsiness, dysphoria, and mental or motor depression the following day. Older nonbenzodiazepine drugs such as chloral hydrate, secobarbital, and pentobarbital continue to be used, but benzodiazepines or one of the newer hypnotics are generally preferred. Daytime sedation is more common with benzodiazepines that have slow elimination rates (e.g., lorazepam) and those that are biotransformed to active metabolites (e.g., flurazepam). Anterograde amnesia occurs to some degree with all hypnotic benzodiazepines. If hypnotics are used nightly, tolerance can occur, which may lead to dose increases by the patient to produce the desired effect. Eszopiclone, zolpidem, and zaleplon have efficacies similar to those of the hypnotic benzodiazepines but cause less daytime cognitive impairment than most benzodiazepines.

Zolpidem is currently the most frequently prescribed hypnotic drug in the United States. Zaleplon acts rapidly, and because of its short half-life, the drug appears to have value in the management of

Table 13–3. Dosages of drugs used commonly for sedation and hypnosis

Sedation		Hypnosis	
Drug	**Dosage (mg)**	**Drug**	**Dosage (mg) (at bedtime)**
Alprazolam	0.25–0.5, 2–3 times daily	Chloral hydrate	500–1000
Buspirone	5–10, 2–3 times daily	Estazolam	0.5–2
Chlordiazepoxide	10–20, 2–3 times daily	Eszopiclone	1–3
Clorazepate	5.0–7.5, twice daily	Flurazepam	15–30
Diazepam	5, twice daily	Lorazepam	2–4
Halazepam	20–40, 3–4 times daily	Quazepam	7.5–15
Lorazepam	1–2, once or twice daily	Secobarbital	100–200
Oxazepam	15–30, 3–4 times daily	Temazepam	7.5–30
Phenobarbital	15–30, 2–3 times daily	Triazolam	0.125–0.5
		Zaleplon	5–20
		Zolpidem	5–10

patients who awaken early in the sleep cycle. The drugs commonly used for sedation and hypnosis are listed in Table 13–3 together with recommended doses.

Other Therapeutic Uses

Table 13–2 summarizes several other important clinical uses of drugs in the sedative-hypnotic class. Drugs used in the management of seizure disorders and as intravenous agents in anesthesia are discussed in Chapters 14 and 15. For sedative and possible amnestic effects during medical or surgical procedures such as endoscopy (e.g., bronchoscopy), as well as for premedication prior to anesthesia, formulations of shorter-acting drugs are preferred. During withdrawal from physiologic dependence on ethanol or other sedative-hypnotics, long-acting drugs such as chlordiazepoxide, diazepam, or, to a lesser extent, phenobarbital are administered in progressively decreasing doses. **Meprobamate** and, more recently, the benzodiazepines have frequently been used as central muscle relaxants, although evidence for general efficacy without accompanying sedation is lacking. A possible exception is diazepam, which has useful relaxant

effects in skeletal muscle spasticity of central origin (Chapter 33).

ADVERSE EFFECTS

Psychomotor Dysfunction

Many of the common adverse effects of drugs in this class result from dose-related depression of CNS functions. Relatively low doses may lead to daytime drowsiness, impaired judgment, and diminished motor skills, sometimes with a significant impact on driving ability, job performance, and personal relationships. These adverse effects are more common with benzodiazepines that have active metabolites with long half-lives (e.g., diazepam, flurazepam). Short-acting hypnotics, especially triazolam, may cause daytime anxiety and amnesia. Anterograde amnesia may occur with benzodiazepines when used at high dosage; they can significantly impair the ability to learn new information, particularly that involving effortful cognitive processes, while leaving the retrieval of previously learned information intact. This effect is utilized to clinical advantage in uncomfortable procedures (e.g., endoscopy) since the appropriate dose leaves the patient able to cooperate during the procedure but amnesic regarding it afterward. The criminal use of benzodiazepines in cases of "date rape" is based on their dose-dependent amnestic effects. Hangover effects are not uncommon following use of hypnotic drugs with long elimination half-lives. Because elderly patients are more sensitive to the effects of sedative-hypnotics, doses approximately half of those used in younger adults are safer and usually as effective. Excessive daytime sedation has been shown to increase the risk of falls and fractures in elderly patients. The most common reversible cause of confusional states in the elderly is overuse of sedative-hypnotics. At higher doses, toxicity may present as lethargy or a state of exhaustion or, alternatively, in the form of gross symptoms equivalent to those of ethanol intoxication. An increased sensitivity to sedative-hypnotics is more common in patients with cardiovascular disease, respiratory disease, or hepatic impairment, and in older patients. Sedative-hypnotics can exacerbate breathing problems in patients with chronic pulmonary disease and in those with symptomatic sleep apnea. The extensive clinical use of triazolam has led to reports of serious CNS effects including behavioral disinhibition, delirium, aggression, and violence. While behavioral disinhibition may occur with sedative-hypnotic drugs, it does not appear to be more prevalent with triazolam than with other benzodiazepines. Disinhibitory reactions during benzodiazepine treatment are more clearly associated with the use of very high doses and the patient's pretreatment level of hostility.

Overdosage

Sedative-hypnotics are the drugs most frequently involved in deliberate overdoses; in part because of their general availability as very commonly prescribed pharmacologic agents. Overdosage can cause severe respiratory and cardiovascular depression; these potentially lethal effects are more likely to occur with alcohols, barbiturates, and carbamates than with benzodiazepines. Management of intoxication requires maintenance of a patent airway and ventilatory support. Flumazenil may reverse CNS depressant effects of benzodiazepines, zolpidem, and zaleplon but has no beneficial action in overdosage with other sedative-hypnotics.

Other Adverse Effects

Adverse effects of the sedative-hypnotics that are not related to their CNS actions occur infrequently. Hypersensitivity reactions, including skin rashes, occur only occasionally with most drugs of this class. Reports of teratogenicity leading to fetal deformation following use of certain benzodiazepines justify caution in the use of these drugs during pregnancy. Barbiturates may precipitate acute intermittent porphyria in susceptible patients.

Alterations in Drug Response

Depending on the dosage and the duration of use, tolerance occurs in varying degrees to many of the pharmacologic effects of sedative-hypnotics. However, it should not be assumed that the degree of tolerance achieved is identical for all pharmacologic effects. There is evidence that the lethal dose range is not altered significantly by the chronic use of sedative-hypnotics. Cross-tolerance between the different sedative-hypnotics, including ethanol, can lead to an unsatisfactory therapeutic response when standard doses of a drug are used in a patient with a recent history of excessive use of these agents. However, there have been few reports of tolerance development when zolpidem or zaleplon was used for less than 4 weeks.

With the chronic use of sedative-hypnotics, especially if doses are increased, a state of physiologic dependence can occur. This may develop to a degree unparalleled by any other drug group, including the opioids. Withdrawal from a sedative-hypnotic in a dependent person can have severe and life-threatening manifestations. Withdrawal symptoms range from restlessness, anxiety, weakness, and orthostatic hypotension to hyperactive reflexes, generalized seizures, and death. The severity of withdrawal symptoms depends to a large extent on the dosage range used immediately prior to discontinuance but also on the particular drug. Symptoms of withdrawal are usually more severe following discontinuance of sedative-hypnotics with shorter half-lives. Eszopiclone, zolpidem, and zaleplon appear to be exceptions to this because withdrawal symptoms are minimal following abrupt discontinuance of these newer agents. Symptoms are less pronounced with the long-acting drugs, which may partly accomplish their own "tapered" withdrawal by virtue of their slow elimination. Cross-dependence, defined as the ability of one drug to suppress abstinence symptoms from discontinuance of another drug, is quite marked among sedative-hypnotics. This provides the rationale for therapeutic regimens in the management of withdrawal states: longer-acting drugs such as chlordiazepoxide, diazepam, and phenobarbital can be used to alleviate withdrawal symptoms of shorter acting drugs, including ethanol.

Drug Interactions

The most frequent drug interactions involving sedative-hypnotics are interactions with other CNS depressant drugs, leading to additive effects. This occurs when sedative-hypnotics are used with other drugs in the class as well as with alcoholic beverages, antihistamines, antipsychotic drugs, opioid analgesics, and tricyclic antidepressants. It should be noted that many oral suspensions and solutions, including over-the-counter cough syrups, contain high concentrations of ethanol.

■ REHABILITATION FOCUS

The prevalence of the use of sedative-hypnotics is high in patients undergoing rehabilitation, although these drugs (with the exception of diazepam) are not used to influence musculoskeletal or other somatic disorders directly. Patients involved in rehabilitation programs may experience increased levels of anxiety related to their physical state of health and well-being. Additionally, hospitalized patients or patients in nursing homes or other long-term care facilities may require some type of sedative-hypnotic for sleep disturbances.

The administration of sedative-hypnotics can have varied clinical consequences. The use of these drugs as antianxiety agents may be beneficial during therapy sessions if they result in the patient being calm and relaxed. However, if their use produces significant CNS depressant effects, therapy sessions requiring active participation by the patient such as gait training or motor control training may be unproductive and potentially hazardous. Sedative-hypnotic use is associated with falls and subsequent trauma especially in older adults.

The use of sedative-hypnotics by patients who are involved in rehabilitation programs may interfere with outcomes at the body function and structure, activity, and participation levels of disability.

■ CLINICAL RELEVANCE FOR REHABILITATION

Adverse Drug Reactions
- Sedation
- Musculoskeletal and other somatic effects

Effects Interfering with Rehabilitation
- Decreased arousal or alertness
- Motor control dysfunction
  - Weakness, increased response time, altered central processing
  - Impaired functional ability

Possible Therapy Solutions
- Explore options with physician regarding the risks and benefits of the medication.
- Schedule therapy when drug levels are the lowest in the system if excessive hangover or sedative effects are problematic.
  - Note: newer hypnotics do not produce excessive hangover effects. Also, for chronic anxiety conditions, antidepressants that are nonsedating like the selective serotonin reuptake inhibitors (SSRIs) may be more appropriate drugs (Chapter 19).

PROBLEM-ORIENTED PATIENT STUDY

Brief History: The patient is a 72-year-old male with a primary diagnosis of lumbar strain secondary to lifting a large generator during an electricity outage associated with a recent tropical hurricane. The patient was initially seen in a QuickCare facility followed by examination by an orthopedic physician who recommended a magnetic resonance image (MRI). Results of the MRI were negative. The orthopedic physician recommended conservative treatment to determine if the patient would respond. The patient was referred to physical therapy for evaluation and treatment as indicated.

Current Status and Drug Therapy: Upon initial examination the patient demonstrated a forward flexed posture with limited trunk range of motion in all planes with pain at end range. The patient had tenderness in the low back paraspinal musculature upon palpation, left more than right. At the activity level, the patient had limited function with sit-to-stand, bed mobility, and stairs, he complained of significant pain with all of these activities. At the participation level, the patient stated he was unable to assist with the clean up of his home and property, and that he felt very useless because he had to rely on others to take care of these issues. He stated this made him very anxious and unable to sleep at night. He stated he was currently taking diazepam at night occasionally to help him sleep and have a restful night. He stated this was medication the QuickCare physician had given him initially and he found it helped him sleep.

Rehabilitation Setting: The patient began a physical therapy treatment intervention consisting of electrical stimulation and thermal pack for pain relief, manual therapy, and therapeutic exercise. On several occasions, the physical therapist noted that when the patient came to therapy early in the morning, he was less attentive to his exercise regimen and seemed very tired. The therapist also noted that he required more time to answer questions and seemed confused at times. Concerned,

the physical therapist questioned him about this behavior. The patient stated that he was sleepy and it was hard for him to concentrate.

Problem/Clinical Options: The therapist questioned the patient again about the medications he was taking, and it became apparent that on the occasions when he had these signs and symptoms, he had taken diazepam the night before to help him sleep and have a restful night. Diazepam has a half-life of approximately 43 hours. Because of the sedative properties of benzodiazepines, it was hypothesized that the patient was having a hangover effect associated with the long half-life of the drug (Box 13–2).

Continued Intervention: The patient was encouraged to contact his regular physician and describe his current problems associated with his sleep disturbance. In the meantime, he was also encouraged to try reducing or eliminating this medication at night for sleep. He was informed that this medication could cause hangover effects such as those he was experiencing even during waking hours, and that these effects could cause possible serious consequences since he was driving himself to therapy.

Outcome: The patient contacted his regular physician, who instructed him not to take this medication for sleeping at night but instead to try other nonpharmacologic therapies including avoiding stimulants before retiring, ensuring a comfortable sleeping environment, and retiring at a regular time each night. The physician also instructed him to take, if needed, an over-the-counter analgesic such as ibuprofen or acetaminophen prior to retiring. The patient followed these recommendations and reported that he was able to get a restful night's sleep and had no more episodes of confusion or lethargy in the morning. The patient continued with his physical therapy program and was eventually discharged from therapy with all goals achieved.

PREPARATIONS AVAILABLE

Benzodiazepines

Alprazolam (generic, Xanax)
Oral: 0.25-, 0.5-, 1-, 2-mg tablets; 0.1, 1 mg/mL solution

Chlordiazepoxide (generic, Librium)
Oral: 5-, 10-, 25-mg capsules; 10-, 25-mg tablets
Parenteral: 100-mg powder for injection

Clonazepam (Klonopin)
Oral: 0.5-, 1-, 2-mg tablets

Clorazepate (generic, Tranxene)
Oral: 3.75-, 7.5-, 15-mg tablets and capsules
Oral sustained release: 11.25-, 22.5-mg tablets

Diazepam (generic, Valium)
Oral: 2-, 5-, 10-mg tablets; 1, 5 mg/mL solutions
Parenteral: 5 mg/mL for injection

Estazolam (generic, ProSom)
Oral: 1-, 2-mg tablets

Flurazepam (generic, Dalmane)
Oral: 15-, 30-mg capsules

Halazepam (Paxipam)
Oral: 20-, 40-mg tablets

Lorazepam (generic, Ativan, Alzapam)
Oral: 0.5-, 1-, 2-mg tablets; 2 mg/mL solution
Parenteral: 2, 4 mg/mL for injection

Midazolam (Versed)
Oral: 2 mg/mL syrup
Parenteral: 1, 5 mg/mL in 1-, 2-, 5-, 10-mL vials for injection

Oxazepam (generic, Serax)
Oral: 10-, 15-, 30-mg capsules, 15-mg tablets

Quazepam (Doral)
Oral: 7.5-, 15-mg tablets

Temazepam (generic, Restoril)
Oral: 7.5-, 15-, 30-mg capsules

Triazolam (generic, Halcion)
Oral: 0.125-, 0.25-mg tablets

Benzodiazepine Antagonist

Flumazenil (Romazicon)
Parenteral: 0.1 mg/mL for IV injection

Barbiturates

Amobarbital (Amytal)
Parenteral: powder in 250-, 500-mg vials to reconstitute for injection

Pentobarbital (generic, Nembutal Sodium)
Oral: 50-, 100-mg capsules; 4 mg/mL elixir
Rectal: 30-, 60-, 120-, 200-mg suppositories
Parenteral: 50 mg/mL for injection

Phenobarbital (generic, Luminal Sodium)
Oral: 15-, 16-, 30-, 60-, 90-, 100-mg tablets; 16-mg capsules; 15, 20 mg/5 mL elixirs
Parenteral: 30, 60, 65, 130 mg/mL for injection

Secobarbital (generic, Seconal)
Oral: 100-mg capsules

Miscellaneous Drugs

Buspirone (BuSpar)
Oral: 5-, 10-, 15-mg tablets

Chloral hydrate (generic, Aquachloral Supprettes)
Oral: 500-mg capsules; 250, 500 mg/5 mL syrups
Rectal: 324-, 500-, 648-mg suppositories

Eszopiclone (Lunesta)
Oral: 1-, 2-, 3-mg tablets

Ethchlorvynol (Placidyl)
Oral: 200-, 500-, 750-mg capsules

Hydroxyzine (generic, Atarax, Vistaril)
Oral: 10-, 25-, 50-, 100-mg tablets; 25-, 50-, 100-mg capsules; 10 mg/5 mL syrup; 25 mg/5 mL suspension
Parenteral: 25, 50 mg/mL for injection

Meprobamate (generic, Equanil, Miltown)
Oral: 200-, 400-mg tablets
Oral sustained release: 200-, 400-mg capsules

Paraldehyde (generic)
Oral, rectal liquids: 1g/ml

Zaleplon (Sonata)
Oral: 5-, 10-mg capsules

Zolpidem (Ambien)
Oral: 5-, 10-mg tablets

REFERENCES

Pharmacology

Bateson AN: The benzodiazepine site of the GABA A receptor: An old target with new potential? *Sleep Med* 2004;5(Suppl 1):S9.

Blednov YA, et al: Deletion of the alpha$_1$ or beta$_2$ subunit of GABA$_A$ receptors reduces actions of alcohol and other drugs. *J Pharmacol Exp Ther* 2003;304:30.

Chouinard G, et al: Metabolism of anxiolytics and hypnotics: Benzodiazepines, buspirone, zopiclone and zolpidem. *Cell Mol Neurobiol* 1999;19:533.

Crestani F, et al: Molecular targets for the myorelaxant action of diazepam. *Mol Pharmacol* 2001;59:442.

Drover DR: Comparative pharmacokinetics and pharmacodynamics of short-acting hypnosedatives: zaleplon, zolpidem and zopiclone. *Clin Pharmacokinet* 2004; 43:227.

Fricchione G: Generalized anxiety disorder. *N Engl J Med* 2004;351:675.

Gottesmann C: GABA mechanisms and sleep. *Neuroscience* 2002;111:231.

Holm KJ, Goa KL: Zolpidem: An update of its pharmacology, therapeutic efficacy and tolerability in the treatment of insomnia. *Drugs* 2000;59:865.

Israel AG, Kramer JA: Safety of zaleplon in the treatment of insomnia. *Ann Pharmacother* 2002;36:852.

Korpi ER, et al: Drug interactions at GABA(A) receptors. *Prog Neurobiol* 2002;67:113.

Kralic JE, et al: GABA(A) receptor alpha-1 subunit deletion alters receptor subtype assembly, pharmacological and behavioral responses to benzodiazepines and zolpidem. *Neuropharmacology* 2002;43:685.

Krystal AD: The changing perspective of chronic insomnia management. *J Clin Psychiatry*. 2004;65(Suppl 8):20.

Mintzer MZ, Griffiths RR: Triazolam and zolpidem: Effects on human memory and attentional processes. *Psychopharmacology* (Berl) 1999;144:8.

Patat A, et al: Pharmacodynamic profile of zaleplon, a new non-benzodiazepine hypnotic agent. *Hum Psychopharmacol* 2001;16:369.

Rosenberg R, et al: An assessment of the efficacy and safety of eszopiclone in the treatment of transient insomnia in healthy adults. *Sleep Med* 2005;6:15.

Rudolph U, et al: GABA(A) receptor subtypes: Dissecting their pharmacological functions. *Trends Pharmacol Sci* 2001;22:188.

Rush CR, et al: Zaleplon and triazolam in humans: Acute behavioral effects and abuse potential. *Psychopharmacology* (Berl) 1999;145:39.

Silber MH: Chronic Insomnia. *N Engl J Med* 2005;353:803.

Stahl SM: Selective actions on sleep or anxiety by exploiting GABA-A/benzodiazepine receptor subtypes. *J Clin Psychiatry* 2002;63:179.

Terzano MG, et al: New drugs for insomnia: Comparative tolerability of zopiclone, zolpidem and zaleplon. *Drug Saf* 2003;26:261.

van Laar MW, Volkerts ER: Driving and benzodiazepine use: Evidence that they do not mix. *CNS Drugs* 1998; 10:383.

Rehabilitation

Leipzig RM, et al: Drugs and falls in older people: A systematic review and meta-analysis: I. Psychotropic drugs. *J Am Geriatr Soc* 1999;47:30.

Neubauer DN: Sleep problems in the elderly. *Am Fam Physician* 1999;59:2551.

Perry SW, Wu A: Rationale for the use of hypnotic agent in a general hospital. *Ann Intern Med* 1984;100:441.

Stoudemire A: Epidemiology and psychopharmacology of anxiety in medical patients. *J Clin Psychiatry* 1996; 57–64.

Verster JC, et al: Residual effects of sleep medication on driving ability. *Sleep Med Rev* 2004;8:309.

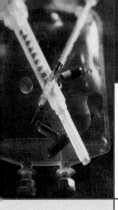

14

ANTISEIZURE DRUGS

Epilepsy comprises a group of chronic syndromes that involve recurrent **seizures.** Approximately 1% of the world's population has **epilepsy;** the second most common neurologic disorder after stroke. Although standard therapy permits control of seizures in 80% of these patients, there are an estimated 500,000 people in the United States who suffer from uncontrolled epilepsy.

Seizures are finite episodes of brain dysfunction resulting from *abnormal transient discharge* of cerebral neurons. The causes of seizures are many. They include the full range of neurologic diseases, such as tumor, head trauma, and stroke. In some patients, the cause of seizures may be less obvious or unknown, such as a congenital abnormality or genetic factor. In other patients, seizures may be caused by an underlying acute toxic or systemic metabolic disorder (e.g., infections, hypoglycemia, hypoxia, poisoning), in which case appropriate therapy is usually directed toward the specific abnormality. Classification of seizure types with clinical descriptions are listed in Table 14–1.

Effective antiseizure drugs have, to varying degrees, selective depressant actions on the abnormal neuronal discharge. However, they vary in their mechanisms of action and in their effectiveness in specific seizure disorders. In most seizure disorders, however, the choice of medication depends on the empiric seizure classification. In this chapter, we will discuss the various drugs used to treat seizures based on their drug class and mechanism of action (Table 14–2) and adverse effects (Table 14–3). We will then discuss their clinical uses in treating epilepsy, based on empiric seizure classification (Figure 14–1).

■ THERAPEUTIC STRATEGIES

For many years it was hoped that a single drug could be developed that would be effective in all forms of epilepsy. However, the causes of epilepsy are extremely diverse, and drug therapy that is effective in one form may be totally ineffective in others. There is, however, some specificity according to seizure type. In addition, owing to varying pharmacokinetic and pharmacodynamic factors, not all patients respond in the same manner to a given antiseizure medication. For this reason, a number of drugs are used to treat epilepsy.

Although seizures are usually self-limiting, even in the absence of drug therapy, uncontrolled recurrence of seizures is not desirable because it is believed that uncontrolled seizures may cause further damage to already injured neurons and may even harm previously healthy neurons. Certain types of seizures can lead to personal injury or even death; at the least, seizures may be personally embarrassing and socially disabling. Consequently, a comprehensive effort is made

Table 14–1. Seizure classification

Seizure Classification	Description
Partial seizures, simple	Consciousness preserved; manifested variously as convulsive jerking, paresthesias, psychic symptoms (altered sensory perception, illusions, hallucinations, affect changes), and autonomic dysfunction
Partial seizures, complex	Impaired consciousness that is preceded, accompanied, or followed by psychologic symptoms
Tonic-clonic seizures, generalized	Tonic phase (less than 1 min) involves abrupt loss of consciousness, muscle rigidity, and respiratory arrest; clonic phase (2–3 min) involves jerking of body muscles, with lip or tongue biting, and fecal and urinary incontinence; formerly called grand mal
Absence seizures, generalized	Impaired consciousness (often abrupt onset and brief), sometimes with automatisms, loss of postural tone, or enuresis; begin in childhood (formerly called petit mal) and usually cease by age 20 years
Myoclonic seizures	Single or multiple myoclonic jerks
Status epilepticus	A series of seizures (usually tonic-clonic) without recovery of consciousness between attacks; it is a life-threatening emergency

to find an effective drug regimen to control or eliminate seizures without causing too many adverse effects (e.g., sedation, lethargy).

BASIC PHARMACOLOGY

Drugs used to treat epilepsy generally inhibit the firing of cerebral neurons by (1) increasing the inhibitory effects of GABA, (2) decreasing the effects of the excitatory amino acids glutamate and aspartate, or (3) by altering the movement of sodium and calcium ions across neuronal membranes. Table 14–2 lists the primary, alternative, and adjunctive drugs used to treat epilepsy according to their drug class and mechanisms of action.

Pharmacokinetics

Antiseizure drugs are commonly used for long periods of time, and consideration of their pharmacokinetic properties is important for avoiding toxicity and drug interactions. For some of these drugs (e.g., phenytoin), determination of plasma levels and clearance in individual patients may be necessary for optimum therapy.

In general, antiseizure drugs are well absorbed orally and have good bioavailability. Most antiseizure drugs are metabolized by hepatic enzymes, and, in some cases, active metabolites are formed. Resistance to antiseizure drugs may involve increased expression of drug transporters at the level of the blood-brain barrier.

Pharmacokinetic drug interactions are common in this drug group. Drugs that inhibit drug metabolism (e.g., cimetidine) or displace anticonvulsants from plasma protein binding sites (e.g., nonsteroidal anti-inflammatory drugs, NSAIDs), may increase plasma concentrations of the antiseizure agents to toxic levels. On the other hand, drugs that induce hepatic drug-metabolizing enzymes (e.g., rifampin) may result in plasma levels of the antiseizure agents that are inadequate for seizure control.

DRUGS USEFUL FOR PARTIAL AND CLONIC-TONIC SEIZURES

Barbiturates

Phenobarbital and other barbiturates such as **mephobarbital** were once considered the safest of

Table 14–2. Drug classification and mechanism of action of common antiseizure drugs

Drug Class or Drug Name	Proposed Mechanism of Action

Barbiturates
  Mephobarbital
  Pentobarbital
  Phenobarbital
  Primidone
	Facilitate the inhibitory effects of GABA; increase the duration of the GABA-gated chloride channel openings. At high concentrations, may also be GABAmimetic

Benzodiazepines
  Clonazepam
  Clorazepate
  Diazepam
  Lorazepam
	Facilitate the inhibitory effects of GABA; increase the frequency of chloride channel opening

Carbamazepine	Blocks sodium channels and inhibits high-frequency repetitive firing in neurons
Felbamate	Mechanism of action is unknown; evidence suggests NMDA receptor blockade via the glycine binding site
Gabapentin	Mechanism of action unknown; may alter GABA metabolism, nonsynaptic GABA release, or reuptake by GABA transporters

Hydantoins
  Ethotoin
  Fosphenytoin
  Mephenytoin
  Phenytoin
	Block sodium channels and inhibit the generation of repetitive action potentials, may also affect other amino acids and neurotransmitters (norepinephrine, GABA, acetylcholine, serotonin)

Lamotrigine	Produces a voltage- and use-dependent inactivation of sodium channels; may also affect voltage activated calcium channels

Succinimides
  Ethosuximide
  Methsuximide
  Phensuximide
	Reduce low-threshold calcium currents primarily in thalamic neurons

Tiagabine	Inhibitor of GABA uptake in both neurons and glia, thus prolonging the inhibitory action of synaptically released GABA
Topiramate	Blocks voltage-dependent sodium channels; may also potentiate the inhibitory effect of GABA (at a site different from benzodiazepine or barbiturate sites)
Valproic acid	Affects sodium currents to block sustained high-frequency repetitive firing of neurons; blockade of NMDA receptor-mediated excitation may also be important
Vigabatrin	Increases the amount of GABA released at synaptic sites; may also potentiate GABA by inhibiting the GABA transporter

GABA = gamma-aminobutyric acid; NMDA = N-methyl-D-aspartate.

Table 14–3. Adverse effects and complications of the use of antiepileptic drugs

Antiepileptic Drug	Adverse Effects
Benzodiazepines	Sedation, tolerance, dependence
Carbamazepine	Diplopia, ataxia, enzyme induction, blood dyscrasias, teratogenic; oxcarbazepine is less toxic
Ethosuximide	Gastrointestinal distress, lethargy, headache
Felbamate	Aplastic anemia, hepatotoxicity
Gabapentin	Sedation, dizziness, behavioral changes
Lamotrigine	Sedation, ataxia, life-threatening rash, Stevens-Johnson syndrome
Levetiracetam	Asthenia, dizziness, sedation
Phenobarbital	Sedation, enzyme induction, tolerance, dependence
Phenytoin	Nystagmus, diplopia, ataxia, sedation, gingival hyperplasia, hirsutism, anemias, enzyme induction, teratogenic
Valproic acid	Gastrointestinal distress, hepatotoxicity (rare but possibly fatal), inhibition of drug metabolism, teratogenic
Vigabatrin	Sedation, weight gain, agitation, confusion, psychosis
Zonisamide	Somnolence, dizziness, agitation, severe rash, Stevens-Johnson syndrome

the antiseizure agents. However, less sedating medications have replaced barbiturates as the drugs of choice for most types of adult seizures. At present, the barbiturates are considered the drugs of choice for seizures only in infants.

Phenobarbital, the prototypic barbiturate, selectively suppresses abnormal neurons, inhibiting the spread and suppressing firing from the focus of discharge. Barbiturates facilitate and prolong the inhibitory effects of gamma-aminobutyric acid (GABA). At therapeutically relevant concentrations, they increase the duration of GABA-mediated chloride channel openings and may block the excitatory transmitter glutamate. At high concentration, sodium channels may also be blocked (Chapter 13). Both the enhancement of GABA-mediated inhibition and the reduction of

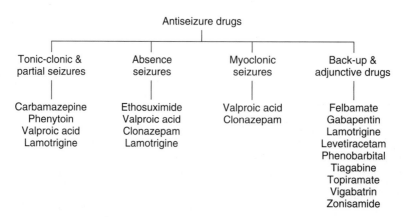

Figure 14–1. Common antiseizure medications categorized by use in seizure types.

glutamate-mediated excitation are seen with therapeutically relevant concentrations of phenobarbital.

Barbiturates are useful in the treatment of partial seizures and generalized tonic-clonic seizures, although they are often tried for virtually every seizure type, especially when attacks are difficult to control. The most common adverse effect is sedation. Also, phenobarbital can produce enzyme induction, tolerance, and dependence.

Hydantoins

Drugs in this class include **phenytoin, ethotoin, mephenytoin,** and **fosphenytoin.** Phenytoin, the prototypic hydantoin, is the oldest nonsedative antiseizure drug, having been introduced in 1938. At therapeutic concentrations, the major action of phenytoin is to block sodium channels and inhibit the generation of repetitive action potentials. This drug class may also decrease neuronal excitability by altering the conductances of potassium and calcium across the nerve membrane.

Phenytoin is one of the most effective drugs against partial seizures and generalized tonic-clonic seizures. Fosphenytoin is a more soluble salt of phenytoin that is used exclusively for parenteral treatment of status epilepticus (see below). Ethotoin and mephenytoin are rarely used. Adverse effects of phenytoin include nystagmus, diplopia, ataxia, sedation, gingival hyperplasia, hirsutism, anemia, enzyme induction, and teratogenesis.

Benzodiazepines

Several members of the benzodiazepine group play prominent roles in the therapy of epilepsy. These drugs facilitate the inhibitory effects of GABA and their antiseizure action is probably mediated through this mechanism (Chapter 13).

Diazepam and **lorazepam** are used in the acute intravenous treatment of status epilepticus. **Clorazepate** is occasionally used as an adjunct in complex partial seizures. **Clonazepam** is a long-acting drug with documented efficacy against absence seizures (see below). It is also an alternative drug choice for myoclonic seizures. Adverse effects of benzodiazepines include sedation, tolerance, and dependence.

Carbamazepine

Carbamazepine is a tricyclic compound closely related to imipramine and similar antidepressants. Its mechanism of action appears to be similar to that of phenytoin. Carbamazepine blocks sodium channels and inhibits high-frequency repetitive firing in neurons. It also acts presynaptically to decrease synaptic transmission. These effects probably account for its anticonvulsant properties.

Carbamazepine is considered a drug of choice for partial seizures and is often used for treatment of generalized tonic-clonic seizures. A derivative, **oxcarbazepine,** is sometimes used. One important clinical advantage of these drugs is that they are not sedative in the usual therapeutic ranges. Adverse effects include diplopia, ataxia, enzyme induction, blood dyscrasias, and teratogenesis.

Felbamate

Felbamate is an adjunct antiseizure agent with severe adverse effects that ultimately limit its clinical use. Although its exact mechanism of action is unknown, evidence suggests blockade of the N-methyl-D-aspartate (NMDA) receptor via the glycine-binding site. While it is effective in some patients with partial seizures and myoclonic seizures, its propensity to cause aplastic anemia and severe hepatotoxicity at unexpectedly high rates diminishes its use.

Gabapentin

Gabapentin, an amino acid derivative originally planned as a spasmolytic, was found to be more effective as an antiseizure drug. Although it has a close structural relationship to GABA, it appears not to act on GABA receptors. It may, however, alter GABA metabolism, its nonsynaptic release, or its reuptake by GABA transporters. An increase in brain GABA concentration is observed in patients.

Gabapentin is effective as an adjunct against partial seizures and generalized tonic-clonic seizures. There is some evidence for its efficacy as monotherapy. It has also been found effective in the treatment of neuropathic pain. The most common adverse effects of gabapentin are sedation, dizziness, behavioral changes, ataxia, headache, and tremor.

Lamotrigine

Lamotrigine is an adjunct drug that produces a voltage- and use-dependent inhibition of presynaptic sodium channels that results in suppression of rapidly firing neurons. This action is most likely responsible for its efficacy in focal epilepsy. Its efficacy in primary generalized absence seizures may involve actions on voltage-activated calcium channels.

Lamotrigine is useful in the treatment of partial seizures and against absence and myoclonic seizures in children. Adverse effects include sedation, ataxia, nausea, dizziness, headache, and life-threatening dermatitis (seen in pediatric patients).

Tiagabine

Tiagabine is an inhibitor of GABA uptake in both neurons and glia, thus prolonging the inhibitory action of synaptically released GABA in the synaptic cleft. Tiagabine is indicated for the adjunctive treatment of partial seizures, although some patients appear to do well with tiagabine monotherapy. The drug is generally well tolerated. Minor adverse events are dose related and include nervousness, dizziness, tremor, difficulty in concentrating, and depression. Excessive confusion, somnolence, or ataxia may require discontinuation. Psychosis occurs rarely.

Topiramate

Topiramate's mechanism of action probably involves blockade of voltage-dependent sodium channels. The drug also appears to potentiate the inhibitory effects of GABA, acting at a site different from benzodiazepine and barbiturate sites. Topiramate also blocks excitatory amino acid receptors. All three of these actions likely contribute to topiramate's anticonvulsant effect. Topiramate is effective as an adjunct against partial and generalized tonic-clonic seizures. Primary adverse effects include sedation, mental dulling, renal stones, and weight loss.

Vigabatrin

Vigabatrin is an irreversible inhibitor of GABA aminotransferase, the enzyme responsible for the degradation of GABA. It apparently acts by increasing the amount of GABA released at synaptic sites, thereby enhancing inhibitory effects. Vigabatrin may also potentiate GABA by inhibiting the GABA reuptake transporter.

Vigabatrin is useful in the treatment of partial seizures and tonic-clonic seizures as an alternative agent. Typical adverse effects include sedation, dizziness, and weight gain. Less common but more troublesome adverse reactions are agitation, confusion, and psychosis.

Other Drugs

Newer drugs used adjunctively in partial and tonic-clonic seizures include **levetiracetam** and **zonisamide.**

■ DRUGS USEFUL IN GENERALIZED (ABSENCE) SEIZURES

Succinimides

This class of drug includes **ethosuximide, phensuximide,** and **methsuximide;** they are primary agents in the treatment of absence seizures. These drugs increase seizure threshold and limit the spread of electrical activity in the brain by reducing low-threshold calcium currents. This effect is seen at therapeutically relevant concentrations in thalamic neurons. Ethosuximide is often used in uncomplicated absence seizures if patients can tolerate its gastrointestinal side effects, including pain, nausea and vomiting. Other adverse effects include lethargy and headache.

Valproic Acid

Valproic acid was originally introduced as a primary agent in the treatment of generalized (absence) seizures, but has proved to also be effective against partial seizures, generalized tonic-clonic seizures, and myoclonic seizures. The drug probably owes its broad spectrum of action to more than one molecular mechanism. Action against partial seizures may be a consequence of the drug's effect on sodium currents, blocking sustained high-frequency firing of neurons. Blockade of NMDA receptor–mediated excitation may also be important. Also, at high concentrations, valproic acid has been shown to increase membrane potassium conductance, thereby hyperpolarizing the resting membrane potential.

Valproic acid is used as a primary agent in the treatment of absence seizures, partial seizures, generalized tonic-clonic seizures, and myoclonic seizures. Gastrointestinal distress, hepatotoxicity, inhibition of drug metabolism, temporary hair loss, and teratogenesis are documented adverse reactions.

CLINICAL MANAGEMENT OF EPILEPSY

Diagnosis of a specific seizure type is important for prescribing the most appropriate antiseizure drug (or combination of drugs). Drug choice is usually based on established efficacy in the specific seizure state that has been diagnosed, the prior responsiveness of the patient, and the anticipated toxicity of the drug.

Treatment may involve combinations of drugs, following the principle of adding known effective agents if the preceding drugs are not sufficient. Table 14–1 lists an empiric seizure classification with descriptions. Table 14–4 lists common types of seizures with the primary, alternative, and adjunct agents used to treat them.

Absence Seizures

Ethosuximide and valproic acid are the preferred drugs used to treat absence seizures because they cause less sedation and tolerance than clonazepam. Ethosuximide is often used in uncomplicated absence seizures if patients can tolerate its gastrointestinal side effects. Valproic acid is particularly useful in patients who have concomitant generalized tonic-clonic or myoclonic seizures. Clonazepam is effective as an alternative drug but has the disadvantages of causing sedation and tolerance. Lamotrigine and topiramate are also approved for use in absence seizures.

Myoclonic Seizures

Myoclonic seizure syndromes are usually treated with valproic acid. Clonazepam can be effective, but the high doses required cause drowsiness. Levetiracetam, lamotrigine, and zonisamide are also used as back-up drugs in myoclonic syndromes. Felbamate has been used adjunctively with the primary drugs but has hematotoxic and hepatotoxic potential.

Table 14–4. Methods of treating the major seizure types

Seizure Type	Primary Agents	Alternative Agents	Adjunct Agents
Absence seizures	Ethosuximide Valproic acid	Clonazepam	Lamotrigine Topiramate
Myoclonic seizures	Valproic acid	Clonazepam Lamotrigine	Felbamate
Partial seizures	Carbamazepine Phenytoin Valproic acid	Phenobarbital Lamotrigine Vigabatrin Primidone	Gabapentin Tiagabine Topiramate Lamotrigine Felbamate
Tonic-clonic seizures	Carbamazepine Phenytoin Valproic acid	Phenobarbital Lamotrigine Vigabatrin Primidone	Gabapentin Tiagabine Topiramate
Status epilepticus	Diazepam (IV) Lorazepam (IV)	Fosphenytoin (IV) Phenytoin (IV) Phenobarbital (especially useful in children)	

IV = intravenous.

Generalized Tonic-Clonic and Partial Seizures

Valproic acid, carbamazepine, and phenytoin are the drugs of choice for generalized tonic-clonic (grand mal) seizures and for most cases of simple and complex partial seizures. Phenobarbital is now considered to be only an alternative agent in adults but continues to be a primary drug in infants. Lamotrigine is another alternative agent, but its usefulness is limited by its toxic potential. Gabapentin may be used adjunctively in refractory cases. Topiramate is approved for adjunctive use with other agents in both tonic-clonic and partial seizures, and vigabatrin may also be useful as a back-up drug. Newer agents approved for use in partial seizures include levetiracetam, tiagabine, and zonisamide.

Status Epilepticus

Intravenous diazepam or lorazepam is usually effective in terminating attacks and providing short-term control. For prolonged therapy, intravenous phenytoin or its more soluble salt, fosphenytoin, are usually used because they are highly effective and less sedating than benzodiazepines or barbiturates. However, phenytoin may cause cardiotoxicity (perhaps because of its solvent propylene glycol), and fosphenytoin is preferred for parenteral use. Phenobarbital has also been used in status epilepticus, especially in children. In very severe status epilepticus that does not respond to these measures, general anesthesia may be used.

Other Clinical Uses

Several antiseizure drugs are effective in the management of **bipolar disorder,** including valproic acid, carbamazepine, phenytoin, and gabapentin. Carbamazepine and oxcarbazepine are drugs of choice for **trigeminal neuralgia.** Gabapentin has efficacy in pain of neuropathic origin, including **postherpetic neuralgia,** and, like phenytoin, may have some value in **migraine.**

◼ SPECIAL CONCERNS

Teratogenicity is a concern for pregnant women taking antiseizure medications. Children born of women taking anticonvulsant drugs have an increased risk of congenital malformations. Spina bifida has been specifically linked to the use of valproic acid and carbamazepine

Children taking antiseizure medications, especially valproic acid, should be closely monitored for **hepatotoxicity.** This risk is greatest for children younger than 2 years but can also occur in patients of any age taking multiple antiseizure drugs.

If withdrawal from antiseizure drugs is contemplated, it should be accomplished gradually to avoid increased seizure frequency and severity. In general, withdrawal from drugs used in absence seizures is more easily accomplished than withdrawal from drugs used in partial or generalized tonic-clonic seizure states. Barbiturates and benzodiazepines are the most difficult to discontinue, sometimes requiring weeks or months to accomplish their complete removal.

◼ REHABILITATION FOCUS

The need for physical therapists to take a thorough medical history is never more relevant than for patients who have a history of seizures and who are taking antiseizure medications. In many instances, a patient will be receiving treatment for a condition unrelated to their epilepsy (e.g., an orthopedic condition or wound therapy) and should be identified for the potential risk for a seizure during therapy. Also, if a patient is receiving therapy for a diagnosis directly related to their seizure activity (e.g., stroke, brain tumor, head trauma), the therapist may help determine the acute efficacy of the antiseizure drug therapy. The primary goal of drug therapy is to control seizure activity without serious adverse effects. The physical therapist may play a vital role in this process by monitoring patient response to medication and informing the medical team of any abnormal findings. In some cases, the drug regimen may be sufficient to control seizure activity but may be causing serious adverse effects. Some of these adverse effects may impact rehabilitation procedures directly; these include sedation, dizziness, ataxia, and gastric disturbances. In cases of ataxia, coordination exercises may need to be added to the rehabilitation program to combat this problem. Finally, some patients with epilepsy are sensitive to environmental stimuli such as sound and light and every attempt should be made to reduce these stimuli during therapy. Physical therapists should be alert for any changes in behavior or functional status (e.g., increase in seizures or increase in adverse reactions) in patients taking antiseizure drugs and report these changes to the appropriate medical personnel.

CLINICAL RELEVANCE FOR REHABILITATION

Adverse Drug Reactions
- Sedation
- Dizziness
- Ataxia; postural imbalance
- Gastrointestinal distress

Effects Interfering with Rehabilitation
- Decreased arousal and alertness
- Postural imbalance due to ataxia
- Uncontrolled seizure activity

Possible Therapy Solutions
- Explore options with physicians regarding the risks versus benefits of the medication as they relate to functional outcomes
- Understand that outcomes may be affected at all levels: body function and structure, activity, and participation.

Potentiation of Functional Outcomes Secondary to Drug Therapy
- Some people with seizures can become seizure-free by using one or more antiseizure medications. In others, antiseizure medications can decrease the frequency and intensity of seizures, enabling patients to meet rehabilitation goals.

PROBLEM-ORIENTED PATIENT STUDY

Brief History: The patient is a 60-year-old male with a primary diagnosis of stroke secondary to a right cerebrovascular accident 15 months prior, with resultant left hemiplegia. The patient initially received rehabilitation in an acute inpatient rehabilitation facility for approximately 8 weeks. He was then transferred to a long-term cognitive rehabilitation facility for approximately 8 weeks. He was discharged to home where he lives with his wife. At the time of discharge home, the patient had made great improvement in his cognitive and speech abilities but was still non-ambulatory. He was subsequently seen by home health providers who felt he had potential for additional functional return and referred him for outpatient rehabilitation therapy.

Current Medical Status and Drug Therapy: The patient was currently medically stable living at home with his wife. His medications included escitalopram (antidepressant), pantoprazole (proton pump inhibitor), amlodipine (calcium channel blocker), warfarin, valproic acid (antiseizure drug), and lamotrigine (antiseizure drug). The patient

stated he developed the seizure disorder poststroke and was initially treated with just valproic acid. He stated that because of breakthrough seizures, a second antiseizure medication, lamotrigine, was added. The patient stated he went every 3 months to have his warfarin and valproic acid levels checked.

Rehabilitation Setting: The patient began outpatient therapy focusing on all three levels of the ICF (International Classification of Functioning) model of functioning and disability (i.e., body functions and structures level, activity level, and participation level) and was making improvements at all three levels.

Problem and Clinical Options: After several months of outpatient therapy, the physical therapist observed that the patient was much more lethargic and very tired on several consecutive sessions. The patient began to require multiple rest periods during treatment sessions. It was also very difficult to communicate with the patient because his speech was soft and muffled. However, there were no new or different sensory or motor neurologic

(continued)

PROBLEM-ORIENTED PATIENT STUDY (*Continued*)

signs that might suggest another stroke. The physical therapist questioned the patient's wife about his behavior and she stated he was indeed much less active at home. The therapist then asked the patient's wife when his blood levels were last checked. She stated it was almost time to have it checked again. The therapist contacted the patient's physician and discussed with him the patient's current clinical findings. The physician scheduled blood

work to be done that day. The physician determined that the patient's blood concentration of valproic acid was elevated above therapeutic levels. He subsequently lowered the patient's daily dose of valproic acid. After several days, the patient began to return to his previous mental and physical status and continued with his therapeutic intervention without further problems.

PREPARATIONS AVAILABLE

Carbamazepine (generic, Tegretol)
Oral: 200-mg tablets; 100-mg chewable tablets; 100 mg/5 mL suspension
Oral extended release: 100-, 200-, 400-mg tablets; 200, 300-mg capsules

Clonazepam (generic, Klonopin)
Oral: 0.5-, 1-, 2-mg tablets

Clorazepate dipotassium (generic, Tranxene)
Oral: 3.75-, 7.5-, 15-mg tablets, capsules
Oral sustained release (Tranxene-SD): 11.25-, 22.5-mg tablets

Diazepam (generic, Valium, others)
Oral: 2-, 5-, 10-mg tablets; 5 mg/5 mL, 5 mg/mL solutions
Parenteral: 5 mg/mL for IV injection
Rectal: 2.5-, 5-, 10-, 15-, 20-mg diazepam viscous rectal solution

Ethosuximide (generic, Zarontin)
Oral: 250-mg capsules; 250 mg/5 mL syrup

Ethotoin (Peganone)
Oral: 250-, 500-mg tablets

Felbamate (Felbatol)
Oral: 400-, 600-mg tablets; 600-mg/5 mL suspension

Fosphenytoin (Cerebyx)
Parenteral: 75 mg/mL for IV or IM injection

Gabapentin (Neurontin)
Oral: 100-, 300-, 400-mg capsules; 600-, 800-mg filmtabs; 50 mg/mL solution

Lamotrigine (Lamictal)
Oral: 25-, 100-, 150-, 200-mg tablets; 2-, 5-, 25-mg chewable tablets

Levetiracetam (Keppra)
Oral: 250-, 500-, 750-mg tablets

Lorazepam (generic, Ativan)
Oral: 0.5-, 1-, 2-mg tablets; 2 mg/mL solution
Parenteral: 2, 4 mg/mL for IV or IM injection

Mephenytoin (Mesantoin)
Oral: 100-mg tablets

Mephobarbital (Mebaral)
Oral: 32-, 50-, 100-mg tablets

Oxcarbazepine (Trileptal)
Oral: 100-, 300-, 600-mg tablets; 60 mg/mL suspension

Pentobarbital sodium (generic, Nembutal)
Parenteral: 50 mg/mL for IV or IM injection

Phenobarbital (generic, Luminal Sodium, others)
Oral: 15-, 16-, 30-, 60-, 90-, 100-mg tablets; 16-mg capsules; 15, 20 mg/5 mL elixirs
Parenteral: 30, 60, 65, 130 mg/mL for IV or IM injection

Phenytoin (generic, Dilantin, others)

Oral (prompt release): 100-mg capsules; 50-mg chewable tablets; 30, 125 mg/5 mL suspension

Oral extended action: 30-, 100-mg capsules

Oral slow release (Phenytek): 200-, 300-mg capsules

Parenteral: 50 mg/mL for IV injection

Tiagabine (Gabitril)

Oral: 4-, 12-, 16-, 20-mg tablets

Topiramate (Topamax)

Oral: 25-, 100-, 200-mg tablets; 15-, 25-mg sprinkle capsules

Trimethadione (Tridione)

Oral: 150-mg chewable tablets; 300-mg capsules; 40 mg/mL solution

Valproic acid (generic, Depakene)

Oral: 250-mg capsules; 250 mg/5 mL syrup (sodium valproate)

Oral sustained release (Depakote): 125-, 250-, 500-mg tablets (as divalproex sodium)

Parenteral (Depacon): 100 mg/mL in 5 mL vial for IV injection

REFERENCES

Backonja MM: Use of anticonvulsants for treatment of neuropathic pain. *Neurology* 2002;59(5 Suppl 2):S14.

Bialer M, et al: Progress report on new antiepileptic drugs: a summary of the Fifth Eiliat Conference. *Epilepsy Res* 2001;43:11.

Duncan JS: The promise of new antiepileptic drugs. *Br J Clin Pharmacol* 2002;53:123.

Hachad H, et al: New antiepileptic drugs: Review on drug interactions. *Ther Drug Monit* 2002;24:91.

Levy RH, et al: *Antiepileptic Drugs*, 5th ed. Philadelphia: Lippincott Williams & Wilkins, 2002.

Löscher W: Basic pharmacology of valproate: A review after 35 years of clinical use for the treatment of epilepsy. *CNS Drugs* 2002;16:669.

Siddiqui A, et al: Association of multidrug resistance in epilepsy with a polymorphism in the drug-transporter gene *ABCB1*. *N Engl J Med* 2002;348:15.

Treiman DM, et al: A comparison of four treatments for generalized convulsive status epilepticus. *N Engl J Med* 1998;339:792.

Wallace SJ: Newer antiepileptic drugs: Advantages and disadvantages. *Brain Dev* 2001;23:277.

Rehabilitation

Chaplin JE, et al: The perceived rehabilitation needs of a hospital-based outpatient sample of people with epilepsy. *Seizure* 1998;7:329.

Fisher RS, et al: The impact of epilepsy from the patient's perspective I. descriptions and subjective perceptions. *Epilepsy Res* 2000;41:39.

Marks WA, et al: Epilepsy: Habilitation and rehabilitation. *Seminars Pediatr Neurol* 2003;10:151.

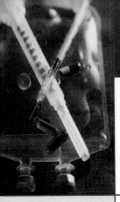

15

GENERAL ANESTHETICS

G eneral anesthesia is a state characterized by analgesia, unconsciousness, amnesia, skeletal muscle relaxation, and inhibition of sensory and autonomic reflexes. The extent to which any individual anesthetic drug can exert these effects varies with the drug, the dosage, and the clinical situation.

Drugs used as general anesthetics are central nervous system (CNS) depressants with actions that can be induced and terminated more rapidly than those of conventional sedative-hypnotics (Chapter 13). An ideal anesthetic drug would induce anesthesia smoothly and rapidly while allowing for prompt recovery after its administration is discontinued. The drug would also possess a wide margin of safety and be devoid of adverse effects. No single anesthetic agent is capable of achieving all of these desirable effects without some disadvantages when used alone. The modern practice of anesthesiology commonly involves the use of combinations of intravenous and inhaled drugs, taking advantage of their individual favorable properties while attempting to minimize adverse reactions. This common practice is known as balanced anesthesia. Classification of drug subgroups and specific drugs used for balanced anesthesia are listed in Figure 15–1 and Table 15–1.

The anesthetic technique will vary depending on the proposed type of diagnostic, therapeutic, or surgical intervention. For minor procedures, so-called monitored anesthesia care or conscious sedation is used, employing oral or parenteral sedatives, often in conjunction with local anesthetics (Chapter 16). These techniques provide profound analgesia, but with retention of the patient's ability to maintain a patent airway and to respond to verbal commands. For more extensive surgical procedures, anesthesia frequently includes the use of preoperative benzodiazepines, induction of anesthesia with intravenous thiopental or propofol, and maintenance of anesthesia with a combination of inhaled and intravenous anesthetic drugs. Such protocols also often include the use of neuromuscular-blocking drugs (Chapter 5). Monitoring of vital signs is the standard method of assessing the depth of anesthesia during surgery.

Although physical therapists are not usually involved in working directly with patients while under general anesthesia, a basic understanding of the mechanism of action and subsequent residual effects of these medications and how they may influence rehabilitation outcomes for several days after their use is important.

STAGES OF ANESTHESIA

Modern anesthetics act very rapidly and achieve deep anesthesia quickly. With older and more slowly-acting anesthetics, the progressively greater depth of central depression associated with

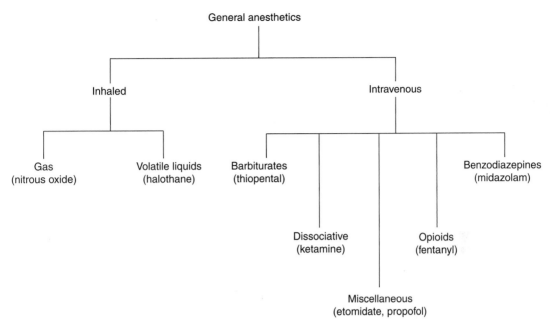

Figure 15–1. Classification of drug subgroups and selected prototype agents used in general anesthesia.

increasing dose or time of exposure is traditionally described as stages of anesthesia.

Stage 1: Analgesia. In this stage, the patient has decreased awareness of pain, sometimes with amnesia. Consciousness may be impaired but is not lost.

Stage 2: Disinhibition. The patient appears to be delirious and excited. Amnesia occurs, reflexes are enhanced, and respiration is typically irregular; retching, vomiting, and incontinence may occur. For these reasons, efforts are made to limit the duration and severity of this stage, which ends with the reestablishment of regular breathing.

Stage 3: Surgical anesthesia. In this stage, the patient is unconscious and has no pain reflexes; respiration is very regular, and blood pressure is maintained.

Stage 4: Medullary depression. The patient develops severe respiratory and cardiovascular depression that requires mechanical and pharmacologic support. Without full circulatory and respiratory support, death rapidly ensues.

Table 15–1. Classification of commonly used general anesthetics

General Anesthetic	Subclass	Prototype	Other Significant Agents
Inhaled anesthetics	Volatile liquids	Halothane	Enflurane, desflurane, isoflurane, sevoflurane
	Gas	Nitrous oxide	
Intravenous anesthetics	Barbiturates	Thiopental	Thiamylal, methohexital
	Opioids	Morphine	Fentanyl, alfentanil, remifentanil
	Phenols	Propofol	
	Benzodiazepines	Midazolam	Diazepam
	Dissociative agent	Ketamine	
	Imidazole	Etomidate	

TYPES OF GENERAL ANESTHESIA

General anesthetics are usually given by inhalation or by intravenous injection. **Nitrous oxide,** a gas at ambient temperature and pressure, continues to be an important component of many anesthesia regimens. **Halothane, enflurane, isoflurane, desflurane, sevoflurane,** and **methoxyflurane** are volatile liquids used as inhaled anesthetics. Several drugs are used intravenously, alone or in combination with other drugs, to achieve an anesthetic state (as components of balanced anesthesia) or to sedate patients in intensive care units who must be mechanically ventilated. These drugs include barbiturates (thiopental, methohexital), benzodiazepines (**midazolam, diazepam**), opioid analgesics (**morphine, fentanyl, sufentanil, alfentanil, remifentanil**), propofol, ketamine, and miscellaneous drugs (**droperidol, etomidate, dexmedetomidine**). Table 15–1 lists the drugs commonly used as inhaled and intravenous anesthetics.

MECHANISMS OF ACTION

The mechanisms of action of general anesthetics are varied. As CNS depressants, these drugs usually increase the threshold for firing of CNS neurons. The potency of inhaled anesthetics is roughly proportionate to their lipid solubility, older hypotheses invoked a nonspecific change in lipid membranes as the mechanism of anesthesia. Current hypotheses regard effects on ion channels and central neurotransmitter mechanisms as primary mechanisms.

Inhaled anesthetics, barbiturates, benzodiazepines, etomidate, and propofol facilitate gamma-aminobutyric acid (GABA)–mediated inhibition at $GABA_A$ receptors. These receptors are sensitive to clinically relevant concentrations of the anesthetic agents. Ketamine does not produce its effects via facilitation of $GABA_A$ receptor functions, but may act via its antagonism of the excitatory neurotransmitter glutamic acid at the N-methyl-D-aspartate (NMDA) receptor. Most inhaled anesthetics also inhibit nicotinic acetylcholine receptor isoforms at moderate to high concentrations. The strychnine-sensitive glycine receptor is another ligand-gated ion channel that may be a target for certain inhaled anesthetics. CNS neurons in different regions of the brain have different sensitivities to general anesthetics; inhibition of neurons involved in pain pathways occurs before inhibition of neurons in the brain stem and midbrain reticular formation (the area for arousal and alertness).

INHALED ANESTHETICS

The inhaled anesthetics, nitrous oxide, and easily vaporized volatile liquids, are administered as gases. Their partial pressure, or "tension," in the inhaled air or in blood or other tissue is a measure of their concentration. Because the standard pressure of the total inhaled mixture is atmospheric pressure (760 mm Hg at sea level), the partial pressure may also be expressed as a percentage of atmospheric pressure. Thus, 50% nitrous oxide in the inhaled air would have a partial pressure of 380 mm Hg.

The speed of induction of anesthesia is a very important characteristic of anesthetic drugs. Speed of induction depends both on drug properties and the patient's clinical condition. Relevant properties include solubility, inspired gas partial pressure, ventilation rate, pulmonary blood flow, and arteriovenous concentration gradient.

1. **Solubility.** The more rapidly a drug equilibrates with the blood, the more quickly the drug passes into the brain to produce anesthetic effects. Drugs with a low blood:gas partition coefficient (e.g., nitrous oxide) equilibrate more rapidly than those with a higher blood solubility (e.g., halothane) and thus have a more rapid onset of action. Partition coefficients for inhalation anesthetics are shown in Table 15–2.

2. **Inspired gas partial pressure.** A high partial pressure of the gas in the lungs results in more rapid achievement of anesthetic levels in the blood. This effect can be exploited by the initial administration of gas concentrations higher than those required for maintenance of anesthesia. A high initial inspired anesthetic concentration will increase the rate of induction of anesthesia by increasing the rate of transfer into the blood. For inhaled anesthetics that have a relatively slow onset of anesthesia (such as halothane or enflurane), a higher percent

concentration (3 to 4%) is administered initially to increase the rate of induction and then reduced (to 1 to 2%) for maintenance when adequate anesthesia is achieved. Adding these agents in combination with an even less soluble agent such as nitrous oxide will further reduce the time required for loss of consciousness.

3. **Ventilation rate.** The greater the ventilation, the more rapid is the rise in alveolar and blood partial pressure of the agent and the onset of anesthesia. High ventilation can be achieved by mechanical or assisted ventilation via an endotracheal tube (i.e., intubated patients).

4. **Pulmonary blood flow.** At high pulmonary blood flows, the gas partial pressure in the blood rises at a slower rate because a larger volume of blood is exposed to the anesthetic gas in the lungs; thus, the onset of anesthesia is delayed. At low flow rates, the rate of rise of arterial tension of inhaled anesthetics is increased and onset of anesthesia is faster. In circulatory shock, this effect may accelerate the rate of onset of anesthesia with agents of high blood solubility.

5. **Arteriovenous concentration gradient.** Uptake of soluble anesthetics into highly perfused tissues may decrease gas tension in mixed venous blood. This can influence the rate of onset of anesthesia because achievement of equilibrium is dependent on the difference in anesthetic tension between arterial and venous blood. The greater the difference in anesthetic tensions between arterial and venous blood, the more has been taken up by viscera, muscle, etc., and the more time it will take to achieve equilibrium with brain tissue.

Termination of Inhaled Anesthetic Action

Inhaled anesthetics are primarily terminated by redistribution of the drug from the brain to the blood and elimination of the drug through the lungs. Like induction of anesthesia, the rate of recovery from anesthesia is faster with drugs with low blood:gas partition coefficients than with anesthetics with high blood solubility. This important property has led to the introduction of several newer inhaled anesthetics (e.g., desflurane, sevoflurane), which, because of their low blood solubility, are characterized by recovery times that are

considerably shorter than is the case with older agents. Some volatile liquids such as halothane and methoxyflurane are also eliminated in part by metabolism in the liver. While metabolism has only a minor influence on the speed of recovery, it can play a significant role in the toxicity of these anesthetics.

Dose-Response Characteristics of Inhaled Anesthetics

The potency of inhaled anesthetics is best measured by the minimum alveolar anesthetic concentration (MAC). MAC is defined as the alveolar concentration required to eliminate the response to a standardized painful stimulus in 50% of patients. The higher the MAC of a given anesthetic, the lower its potency. Each anesthetic has a defined average MAC (Table 15–2), but this value may vary among different patients depending on age, cardiovascular status, and use of adjuvant drugs. Estimations of MAC value suggest a relatively steep dose-response relationship for inhaled anesthetics. MACs for infants and elderly patients are lower than those for adolescents and young adults. When several anesthetic agents are used simultaneously, their MAC values are additive.

Clinical Use of Inhaled Anesthetics

Volatile anesthetics are rarely used as the sole agents for induction and maintenance of anesthesia. More commonly, they are combined with intravenous agents in balanced anesthesia regimens. Of the inhaled anesthetics, nitrous oxide, desflurane, sevoflurane, and isoflurane are the most commonly used in the United States. Use of the more soluble volatile anesthetics has declined during the last decade as more surgical procedures are performed on an outpatient ("short-stay") basis. The low blood:gas coefficients of desflurane and sevoflurane afford more rapid recovery and fewer postoperative adverse effects than halothane or isoflurane (Table 15–2). Although halothane is still used in pediatric anesthesia, sevoflurane is rapidly replacing halothane in this setting. As indicated previously, nitrous oxide lacks sufficient potency to produce surgical anesthesia by itself and is used with volatile or intravenous anesthetics to produce a general anesthetic state.

Table 15–2.	Properties of some inhaled anesthetics		
Anesthetic	Blood: Gas Partition Coefficient[1]	Minimal Alveolar Conc. (MAC) (%)[2]	Comments
Nitrous oxide	0.47	>100	Incomplete anesthetic; rapid onset and recovery
Desflurane	0.42	6–7	Low volatility; poor induction agent; rapid recovery
Sevoflurane	0.69	2.0	Rapid onset and recovery; unstable in soda-lime
Isoflurane	1.40	1.4	Medium rate of onset and recovery
Enflurane	1.80	1.7	Medium rate of onset and recovery
Halothane	2.30	0.75	Medium rate of onset and recovery
Methoxyflurane	12	0.16	Slow onset and recovery

[1]Partition coefficients (at 37°C) are from multiple literature sources.
[2]MAC is the anesthetic concentration that produces immobility in 50% of patients exposed to a noxious stimulus.

Adverse Effects

Central Nervous System

The goal of anesthesia practice is to produce analgesia, loss of consciousness, amnesia, and muscle relaxation with loss of reflexes. This is achieved by CNS depression. There are, however, other CNS effects that are considered adverse or undesired. These include a reduction in vascular resistance resulting in increased cerebral blood flow, which can lead to an increase in intracranial pressure.

Cardiovascular System

Most inhaled anesthetics (except nitrous oxide) decrease arterial blood pressure moderately. Of the volatile gases, enflurane and halothane are myocardial depressants that decrease cardiac output, whereas isoflurane causes peripheral vasodilation. Unfortunately, blood flow to the liver and kidney is also decreased by most inhaled agents. Halothane sensitizes the myocardium to endogenous and exogenous catecholamines and can lead to ventricular arrhythmias.

Respiratory System

In the respiratory system, rate of respiration may be increased by inhaled anesthetics, but tidal volume and minute ventilation are decreased, leading to an increase in arterial CO_2 tension. Inhaled anesthetics decrease ventilatory response to hypoxia even at subanesthetic concentrations (e.g., during recovery). Nitrous oxide has the smallest effect on respiration. Most inhaled anesthetics are bronchodilators, but desflurane is a pulmonary irritant and may cause bronchospasm requiring the use of an adjuvant agent to control secretions.

Other

Although rare, severe toxicities are sometimes associated with inhaled anesthetics. Postoperative hepatitis can occur following the use of halothane. Malignant hyperthermia may occur when inhaled anesthetics are used together with neuromuscular blockers, especially succinylcholine (Chapter 5). Malignant hyperthermia is characterized by the uncontrolled release of calcium by the sarcoplasmic reticulum of skeletal muscle leading to muscle spasm, hyperthermia, and autonomic lability. **Dantrolene** (Chapter 33), with supportive management, is indicated for the treatment of this life-threatening condition.

■ INTRAVENOUS ANESTHETICS

With changes in health-care delivery systems in the last 20 years, there has been increasing use of intravenous drugs in anesthesia, both as adjuncts to inhaled

Table 15–3.	Characteristics of intravenous anesthetics	
Drug	**Induction and Recovery**	**Comments**
Etomidate	Rapid onset and moderately fast recovery	Cardiovascular stability; decreased steroidogenesis; involuntary muscle movements
Fentanyl	Slow onset and recovery; naloxone reversal available	Used in balanced anesthesia and conscious sedation; marked analgesia
Ketamine	Moderately rapid onset and recovery	Cardiovascular stimulation; increased cerebral blood flow; emergence reactions impair recovery
Midazolam	Slow onset and recovery; flumazenil reversal available	Used in balanced anesthesia and conscious sedation; cardiovascular stability; marked amnesia
Propofol	Rapid onset and rapid recovery	Used in induction and for maintenance; hypotension; useful antiemetic action
Thiopental	Rapid onset and rapid recovery (bolus dose); slow recovery following infusion	Standard induction agent; cardiovascular depression; avoid in porphyrias

anesthetics and in techniques that do not include inhaled anesthetics (e.g., total intravenous anesthesia). Unlike inhaled anesthetics, intravenous agents do not require specialized vaporizer equipment for their delivery or expensive facilities for the recovery and disposal of exhaled gases. Intravenous drugs such as thiopental, etomidate, ketamine, and propofol have an onset of anesthetic action faster than the fastest of the inhaled gaseous agents such as desflurane and sevoflurane. Therefore, intravenous agents are commonly used for induction of anesthesia. Recovery is sufficiently rapid with many intravenous drugs to permit short ambulatory (outpatient) surgical procedures. In the case of propofol, recovery times are similar to those seen with the shortest-acting inhaled anesthetics. The anesthetic potency of intravenous anesthetics, including thiopental, ketamine, and propofol, is adequate to permit their use as the sole anesthetic in short surgical procedures when combined with nitrous oxide and opioid analgesics. Adjunctive use of potent opioids (e.g., fentanyl and related compounds) contributes cardiovascular stability, enhanced sedation, and profound analgesia. Other intravenous agents such as the benzodiazepines (e.g., midazolam, diazepam) have slower onset and recovery features and are rarely used for induction of anesthesia. However, preanesthetic administration of

benzodiazepines can be used to provide a basal level of sedation and amnesia when used in conjunction with other anesthetic agents. The characteristics of selected intravenous anesthetics are summarized in Table 15–3.

Barbiturates

Thiopental and **methohexital** have high lipid solubility, which promotes rapid entry into the brain and results in surgical anesthesia in one circulation time (<1 minute). These drugs are used for induction of anesthesia and for short surgical procedures. Their anesthetic effects are terminated by redistribution from the brain to other highly perfused tissues (Figure 15–2), but hepatic metabolism is required for elimination from the body. Barbiturates are respiratory and circulatory depressants and because they depress cerebral blood flow, they can also decrease intracranial pressure. (Refer to Chapter 13 for a more complete discussion.)

Benzodiazepines

Midazolam is often used with inhaled anesthetics and intravenous opioids. The onset of its CNS effects is slower than that of thiopental, and it has a longer duration of action. Cases of severe postoperative respiratory depression have occurred but the benzodiazepine

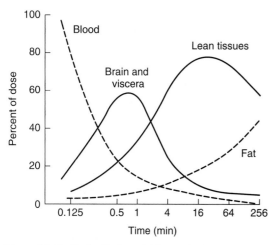

Figure 15–2. Redistribution of thiopental after intravenous bolus administration.

receptor antagonist **flumazenil** can be used to accelerate recovery. Prolonged sedation is often problematic during recovery. (Refer to Chapter 13 for a more complete discussion.)

Etomidate

This intravenous anesthetic affords rapid induction with minimal change in cardiac function or respiratory rate and it has a short duration of action. The drug is not analgesic, and its primary advantage is in anesthesia for patients with limited cardiac or respiratory reserve. Etomidate may cause local pain and myoclonus on injection, and nausea and vomiting postoperatively. Prolonged administration may cause adrenal suppression. In critically ill patients, prolonged infusion may result in hypotension and electrolyte imbalance.

Ketamine

This drug produces a state of *"dissociative anesthesia"* in which the patient remains conscious but has marked catatonia, analgesia, and amnesia. Ketamine is a chemical congener of the psychotomimetic agent phencyclidine (PCP). The drug is the only intravenous anesthetic that is a cardiovascular stimulant, and this action may lead to an increase in intracranial pressure. In most patients, ketamine decreases the respiratory rate. However, upper airway muscle tone is well maintained, and airway reflexes are usually preserved. Emergence reactions, including disorientation, excitation, and hallucinations, which occur during recovery from ketamine anesthesia, can be reduced by the preoperative use of benzodiazepines. Because of the high incidence of postoperative psychic phenomena associated with its use, ketamine is not commonly used in general surgery in the United States, but it is considered useful for poor-risk geriatric patients and in unstable patients (e.g., cardiogenic or septic shock) because of its cardiostimulatory properties. It is also used in low doses for outpatient anesthesia in combination with propofol and in children undergoing painful procedures (e.g., dressing changes for burns).

Opioids

Morphine and **fentanyl** are used with other CNS depressants (nitrous oxide, benzodiazepines) in anesthesia regimens and are especially valuable in high-risk patients who might not survive a full general anesthetic. Intravenous opioids may cause chest wall rigidity that can impair ventilation. Respiratory depression with these drugs may be reversed postoperatively with naloxone. **Alfentanil** and **remifentanil** have been used for induction of anesthesia. Recovery from the actions of remifentanil is faster than recovery from other opioids used in anesthesia because of its rapid metabolism by blood and tissue esterases.

Neuroleptanesthesia is a state of analgesia and amnesia produced when fentanyl is used with droperidol and nitrous oxide. Newer opioids related to fentanyl have been introduced for intravenous anesthesia.

Opioid analgesics are also used at low doses by epidural and spinal routes of administration to produce excellent postoperative analgesia. (Refer to Chapter 20 for a more complete discussion.)

Propofol

Propofol is the most commonly used intravenous anesthetic in the United States. It produces anesthesia as rapidly as the intravenous barbiturates, and recovery is more rapid. Propofol has antiemetic actions, and recovery is not delayed after prolonged infusion. It is used for induction and maintenance of anesthesia in balanced anesthesia and as the primary anesthetic in outpatient surgery. Propofol may cause marked hypotension during induction of anesthesia, primarily through decreased peripheral resistance. Total body clearance of propofol is greater than hepatic blood flow, suggesting that its elimination includes other mechanisms in addition to metabolism by liver enzymes.

REHABILITATION FOCUS

The primary concern for the physical therapist when treating patients who have been under general anesthesia is the lingering postoperative effect of these agents. Because of changing health-care policies and current advances in surgical procedures, many patients requiring general anesthesia for minor surgery go home that same day. This can be problematic, especially when the patient requires physical therapy for immediate mobilization (e.g., crutch training, upright activity).

Common adverse effects that may interfere with immediate therapeutic intervention include sedation, confusion, and muscle weakness (especially if neuromuscular-blocking agents have been used). The elderly or debilitated patient with impaired drug metabolism and elimination mechanisms may continue to show some anesthetic effects (hypotension, respiratory depression, ataxia) for several days after the discontinuance of the anesthetic agents. The physical therapist may assist in the recovery of the patient who has received general anesthesia by providing early mobilization and implementing pulmonary hygiene activities such as chest percussion, postural drainage positioning, and breathing exercises to combat pulmonary problems associated with the use of general anesthetics. General anesthetics depress mucociliary clearance in the airway, leading to an increase in bronchial secretions and pooling of mucus in the lungs which can lead to atelectasis and respiratory infections.

CLINICAL RELEVANCE FOR REHABILITATION

Adverse Drug Reactions
- Sedation
- Confusion
- Muscle weakness, ataxia
- Respiratory compromise

Effects Interfering with Rehabilitation
- Sedation
- Altered mental status
- Muscle weakness, ataxia
- Altered physiological functioning such as respiratory depression and hypotension

Possible Therapy Solutions
- Time: Usually passage of time will allow for the effects of the anesthesia to wear off.
- Contact physician if any adverse effects continue for a prolonged period of time.

PROBLEM-ORIENTED PATIENT STUDY

Brief History: The patient is a 72-year-old female who sustained a right proximal femoral shaft fracture secondary to a fall down eight concrete steps outside a medical office building. The patient stated she was on her way to see her physician for a yearly check-up and lost her balance stepping onto the top step going into the building. Three months ago, she had a total knee replacement (TKR) of the right knee. The patient was admitted to the hospital and required open reduction internal fixation of the right femur. The patient is 5 feet, 2 inches tall with a body mass index of 31.

Current Medical Status and Drug Therapy: The patient was referred to rehabilitation services

(continued)

PROBLEM-ORIENTED PATIENT STUDY (*Continued*)

24 hours after surgery for mobilization, out-of-bed activity, and gait training with non-weight-bearing status on the right. Upon chart review, the physical therapist noted that the operation report was unremarkable. The anesthesia report showed the patient received balanced anesthesia of inhaled nitrous oxide for induction followed by enflurane, intravenous anesthetics including thiopental and fentanyl, and the oral sedative-hypnotic diazepam. The patient is currently receiving pain medications as needed.

Rehabilitation Setting: Upon initial examination day 1 postsurgery by the acute care physical therapist, the patient was very lethargic and extremely difficult to arouse. Nursing stated the patient had a restful evening with no major complaints, and that she had not requested any additional pain medications. The physical therapist made several attempts to sit the patient on the edge of the bed but was unsuccessful. The physical therapist, with assistance of three aides, transferred the patient by a full-body-dependent transfer to a cardiac chair for slow mobilization to an upright posture. During this activity, the patient was still hard to arouse

and unable to carry on a conversation with the physical therapist. The patient was returned to bed with the same type of transfer. The physical therapist noted the difficulty in arousing the patient and her difficulty in following commands in the patient's chart. On day 2 postsurgery, the patient was again seen by the physical therapist for out-of-bed activities and gait training. On this date, the patient was alert and very willing to assist the physical therapist with all activities. The patient stated that she did not remember the physical therapist coming the day before.

Problem/Clinical Options: It was concluded that the patient was still recovering from the effects of her balanced anesthesia. The prolonged effects may have been due to the type of balanced anesthesia she received or to a prolonged elimination time due to redistribution of the drugs into body tissues (diazepam is a highly lipid-soluble benzodiazepine). The patient ultimately was able to become independent with all transfers, underwent gait training with non-weight-bearing on the right, and was discharged home with home health services.

PREPARATIONS AVAILABLE[1]

Desflurane (Suprane)
Liquid: 240 mL for inhalation

Dexmedetomidine (Precedex)
Parenteral: 100 mcg/mL for IV infusion

Diazepam (generic, Valium)
Oral: 2-, 5-, 10-mg tablets; 5 mg/5 mL and 5 mg/mL solution
Oral sustained release: 15-mg capsules
Parenteral: 5 mg/mL for injection

Droperidol (generic, Inapsine)
Parenteral: 2.5 mg/mL for IV or IM injection

Enflurane (Enflurane, Ethrane)
Liquid: 125, 250 mL for inhalation

Etomidate (Amidate)
Parenteral: 2 mg/mL for injection

Halothane (generic, Fluothane)
Liquid: 125, 250 mL for inhalation

Isoflurane (Isoflurane, Forane)
Liquid: 100 mL for inhalation

Ketamine (generic, Ketalar)
Parenteral: 10, 50, 100 mg/mL for injection

Lorazepam (generic, Ativan)
Oral: 0.5-, 1-, 2-mg tablets; 2 mg/mL solution
Parenteral: 2, 4 mg/mL for injection

Methohexital (Brevital Sodium)
Parenteral: 0.5-, 2.5-, 5-g powder to reconstitute for injection

Methoxyflurane (Penthrane)
Liquid: 15, 125 mL for inhalation

Midazolam (generic, Versed)
Parenteral: 1, 5 mg/mL for injection in 1-, 2-, 5-, 10-mL vials
Oral: 2 mg/mL syrup

Nitrous oxide (gas, supplied in blue cylinders)

Propofol (generic, Diprivan)
Parenteral: 10 mg/mL for IV injection

Sevoflurane (Ultane)
Liquid: 250 mL for inhalation

Thiopental (generic, Pentothal)
Parenteral: powder to reconstitute 20, 25 mg/mL for IV injection

[1]See Chapter 20 for formulations of opioid agents used in anesthesia.

REFERENCES

Abraham RB, et al: Malignant hyperthermia. *Postgrad Med J* 1998;74:11.

Angelini G, et al: Use of propofol and other nonbenzodiazepine sedatives in the intensive care unit. *Crit Care Clin* 2001;17:863.

Beaussier M, et al: Comparative effects of desflurane and isoflurane on recovery after long lasting anaesthesia. *Can J Anaesth* 1998;45:429.

Campagna JA, et al: Mechanisms of actions of inhaled anesthetics. *N Engl J Med* 2003;348:2110.

Dickinson R: Selective synaptic actions of thiopental and its enantiomers. *Anesthesiology* 2002;96:884.

Eger EI II, et al: Minimum alveolar anesthetic concentration: A standard of anesthetic potency. *Anesthesiology* 1965;26:756.

Eger EI II: Uptake and distribution. In: *Anesthesia*, 4th ed. Miller RD (ed). Churchill Livingstone, 1994.

Kang TM: Propofol infusion syndrome in critically ill patients. *Ann Pharmacother* 2002;36:1453.

Nelson LE, et al: The sedative component of anesthesia is mediated by GABA$_A$ receptors in an endogenous sleep pathway. *Nat Neurosci* 2002;5:979.

Park KW: Cardiovascular effects of inhalational anesthetics. *Int Anesthesiol Clin* 2002;40:1.

Patel S: Cardiovascular effects of intravenous anesthetics. *Int Anesthesiol Clin* 2002;40:15.

Rosen MA: Management of anesthesia for the pregnant surgical patient. *Anesthesiology* 1999;91:1159.

Trapani G, et al: Propofol in anesthesia. Mechanism of action, structure-activity relationships, and drug delivery. *Curr Med Chem* 2000;7:249.

Trudell JR, Bertaccini E: Molecular modelling of specific and non-specific anaesthetic interactions. *Br J Anaesth* 2002;89:32.

White PF (ed): *Textbook of Intravenous Anesthesia*. Baltimore: Williams & Wilkins, 1997.

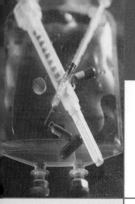

16

LOCAL ANESTHETICS

Local anesthesia is the condition that results when sensory transmission from a local area of the body to the central nervous system (CNS) is blocked. The local anesthetics constitute a group of chemically similar agents that block the sodium channels of excitable membranes. Because these drugs can be administered by topical application or by injection in the target area, the anesthetic effect can be restricted to a localized area (e.g., cornea, arm, foot). Even when these drugs are given in the vicinity of the spinal cord, it is still considered a form of local anesthesia because only a specific level of cord impulse transmission is blocked. When given intravenously, however, these drugs can have effects on other tissues.

Local anesthetics are used for a variety of purposes, including localized surgical procedures, labor and delivery, and joint manipulations. They can also be used for short-term pain relief in conditions such as tendonitis or in long-term situations such as pain associated with cancer. Table 16–1 presents some of the methods of delivery of local anesthetics and the common clinical uses of each method.

CHEMISTRY AND PHARMACOKINETICS

Most local anesthetics in current use are esters or amides. In addition, they are amines with the ability to bind a proton (H^+ ion) and become charged under acidic conditions. They differ in potency, duration of action, and surface activity (Figure 16–1). Many short-acting local anesthetics are readily absorbed into the bloodstream from the injection site after administration. Therefore, the duration of local action is limited unless blood flow to the area is reduced. This can be accomplished by coadministration of a vasoconstrictor (usually an alpha [α] agonist sympathomimetic such as **epinephrine** or **phenylephrine**) with the local anesthetic agent. The vasoconstrictor retards the removal of the drug from the injection site and may reduce the potential for CNS toxicity. **Cocaine** is an important exception because it has intrinsic sympathomimetic action (Chapter 6). The longer-acting agents (e.g., **tetracaine** and **bupivacaine**) are also less dependent on the coadministration of vasoconstrictors. Surface activity (ability to reach superficial nerves when applied to the surface of the skin or mucous membranes) is a property of only a few local anesthetics (e.g., cocaine and **benzocaine**).

Metabolism of ester local anesthetics is carried out by plasma cholinesterases and occurs rapidly. **Procaine**, the prototypic ester local anesthetic, has a half-life of 1 to 2 minutes. The amides are metabolized in the liver with half-lives of 2 to 6 hours.

Table 16–1.   Methods of delivery and clinical uses of local anesthetics

Method of Administration	Descriptions	Clinical Use
Topical administration	Drug is applied directly to the surface of the skin, mucous membrane, cornea, and other regions to produce analgesia	Minor surface irritation or injury (minor burn, abrasions, inflammation); minor surgical procedures (wound cleansing, piercing, circumcision); hypertonicity
Transdermal administration	Drug is applied to the surface of the skin or other tissue with the intent that the drug will be absorbed into underlying tissues. May be enhanced by the use of electrical current (iontophoresis) or ultrasound (phonophoresis)	Painful subcutaneous structures (tendons, bursae, soft tissue); dermatologic surgeries
Infiltration anesthesia	Drug is injected directly into the selected tissue and allowed to diffuse to sensory nerve endings within that tissue	Suturing of lacerated skin
Peripheral nerve block	Drug is injected close to the nerve trunk so that transmission along the peripheral nerve is interrupted	Dental procedures; minor surgical procedures; some chronic conditions such as rheumatoid arthritis; specific nerve pain
Central nerve blockade	Drug injected within the spaces surrounding the spinal cord for epidural nerve blockade or spinal nerve blockade	Obstetric procedures; alternative to general anesthesia for lumbar surgery and hip and knee arthroplasty; relief of acute or chronic pain
Sympathetic block	Selective interruption of sympathetic efferent discharge (anesthetic is not used to provide analgesia)	Reflex sympathetic dystrophy syndrome
Intravenous regional anesthesia (Bier block)	Anesthetic is injected into a peripheral distal vein located in a selected arm or leg with a proximally placed tourniquet to isolate the limb circulation	Used for short surgical procedures of less than 45 min

■ MECHANISM OF ACTION

Local anesthetics block voltage-dependent sodium channels and reduce the influx of sodium ions, thereby preventing depolarization of the membrane and blocking conduction of the action potential. Local anesthetics gain access to their receptors on the channels from the cytoplasm or the membrane (Figure 16–2). Because the drug molecule must cross the lipid membrane to reach the cytoplasm, the more lipid-soluble (nonionized, uncharged) form reaches effective intracellular concentrations more rapidly than does the ionized form.

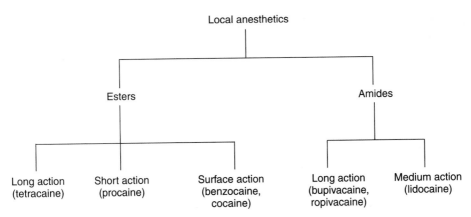

Figure 16–1. Common local anesthetics subdivided by class and duration of action.

On the other hand, once inside the axon, the ionized (charged) form of the drug is the more effective blocking entity. Thus, both the nonionized and the ionized forms of the drug play important roles, the first in reaching the receptor site and the second in causing the effect. The affinity of the receptor site within the sodium channel for the local anesthetic is a function of the state of the channel, whether it is resting, open, or inactivated, and therefore is both voltage- and time-dependent, following the same rules of sodium channel blocking as antiarrhythmic drugs (Chapter 10). More rapidly firing nerve fibers (e.g., sensory fibers) are usually blocked before more slowly firing fibers (e.g., motor fibers).

When the local anesthetic is bound to the receptor site on the sodium channel, the channel is maintained in a blocked condition. By blocking a sufficient number of channels, the anesthetic prevents action

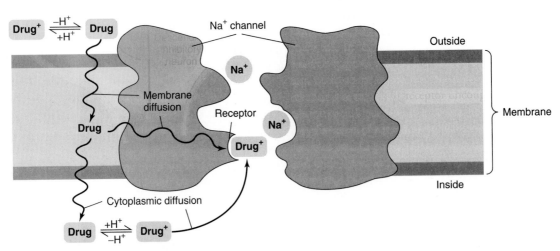

Figure 16–2. Schematic diagram of the sodium channel in an axon and the pathways by which a local anesthetic molecule (Drug) may reach its receptor. Sodium ions are not able to pass through the channel when the drug is bound to the receptor. The local anesthetic diffuses within the membrane in its uncharged form. In the aqueous extracellular and intracellular spaces, the charged form is also present.

potential propagation along the affected portion of the nerve axon. Other ions can influence local anesthetic action. For example, high concentrations of extracellular K^+ enhance local anesthetic activity, whereas elevated extracellular Ca^{2+} antagonizes blockade.

PHARMACOLOGIC EFFECTS

The differences in sensitivity of various types of nerve fibers to local anesthetics depend on fiber diameter, myelination, physiologic firing rate, and anatomic location (Table 16–2). In general, smaller fibers are blocked more easily than larger fibers, and myelinated fibers are blocked more easily than unmyelinated fibers. Activated pain fibers fire rapidly; therefore, pain sensation appears to be blocked by lower concentrations of local anesthetics. Fibers located in the periphery of a thick nerve bundle are blocked sooner than those in the core because they are exposed earlier to higher concentrations of the anesthetic.

CLINICAL USES

The local anesthetics are commonly used for minor skin injuries or irritations and various surgical procedures. Local anesthetics are also used in spinal anesthesia by injection of the drug into the epidural or subarachnoid space surrounding the spinal cord (Figure 16–3). They can be used to produce temporary autonomic blockade in ischemic conditions in the limbs. Slow epidural infusion at low concentrations has been used successfully for postoperative analgesia (in the same way as postoperative epidural opioid infusion; i.e., patient-controlled analgesia [PCA], refer to Chapter 20). However, repeated epidural injection in anesthetic doses may lead to tachyphylaxis. See Table 16–1 for a list of clinical uses of local anesthetics.

ADVERSE EFFECTS

The intended effect of any administered local anesthetic is to produce a regional response by affecting specifically targeted nerves. However, these drugs can be absorbed into the general circulation and have effects on other tissues and organs. Systemic effects are most likely to occur if an excess of drug is used, if there is greater absorption of the drug than anticipated, or if the drug is unintentionally injected directly into the systemic circulation.

The most important toxic effects of most local anesthetics are in the CNS. All local anesthetics are capable of producing a spectrum of central effects,

Table 16–2.	**Relative size and susceptibility of types of nerve fibers to local anesthetics**				
Fiber Type	Function	Diameter (μm)	Myelination	Conduction Velocity (m/s)	Sensitivity to Block
Type A					
Alpha	Proprioception, motor	12–20	Heavy	70–120	+
Beta	Touch, pressure	5–12	Heavy	30–70	++
Gamma	Muscle spindles	3–6	Heavy	15–30	++
Delta	Pain, temperature	2–5	Heavy	12–30	+++
Type B	Preganglionic autonomic	<3	Light	3–15	++++
Type C					
Dorsal root	Pain	0.4–1.2	None	0.5–2.3	++++
Sympathetic	Postganglionic	0.3–1.3	None	0.7–2.3	++++

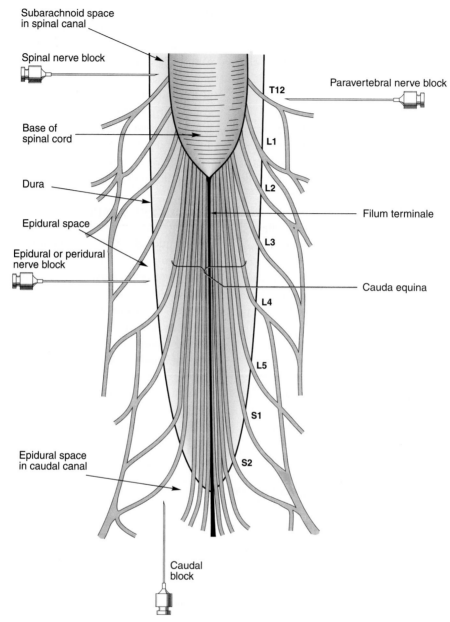

Figure 16–3. Schematic diagram of injection sites for local anesthetics in and near the spinal canal.

including lightheadedness, sedation, restlessness, confusion, agitation, nystagmus, and, at very high doses, tonic-clonic convulsions. Convulsions may be followed by coma with respiratory and cardiovascular depression. Thus, CNS excitation may be followed by CNS depression. This depression may impair respiratory function and death from respiratory failure may occur.

With the exception of cocaine, all local anesthetics are vasodilators. Patients with preexisting cardiovascular disease may develop heart block and other disturbances of cardiac electrical function at high plasma levels of local anesthetics. The direct cardiovascular effects associated with local anesthetics (except cocaine) include vasodilation, decreased heart rate, decreased force of contraction, and decreased cardiac excitability and conduction. These depressant effects on the heart can occur if sufficient amounts of the local anesthetic reach the systemic circulation. They may be opposed by baroreceptor reflex responses evoked by hypotension. **Bupivacaine** may produce severe cardiovascular toxicity, including arrhythmias and hypotension, if given intravenously.

The ability of cocaine to block norepinephrine reuptake at sympathetic neuroeffector junctions and the vasoconstricting actions of the drug contribute to cardiovascular toxicity. When used as a drug of abuse, the cardiovascular toxicity of cocaine includes severe hypertension with cerebral hemorrhage, cardiac arrhythmias, and myocardial infarction.

Severe local anesthetic toxicity is treated symptomatically; there are no specific antidotes. Convulsions are usually managed with intravenous **diazepam** or a short-acting barbiturate such as **thiopental**. Hyperventilation with oxygen is helpful. Occasionally, a neuromuscular-blocking drug may be used to control violent convulsive activity. The cardiovascular toxicity of bupivacaine overdose is difficult to treat and has caused fatalities in healthy young adults.

REHABILITATION FOCUS

Local anesthetics have applications in many different clinical conditions. For this reason, there are multiple patient situations where physical therapists may encounter their use both directly and indirectly. Patients suffering from minor skin injuries or irritations may be using a topical anesthetic. Therapists may be involved in administering the local anesthetic either topically or transdermally for the treatment of hypertonicity (i.e., increased resistance to passive stretch secondary to an upper motor neuron lesion) or musculoskeletal disorders (tendonitis, bursitis), respectively. Some patients involved in rehabilitation programs may have received central nerve blocks for severe and chronic pain and have been referred for comprehensive therapy programs to improve their overall functional status. Patients who have received autonomic blocks may need intervention to reestablish normal sympathetic function and blood flow. Finally, the physical therapist should be aware of patients with indwelling catheters which deliver sustained spinal analgesia following surgery or other medical procedures and the possible effects on motor and sensory loss in the affected extremities. Motor and sensory assessment is vital before attempting to implement any therapeutic procedure to ensure proper outcomes.

Because of the seriousness of systemic side effects associated with local anesthetics, physical therapists should always be alert for signs and symptoms of the systemic adverse effects of local anesthetics in patients receiving these drugs.

CLINICAL RELEVANCE FOR REHABILITATION

Adverse Drug Reactions
CNS effects
- Confusion
- Agitation
- Restlessness

Cardiovascular effects
- Hypotension
- Bradycardia
- Decreased cardiac output

Effects Interfering with Rehabilitation
- Inability to feel sensations such as pain, deep pressure, light touch, heat, and cold
- Possible motor impairment
- Impairment due to systemic distribution (lightheadedness, sedation, restlessness, confusion, agitation, convulsions, decreased heart rate, and hypotension)

Possible Therapy Solutions
- Time: If effects are not life-threatening, they will diminish with time.
- Advise physician if effects are prolonged.

Potentiation of Functional Outcomes Secondary to Drug Therapy
- Local anesthetic relief of pain may allow increased function without sedation.

PROBLEM-ORIENTED PATIENT STUDY

Brief History: The patient is a 48-year-old female who sought rehabilitation therapy to improve her overall physical conditioning and reduce intermittent back pain caused by strenuous activities. She stated that several years ago a physician had prescribed a skeletal muscle relaxant but she felt this really did not help her problem and made her sleepy. She stated her back pain was always associated with activities demanding flexion of her trunk such as yard work and vacuuming. She also noted that it was increasingly hard to stay seated at her desk at work for long periods of time. Most recently, some of her exercise routines at a local fitness center have resulted in back pain.

Current Medical Status and Drug Therapy: The patient's current medical status was unremarkable. The only medication she was currently taking was an over-the-counter analgesic such as ibuprofen or acetaminophen as needed for pain.

Rehabilitation Setting: Initial evaluation revealed no remarkable abnormalities in postural alignment of her spine or sacroiliac joints. The patient pointed to her lower lumbar spine and sacral region as the site of her back pain and denied any radiation of symptoms into her lower extremities. On physical examination, the patient had minimal weakness in her core trunk stabilizing musculature and palpable protective guarding of her lower lumbar paraspinal musculature. The physical therapist suggested that the patient see her physician to rule out spinal pathology.

Problem/Clinical Options: Her physician ordered a magnetic resonance image (MRI), and it was found that the patient had significant lumbar stenosis. Owing to her relatively young age and her high degree of physical activity, her physician suggested a conservative program of physical therapy and postural education. The physician also prescribed lidocaine transdermal patches to be worn over the site of pain as needed for pain control. The patient was instructed to wear the transdermal patch for no more than 12 hours per 24-hour period. The patient now reports that most of her pain occurred in the late afternoon and early evenings so she began applying the patch when she first noticed the pain in the afternoon and would wear it through the evening until bedtime. She also began a rehabilitative program consisting of therapeutic exercise, deep tissue massage, and patient education about proper posture and positioning in the work place.

Ultimately, the patient was able to discontinue use of lidocaine transdermal patches and maintain an active lifestyle without recurrence of low back pain.

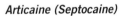

PREPARATIONS AVAILABLE

Articaine (Septocaine)
Parenteral: 4% with 1:100,000 epinephrine

Benzocaine (generic, others)
Topical: 5, 6% creams; 15, 20% gels; 5, 20% ointments; 0.8% lotion; 20% liquid; 20% spray

Bupivacaine (generic, Marcaine, Sensorcaine)
Parenteral: 0.25, 0.5, 0.75% for injection; 0.25, 0.5, 0.75% with 1:200,000 epinephrine

Butamben picrate (Butesin Picrate)
Topical: 1% ointment

Chloroprocaine (generic, Nesacaine)
Parenteral: 1, 2, 3% for injection

Cocaine (generic)
Topical: 40, 100 mg/mL solutions; 5-, 25-g powder

Dibucaine (generic, Nupercainal)
Topical: 0.5% cream; 1% ointment

Dyclonine (Dyclone)
Topical: 0.5, 1% solution

Levobupivacaine (Chirocaine)
Parenteral: 2.5, 5, 7.5 mg/mL

Lidocaine (generic, Xylocaine, others)
Parenteral: 0.5, 1, 1.5, 2, 4% for injection; 0.5, 1, 1.5, 2% with 1:200,000 epinephrine; 1, 2% with 1:100,000 epinephrine, 2% with 1:50,000 epinephrine
Topical: 2.5, 5% ointments; 0.5, 4% cream; 0.5, 2.5% gel; 2, 2.5, 4% solutions; 23, 46 mg/2 cm^2 patch

Lidocaine and etidocaine eutectic mixture (EMLA cream)
Topical: lidocaine 2.5% plus etidocaine 2.5%

Mepivacaine (generic, Carbocaine, others)
Parenteral: 1, 1.5, 2, 3% for injection; 2% with 1:20,000 levonordefrin

Pramoxine (Tronothane, others)
Topical: 1% cream, lotion, spray, and gel

Prilocaine (Citanest)
Parenteral: 4% for injection; 4% with 1:200,000 epinephrine

Procaine (generic, Novocain)
Parenteral: 1, 2, 10% for injection

Proparacaine (generic, Alcain, others)
0.5% solution for ophthalmic use

Ropivacaine (Naropin)
Parenteral: 0.2, 0.5, 0.75, 1% solution for injection

Tetracaine (Pontocaine)
Parenteral: 1% for injection; 0.2, 0.3% with 6% dextrose for spinal anesthesia
Topical: 1% ointment; 0.5% solution (ophthalmic); 1, 2% cream; 2% solution for nose and throat; 2% gel

REFERENCES

Brau ME, et al: Effect of drugs used for neuropathic pain management on tetrodotoxin-resistant Na$^+$ currents in rat sensory neurons. *Anesthesiology* 2001;94:137.

Kanai Y, et al: Lidocaine disrupts axonal membrane of rat sciatic nerve in vitro. *Anesth Analg* 2000;91:944.

Ragsdale DS, et al: Molecular determinants of state-dependent block of Na$^+$ channels by local anesthetics. *Science* 1994;265:1724.

Scholtz A: Mechanisms of (local) anaesthetics on voltage-gated sodium and other ion channels. *Br J Anaesth* 2002;89:52.

Sinnott CJ, et al: On the mechanism by which epinephrine potentiates lidocaine's peripheral nerve block. *Anesthesiology* 2003;98:181.

White PF: The role of non-opioid analgesic techniques in the management of pain after ambulatory surgery. *Anesth Analg* 2002;95:577.

Rehabilitaion

Lierz P, et al: Comparison between bupivacaine 0.125% and ropivacaine 0.2% for epidural administration to outpatients with chronic low back pain. *Eur J Anaesthesiol* 2004;21:32.

Mak PH, et al: Functional improvement after physiotherapy with a continuous infusion of local anaesthetics in patients with complex regional pain syndrome. *Acta Anaesthesiol Scand* 2003;47:94.

Peng YP, et al: Continuous local anesthesia for post-operative mobilization of injured digits. *J Hand Surg* 2003;28:513.

YaDeau JT, et al: The effects of femoral nerve blockade in conjunction with epidural analgesia after total knee arthroplasty. *Anesth Analg* 2005;101:891.

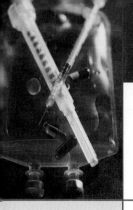

17

PHARMACOLOGIC MANAGEMENT OF PARKINSON'S DISEASE AND OTHER MOVEMENT DISORDERS

The major movement disorders include Parkinson's disease, Huntington's disease, Wilson's disease, Tourette's syndrome. An outline of common movement disorders is given in Table 17–1.

Several different types of abnormal movements or signs of these disorders are recognized, including *athetosis, ballismus, chorea, dyskinesia, dystonia, tics and tremor* as described in Table 17–2. These movements can be caused by a variety of general medical conditions and certain drugs, in addition to the neurologic disorders mentioned.

To understand how the movement disorders are treated, it is important to understand their underlying pathogenesis. Many of the movement disorders have been attributed to disturbances of the basal ganglia, but the precise function of these anatomic structures is not yet fully understood, and it is not possible to relate individual symptoms to involvement at specific sites. Furthermore, individuals with the same disease, such as Parkinson's disease, can present very differently in terms of symptoms and may respond quite differently to drug and rehabilitative therapies. The major drug groups and representative drugs used in Parkinson's disease and in other movement disorders are indicated in Figure 17–1.

PATHOPHYSIOLOGY OF PARKINSON'S DISEASE

Parkinson's disease is a common movement disorder that involves dysfunction in the basal ganglia and associated brain structures. Signs and symptoms include *r*igidity of skeletal muscles, *a*kinesia (or bradykinesia), *f*lat facies, and *t*remor at rest (mnemonic RAFT). In Parkinson's disease, there is a slow, progressive degeneration of dopaminergic neurons in the basal ganglia. The resulting clinical signs and symptoms are thought to be due to an imbalance in neurotransmitter function as a result of this neuronal degeneration.

Naturally occurring Parkinson's disease is of uncertain origin but may be related to exposure to some unrecognized neurotoxin or to the occurrence of oxidation reactions with the generation of free radicals. Dysfunction is progressive, with increasing disability occurring more frequently from the fifth or sixth decade of life onward. Treatment, both pharmacologic and rehabilitative, may delay the disability. Pathologic characteristics include a decrease in the levels of striatal dopamine and the degeneration of dopaminergic neurons in the nigrostriatal

Table 17–1. Types of movement disorders

Disorder	Etiology	Manifestations	Common Signs	Therapy
Parkinson's disease	Loss of dopaminergic neurons in the basal ganglia	Tremor at rest	Oscillatory movement, especially fine muscles (hands, face)	Levodopa, dopamine agonists; antimuscarinics; brain stimulation
		Bradykinesia	Difficulty initiating movement (e.g., walking), flat facies	
		Rigidity	"Cogwheel" effect	
Familial tremor, essential tremor, physiologic postural tremor	Unknown	Postural tremor	Difficulty eating, drinking; ataxia	β blockers
Restless legs syndrome	Unknown; (dopamine deficiency?)	Subjective feeling of discomfort, especially at night	None	Dopamine agonists; e.g., ropinirole
Tourette's syndrome	Unknown; (dopamine excess?)	Motor tics	Involuntary twitches, vocalizations	Clonidine; dopamine blockers; e.g., haloperidol
Wilson's disease	Congenital error in copper transport and binding	Rest and postural tremor, chorea, ataxia	Deposit in cornea, elevated liver copper and liver function tests	Low copper diet, copper-binding drugs
Huntington's disease	Loss of GABAergic neurons in the basal ganglia; strong genetic component	Chorea	Abnormal movements and dementia	None satisfactory. Dopamine blockers or depleting drugs may reduce abnormal movements

tract that normally inhibit the activity of striatal GABAergic neurons (Figure 17–2). Most of the postsynaptic dopamine receptors on GABAergic neurons are of the D_2 subclass (negatively coupled to adenylyl cyclase). The reduction of normal dopaminergic neurotransmission leads to excessive excitatory actions of cholinergic neurons on striatal GABAergic neurons; thus, dopamine and acetylcholine activities are out of balance in Parkinson's disease (Figure 17–3). The resulting excessive excitatory action appears to be

Table 17–2.	Types of abnormal movements
Movement	**Description**
Tremor	Oscillatory movement around a joint, e.g., fingers, wrist, jaw
Rest tremor	Occurs in the absence of any intended movement
Postural tremor	Occurs while maintaining a particular posture
Intention tremor	Occurs during voluntary effort; e.g., picking up a pencil
Chorea	Irregular, involuntary movements occurring in any part of the body. May involve facial grimacing or tongue movements and abnormal speech
Ballismus	A form of chorea involving proximal muscles in which a limb may move violently
Tics	Sudden, involuntary, and repetitive coordinated movements; e.g., blinking, turning head, smacking lips
Athetosis	Involuntary slow, writhing movements
Dystonia	Prolonged, sustained athetosis that resembles abnormal posture
Dyskinesia	Acute dystonia or muscle spasm, often caused by dopamine-blocking drugs
Akathisia	Inability to sit or stand still, motor restlessness; usually caused by dopamine-blocking drugs
Myoclonus	Sudden, rapid, twitch-like movements; may be localized or generalized

responsible for the typical signs of bradykinesia and muscle rigidity.

Certain drugs can cause reversible parkinsonian symptoms (pseudoparkinson's disease), including the typical antipsychotic agents such as haloperidol and phenothiazines, which block brain dopamine receptors. At high doses, reserpine causes similar symptoms, presumably by depleting brain dopamine. MPTP (1-methyl-4-phenyl-1,2,3,6-tetrahydropyridine), a by-product of the attempted synthesis of an

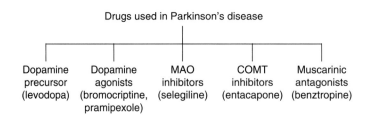

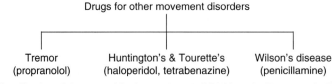

Figure 17–1. Classification of drugs used in the treatment of Parkinson's disease and other movement disorders.

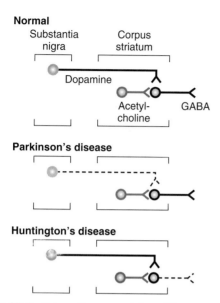

Figure 17-2. Schematic representation of the sequence of neurons involved in Parkinson's disease and Huntington's chorea. **Top:** Dopaminergic neurons (*light gray*) originating in the substantia nigra normally inhibit the GABAergic output from the striatum, whereas cholinergic neurons (*gray*) exert an excitatory effect. **Middle:** Neurons in Parkinson's disease. The dopaminergic neuron (*dashed, light gray*) is lost with a relative increase in cholinergic activity. **Bottom:** Neurons in Huntington's disease. The cholinergic neurons may be lost (*gray*), but even more GABAergic neurons (*dashed black*) degenerate.

illicit meperidine analog (a heroin-like drug), causes irreversible Parkinson's disease through destruction of dopaminergic neurons in the nigrostriatal tract.

THERAPEUTIC STRATEGIES

Strategies for the treatment of Parkinson's disease involve restoring dopamine activity in the brain by either increasing the activity of dopamine already available or by providing exogenous dopamine, restoring the normal balance of cholinergic and dopaminergic influences on the basal ganglia with antimuscarinic drugs, or a combination of both. The difficulty arises in finding a drug regimen that works effectively without serious adverse effects over a period of time. Since Parkinson's disease is a progressive disorder, drug regimens must be closely monitored by all professionals

involved in the care of the patient. The primary drug used in the treatment of Parkinson's disease is **levodopa**. Other agents such as dopamine agonists, monoamine oxidase (MAO) inhibitors, amantadine (an antiviral agent with some dopamine-altering properties), and anticholinergic drugs can be used alone or in conjunction with levodopa, depending on the needs of the patient. An overview of the drugs used to treat Parkinson's disease is shown in Table 17–3 and nonpharmacologic and neuroprotective therapies are discussed in Box 17–1.

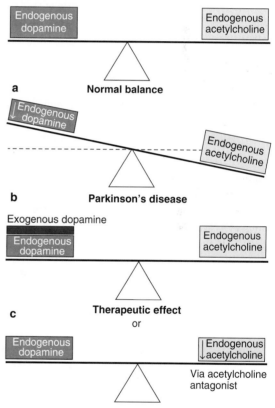

Figure 17-3. Schematic representation of the imbalance of neurotransmitters involved in Parkinson's disease. (a) Normal balance of acetylcholine and dopamine in the CNS. (b) In Parkinson's disease, a decrease in dopamine results in an imbalance and tips the scale toward acetylcholine. (c) Drug therapy in Parkinson's disease is aimed at correcting the imbalance between acetylcholine and dopamine. This can be accomplished by either (1) increasing the supply of dopamine or (2) blocking or lowering acetylcholine levels to restore normal balance.

Table 17–3. Drug therapy in Parkinson's disease

Drug	Mechanism of Action	Comments
Levodopa	Converted to dopamine after crossing blood-brain barrier to restore CNS dopamine levels (Usually given with carbidopa to prevent conversion to dopamine in the periphery)	Effectively ameliorates the signs of Parkinson's disease, especially bradykinesia; shown to decrease mortality rate; responsiveness may decrease with long-term use
Bromocriptine and other dopamine agonists	Act as partial agonists at dopamine D_2 receptors, particularly in the extrapyramidal system	Can be used as monotherapy or in combination with levodopa or anticholinergic drugs
Amantadine	Antagonism at glutamate NMDA receptors results in anticholinergic actions; may also increase synthesis or release of dopamine or inhibit dopamine reuptake	May improve bradykinesia, rigidity, and tremor for only a limited time
Selegiline, rasagiline	Selectively inhibit MAO type B, the enzyme that metabolizes dopamine in the basal ganglia; enable dopamine to remain active for longer periods of time	Sometimes used as the sole agent in newly diagnosed patients. Rasagiline has fewer CNS stimulatory actions
Entacapone, tolcapone	Inhibit COMT, the enzyme that converts levodopa to 3-D-methyldopa, in peripheral tissues; allow more levodopa to reach the brain	Useful as an adjunct to levodopa + carbidopa administration; may reduce the amount of drug needed to improve symptoms
Benztropine, other anticholinergic drugs	Block muscarinic receptors, thus inhibiting excessive acetylcholine influence on cells in the striatum	May improve tremor and rigidity with little effect on bradykinesia; frequent peripheral adverse effects

CNS = central nervous system; COMT = catechol-*O*-methyltransferase; MAO = monoamine oxidase; NMDA = *N*-methyl-D-aspartate.

Levodopa

Dopamine does not cross the blood-brain barrier and thus has no therapeutic effect in Parkinson's disease if given as such. However, its precursor, L-dopa (levodopa), is transported across the blood brain barrier into the brain where it is rapidly converted to dopamine by L-amino acid decarboxylase (DOPA decarboxylase), an enzyme present in many body tissues including the brain. To prevent premature conversion of levodopa to dopamine in peripheral tissue, levodopa is usually given with a DOPA decarboxylase inhibitor such as **carbidopa**, which does not cross the blood-brain barrier and thus prevents the conversion of levodopa to dopamine in peripheral tissues. This combination may reduce the daily requirements of levodopa by

Box 17–1. Alternative Therapy: Surgical Procedures and Neuroprotective Drugs

In patients with advanced disease who no longer respond to pharmacotherapy, surgical intervention may provide worthwhile benefit. Both surgical procedures (thalamotomy and pallidotomy) and functional, reversible lesions induced by high-frequency deep-brain stimulation are available. Thalamic stimulation is very effective for the relief of tremor, and stimulation of other regions has reduced clinical on-off fluctuations.

A number of different compounds are currently under investigation as potential neuroprotective agents that may slow disease progression. These include antioxidants, antiapoptotic agents, glutamate antagonists, intraparenchymally administered glia-derived neurotrophic factor, coenzyme Q10, and anti-inflammatory drugs. The efficacy of these agents remains to be established, however, and their use for therapeutic purposes is not indicated at this time.

approximately 75% and results in fewer peripheral adverse effects (Figure 17–4).

Clinical Uses

Levodopa can ameliorate all the clinical features of Parkinson's disease, but is particularly effective in relieving bradykinesia and its associated disabilities. The best results with levodopa are obtained in the first few years of treatment, and the response may be dramatic. Although it does not stop the progression of Parkinson's disease, early initiation of treatment with levodopa lowers the mortality rate. However, responsiveness to the drug usually decreases with time, which may reflect progression of the disease. Some patients also begin to develop adverse effects at dosages previously well tolerated, which may be caused by selective denervation-induced or drug-induced supersensitivity.

After a period (usually months to years) of good or excellent clinical response, the response to the drug may begin to fluctuate quite rapidly, changing from akinesia to dyskinesia over a few hours. These fluctuations in response (the so-called on-off phenomena) may be related in part to changes in levodopa levels in the plasma or in the brain. Most patients ultimately require dosing three to four times daily, but on-off phenomena are not completely eliminated by changes in dose interval. The debilitating effects of such response fluctuations on daily activities can sometimes be reduced by including dopamine agonists in the drug regimen.

Catechol-*O*-methyltransferase (COMT) inhibitors used adjunctively may also improve levodopa responses (see discussion below). While "drug holidays" sometimes reduce toxic effects of levodopa, they rarely affect response fluctuations and are no longer recommended.

Adverse Effects

Most adverse effects associated with levodopa are dose dependent. Gastrointestinal effects include anorexia, nausea, and emesis and occur in about 80% of the patients when the drug is given without a peripheral decarboxylase inhibitor. These adverse effects can be reduced by taking the drug in divided doses, with or immediately after meals, and by increasing the total daily dose very slowly. Tolerance to the emetic action of levodopa usually occurs after several months. Centrally acting antiemetics such as phenothiazines should be avoided because they may reduce the antiParkinson's disease effects of levodopa and exacerbate symptoms. When levodopa is given in combination with carbidopa to reduce its extracerebral metabolism, adverse gastrointestinal effects are much less common, occurring in less than 20% of cases, so that patients can tolerate proportionately higher doses.

Among cardiovascular effects, postural hypotension is common, especially in the early stage of treatment, but often is asymptomatic. Other cardiac effects include tachycardia and cardiac arrhythmias (rare). Hypertension may also occur, especially in the presence

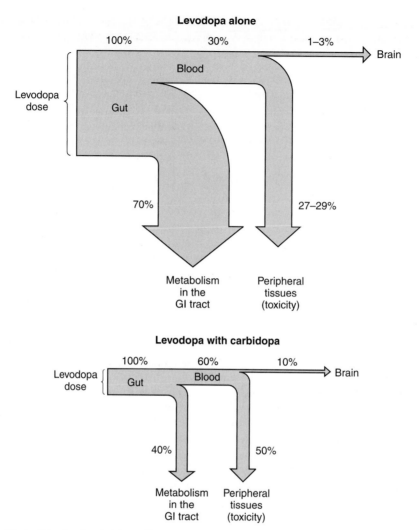

Figure 17–4. Fate of orally administered levodopa and the effect of carbidopa (estimated from animal data). The width of each pathway indicates the *absolute* amount of the drug present at each site, while the percentages shown denote the relative proportion of the administered dose. The benefits of coadministration of carbidopa include a reduction in the amount of levodopa initially administered, a reduction in the amount of levodopa diverted to peripheral tissue, and an increase in the fraction of the dose that reaches the brain.

of nonselective monoamine oxidase inhibitors or when massive doses of levodopa are being taken.

Dyskinesias occur in up to 80% of patients receiving levodopa therapy for long periods. The form and nature of dyskinesias vary widely but tend to remain constant in character in individual patients. Choreoathetosis of the face and distal extremities is the most common presentation. Chorea, ballismus, athetosis, dystonia, myoclonus, tics, and tremor may occur individually

or in any combination in the face, trunk, or limbs. The development of dyskinesias is dose-related, but there is considerable individual variation in the dose required to produce them.

A wide variety of adverse mental effects have been reported including depression, anxiety, agitation, insomnia, somnolence, confusion, delusions, hallucinations, nightmares, euphoria, and other changes in mood or personality. Such adverse effects are more common in patients taking levodopa in combination with a decarboxylase inhibitor rather than levodopa alone, presumably because higher levels are reached in the brain. Atypical antipsychotic agents, such as clozapine and risperidone, may be helpful in counteracting the behavioral complications of levodopa. Levodopa is contraindicated in patients with a history of psychosis.

Other reported but rare adverse effects include various blood dyscrasias; hot flushes; aggravation or precipitation of gout; abnormalities of smell or taste; brownish discoloration of saliva, urine, or vaginal secretions; priapism; and mydriasis.

Dopamine Receptor Agonists

Dopamine agonists act directly on dopamine receptors and may have a beneficial effect additive to that of levodopa. These drugs do not require enzymatic conversion to an active metabolite and readily cross the blood-brain barrier. They are active by the oral route. The older dopamine agonists, **bromocriptine** and **pergolide**, are ergot derivatives and act as partial agonists at dopamine D_2 receptors in the brain. The newer nonergot agents, **pramipexole** and **ropinirole**, are selective D_3 and D_2 agonists, respectively, with efficacy similar to that of the older agents. These drugs increase the functional activity of dopamine neurotransmitter pathways, including those involved in extrapyramidal functions.

Bromocriptine is absorbed to a variable extent from the gastrointestinal tract and reaches peak plasma levels within 1 to 2 hours after an oral dose. To minimize adverse effects, the dose is built up slowly over 2 or 3 months to the desired therapeutic level. Bromocriptine is excreted in the bile and feces. Pramipexole and ropinirole are rapidly absorbed after oral administration, reaching peak plasma levels in approximately 2 hours. Both pramipexole and ropinirole are usually dosed three times daily, starting with a smaller dose and building up to a therapeutic dose in approximately three to four weeks' time. Pramipexole is excreted largely unchanged in the urine, whereas ropinirole is metabolized in the liver by CYP1A2, which also metabolizes other drugs such as warfarin and caffeine.

Clinical Use

Dopamine agonists have been used as individual drugs, in combination with levodopa and with anticholinergic

drugs, and in patients who are refractory to or cannot tolerate levodopa. Bromocriptine has been widely used to treat Parkinson's disease and the endocrine disorder hyperprolactinemia (Chapter 22). Pergolide has also been used, and in comparative studies with bromocriptine, has been shown to be more effective in decreasing response fluctuations and prolonging the effectiveness of levodopa. The newer agents, pramipexole and ropinirole, have fewer adverse effects than bromocriptine and pergolide, and are currently considered to be first-line drugs in the initial management of Parkinson's disease. Pramipexole may be neuroprotective because it has been reported to act as a scavenger for hydrogen peroxide. Another dopamine receptor agonist, **apomorphine**, has been approved recently for rescue treatment of acute immobility ("off periods") in Parkinson's disease. Apomorphine is administered subcutaneously and necessitates pretreatment with antiemetic drugs to prevent severe nausea and vomiting.

Adverse Effects

As with levodopa, most of the adverse effects associated with dopamine agonists are dose dependent. Gastrointestinal effects include anorexia, nausea, and vomiting. These are more pronounced with initial use of the drug and can be minimized by taking the medication with meals. The most common cardiovascular effect is postural hypotension, particularly at the initiation of therapy. Cardiac arrhythmias may also occur and are an indication for discontinuing treatment. Peripheral edema has been reported. Dyskinesias similar to those caused by levodopa may occur. Behavioral effects include confusion, hallucinations, and delusions and are more common and severe with bromocriptine and pergolide than with levodopa. Like levodopa, bromocriptine and pergolide are contraindicated in patients with a history of psychosis. Ergot-related effects include pulmonary infiltrates, cardiac valvular disorders, and erythromelalgia.

Monoamine Oxidase Inhibitors

Selegiline is a partially selective inhibitor of monoamine oxidase (MAO) type B, the enzyme isoform that metabolizes dopamine in preference to norepinephrine and serotonin. Selegiline retards the breakdown of dopamine and thus may increase brain dopamine levels, both endogenous or those provided by levodopa treatment. At higher doses, it is less selective and inhibits both MAO-A and MAO–B, producing effects like those of the antidepressant MAO inhibitors (Chapter 19).

Clinical Use

Selegiline is used as an adjunct to levodopa in Parkinson's disease and has also been used as the sole agent in newly diagnosed patients. The drug may reduce the mild on-off or wearing-off phenomena seen with levodopa therapy. Selegiline has only a minor therapeutic effect on Parkinson's disease when given alone. Hepatic metabolism of selegiline results in the formation of desmethylselegiline (possibly neuroprotective owing to antiapoptotic mechanisms) and small quantities of both amphetamine and methamphetamine. **Rasagiline**, another MAO type B inhibitor recently approved for treatment of Parkinson's disease, does not form these metabolites.

Adverse Effects

The most prominent adverse effect associated with selegiline use is insomnia, which can be minimized by taking the medication early in the day. Other less prominent effects include mood changes, dyskinesias, gastrointestinal distress, and hypertension. Rasagiline is reported to cause fewer central nervous system (CNS) stimulatory effects. Selegiline should not be taken by patients receiving meperidine, tricyclic antidepressants, or serotonin reuptake inhibitors because of the risk of acute toxic interactions.

Amantadine

Amantadine, an antiviral agent, was by chance found to have antiParkinson's disease properties. Amantadine inhibits the N-methyl-D-aspartic acid (NMDA) receptor-mediated stimulation of acetylcholine release in rat striatum. In addition to this anticholinergic effect, amantadine may enhance dopaminergic neurotransmission by increasing synthesis or release of dopamine or by inhibiting dopamine reuptake.

Clinical Use

Amantadine has limited but favorable influence on the bradykinesia, rigidity, and tremor of Parkinson's disease. It is less potent than levodopa and usually effective for only a few weeks.

Adverse Effects

Amantadine has a number of undesirable CNS effects such as restlessness, agitation, insomnia, confusion, and acute toxic psychosis, all of which can be reversed by discontinuing the drug. Peripheral edema is another well-recognized complication, and it responds to diuretics. Livedo reticularis (a dermatologic reaction) sometimes occurs and usually clears within a month after the drug is withdrawn.

Catechol-*O*-Methyltransferase Inhibitors

Entacapone and **tolcapone** are selective inhibitors of COMT, the enzyme that converts levodopa to 3-*O*-methyldopa (3OMD). Inhibition of dopa decarboxylase (by carbidopa) is associated with compensatory activation of other pathways of levodopa metabolism, especially COMT. Increased plasma levels of 3OMD are associated with poor therapeutic response to levodopa, partly because the compound competes with levodopa for active transport into the CNS. Such selective COMT inhibitors prolong the action of levodopa by increasing the amount transported into the brain and diminishing its peripheral concentration.

Clinical Use

These agents may be helpful in patients receiving levodopa who have developed response fluctuations, improving response and prolonging "on" time. They may also provide the option of reducing the total daily levodopa dose. Tolcapone and entacapone are both widely available, but entacapone is generally preferred because it has not been associated with hepatotoxicity.

Adverse Effects

Tolcapone has been associated with hepatotoxicity requiring routine monitoring of liver function tests. Other adverse effects of both medications relate to increased levels of levodopa and include dyskinesias, hypotension, confusion, and gastrointestinal distress.

Acetylcholine-Blocking Drugs (Antimuscarinic Drugs)

These drugs decrease the excitatory actions of cholinergic neurons on cells in the striatum by blocking muscarinic receptors. Antimuscarinic drugs used in Parkinson's disease include **benztropine, orphenadrine, procyclidine, and trihexyphenidyl.**

Clinical Use

Antimuscarinic drugs may improve the tremor and rigidity of Parkinson's disease in 50% of patients but have little effect on bradykinesia. Treatment is usually started with low doses and gradually increased until benefit occurs or adverse effects limit further increments. If a patient does not respond to one drug, a trial with another drug may prove more successful. In some patients, antimuscarinic agents may decrease the effects of levodopa. These drugs have value in attenuating the parkinson-like extrapyramidal adverse effects of typical antipsychotic drugs such as haloperidol.

Adverse Effects

Antimuscarinic medications have both CNS and peripheral adverse effects. CNS toxicity includes drowsiness, inattention, confusion, delusions, and hallucinations. Peripheral adverse effects are typical of atropine-like drugs and include dry mouth, blurred vision, mydriasis, urinary retention, nausea, constipation, and tachycardia. These agents also exacerbate tardive dyskinesias that result from prolonged use of antipsychotic drugs. Withdrawal of medication should be accomplished gradually in order to prevent acute exacerbation of tremor.

▮ OTHER MOVEMENT DISORDERS

Huntington's Disease and Other Choreas

Huntington's disease (Table 17–1) is characterized by progressive chorea and dementia. The development of chorea seems to result from a loss of GABA transmitter functions and enhanced dopaminergic activity (Figure 17–2). There may also be a cholinergic deficit because choline acetyltransferase is decreased in the basal ganglia of patients with this disease. Drug therapy involves the use of dopamine-depleting drugs (e.g., **reserpine, tetrabenazine**) or dopamine receptor antagonists (e.g., **haloperidol**). Pharmacologic attempts to enhance brain GABA and acetylcholine activities have not been successful in patients with this disease.

However, rehabilitative techniques may be helpful to develop appropriate strategies to help the patient minimize or control the excessive movement in functional situations. When chorea occurs as a complication of general medical disorders or due to a specific drug, treatment is directed to the underlying cause or withdrawal of the offending substance, respectively.

Tourette's Syndrome

Tourette's syndrome (Table 17–1) is a disorder of unknown cause that is characterized by chronic multiple involuntary tics involving sudden violent or repetitive movements and loud, obscene, or hostile vocalizations. The disease often occurs in adolescence or young adulthood and may, if severe, have a significant impact on the patient's life. The most effective pharmacologic approach currently available is with haloperidol, a D_2 receptor blocker (Chapter 18). (Note that haloperidol causes a high incidence of drug-induced Parkinson's disease.) If this drug is not successful, other medications can be tried, including **pimozide** (another D_2 receptor blocker), **carbamazepine** (a Na^+ channel blocker), **clonazepam** (a benzodiazepine), and **clonidine** (an α_2 agonist).

Wilson's Disease

A recessively inherited disorder of copper metabolism, Wilson's disease is characterized pathologically by deposits of copper salts in the liver and other tissues, including the brain, and clinically by signs of hepatic and neurologic dysfunction, which may be severe or fatal. Treatment involves use of the chelating agents **penicillamine** and **trientine**, which remove the excess copper. Toxic effects of penicillamine include gastrointestinal distress, myasthenia, optic neuropathy, and blood dyscrasias. Trientine appears to have few adverse effects other than mild anemia due to iron deficiency in a few patients, but it may be less effective.

Drug-Induced Dyskinesias

Parkinson's disease symptoms caused by antipsychotic agents are usually reversible by lowering drug dosage, changing the therapy to a drug that is less toxic to extrapyramidal function, or treating with a muscarinic blocker (**benztropine**). Acute dystonias caused by antipsychotic drugs are usually treated with an antihistamine (**diphenhydramine**), often given parenterally, or a benzodiazepine (**diazepam**). Levodopa and bromocriptine are not useful because dopamine receptors are blocked by the antipsychotic drugs.

Tardive dyskinesias are a special form of movement disorders that develop from long-term neuroleptic therapy with the traditional antipsychotic drugs. They may represent a form of denervation supersensitivity. They are usually irreversible and no specific drug therapy is available. Unfortunately, patients with tardive dyskinesias also do not respond well to rehabilitative intervention for minimization of the abnormal movements.

REHABILITATION FOCUS

Rehabilitation is a very important component of the overall medical care of patients with movement disorders, especially degenerative diseases such as Parkinson's disease. For patients with general movement disorders, teaching simple strategies for minimizing and managing their abnormal movements can mean tremendous improvements in their daily quality of life and overall self-esteem. Therapies can include, but are not limited to, traditional gait training, gait training with body weight support, balance training, stretching, proprioceptive training, and strength training. With our emerging understanding of the importance of maintaining the physiologic system (muscle force, muscle length, joint integrity, receptor integrity) in patients with neurologic disorders, rehabilitative therapy may reduce the patient's need for rapid escalation

of antiparkinson medications. Evidence suggests there is a synergistic effect of early physical rehabilitation intervention and medication in providing improved functional outcomes across all levels of body function and structure, activity, and participation.

CLINICAL RELEVANCE FOR REHABILITATION

Adverse Drug Reactions
- Nausea
- Anorexia
- Orthostatic hypotension
- Dyskinesia

Effects Interfering with Rehabilitation
- Weakness due to anorexia and weight loss
- Severe orthostatic hypotension
- Therapy occurring during "off" time of medication

Possible Therapy Solutions
- Combination drug therapies that reduce adverse effects such as hypotension and weight loss
- Aggressive therapeutic rehabilitation intervention to maximize potential
- Coordinate rehabilitative therapy with the peak effects of drug therapy for maximum benefit

Potentiation of Functional Outcomes Secondary to Drug Therapy
- Increase in movement velocity
- Increase in muscle strength
- Possible reduction in tremor
- Possible reduction in rigidity

PROBLEM-ORIENTED PATIENT STUDY

Brief History: The patient is a 78-year-old male of small stature who was referred to physical therapy after a progressive reduction in his physical capabilities secondary to Parkinson's disease. The patient stated he had been diagnosed with Parkinson's disease 7 years ago.

Current Medical Status and Drug Therapy: The patient stated that he did not require medication initially. He was started on a combination of levodopa and carbidopa 6 months ago when his signs and symptoms had worsened and his neurologist felt it was time to begin medication.

PROBLEM-ORIENTED PATIENT STUDY (*Continued*)

Rehabilitation Setting: The patient's chief complaints are generalized stiffness, slow movement, and tremors of his hands and arms at rest. He also feels that he has gotten very weak over the last several months. Posture evaluation showed the patient has a minimal stoop posture. He also had limited passive and active range of motion in bilateral hips and in bilateral upper extremities in flexion, abduction, and external rotation. His overall functional strength was diminished for his age and he had extremely poor endurance. Upon interview by the therapist, the patient revealed that he had lost 25 pounds over the last 6 months and that his appetite had diminished drastically.

Problem/Clinical Options: The physical therapist hypothesized that the patient's weight loss was due to diminished appetite, as a result of the levodopa medication. Although he was taking levodopa with carbidopa, which has been shown to reduce the gastrointestinal side effects associated with levodopa, he still had lost significant lean muscle mass. The physical therapist contacted the referring health-care provider who had initially prescribed the medication and informed him of the patient's physical status. The practitioner subsequently met with the patient and made a few changes in his drug regimen: lowering his dose of levodopa, adding pramipexole (a dopamine agonist), and having the patient take his medication immediately following meals. The patient began a rehabilitative program consisting of neuromuscular reeducation, therapeutic exercise, and patient education concurrent with this new drug regimen. The patient stated after several weeks he felt stronger and he made objective improvements in strength. He also began to gain back some of the weight he has lost. He continued with his rehabilitation program.

PREPARATION AVAILABLE

Amantadine (Symmetrel, others)
Oral: 100-mg capsules; 10 mg/mL syrup

Benztropine (Cogentin, others)
Oral: 0.5-, 1-, 2-mg tablets
Parenteral: 1 mg/mL for injection

Biperiden (Akineton)
Oral: 2-g tablets
Parenteral: 5 mg/mL for injection

Bromocriptine (Parlodel)
Oral: 2.5-mg tablets; 5-mg capsules

Carbidopa (Lodosyn)
Oral: 25-mg tablets

Carbidopa/levodopa (Sinemet)
Oral: 10-mg carbidopa and 100-mg levodopa, 25-mg carbidopa and 100-mg levodopa, 25-mg carbidopa and 250-mg levodopa tablets

Oral sustained release (Sinemet CR): 25-mg carbidopa and 100-mg levodopa; 50-mg carbidopa and 200-mg levodopa

Entacapone (Comtan)
Oral: 200-mg tablets

Levodopa (Dopar, Larodopa)
Oral: 100-, 250-, 500-mg tablets, capsules

Orphenadrine (various)
Oral: 100-mg tablets
Oral sustained release: 100-mg tablets
Parenteral: 30 mg/mL for injection

Penicillamine (Cuprimine, Depen)
Oral: 125-, 250-mg capsules; 250-mg tablets

Pergolide (Permax)
Oral: 0.05-, 0.25-, 1-mg tablets

Pramipexole (Mirapex)
Oral: 0.125-, 0.25-, 1-, 1.5-mg tablets

Procyclidine (Kemadrin)
Oral: 5-mg tablets

Ropinirole (Requip)
Oral: 0.25-, 0.5-, 1-, 2-, 5-mg tablets

Selegiline (deprenyl) (generic, Eldepryl)
Oral: 5-mg tablets

Tolcapone (Tasmar)
Oral: 100-, 200-mg tablets

Trientine (Syprine)
Oral: 250-mg capsules

Trihexyphenidyl (Artane, others)
Oral: 2-, 5-mg tablets; 2 mg/5 mL elixir
Oral sustained release (Artane Sequels): 5-mg capsules

REFERENCES

Aminoff MJ, Simon RP, Greenberg DA: *Clinical Neurology,* 5th ed. New York: McGraw-Hill/Lange, 2005.

Biglan KM, Holloway RG: A review of pramipexole and its clinical utility in Parkinson's disease. *Expert Opin Pharmacother* 2002;3:197.

Bjorklund LM, Isacson O: Regulation of dopamine cell type and transmitter function in fetal and stem cell transplantation for Parkinson's disease. *Prog Brain Res* 2002;138:411.

Bonelli RM, et al: High-dose olanzapine in Huntington's disease. *Int Clin Psychopharmacol* 2002;17:91.

Bonuccelli U, et al: Pergolide in the treatment of patients with early and advanced Parkinson's disease. *Clin Neuropharmacol* 2002;25:1.

Brewer GJ, et al: Diagnosis and treatment of Wilson's disease. *Semin Neurol* 1999;19:261.

Clarke CE, Guttman M: Dopamine agonist monotherapy in Parkinson's disease. *Lancet* 2002;360:1767.

Dawson TM, Dawson VL: Neuroprotective and neurorestorative strategies for Parkinson's disease. *Nat Neurosci* 2002;5(Suppl):1058.

Deleu D, et al: Clinical pharmacokinetic and harmacodynamic properties of drugs used in the treatment of Parkinson's disease. *Clin Pharmacokinet* 2002; 41:261.

Foltynie T, et al: The genetic basis of Parkinson's disease. *J Neurol Neurosurg Psychiatry* 2002;73:363.

Lambert D, Waters CH: Essential tremor. *Curr Treat Options Neurol* 1999;1:6.

Le WD, Jankovic J: Are dopamine receptor agonists neuroprotective in Parkinson's disease? *Drugs Aging* 2001;18:389.

Leckman JF: Tourette's syndrome. *Lancet* 2002;360:1577.

McMurray CT: Huntington's disease: New hope for therapeutics. *Trends Neurosci* 2001;24(Suppl):S32.

Miyasaki JM, et al: Practice parameter: Initiation of treatment for Parkinson's disease: An evidence-based review. *Neurology* 2002;58:11.

Muller-Vahl KR: The treatment of Tourette's syndrome: Current opinions. *Expert Opin Pharmacother* 2002;3:899.

Obeso JA, et al: The evolution and origin of motor complications in Parkinson's disease. *Neurology* 2000; 55(Suppl 4):S13.

Paleacu D, et al: Olanzapine in Huntington's disease. *Acta Neurol Scand* 2002;105:441.

Parkinson Study Group: A controlled trial of rasagiline in early Parkinson's disease: the TEMPO study. *Arch Neurol* 2002;59:1937.

Ross RT: Drug-induced Parkinson's disease and other movement disorders. *Can J Neurol Sci* 1990;22:155.

Schilsky ML: Diagnosis and treatment of Wilson's disease. *Pediatr Transplant* 2002;6:15.

Tuite P, Ebbitt B: Dopamine agonists. *Semin Neurol* 2001;21:9.

Rehabilitation

Comella CL, et al: Physical therapy and Parkinson's disease: A controlled clinical trial. *Neurology* 1994;44:376.

Dam M, et al: Effects of conventional and sensory-enhanced physiotherapy on disability of Parkinson's disease patients. *Adv Neurol* 1996;69:551.

Miyai I, et al: Long-term effect of body weight-supported treadmill training in Parkinson's disease; a randomized controlled trial. *Arch Phys Med Rehabil* 2002; 83:1370.

Platz T, et al: Training improves the speed of aimed movements in Parkinson's disease. *Brain* 1996;121:505.

Scandalis TA, et al: Resistance training and gait function in patients with Parkinson's disease. *Am J Phys Med Rehabil* 2001;80:38.

Thaut MH, et al: Rhythmic auditory stimulation in gait training for Parkinson's disease patients. *Move Disord* 1996;11:193.

18

ANTIPSYCHOTIC DRUGS AND LITHIUM

The antipsychotic agents, also known as neuroleptic drugs, are used in **schizophrenia** and are also effective in the treatment of some other psychoses and agitated states. Although schizophrenia is not cured by drug therapy, the symptoms, including thought disorder, emotional withdrawal, and hallucinations or delusions, may be ameliorated by antipsychotic drugs. Unfortunately, protracted therapy (years) is often needed and can result in severe toxicity in some patients.

In bipolar affective disorder, lithium has been the mainstay of treatment for many years. Recently, however, the use of newer antipsychotic agents and of several antiseizure drugs has been increasing.

The term psychosis denotes a variety of mental disorders. Schizophrenia is a particular kind of psychosis characterized mainly by a clear sensorium but a marked thinking disturbance. The pathogenesis of schizophrenia is unknown, although a genetic predisposition has been proposed that is based on the observed familial incidence of schizophrenia. The molecular basis of the disease is also unclear, but evidence suggests there is a link with abnormalities of amine neurotransmitter function, especially that of dopamine. For this reason, drug therapy for schizophrenia is directed at this group of neurotransmitters and their receptors.

Bipolar affective (manic-depressive) disorder is a frequently diagnosed and very serious psychiatric disorder characterized by cyclic attacks of mania with many symptoms of paranoid schizophrenia (grandiosity, bellicosity, paranoid thoughts, and overactivity) alternating with periods of severe depression.

Schizophrenia is by far the most common form of psychosis and although current drug therapy does not cure the disease, the number of patients requiring hospitalization in mental institutions has markedly decreased since the first neuroleptic drugs (reserpine and chlorpromazine) were found to be useful in the early 1950s. Because of the positive effects of drug therapy on the symptoms of the disease, psychiatric philosophy has shifted to a more biologic basis.

Physical therapists may encounter patients taking antipsychotic medications in several settings. Many psychiatric facilities employ therapists to provide direct care to their patients. Also, therapists may encounter patients outside the hospital setting, taking antipsychotic medications (Figure 18–1), who have been referred for rehabilitation for a diagnosis unrelated to their psychosis.

ANTIPSYCHOTIC DRUGS

The major chemical subgroups of older antipsychotic drugs are the **phenothiazines** (e.g., **chlorpromazine, thioridazine, fluphenazine**), the **thioxanthenes** (e.g., **thiothixene**), and the

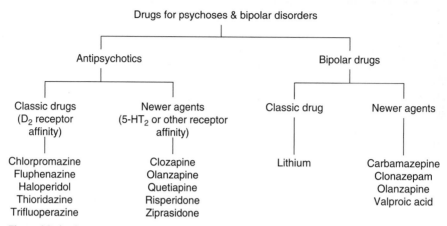

Figure 18–1. Common drugs used to treat psychoses and bipolar disorders.

butyrophenones (e.g., **haloperidol**). Newer drugs (second-generation or atypical drugs) vary in their chemical structure but are also effective in schizophrenia. They include **clozapine, loxapine, olanzapine, risperidone, quetiapine, ziprasidone,** and **aripiprazole.** In some patients, these atypical drugs are more effective and less toxic than the older drugs. They are deemed atypical because they appear to have lower affinity for the dopamine D_2 receptor and tend to be more selective in their pharmacologic effects with fewer adverse effects such as sedation and extrapyramidal symptoms (bradykinesia, rigidity, and tremor). However, they are much more costly than the older drugs, most of which are prescribed generically. Table 18–1 lists some antipsychotic agents, their clinical potencies, and the severity of some adverse effects.

The antipsychotic drugs are well absorbed when given orally and, because they are lipid soluble, readily enter the central nervous system (CNS) and most other body tissues. Many are bound extensively to

Table 18–1.	Antipsychotic drugs: potency and toxicities			
Drug	**Clinical Potency**	**Extrapyramidal Toxicity**	**Sedative Action**	**Hypotensive Actions**
Chlorpromazine	Low	Medium	High	High
Fluphenazine	High	High	Low	Very low
Thiothixene	High	Medium	Medium	Medium
Haloperidol	High	Very high	Low	Very low
Clozapine	Medium	Very low	Low	Medium
Risperidone	High	Low[1]	Low	Low
Olanzapine	High	Very low	Medium	Low
Quetiapine	Low	Very low	Medium	Low to medium
Ziprasidone	Medium	Very low	Low	Very low
Aripiprazole	High	Very low	Very low	Low

[1]At dosages below 8 mg/day.

plasma proteins. These drugs require metabolism by liver enzymes before elimination and have long plasma half-lives that permit once-daily dosing. Parenteral forms of some agents are available for both rapid initiation of therapy and depot treatment, the latter helping to improve drug compliance, a major problem for patients who suffer from schizophrenia.

Mechanism of Action

The mechanism of action of antipsychotic agents most commonly related to the treatment of schizophrenia is based on the *dopamine hypothesis of schizophrenia*. This hypothesis proposes that the disorder is caused by a relative excess of functional activity of the neurotransmitter dopamine in specific neuronal tracts in the brain. The hypothesis is based on the observations that many antipsychotic drugs block brain dopamine receptors (especially D_2 receptors) and dopamine agonist drugs (e.g., amphetamine, levodopa) exacerbate schizophrenia. Also, an increased density of dopamine receptors has been detected in certain brain regions of untreated patients diagnosed with schizophrenia. The dopamine hypothesis of schizophrenia is not fully satisfactory because antipsychotic drugs are only partially effective in most patients and because many effective

drugs have a much higher affinity for other receptors than for D_2 receptors.

There are five recognized dopamine receptors (D_1 to D_5). Each is a member of the G protein–coupled receptor class. The D_2 receptor, found in the caudate putamen, nucleus accumbens, cerebral cortex, and hypothalamus, is negatively coupled to adenylyl cyclase via a G_i protein. The therapeutic efficacy of most of the older antipsychotic drugs correlates with their relative affinity for the D_2 receptor. Unfortunately, blockade of D_2 receptors also correlates strongly with extrapyramidal dysfunction. Most of the newer atypical antipsychotic agents have higher affinities for other receptors than for the D_2 receptor. For example, α adrenoceptor-blocking action correlates well with antipsychotic effect for several of the drugs (Table 18–2). Clozapine, a drug with significant D_4 and serotonin (5-HT) type 2 receptor-blocking actions, has low affinity for D_2 receptors. Several of the newer atypical drugs (e.g., olanzapine, aripiprazole, and risperidone) have high affinity for 5-HT_{2A} receptors, although they may also interact with D_2 and other receptors. Ziprasidone is an antagonist at the D_2, 5-HT_{2A}, and 5-HT_{1D} receptors and an agonist at the 5-HT_{1A} receptor. The newest antipsychotic agent, aripiprazole, is a partial

Table 18–2.	Relative receptor-blocking actions of neuroleptic drugs					
Drug	D_2 **Block**	D_4 **Block**	**Alpha$_1$ Block**	**5-HT$_2$ Block**	**M Block**	**H$_1$ Block**
Most phenothiazines and thioxanthines	++	–	++	+	+	+
Thioridazine	++	–	++	+	+++	+
Haloperidol	+++	–	+	–	–	–
Clozapine	–	++	++	++	++	+
Molindone	++	–	+	–	+	+
Olanzapine	+	–	+	++	+	+
Quetiapine	+	–	+	++	+	+
Risperidone	++	–	+	++	+	+
Ziprasidone	++	–	++	++	–	+
Aripiprazole[1]	+	+	+	++	–	+

[1]Partial agonist at D_2 and 5-HT_{1A} receptors and antagonist activity at 5-HT_{2A} receptors.

+, blockade; –, no effect. The number of plus signs indicates the intensity of receptor blockade.

D, dopamine; M, muscarinic; H, histamine; 5-HT, serotonin.

agonist at D_2 and 5-HT$_{1A}$ receptors, but is a strong antagonist at 5-HT$_{2A}$ receptors. Most of the atypical drugs cause less extrapyramidal dysfunction than standard drugs. With the exception of haloperidol, all antipsychotic drugs block H$_1$ histamine receptors to some degree.

Dopamine receptor blockade is the major effect that correlates with therapeutic benefit for older antipsychotic drugs. Dopaminergic tracts in the brain include the mesocortical-mesolimbic pathways (regulating mentation and mood), nigrostriatal tract (extrapyramidal function), tuberoinfundibular pathways (control of prolactin release), and chemoreceptor trigger zone (emesis). Mesocortical-mesolimbic dopamine receptor blockade presumably underlies antipsychotic effects, and a similar action on the chemoreceptor trigger zone leads to the useful antiemetic properties of some antipsychotic drugs. Adverse effects resulting from receptor blockade in the other dopaminergic tracts, a major problem with older antipsychotic drugs, include extrapyramidal dysfunction and hyperprolactinemia (see section on Adverse Effects below).

Clinical Use

The primary clinical use of antipsychotic drugs is for the treatment of schizophrenia. These agents reduce some of the positive symptoms of schizophrenia, including hyperactivity, bizarre ideation, hallucinations, and delusions. Consequently, antipsychotic drugs can facilitate functioning in individual activity and social participation in both inpatient and outpatient environments. Beneficial effects may take several weeks to develop. Newer atypical drugs also improve some of the negative symptoms of schizophrenia, including emotional blunting and social withdrawal. Older drugs are still commonly used; in part because of their low cost in comparison with newer agents. However, none of the traditional drugs has much effect on these negative symptoms. A representative group of antipsychotic drugs, both older typical agents and newer atypical agents, with selective advantages and disadvantages is presented in Table 18–3.

Antipsychotic drugs are often used with lithium in the initial treatment of mania (discussed below). Olanzapine has been used as the sole agent in the manic phase and acts as a mood stabilizer in bipolar disorder. The antipsychotic drugs are also used in the management of psychotic symptoms of schizoaffective disorders, in Tourette's syndrome, and for management of toxic psychoses caused by overdosage of certain CNS stimulants. **Molindone**, although rarely used in schizophrenia, is effective in treating Tourette's syndrome. The newer atypical antipsychotics have been used to allay psychotic symptoms in patients with Alzheimer's disease or Parkinson's disease.

In addition, most phenothiazines have antiemetic actions related to D_2 and H$_1$ receptor blockade. The latter also contributes to their use as antipruritics and sedatives.

Adverse Effects

Most of the unwanted effects of antipsychotics are extensions of their known pharmacologic actions (Tables 18–1 and 18–4). A few are due to allergic and idiosyncratic reactions.

Extrapyramidal Symptoms

A Parkinson-like syndrome with bradykinesia, rigidity, and tremor is an extremely common adverse effect occurring early during treatment with older agents. These dose-dependent extrapyramidal effects are reversible by decreasing the dose of the drug or by treating the symptoms with conventional antiparkinsonism drugs of the antimuscarinic type (Chapter 17). Extrapyramidal toxicity occurs most frequently with haloperidol and the more potent phenothiazines (e.g., fluphenazine, trifluoperazine). Pseudoparkinsonism occurs infrequently with clozapine and the newer drugs. Other reversible neurologic dysfunctions that occur more frequently with older agents include akathisia and dystonias; these usually respond to treatment with diphenhydramine or muscarinic-blocking agents.

Tardive dyskinesia is a disorder characterized by choreoathetoid movements of the muscles of the lips, tongue, and jaw. This important toxicity may be irreversible. Tardive dyskinesias tend to develop after several years of antipsychotic drug therapy but have appeared as early as 6 months. Antimuscarinic drugs that usually ameliorate other extrapyramidal effects generally *increase* the severity of tardive dyskinesia

Table 18–3.   Some representative antipsychotic drugs

Drug Class	Drug	Advantages	Disadvantages
Traditional Agents			
Phenothiazines	Chlorpromazine[1]	Generic, inexpensive	Many adverse effects, especially autonomic
	Thioridazine[2]	Slight extrapyramidal syndrome; generic	800 mg/day limit; no parenteral form; cardiotoxicity
	Fluphenazine[3]	Depot form also available (enanthate, decanoate)	(?) Increased tardive dyskinesia
Thioxanthene	Thiothixene	Parenteral form also available; (?) decreased tardive dyskinesia	Uncertain
Butyrophenone	Haloperidol	Parenteral form also available; generic	Severe extrapyramidal syndrome
Dibenzoxazepine	Loxapine	(?) No weight gain	Uncertain
Atypical Agents			
	Clozapine	May benefit treatment-resistant patients; little extrapyramidal toxicity	May cause agranulocytosis in up to 2% of patients
	Risperidone	Broad efficacy; little or no extrapyramidal system dysfunction at low doses	Extrapyramidal system dysfunction and hypotension with higher doses
	Olanzapine	Effective against negative as well as positive symptoms; little or no extrapyramidal system dysfunction	Weight gain
	Quetiapine	Similar to risperidone; perhaps less weight gain	Dose must be adjusted if there is associated hypotension; short $t_{1/2}$ and twice-daily dosing
	Ziprasidone	Perhaps less weight gain than clozapine, parenteral form available	QT_c prolongation
	Aripiprazole	Lower weight gain liability, long half-life, novel mechanism potential	Uncertain, novel toxicities possible

[1]Other aliphatic phenothiazines: promazine, triflupromazine.

[2]Other piperidine phenothiazine: mesoridazine.

[3]Other piperazine phenothiazines: perphenazine, prochlorperazine, trifluoperazine.

Table 18–4.	Adverse pharmacologic effects of antipsychotic drugs	
Type	**Manifestations**	**Mechanism**
Autonomic nervous system	Loss of accommodation, dry mouth, difficulty urinating, constipation	Muscarinic cholinoceptor blockade
	Orthostatic hypotension, impotence, failure to ejaculate	Alpha adrenoceptor blockade
Central nervous system	Pseudoparkinsonism, akathisia, dystonias	Dopamine receptor blockade
	Tardive dyskinesia	Supersensitivity of dopamine receptors
	Toxic-confusional state	Muscarinic blockade
Endocrine system	Amenorrhea-galactorrhea, infertility, impotence	Dopamine receptor blockade resulting in hyperprolactinemia
Other	Weight gain	Possibly combined H_1 and $5-HT_2$ blockade

symptoms. There is no effective drug treatment for tardive dyskinesia. Switching to clozapine does not exacerbate the condition. Tardive dyskinesia may be attenuated *temporarily* by increasing neuroleptic dosage; this suggests that tardive dyskinesia may be caused by dopamine receptor sensitization.

Autonomic Effects
Autonomic effects result from blockade of peripheral muscarinic receptors and α adrenoceptors and are more difficult to manage in elderly patients. Tolerance to some of the autonomic effects occurs with continued therapy. Thioridazine has the strongest autonomic effects and haloperidol the weakest. Clozapine and most of the atypical drugs have intermediate autonomic effects (Table 18–2).

Muscarinic receptor blockade, with atropine-like effects (dry mouth, constipation, urinary retention, and visual problems), are often pronounced with the use of thioridazine and phenothiazines (e.g., chlorpromazine). These effects also occur with clozapine and most of the atypical drugs but not with ziprasidone or aripiprazole. Antimuscarinic CNS effects may include a toxic confusional state similar to that produced by atropine and the tricyclic antidepressants (Table 18–4).

Alpha receptor blockade, which manifests as postural hypotension, is a common adverse effect of many of these drugs, especially phenothiazines. In the elderly, measures must be taken to avoid falls resulting from postural fainting. All of the atypical drugs can cause orthostatic hypotension. Failure to ejaculate is common in men treated with the phenothiazines (Table 18–4).

Metabolic and Endocrine Effects
Weight gain is very common, especially with several of the atypical agents including clozapine and olanzapine. Monitoring of food intake, especially carbohydrates, may be necessary. Hyperglycemia may develop, but whether secondary to weight gain–associated insulin resistance or due to other potential mechanisms remains to be clarified. Hyperprolactinemia in women results in the amenorrhea-galactorrhea syndrome and infertility; in men, loss of libido, impotence, and infertility may result.

Most of these endocrine side effects are predictable manifestations of dopamine D_2 receptor blockade in the pituitary; dopamine is the normal inhibitory regulator of prolactin secretion.

Neuroleptic Malignant Syndrome
Patients who are particularly sensitive to the extrapyramidal effects of antipsychotic drugs may develop a life-threatening malignant hyperthermic syndrome. The symptoms include muscle rigidity, impairment of

sweating, hyperpyrexia, and autonomic instability. Drug treatment involves the prompt use of dantrolene and perhaps dopamine agonists.

Sedation

The sedative properties of antipsychotic drugs are variable (Table 18–1). They are more marked with phenothiazines (especially chlorpromazine) than with other antipsychotics. Although it was previously thought that sedation enhanced the efficacy of these drugs, current practice indicates that these effects offer no benefit and can be detrimental in withdrawn patients with psychosis. Fluphenazine and haloperidol are the least sedating of the older drugs; aripiprazole appears to be the least sedating of the newer agents.

Miscellaneous Effects

Visual impairment caused by retinal deposits has occurred with thioridazine. At high doses, thioridazine may also cause severe conduction defects in the heart resulting in fatal ventricular arrhythmias. Ziprasidone prolongs the QT interval of the electrocardiogram, which may lead to cardiac arrhythmias (e.g., torsade de pointes). Clozapine causes a small but important (1 to 2%) incidence of agranulocytosis, and at high doses has caused seizures.

LITHIUM AND OTHER DRUGS USED IN BIPOLAR DISORDER

Bipolar affective (manic-depressive) disorder is a very serious psychiatric condition characterized by cyclic attacks of mania with many symptoms of paranoid schizophrenia. The episodes of mood swings characteristic of this condition are generally unrelated to life events. Although the exact biologic disturbance has not been identified, a preponderance of catecholamine-related activity is thought to be present during the manic phase. Drugs that increase this activity tend to exacerbate mania, whereas those that reduce activity of dopamine or norepinephrine relieve mania. Acetylcholine or glutamate may also be involved. The nature of the abrupt switch from mania to depression experienced by some patients is uncertain. Bipolar disorder has a strong familial component, and genetic studies have identified at least three possible linkages to different chromosomes.

Lithium is often referred to as an "antimanic" drug, but is more properly considered a "mood-stabilizing" agent because its primary action is to prevent mood swings. **Carbamazepine** has also been recognized as effective in some manic-depressive patients despite not being formally approved for such use. **Valproic acid** has recently been approved for the treatment of mania, and is being evaluated as a mood stabilizer. Atypical antipsychotics, beginning with olanzapine, are being investigated and approved as antimanic agents and potential mood stabilizers (Figure 18–1).

Lithium is absorbed rapidly and completely from the gut. The drug is distributed throughout the body water. Lithium is not metabolized and is cleared by the kidneys at a rate one-fifth that of creatinine. The half-life of lithium is about 20 hours. Plasma levels should be monitored, especially during the first weeks of therapy, to establish an effective and safe dosage regimen. Major problems can arise with lithium use if it accumulates within the body. The therapeutic plasma concentration range is 0.6 to 1.4 mEq/L. Plasma levels of the drug may be altered by changes in body water. Dehydration, or treatment with thiazide diuretics, may result in an increase of lithium in the blood to toxic levels. Theophylline increases the renal clearance of lithium. The pharmacokinetics of lithium are characterized in Table 18–5.

Mechanism of Action

The mechanism of action of lithium is not well defined. Three major possibilities exist: (1) an effect on electrolyte and ion transport, (2) an effect on neurotransmitters and their release, and (3) an effect on second messengers and intracellular enzymes that mediate transmitter actions.

Lithium is closely related to sodium in its properties and can substitute for sodium in generating action potentials and in Na^+-Na^+ exchange across membranes, inhibiting this process. Lithium also appears to enhance some of the actions of serotonin and may decrease norepinephrine and dopamine turnover. It may also augment the synthesis of acetylcholine. However, one of the best-defined actions of lithium is its effect on inositol phosphates. The drug inhibits the recycling of neuronal membrane phosphoinositides

Table 18–5.	Pharmacokinetics of Lithium
Absorption	Virtually complete within 6–8 h; peak plasma levels in 30 min to 2 h
Distribution	In total body water; slow entry into intracellular compartment. Initial volume of distribution is 0.5 L/kg, rising to 0.7–0.9 L/kg; some sequestration in bone. No protein binding.
Metabolism	None
Excretion	Virtually entirely in urine. Lithium clearance about 20% of creatinine. Plasma half-life about 20 h.
Target plasma concentration	0.6–1.4 mEq/L

involved in the generation of inositol trisphosphate (IP_3) and diacylglycerol (DAG). These second messengers are important in amine neurotransmission, including that mediated by central adrenoceptors and muscarinic receptors (Figure 18–2). It is hypothesized that the activity in phosphatidylinositol 4,5-bisphosphate (PIP_2)–dependent pathways is abnormally increased in manic episodes and that lithium causes a selective depression of the overactive circuits.

Clinical Use

Lithium carbonate is used in the treatment of bipolar disorder. Maintenance therapy with lithium decreases manic behavior and reduces both the frequency and the magnitude of mood swings. Neuroleptics or benzodiazepines are commonly required at the initiation of treatment because lithium has a slow onset of action. Antidepressant drugs are often required concurrently during maintenance. Alternative drugs of value in bipolar disorder include olanzapine and valproic acid and several other antiseizure drugs (e.g., clonazepam, gabapentin, lamotrigine).

Lithium may also be used in conjunction with antipsychotic agents for the treatment of schizophrenia in patients who might otherwise be treatment resistant with regular antipsychotic agents. Another interesting application of lithium is as an adjunct to tricyclic antidepressants and selective serotonin reuptake inhibitors in patients with unipolar depression who do not respond fully to monotherapy with the antidepressant. For this application, concentrations of lithium at the lower end of the recommended range for manic depressive illness appear to be adequate.

Adverse Effects

Adverse neurologic effects of lithium at therapeutic levels include tremor, sedation, ataxia, and aphasia. Any marked changes in mental behavior such as confusion or withdrawal or bizarre motor movements may indicate drug toxicity and serum concentrations should be evaluated. Thyroid enlargement may occur, but thyroid dysfunction is rare. Reversible nephrogenic diabetes insipidus occurs commonly at therapeutic drug levels. Edema is a frequent adverse effect of lithium therapy and may be related to some effect of lithium on sodium retention. Transient acneiform skin

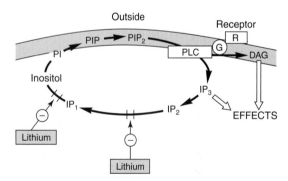

Figure 18–2. Effect of lithium on the inositol trisphosphate (IP_3) and diacylglycerol (DAG) second-messenger system. The schematic diagram shows the synaptic membrane of a neuron in the brain. (PLC = phospholipase C; G = coupling protein; R = receptor; EFFECTS = activation of protein kinase C, mobilization of intracellular Ca^{2+}, etc.) By interfering with the recycling of inositol substrates, lithium may cause depletion of the second-messenger source PIP_2 and reduce the release of IP_3 and DAG. Lithium may also act by other mechanisms.

eruptions have been noted early in lithium treatment. Leukocytosis is always present during lithium treatment. The use of lithium during pregnancy may increase the incidence of congenital cardiac anomalies (Ebstein's anomaly). Lithium is contraindicated in nursing mothers.

REHABILITATION FOCUS

Antipsychotic drugs have had a major impact on psychiatric treatment over the last 50 years. They have shifted the care of patients from mental institutions to the community. For many patients, this shift has provided a better quality of life. As a result, many physical therapists will have the opportunity to treat such patients. Regardless of the reason for which they have been referred for rehabilitation, they will benefit from these agents by improved behavior and reality perception, which will ultimately improve their rehabilitation outcomes.

The medical staff must always weigh the risk of side effects with the benefits of the antipsychotic drugs. Some adverse effects such as sedation, dry mouth, and constipation are only symptomatic and can usually be tolerated. Physical therapists must be aware of orthostatic hypotension and the potential risk of falls and should educate the patient regarding such events. The major adverse effects associated with the use of the older antipsychotic agents are the extrapyramidal effects of bradykinesia, tremor, and rigidity. Therapists should be aware of any changes in balance, posture, or involuntary movements and report these to the attending physician.

CLINICAL RELEVANCE FOR REHABILITATION

Adverse Drug Reactions
- Sedation
- Orthostatic hypotension
- Extrapyramidal effects

Effects Interfering with Rehabilitation
- Sedation
- Bradykinesia, tremor, rigidity
- Balance and posture problems
- Tardive dyskinesia

Possible Therapy Solutions
- Orthostatic hypotension: compressive garments, tilt table, allow sufficient time for the patient's blood pressure to adjust to postural changes; monitor response to exercise.

Potentiation of Functional Outcomes Secondary to Drug Therapy
- In many cases, these medications can help with functional outcomes at both the activity and participation levels.

PROBLEM-ORIENTED PATIENT STUDY

Brief History: The patient is a 56-year-old male who was referred to rehabilitation by his family physician after several reported falls and increasing problems with balance as per his wife's observation. The patient has a history of schizophrenia that has been well controlled with medication. Hesitantly, the patient also reports several recent episodes of being lightheaded. He states he has begun to feel extremely stiff at times and has a hard time moving.

Current Medical Status and Drug Therapy: The patient has no current medical problems. Recent neurologic diagnostic tests have ruled out any CNS pathology. The patient is currently taking pantoprazole (a proton pump inhibitor) and risperidone. The patient states that his prescribing practitioner recently increased his dose of risperidone after a recent psychotic episode.

Rehabilitation Setting: The patient presented in no acute physical distress. Evaluation revealed that

(continued)

PROBLEM-ORIENTED PATIENT STUDY (*Continued*)

the patient suffered from orthostatic hypotension evident by a rapid fall in blood pressure with positional changes. The patient also presented with postural rigidity evident by resistance to passive stretch in both the upper extremities and lower extremities; it was more severe in the lower extremities. The patient did not demonstrate a resting tremor. Balance testing using the Clinical Test for Sensory Integration and Balance revealed increased sway in conditions with absent or impaired vision and impaired somatosensory input.

Problem/Clinical Options: Consultation between the physical therapist and the patient's prescribing health-care provider determined that the patient may be experiencing adverse effects of postural hypotension and extrapyramidal system dysfunction that can be associated with the use of risperidone at high doses. Since this dose of medication was controlling the patient's psychosis, the prescribing practitioner was reluctant to make any abrupt changes in the patient's medication. Therefore, the physical therapist educated the patient and his wife about postural hypotension and how to prevent episodes of syncope. The patient also began a program of stretching and functional balance training. The patient, the physical therapist, and prescribing practitioner agreed to follow the patient's symptoms closely. The patient's condition would be reevaluated in 3 months.

PREPARATIONS AVAILABLE

Antipsychotic Agents

Aripiprazole (Abilify)
Oral: 10-, 15-, 20-, 30-mg tablets

Chlorpromazine (generic, Thorazine, others)
Oral: 10-, 25-, 50-, 100-, 200-mg tablets; 10 mg/5 mL syrup; 30, 100 mg/mL concentrate
Oral sustained release: 30-, 75-, 150-mg capsules
Rectal: 25-, 100-mg suppositories
Parenteral: 25 mg/mL for IM injection

Clozapine (generic, Clozaril)
Oral: 25-, 100-mg tablets

Fluphenazine (generic, Permitil, Prolixin)
Oral: 1-, 2.5-, 5-, 10-mg tablets; 2.5 mg/5 mL elixir; 5 mg/mL concentrate
Parenteral: 2.5 mg/mL for IM injection

Fluphenazine esters (generic [decanoate only], Prolixin Enanthate, Prolixin Decanoate)
Parenteral: 25 mg/mL

Haloperidol (generic, Haldol)
Oral: 0.5-, 1-, 2-, 5-, 10-, 20-mg tablets; 2 mg/mL concentrate
Parenteral: 5 mg/mL for IM injection

Haloperidol ester (Haldol Decanoate)
Parenteral: 50-, 100-mg/mL for IM injection

Loxapine (Loxitane)
Oral: 5-, 10-, 25-, 50-mg capsules; 25 mg/mL concentrate
Parenteral: 50 mg/mL for IM injection

Mesoridazine (Serentil)
Oral: 10-, 25-, 50-, 100-mg tablets; 25 mg/mL concentrate
Parenteral: 25 mg/mL for IM injection

Molindone (Moban)
Oral: 5-, 10-, 25-, 50-, 100-mg tablets; 20-mg/mL concentrate

Olanzapine (Zyprexa)
Oral: 2.5-, 5-, 7.5-, 10-, 15-, 20-mg tablets; 5-, 10-, 15-, 20-mg orally disintegrating tablets

Perphenazine (generic, Trilafon)
Oral: 2-, 4-, 8-, 16-mg tablets; 16 mg/5 mL concentrate
Parenteral: 5 mg/mL for IM or IV injection

Pimozide (Orap)
Oral: 1-, 2-mg tablets

Prochlorperazine (generic, Compazine)
Oral: 5-, 10-mg tablets; 5 mg/5 mL syrup
Oral sustained release: 10-, 15-mg capsules
Rectal: 2.5-, 5-, 25-mg suppositories
Parenteral: 5 mg/mL for IM injection

Promazine (generic, Sparine)
Oral: 25-, 50-mg tablets
Parenteral: 25-, 50-mg/mL for IM injection

Quetiapine (Seroquel)
Oral: 25-, 100-, 200-, 300-mg tablets

Risperidone (Risperdal)
Oral: 0.25-, 0.5-, 1-, 2-, 3-, 4-mg tablets; 1 mg/mL oral solution

Thioridazine (generic, Mellaril, others)
Oral: 10-, 15-, 25-, 50-, 100-, 150-, 200-mg tablets; 30, 100-mg/mL concentrate; 25, 100 mg/5 mL suspension

Thiothixene (generic, Navane)
Oral: 1-, 2-, 5-, 10-, 20-mg capsules; 5 mg/mL concentrate

Trifluoperazine (generic, Stelazine)
Oral: 1-, 2-, 5-, 10-mg tablets; 10 mg/mL concentrate
Parenteral: 2 mg/mL for IM injection

Triflupromazine (Vesprin)
Parenteral: 10, 20 mg/mL for IM injection

Ziprasidone (Geodon)
Oral: 20-, 40-, 60-, 80-mg capsules
Parenteral: 20-mg/mL for IM injection

Mood Stabilizers

Carbamazepine (generic, Tegretol, others)
Oral: 200-mg tablets, 100-mg chewable tablets; 100 mg/5 mL oral suspension.
Oral extended release: 100-, 200-, 400-mg tablets; 200-, 300-mg capsules

Divalproex (Depakote)
Oral: 125-, 250-, 500-mg delayed-release tablets

Lithium carbonate (generic, Eskalith) (Note: 300-mg lithium carbonate = 8.12 mEq Li$^+$)
Oral: 150-, 300-, 600-mg capsules; 300-mg tablets; 8 mEq/5 mL syrup
Oral sustained release: 300-, 450-mg tablets

Valproic acid (generic, Depakene)
Oral: 250-mg capsules; 250 mg/5 mL syrup

REFERENCES

Antipsychotics

Bilder RM, et al: Neurocognitive effects of clozapine, olanzapine, risperidone, and haloperidol in patients with chronic schizophrenia or schizoaffective disorder. *Am J Psychiatry* 2002;159:1018.

Breier A, Berg PH: The psychosis of schizophrenia: Prevalence, response to atypical antipsychotics, and prediction of outcome. *Biol Psychiatry* 1999;46:361.

Carlsson A, et al: Neurotransmitter interactions in schizophrenia—therapeutic implications. *Biol Psychiatry* 1999;46:1388.

Dickey W: The neuroleptic malignant syndrome. *Prog Neurobiol* 1991;36:423.

Freudenreich O, Goff DC: Antipsychotic combination therapy in schizophrenia. A review of efficacy and risks of current combinations. *Acta Psychiatr Scand* 2002;106:323.

Haddad PM, Anderson IM: Antipsychotic-related QT$_c$ prolongation, torsade de pointes and sudden death. *Drugs* 2002;62:1649.

Hugenholtz GW, et al: Short-acting parenteral antipsychotics drive choice for classical versus atypical agents. *Eur J Clin Pharmacol* 2003;58:757.

McGavin JK, Goa KL: Aripiprazole. *CNS Drugs* 2002;779:786.

Seeman P: Dopamine receptors and the dopamine hypothesis of schizophrenia. *Synapse* 1987;1:133.

Stefansson H, et al: Neuregulin 1 and susceptibility to schizophrenia. *Am J Hum Genet* 2002;71:877.

Mood Stabilizers

Bowden CL: Valproate in mania. In Bipolar Medications: Mechanisms of Action. Manji HK, Bowden CL, Belmaker RH (eds). Arlington, VA: American Psychiatric Press, 2000.

Bowden CL, et al: Efficacy of divalproex vs lithium, placebo in the treatment of mania. *JAMA* 1994;271:918.

Goodwin FK, Ghaemi SN: Bipolar disorder: state of the art. *Dialogues Clin Neurosci* 1999;1:41.

Jope RS: Anti-bipolar therapy: mechanism of action of lithium. *Mol Psychiatry* 1999;4:117.

Manji HK, Chen G: PKC, MAP kinases and the bcl-2 family of proteins as long-term targets for mood stabilizers. *Mol Psychiatry* 2002;(7 Suppl 1):S46.

Schou M: Lithium treatment at 52. *J Affect Disord* 2001; 67:21.

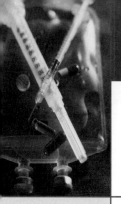

19

ANTIDEPRESSANT AGENTS

Major depression is one of the most common forms of mental illness in the United States with as many as 6% of the population depressed at any given moment (point prevalence), and an estimated 10% of people becoming depressed during their lifetime (lifetime prevalence). The symptoms of depression can be both psychologic and physiologic, and are often subtle and unrecognized by patients and health-care professionals. Symptoms may include intense feelings of sadness and despair, sleep disturbances (too much or too little), anorexia, fatigue, somatic complaints, and suicidal thoughts.

Depression is a heterogeneous disorder that has been classified as (1) "reactive" or "secondary" depression (most common), occurring in response to stimuli such as grief or illness; (2) "endogenous" depression or major depressive disorder, a genetically determined biochemical disorder of depressed mood without any obvious medical or situational causes, manifested by an inability to experience ordinary pleasure or to cope with ordinary life events; and (3) depression associated with bipolar affective (manic-depressive) disorder.

Physical therapists may encounter patients taking antidepressant medications under a number of circumstances. Many patients who have experienced life-changing disabilities become depressed and may require medication for a limited time to control their depression. Other patients may have a history of chronic depression not related to their therapy diagnosis and require long-term treatment. Drugs used in treating depressive disorders are highly effective in some patients but only modestly, or not at all, effective in others. No patients are cured. The major subclasses of antidepressant drugs are outlined in Figure 19–1.

▪ PATHOGENESIS OF MAJOR DEPRESSION

The *amine hypothesis of mood* postulates that brain amines, particularly norepinephrine (NE) and (serotonin, 5-HT), are neurotransmitters in pathways that function in the expression of mood. According to the hypothesis, a functional decrease in the activity of such amines is thought to result in depression; a functional increase in activity results in mood elevation. The amine hypothesis is largely based on studies showing that drugs (such as reserpine) that deplete central amines cause depression, and that most drugs capable of alleviating the symptoms of a major depressive disorder enhance the actions of the neurotransmitters 5-HT and NE in central synapses. Difficulties with this hypothesis include the facts that (1) postmortem studies do not reveal any decreases in the brain levels of NE or 5-HT in untreated patients suffering from endogenous depression; (2) although antidepressant drugs may cause biochemical changes in

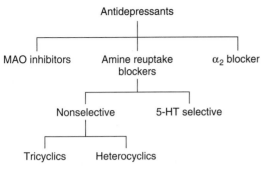

Figure 19–1. Major subclasses of antidepressants.

brain amine activity within hours, weeks may be required for them to achieve clinical effects; (3) with chronic use, most antidepressants ultimately cause a *down*-regulation of amine receptors; and (4) at least one effective antidepressant, bupropion, has minimal effects on brain NE or 5-HT.

While the amine hypothesis is undoubtedly too simplistic, it has provided the major experimental models for the discovery of new antidepressant drugs. As a result, all the currently available antidepressant drugs—except bupropion—have significant actions on the metabolism or reuptake of these amines, or are antagonists at presynaptic serotonin or norepinephrine receptors or both.

◼ DRUG CLASSIFICATION

Drugs that have been found to have antidepressant activity are grouped into categories based on their chemical structures or purported mechanisms of action. The categories include the **tricyclic antidepressants** (TCAs), heterocyclics (second- and third-generation drugs that followed the TCAs), **monoamine oxidase inhibitors** (MAOIs), and **selective serotonin reuptake inhibitors** (SSRIs). Table 19–1 is a selective list of common antidepressant drugs.

Tricyclic Antidepressants

Tricyclic antidepressants (e.g., **imipramine, amitriptyline**) were the first successful antidepressants. They are structurally related to the phenothiazine antipsychotics and share certain of their pharmacologic effects. The

Table 19–1.	List of common antidepressant drugs

Drug

Tricyclics
    Amitriptyline
    Clomipramine
    Desipramine
    Doxepin
    Imipramine
    Nortriptyline
    Protriptyline
    Trimipramine
Second-Generation and Subsequent Drugs
    Amoxapine
    Bupropion
    Duloxetine
    Maprotiline
    Mirtazapine
    Nefazodone
    Trazodone
    Venlafaxine
Monoamine Oxidase Inhibitors
    Phenelzine
    Tranylcypromine
Selective Serotonin Reuptake Inhibitors
    Citalopram
    Escitalopram
    Fluoxetine
    Fluvoxamine
    Paroxetine
    Sertraline

TCAs are well absorbed orally but may undergo first-pass metabolism. They have high volumes of distribution and are not readily dialyzable. Extensive hepatic metabolism is required for their elimination; plasma half-lives of 8 to 36 hours usually permit once-daily dosing. Both amitriptyline and imipramine form active metabolites, **nortriptyline** and **desipramine**, respectively.

Heterocyclic Antidepressants

These drugs have varied structures and include second-generation antidepressants (e.g., **amoxapine, bupropion,** maprotiline, trazodone) and newer, third-generation drugs (duloxetine, mirtazapine, nefazodone, venlafaxine). The pharmacokinetics of most of these agents are similar to those of the TCAs. Nefazodone and trazodone are exceptions; their half-lives are quite short and usually require administration two or three times daily.

Monoamine Oxidase Inhibitors

The MAOIs (e.g., phenelzine, tranylcypromine) are structurally related to amphetamines and are orally active. They inhibit both MAO-A, which metabolizes NE, 5-HT, and tyramine, and MAO-B, which metabolizes dopamine. Tranylcypromine is the fastest in onset of effect but has a shorter duration of action (about 1 week) than other MAOIs (2 to 3 weeks). In spite of these prolonged actions, the MAOIs are given daily. It is prudent to assume that the drug effect will persist from 7 days (tranylcypromine) to 2 or 3 weeks (phenelzine) after *discontinuance* of the drug.

These drugs are inhibitors of hepatic drug-metabolizing enzymes and cause many drug interactions.

Selective Serotonin Reuptake Inhibitors

Fluoxetine is the prototype of a group of drugs that are SSRIs. All of them require hepatic metabolism and have half-lives of 18 to 24 hours. However, fluoxetine forms an active metabolite with a half-life of several days (the basis for a once-weekly formulation). Other members of this group (e.g., sertraline, citalopram, escitalopram, fluvoxamine, paroxetine) do not form long-acting metabolites.

■ MECHANISMS OF ACTION

Potential sites of action of antidepressants at CNS synapses are shown in Figure 19–2. Most antidepressant drugs appear to cause potentiation of the neurotransmitter actions of norepinephrine, serotonin, or

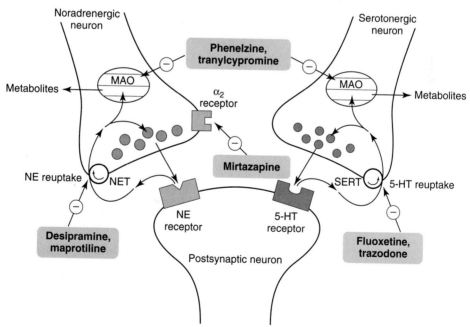

Figure 19–2. Possible sites of action of antidepressant drugs. Inhibition of neuronal reuptake of norepinephrine (NE) and serotonin (5-HT) increases the synaptic activities of these neurotransmitters. Inhibition of monoamine oxidase increases the presynaptic stores of both NE and 5-HT, which leads to increased neurotransmitter effects. Blockade of the presynaptic α_2 autoreceptor prevents feedback inhibition of the release of NE. (NET = NE transporter; SERT = 5-HT transporter.) NOTE: These are acute actions of antidepressants.

both. The only exception is bupropion, which has an unknown mechanism of action. Long-term use of tricyclics and MAOIs, but not SSRIs, leads to *down-regulation* of β-adrenergic receptors.

Tricyclic Antidepressants

The acute effect of tricyclic drugs is to inhibit the reuptake mechanisms (*NET* [NE transporter] and *SERT* [serotonin transporter]) responsible for the termination of the synaptic actions of NE and 5-HT in the brain. This presumably results in potentiation of their neurotransmitter actions at postsynaptic receptors.

Heterocyclic Antidepressants

Some second-generation drugs inhibit the reuptake of NE (e.g., maprotiline); others have more effect on 5-HT reuptake (e.g., trazodone). The third-generation drug venlafaxine, although not a tricyclic, is a potent inhibitor of the 5-HT transporter and, at higher doses, of the NE transporter as well. Mirtazapine has a unique action; it increases amine release from nerve endings by antagonism of presynaptic α_2 adrenoceptors involved in feedback inhibition. However, antagonism of presynaptic 5-HT_{2A} and 5-HT_{2C} receptors has also been implicated in the antidepressant actions of mirtazapine, nefazodone, and trazodone.

Monoamine Oxidase Inhibitors

The MAOIs increase brain amine levels by interfering with their metabolism in the nerve endings, resulting in an increase in the vesicular stores of NE and 5-HT. When neuronal activity discharges the vesicles, increased amounts of the amines are released, presumably enhancing their actions.

Selective Serotonin Reuptake Inhibitors

The acute effect of the SSRIs is a highly selective action on 5-HT transporters. They block the reuptake of 5-HT without affecting reuptake of other amine neurotransmitters. Because of their selectivity, they produce fewer and less troublesome adverse effects than nonselective antidepressant drugs.

CLINICAL USES

The major indication for these drugs is to treat depression, but a number of other uses have been established by clinical experience and controlled trials.

Depression

Patients with major depression typically vary in their responsiveness to individual agents. Because of more tolerable adverse effects and greater safety in overdose (see discussion below), the newer drugs (SSRIs, certain heterocyclics) are now the most widely prescribed antidepressants. However, none of the newer antidepressants has been shown to be more effective overall than tricyclic drugs. As alternative agents, tricyclic drugs continue to be most useful in patients with psychomotor retardation, sleep disturbances, poor appetite, and weight loss. MAOIs may be most useful in patients with significant anxiety, phobic features, and hypochondriasis. SSRIs may decrease appetite and overweight patients often lose weight on these drugs, at least during the first 6 to 12 months of treatment.

Panic Disorder

Imipramine, a TCA, was first shown in 1962 to have a beneficial effect in the acute episodes of anxiety that have come to be known as panic attacks. Recent studies have shown imipramine to be as effective as MAOIs and benzodiazepines. It has also been demonstrated that SSRIs are effective in panic disorder. In some instances, benzodiazepines are preferred, as they are well tolerated and their clinical effects become evident promptly. Alternatively, if one wishes to avoid the physiologic dependence associated with chronic benzodiazepine use, SSRIs are acceptable for many patients, although they require several weeks to produce full therapeutic effects.

Obsessive-Compulsive Disorder

The SSRIs have been shown to be uniquely effective for treating this disorder. Recent studies have focused on fluoxetine and other SSRIs although clomipramine, a mixed serotonin and norepinephrine uptake inhibitor, may be more potent. Fluvoxamine is marketed exclusively for obsessive-compulsive disorder in the United States.

Chronic Pain

Clinicians in pain clinics have found tricyclics to be useful for treating a variety of chronically painful states that often cannot be definitively diagnosed. Whether such painful states represent depressive equivalents or whether such patients become secondarily depressed after some initial pain-producing insult is not clear. It is even possible that the tricyclics work directly on pain pathways.

Controlled studies of higher doses of venlafaxine and duloxetine, which inhibit both norepinephrine and serotonin uptake, also show efficacy in pain states. SSRIs, however, are not effective for chronic pain.

Other Clinical Uses

TCAs are also used in the treatment of bipolar affective disorders, enuresis, and attention deficit hyperkinetic disorder. In addition to their common use in depressive disorders, the SSRIs are also effective in patients who suffer from generalized anxiety disorders, social phobias, bulimia, and premenstrual dysphoric disorder and may also be useful in the treatment of alcohol dependence. Trazodone is frequently prescribed for insomnia. Bupropion is used for management of patients attempting to withdraw from nicotine dependence.

ADVERSE EFFECTS

Most common unwanted effects of antidepressant drugs are minor, but they may seriously affect patient compliance. The more seriously depressed the patient is, the more likely it is that unwanted effects will be tolerated. Adverse effects of various antidepressants are summarized in Table 19–2.

Table 19–2.	Adverse effects of antidepressant drugs
Drug/Drug Class	**Adverse Effects**
Tricyclics	Sedation (sleepiness, additive effects with other sedative drugs) Sympathomimetic (tremor, insomnia) Antimuscarinic (blurred vision, constipation, urinary hesitancy, confusion) Cardiovascular (orthostatic hypotension, conduction defects, arrhythmias) Psychiatric (aggravation of psychosis, withdrawal syndrome) Neurologic (seizures) Metabolic-endocrine (weight gain, sexual disturbances)
Monoamine oxidase inhibitors	Sleep disturbances, weight gain, postural hypotension, sexual disturbances (phenelzine)
Amoxapine	Similar to the tricyclics with the addition of some effects associated with the antipsychotics
Maprotiline	Similar to tricyclics; seizures are dose-related
Mirtazapine	Somnolence, increased appetite, weight gain, dizziness
Trazodone, nefazadone	Drowsiness, dizziness, insomnia, nausea, agitation
Venlafaxine	Nausea, somnolence, sweating, dizziness, sexual disturbances, hypertension, anxiety
Bupropion	Dizziness, dry mouth, sweating, tremor, aggravation of psychosis, potential for seizures at high doses
Fluoxetine and other serotonin reuptake inhibitors	Gastrointestinal symptoms, decreased libido, sexual dysfunction, anxiety (acutely), insomnia, tremor

Tricyclic Antidepressants

Some of the adverse effects of TCAs are predictable from their pharmacodynamic actions. These include (1) excessive sedation, lassitude, fatigue, and, occasionally, confusion; (2) sympathomimetic effects, including tachycardia, agitation, sweating, and insomnia; (3) antimuscarinic effects (especially amitriptyline); (4) orthostatic hypotension, electrocardiographic abnormalities, and cardiomyopathies; (5) tremor and paresthesias; and (6) weight gain. Overdosage with tricyclics is extremely hazardous, and the ingestion of as little as a 2-week supply has been lethal. Manifestations of overdose include (1) agitation, delirium, neuromuscular irritability, convulsions, and coma; (2) respiratory depression and circulatory collapse; (3) hyperpyrexia; and (4) cardiac conduction defects and severe arrhythmias. The "3 Cs"—coma, convulsions, and cardiotoxicity—are characteristic.

Heterocyclic Antidepressants

These second- and third-generation drugs have varied adverse effects. Mirtazapine causes weight gain and is markedly sedating, as is trazodone. Amoxapine, maprotiline, mirtazapine, and trazodone cause some autonomic effects. Amoxapine is also a dopamine receptor blocker and may cause akathisia, pseudoparkinsonism, and the amenorrhea-galactorrhea syndrome. Adverse effects of bupropion include dizziness, dry mouth, aggravation of psychosis, and, at high doses, seizures. Seizures and cardiotoxicity are prominent features of overdosage with amoxapine and maprotiline. Venlafaxine causes asthenia and somnolence and overdosage is cardiotoxic. Nefazodone is hepatotoxic, and patients and caregivers are advised to be alert for signs and symptoms of liver dysfunction such as anorexia, gastrointestinal complaints, and jaundice.

Selective Serotonin Reuptake Inhibitors

Fluoxetine and the other SSRIs may cause nausea, headache, anxiety, agitation, insomnia, and sexual dysfunction. Jitteriness can be alleviated by starting with low doses or by adjunctive use of benzodiazepines or low-dose trazodone. Extrapyramidal effects early in treatment may include akathisia, dyskinesias, and dystonic reactions. Seizures are a consequence of gross overdosage. A withdrawal syndrome has been described for SSRIs that includes nausea, dizziness, anxiety, tremor, and palpitations.

Monoamine Oxidase Inhibitors

Adverse effects of the MAOIs include hypertensive reactions in response to sympathomimetics, hyperthermia, and CNS stimulation leading to agitation and convulsions. Hypertensive crisis may occur in patients taking MAOIs who consume food or medications that contain high concentrations of sympathomimetics such as tyramine (Table 19–3).

In the absence of sympathomimetics, MAOIs typically *lower* blood pressure; overdosage with these drugs may result in shock, hyperthermia, and seizures.

■ ANTIDEPRESSANTS IN CHILDREN AND ADOLESCENTS

Studies suggesting an increased risk of suicide in children and adolescents taking antidepressants have received heavy media attention. While it is not clear that the drugs (rather than the disease) are responsible, the incidence of suicide is increased in untreated as well as treated depressed individuals. For this reason, parents, other family, and caregivers of children and adolescents being treated with antidepressants should be aware of potential warning signs such as agitation, irritability, and unusual changes in behavior, and any other indicators of suicidal tendencies. Monitoring should be done on a daily basis and any changes should be reported to the prescribing practitioner immediately.

■ DRUG INTERACTIONS

Patients may have both pharmacodynamic and pharmacokinetic interactions when taking antidepressants with other drugs. Tricyclic drug interactions include additive depression of the CNS with other central depressants, including ethanol, barbiturates, benzodiazepines, and opioids. Tricyclics may also cause reversal of the antihypertensive action of guanethidine by blocking its transport into sympathetic nerve endings.

Table 19–3.   Foods, beverages, and over-the-counter medications to avoid in patients taking monoamine oxidase inhibitors

Meat and Fish
  Pickled herring
  Liver
  Dry sausage (Genoa salami, hard salami, pepperoni, and Lebanon bologna)
Vegetables
  Broad bean pods (fava bean pods)
  Sauerkraut
Dairy Products
  Cheese (cottage cheese and cream cheese are allowed)
  Yogurt
Beverages
  Beer and wine
  Alcohol-free and reduced-alcohol beer and wine products
Miscellaneous
  Yeast extract
  Meat extract
  Excessive amounts of chocolate and caffeine
  Spoiled or improperly refrigerated, handled, or stored protein-rich foods such as meats, fish and dairy
    products, including foods that may have undergone protein changes by aging, pickling, fermentation, or
    smoking to improve flavor should be avoided
Over-the-Counter Medications
  Cold and cough preparations (including those containing dextromethorphan)
  Nasal decongestants (tablets, drops, or spray)
  Hay-fever medication
  Sinus medications
  Asthma inhalant medications
  Antiappetite medications

Less commonly, tricyclics may interfere with the antihypertensive actions of methylnorepinephrine (the active metabolite of methyldopa) and clonidine.

Of the heterocyclic drugs, both nefazodone and venlafaxine are inhibitors of cytochrome P450 isozymes. Through this action, nefazodone inhibits the metabolism of alprazolam and triazolam, and venlafaxine inhibits the metabolism of haloperidol.

The SSRIs are also inhibitors of hepatic cytochrome P450 isozymes, an action that has led to increased activity of other drugs, including TCAs and warfarin.

Citalopram and escitalopram cause fewer drug interactions than other SSRIs. A **serotonin syndrome** was first described for an interaction between fluoxetine and an MAOI. This life-threatening syndrome includes severe muscle rigidity, myoclonus, hyperthermia, cardiovascular instability, and marked CNS stimulatory effects, including seizures. Drugs implicated include MAOIs, TCAs, meperidine, and possibly illicit recreational drugs such as methylenedioxymethamphetamine (MDMA; "ecstasy"). Antiseizure drugs, muscle relaxants, and blockers of 5-HT receptors have been

Table 19–4.   Drug interactions observed with antidepressant medications

Antidepressant	Taken With	Consequence
Fluoxetine	Lithium, tricyclics, warfarin	Increased blood levels of the second drug; doses may need to be decreased
Fluvoxamine	Alprazolam, theophylline, tricyclics, warfarin	Increased blood levels of the second drug; doses may need to be decreased
MAOIs	Sympathomimetics, tyramine, SSRIs	Hypertensive crisis; serotonin syndrome
Nefazodone	Alprazolam, triazolam	Increased blood levels of the second drug; doses may need to be decreased
Paroxetine	Procyclidine, theophylline, tricyclics, warfarin	Increased blood levels of the second drug; doses may need to be decreased
Sertraline	Tricyclics, warfarin	Increased effects; doses may need to be decreased
Tricyclics	CNS depressants (e.g., ethanol, sedative-hypnotics)	Additive CNS depression[1]
	Clonidine, guanethidine, methyldopa	Decreased antihypertensive effects

CNS = central nervous system; MAOIs = monoamine oxidase inhibitors; SSRIs = selective serotonin reuptake inhibitors.
[1]Includes tricyclics and heterocyclics with sedative actions (e.g., mirtazapine, nefazodone, and trazodone).

used in the management of the syndrome. Table 19–4 outlines drug interactions observed with antidepressant medications.

REHABILITATION FOCUS

Antidepressant drugs are frequently prescribed to patients suffering from stroke, multiple sclerosis, spinal cord injury, amputation, and severe trauma. Therapists treating patients who have sustained a catastrophic injury or illness are therefore likely to encounter the use of antidepressant agents to improve the patient's mood and feeling of well-being. There is some evidence to suggest that use of these agents early in the rehabilitation process may improve functional gains and outcomes. Effective treatment of depression is however a difficult clinical task. Even with appropriate pharmacologic and psychologic treatment, some patients do not respond. Treatment of 1 month or more may be required before the benefits of drug treatment are realized. Also, the adverse effects of drug treatment

vary from individual to individual. Adverse effects must be monitored closely and changes in the drug regimen made until the optimal drug for each individual is identified.

CLINICAL RELEVANCE FOR REHABILITATION

Adverse Drug Reactions
Tricyclics/Heterocyclics
- Sedation
- Orthostatic hypotension
- Sympathomimetic effects (tremor)
- Antimuscarinic effects (constipation, urinary hesitancy, blurred vision)

SSRIs
- Insomnia, agitation (the "jitters")
- Nausea and diarrhea

MAOIs
- CNS excitation and possible hypertensive crisis
- Postural hypotension

Effects Interfering with Rehabilitation
- Sedation
- Cardiovascular considerations
  - Orthostatic hypotension
  - Hypertensive crisis

Possible Therapy Solutions
- Orthostatic hypotension: compressive garments, tilt table, allow patient's BP time to adjust to postural changes; monitor response to exercise.

Potentiation of Functional Outcomes Secondary to Drug Therapy
- In many cases, antidepressant medications can help with overall functional outcomes at both the activity and participation levels owing to their psychologic effects.

PROBLEM-ORIENTED PATIENT STUDY

Brief History: The patient is a 44-year-old male with a primary diagnosis of amputation of the right lower leg secondary to trauma sustained in a motor vehicle accident. The patient was initially treated at a hospital with level 1 trauma status. The patient underwent surgery to remove his leg and foot. The patient was left with an 8-inch stump distal to the knee. While in the hospital, he received standard physical therapy, occupational therapy, and social services. He was discharged to outpatient therapy for further intervention and permanent prosthesis training.

Current Status and Drug Therapy: Upon initial examination at the body functions and structures level, the patient demonstrated moderate weakness in his right lower extremity. The patient had tenderness and increased sensitivity in the residual limb. At the activity level, the patient had limited function with sit-to-stand transfers, gait, and stairs, complaining of significant pain in his right residual limb with all weight-bearing activities. At the participation level, the patient stated he was unable to work and was very concerned since he was self-employed with a lawn and landscaping service. He stated this made him very anxious and unable to sleep at night. He was occasionally taking diazepam at night to help him sleep and tramadol as needed for pain.

Rehabilitation Setting: The patient began rehabilitation intervention consisting of therapeutic exercise, gait training, and activities of daily living training. On several occasions, the therapist noted that the patient complained of not being able to take a deep breath and a burning and "squeezing" feeling in his chest. Upon questioning, he stated that this happened almost every night in the early evening and occasionally during the day. He also stated that he was having a hard time sleeping at night but did not like taking the diazepam as it made him feel "sleepy" in the morning.

Problem/Clinical Options: With the patient's approval, the physical therapist contacted the patient's physician to inform him of the patient's major complaints. The patient subsequently had a complete cardiac work-up that proved negative. The patient's physician, hypothesizing that he was suffering from secondary depression, prescribed paroxetine twice a day and esomeprazole daily.

Outcome: The patient tolerated this drug regimen with no major adverse reactions. He continued with rehabilitation therapy, and over the next several weeks, he reported an improvement in his sleep pattern as well as a cessation of the burning

(*continued*)

PROBLEM-ORIENTED PATIENT STUDY (*Continued*)

and squeezing feeling in his chest. The therapist noted an improvement in the patient's attitude toward rehabilitation and compliance with his home exercise program and prosthetic training.

The patient continued with his therapy program and was eventually discharged as independent with all functional activities. He was eventually able to return to work.

PREPARATIONS AVAILABLE

Tricyclics

Amitriptyline (generic, Elavil, others)
Oral: 10-, 25-, 50-, 75-, 100-, 150-mg tablets
Parenteral: 10 mg/mL for IM injection

Clomipramine (generic, Anafranil; labeled only for obsessive-compulsive disorder)
Oral: 25-, 50-, 75-mg capsules

Desipramine (generic, Norpramin, Pertofrane)
Oral: 10-, 25-, 50-, 75-, 100-, 150-mg tablets

Doxepin (generic, Sinequan, others)
Oral: 10-, 25-, 50-, 75-, 100-, 150-mg capsules;
10 mg/mL concentrate

Imipramine (generic, Tofranil, others)
Oral: 10-, 25-, 50-mg tablets (as hydrochloride);
75-, 100-, 125-, 150-mg capsules (as pamoate)
Parenteral: 25 mg/2 mL for IM injection

Nortriptyline (generic, Aventyl, Pamelor)
Oral: 10-, 25-, 50-, 75-mg capsules; 10 mg/5 mL solution

Protriptyline (generic, Vivactil)
Oral: 5-, 10-mg tablets

Trimipramine (Surmontil)
Oral: 25-, 50-, 100-mg capsules

Second-Generation and Subsequent Drugs

Amoxapine (generic, Asendin)
Oral: 25-, 50-, 100-, 150-mg tablets

Bupropion (generic, Wellbutrin)
Oral: 75-, 100-mg tablets; 100-, 150-mg sustained-release tablets

Duloxetine (Cymbalta)
Oral: 20-, 30-, 60-mg capsule

Maprotiline (generic, Ludiomil)
Oral: 25-, 50-, 75-mg tablets

Mirtazapine (Remeron)
Oral: 15-, 30-, 45-mg tablets

Nefazodone (Serzone)
Oral: 50-, 100-, 150-, 200-, 250-mg tablets

Trazodone (generic, Desyrel)
Oral: 50-, 100-, 150-, 300-mg tablets

Venlafaxine (Effexor)
Oral: 25-, 37.5-, 50-, 75-, 100-mg tablets;
37.5-, 75-, 150-mg extended-release tablets

Selective Serotonin Reuptake Inhibitors

Citalopram (Celexa)
Oral: 20-, 40-mg tablets

Escitalopram (Lexapro)
Oral: 5-, 10-, 20-mg tablets

Fluoxetine (generic, Prozac)
Oral: 10-, 20-mg pulvules; 10-mg tablets; 20 mg/5 mL liquid
Oral delayed release (Prozac Weekly): 90-mg capsules

Fluvoxamine (Luvox, labeled only for obsessive-compulsive disorder)
Oral: 25-, 50-, 100-mg tablets

Paroxetine (Paxil)
Oral: 10-, 20-, 30-, 40-mg tablets; 10 mg/5 mL suspension; 12.5-, 25-, 37.5-mg controlled-release tablets

Sertraline (Zoloft)
Oral: 25-, 50-, 100-mg tablets

Monoamine Oxidase Inhibitors

Phenelzine (Nardil)
Oral: 15-mg tablets

Tranylcypromine (Parnate)
Oral: 10-mg tablets

Other

Atomoxetine (Strattera)
Oral: 10-, 18-, 25-, 40-, 60-mg capsule

REFERENCES

American Psychiatric Association: *Diagnostic and Statistical Manual of Mental Disorders,* 4th ed. Arlington, VA, 1994.

American Psychiatric Association: APA practice guideline for major depressive disorder in adults. *Am J Psychiatry* 1993;150(Suppl):1.

Anderson IM, Tomenson BM: Selective serotonin reuptake inhibitors versus tricyclic antidepressants: A meta-analysis of efficacy and tolerability. *J Affect Disord* 2000;58:19.

Boyer EW, Shannon M: The serotonin syndrome. *N Engl J Med* 2005;352(11):1112.

Briley M: New hope in the treatment of painful symptoms in depression. *Curr Opin Investig Drugs* 2003;4:42.

Duman RS, et al: A molecular and cellular theory of depression. *Arch Gen Psychiatry* 1997;54:597.

Ernst CL, Goldberg JF: Antidepressant properties of anticonvulsant drugs for bipolar disorder. *J Clin Psychopharmacol* 2003;23:182.

Geddes JR, et al: Relapse prevention with antidepressant drug treatment in depressive disorders: A systematic review. *Lancet* 2003;361:653.

Gillman PK: A review of serotonin toxicity data: Implications for the mechanisms of antidepressant drug action. *Biol Psychiatry* 2006;59(11):1046.

Harvey AT, et al: Evidence of the dual mechanisms of action of venlafaxine. *Arch Gen Psychiatry* 2000;57:503.

Leslie LK, et al: The Food and Drug Administration's Deliberations on Antidepressant Use in Pediatric Patients. *Pediatrics* 2005;116:195.

Mann JJ: The medical management of depression. *N Engl J Med* 2005;353:1819.

Merikangas KR, et al: Workgroup Reports: NIMH Strategic Plan for Mood Disorders Research, Future of Genetics of Mood Disorders Research. *Biol Psychiatry* 2002;52:457.

Meyer JH, et al: Occupancy of serotonin transporters by paroxetine and citalopram during treatment of depression: A [(11)C]DASB PET imaging study. *Am J Psychiatry* 2001;158:1843.

Nestler EJ, et al: Preclinical models: Status of basic research in depression. *Biol Psychiatry* 2002;52:503.

Rush JA, Ryan ND: Current and emerging therapeutics for depression. In *Neuropsychopharmacology: The Fifth Generation of Progress.* Davis KL, et al, ed. Philadelphia: Lippincott Williams & Wilkins, 2002.

Schatzberg I, et al: Molecular and cellular mechanisms in depression. In *Neuropsychopharmacology: The Fifth Generation of Progress.* Davis KL, et al, ed. Philadelphia: Lippincott Williams & Wilkins, 2002.

Simon GE, et al: Suicide risk during antidepressant treatment. *Am J Psychiatry* 2006;163:41.

Stahl SM, et al: Comparative efficacy between venlafaxine and SSRIs: A pooled analysis of patients with depression. *Biol Psychiatry* 2002;52:1166.

Rehabilitation

Allen BP, et al: Minor depression and rehabilitation outcome for older adults in subacute care. *J Behav Health Serv Res* 2004;31:189.

Hosaka T, et al: Pschiatric evaluation of rehabilitation patients. *Tokai J Exp Clin Med* 1994;19:11.

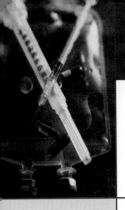

20

OPIOID ANALGESICS AND ANTAGONISTS

Derivatives of the opium poppy have been used to relieve severe pain for hundreds (possibly thousands) of years. **Morphine**, the prototypic opioid agonist, does so with remarkable efficacy. This alkaloid (named after Morpheus, the Greek god of dreams) is extracted from crude opium, which is obtained from the opium poppy seed pod. Morphine remains the standard against which all drugs that have strong analgesic action are compared in terms of efficacy and potency. These drugs are collectively known as opioid analgesics and include not only the natural opium alkaloids and semisynthetic alkaloid derivatives from opium, but also synthetic surrogates (opioid-like analgesic drugs whose actions are blocked by the nonselective antagonist **naloxone**), and endogenous peptides that interact with several opioid receptor subtypes. Opioid analgesics are characterized by their ability to relieve moderate to severe pain. Many opioids also have useful antitussive or antidiarrheal effects.

Analgesic drug therapy and many physical therapy interventions are aimed at the same outcome: pain relief. For this reason, analgesic drugs are among the most frequently prescribed medications for patients receiving rehabilitative therapy. It is essential for physical therapists to be familiar with the intended uses and common adverse effects of opioid analgesics to effectively monitor patient outcomes. The opioid medications are classified as controlled substances because of their potential for abuse; therefore, an understanding of the clinical signs of physical dependence and tolerance is also needed. The major subclasses of opioid agonist and antagonist drugs are outlined in Figure 20–1.

The other major group of analgesic drugs comprises aspirin and the other nonsteroidal anti-inflammatory drugs (NSAIDs). The NSAIDs have a significantly lower maximal efficacy than the opioids and have no addiction liability. Therefore, they are not considered narcotics and are available with an ordinary prescription or even over-the-counter. The NSAIDs are discussed in Chapter 34.

ENDOGENOUS OPIOID PEPTIDES

Although they are not peptides, opioid alkaloids (e.g., morphine) produce analgesia through actions in regions of the brain that contain endogenous peptides which have opioid-like pharmacologic properties. The general term currently used for these substances is endogenous opioid peptides, which replaces the previous term *endorphins*. Three families of endogenous opioid peptides have been described: **enkephalins**, **dynorphans**, and **endorphins**. These

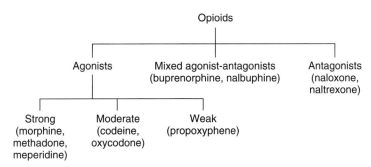

Figure 20–1. Major subclasses of opioid agonists and antagonists.

peptides are synthesized in the soma of neurons and transported to the nerve endings where they accumulate in synaptic vesicles and are released from nerve terminals. Although chemically quite different from the opioid alkaloids, these endogenous peptides bind to opioid receptors and modulate transmission in the brain and spinal cord, and at the primary afferents. It remains unclear whether these peptides function as classic neurotransmitters or as modulator neuropeptides. Opioid peptides are also found in the adrenal medulla and the neural plexus (enteric nervous system) of the gut.

DRUG CLASSIFICATION

The opioid analgesics and related drugs are derived from several chemical subgroups and may be classified in several ways. Opioid drugs can be subdivided according to their major therapeutic uses; that is, analgesics, antitussives, and antidiarrheal drugs. A second method of classification is according to their strength of analgesia: strong, moderate, or weak agonists. Partial agonists are opioids that exert less analgesia than morphine, a strong full agonist. Another clinically useful way to classify these drugs is based on their ratio of agonist to antagonist effects. Thus, opioid drugs may be classified as pure agonists (receptor activators [strong or mild to moderate]), pure antagonists (receptor blockers), or mixed agonist-antagonists, which are capable of activating one opioid receptor subtype and blocking another subtype (Table 20–1).

PHARMACOKINETIC PROPERTIES

Most drugs in this class are well absorbed when given by the subcutaneous, intramuscular, and oral routes. However, because of extensive first-pass metabolism, the oral dose of some opioids such as morphine, hydromorphone, and oxymorphone may need to be much higher than the parenteral dose to elicit a therapeutic effect. Nasal insufflation of certain opioids can result in higher bioavailability by avoiding first-pass metabolism. Additionally, sustained-release forms of some drugs are now available, including morphine and oxycodone. Other routes of opioid administration include oral mucosal, iontophoresis, and transdermal patch, which can provide delivery of potent analgesics over days. The epidural and intrathecal routes are usually used for postsurgical analgesia.

Opioid drugs are widely distributed to body tissues, but localize in highest concentrations in tissues that are highly perfused such as the brain, lungs, liver, kidneys, and spleen. Drug concentrations in skeletal muscle may be lower, but this tissue serves as the main reservoir because of its greater bulk. Even though blood flow to fatty tissue is much lower than to the highly perfused tissues, accumulation can be very important, particularly after frequent high-dose administration or continuous infusion of highly lipophilic opioids that are slowly metabolized (e.g., fentanyl). Opioids cross the placental barrier and exert effects that can result in both respiratory depression and, with continuous exposure, physical dependence in neonates.

Table 20–1.	Common opioid analgesics	

Generic Name	Route of Administration	Duration (h)
Strong Agonists		
Morphine[1]	Oral, IM, IV, SQ	4–5
	Epidural, intrathecal	Up to 24
Hydromorphone	Oral, IM, IV, SQ	2–4
Oxymorphone	IM, IV, SQ, rectal	3–6
Methadone	Oral, IM, IV	4–6
Meperidine	Oral, IM, IV, SQ	2–4
Fentanyl	IM	1–2
	IV	0.5–1
Sufentanil	IV	1–1.5
Alfentanil	IV	0.25–0.75
Levorphanol	Oral, IM, IV, SQ	4–5
Mild-to-Moderate Agonists		
Codeine	Oral, IM, SQ	4
Hydrocodone[2]	Oral	4–6
Oxycodone[1,3]	Oral	3–4
Propoxyphene	Oral	4–6
Partial Agonist		
Buprenorphine	Oral, IM, IV	4–8
Mixed Agonist-Antagonist		
Pentazocine	Oral	3
	IM, IV, SQ	2–3
Nalbuphine	IM, IV, SQ	3–6
Butorphanol	IM	3–4
	IV	2–4

IM = intramuscular; IV = intravenous; SQ = subcutaneous.

[1]Available in sustained-release forms for morphine and oxycodone.

[2]Available in tablets containing acetaminophen.

[3]Available in tablets containing acetaminophen; aspirin.

With few exceptions, the opioids are metabolized by hepatic enzymes, usually to inactive polar metabolites (mostly glucuronide conjugates) before their elimination by the kidney. However, morphine-6-glucuronide, a metabolite of morphine, has analgesic activity equivalent to that of morphine, and morphine-3-glucuronide (the primary metabolite) has neuroexcitatory effects. Some degree of metabolism also occurs in other

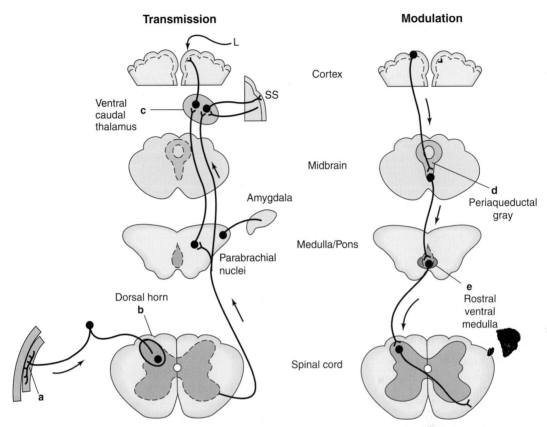

Figure 20–2. Putative sites of action of opioid analgesics. On the left, sites of action on the ascending pain transmission pathway from the periphery to the higher centers are shown. (a) Direct action of opioids on inflamed peripheral tissues. (b) Inhibition occurs in the spinal cord. (c) Possible site of action in the thalamus. Different thalamic regions project to somatosensory (SS) or limbic (L) cortex. Parabrachial nuclei (medulla/pons) project to the amygdala. On the right, sites of action on the descending pain transmission pathway (modulation) are shown. Actions of opioids on pain-modulating neurons in the midbrain (d) and medulla (e) indirectly control pain transmission pathways.

tissues, such as the lungs, kidneys, and central nervous system.

MECHANISM OF ACTION

Opioid agonists produce analgesia by binding to specific G protein–coupled receptors, located primarily in brain and spinal cord, and altering the transmission and modulation of pain.

Receptors

Opioid receptors are located on primary afferents and spinal cord pain transmission neurons (ascending pathways) and on neurons in the midbrain and medulla (descending pathways) that function in pain modulation (Figure 20–2). Other opioid receptors that may be involved in altering reactivity to pain are located on neurons in the basal ganglia, the hypothalamus, the limbic structures, and the cerebral cortex.

Three major opioid receptor subtypes have been extensively characterized: μ **(mu)**, δ **(delta), and** κ **(kappa) receptors.** All three receptor subtypes appear to be involved in analgesic mechanisms (Table 20–2). The μ-receptor activation plays a major role in the respiratory depressant actions of opioids and κ-receptor activation appears to be involved in sedative actions.

Table 20–2.	Opioid receptor subtypes, some of their functions, and endogenous opioid peptide affinity	
Receptor Subtype	**Functions**	**Endogenous Opioid Peptide Affinity**
μ (mu)	Supraspinal and spinal analgesia; sedation; inhibition of respiration; slowed GI transit; modulation of hormone and neurotransmitter release	Endorphins > enkephalins > dynorphins
δ (delta)	Supraspinal and spinal analgesia; modulation of hormone and neurotransmitter release	Enkephalins >> endorphins and dynorphins
κ (kappa)	Supraspinal and spinal analgesia; psychotomimetic effects; slowed GI transit	Dynorphins >> endorphins and enkephalins

GI = gastrointestinal.

Ionic Mechanisms

Opioid analgesics *inhibit* synaptic activity partly through direct activation of opioid receptors and partly through release of the endogenous opioid peptides, which are themselves inhibitory to neurons. All three major opioid receptors are coupled to their effectors by G proteins and activate phospholipase C or inhibit adenylyl cyclase. At the postsynaptic level, activation of these receptors can open K^+ ion channels to cause membrane hyperpolarization (inhibitory postsynaptic potentials). At the presynaptic level, opioid receptor activation can close voltage-gated Ca^{2+} ion channels to inhibit neurotransmitter release. Figure 20–3 schematically illustrates the presynaptic action at all three receptor types and the postsynaptic effect at μ receptors on nociceptive afferents in the spinal cord. The presynaptic action—depressed transmitter release—has been demonstrated for a large number of neurotransmitters including glutamate, the principle excitatory amino acid released from nociceptive nerve terminals, as well as acetylcholine, norepinephrine, serotonin, and substance P.

Receptor Distribution and Neural Mechanisms of Analgesia

Opioid receptor-binding sites have been localized autoradiographically for each receptor subtype. All three major receptors are present in high concentrations in the dorsal horn of the spinal cord (Figure 20–2b). Receptors are present both on spinal cord pain transmission neurons and on the primary afferents that relay the nociceptive signal to them (Figure 20–2, left side). Opioid agonists inhibit the release of excitatory transmitters from these primary afferents, and they directly inhibit dorsal horn pain transmission neurons. Thus, opioids exert a powerful analgesic effect directly upon the spinal cord. This spinal action has been exploited clinically by direct application of opioid agonists to the spinal cord, which provides a regional analgesic effect while reducing the unwanted respiratory depression, nausea and vomiting, and sedation that may occur from the supraspinal actions of systemically administered opioids.

Under most circumstances, opioids are given systemically and thus act simultaneously at both spinal and supraspinal sites; interaction in these two areas tends to increase their overall analgesic efficacy. Different combinations of opioid receptors are found in the supraspinal regions implicated in pain transmission and modulation (Figure 20–2). Of particular importance are opioid binding sites in pain-modulating descending pathways (Figure 20–2, right), including the rostral ventral medulla, the locus ceruleus, and the midbrain periaqueductal gray area. At these sites as at others, opioids are inhibitory, yet neurons that send

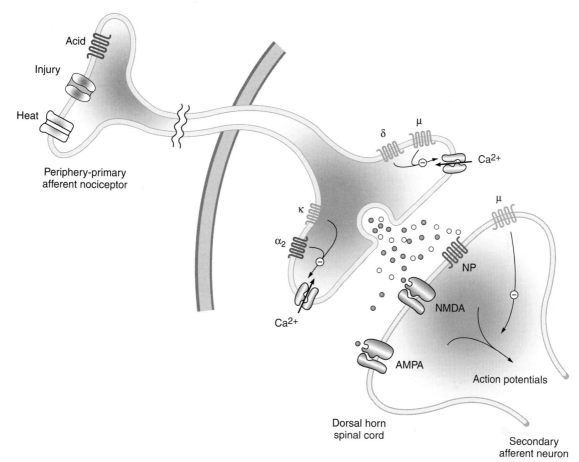

Figure 20–3. Spinal sites of opioid action and some other analgesic agents. The μ, κ, and δ agonists reduce transmitter release (often glutamate and excitatory neuropeptides) from presynaptic terminals of nociceptive primary afferents. The μ agonists also hyperpolarize second-order pain transmission neurons by increasing K+ conductance, evoking an inhibitory postsynaptic potential. Alpha$_2$ agonists appear to act on adrenoceptors on the presynaptic terminal of the primary afferent neuron. AMPA, NMDA = glutamate receptors; NP = neuro peptide.

processes to the spinal cord to inhibit pain transmission neurons are activated by the drugs. This activation has been shown to result from the inhibition of inhibitory neurons in several locations (Figure 20–4).

When pain-relieving opioid drugs are given systemically, they presumably act upon brain circuits normally regulated by endogenous opioid peptides. Part of the pain-relieving action of exogenous opioids involves the release of endogenous opioid peptides. An exogenous opioid agonist (e.g., morphine) may act primarily and directly at the μ receptor, but this action may evoke the release of endogenous opioids that additionally act at δ and κ receptors. Thus, even a receptor-selective ligand can initiate a complex sequence of events involving multiple synapses, transmitters, and receptor types.

Animal and human clinical studies demonstrate that both endogenous and exogenous opioids can also produce opioid-mediated analgesia at sites *outside* the central nervous system (CNS). Pain associated with inflammation seems especially sensitive to these peripheral opioid actions. The identification of functional μ receptors on the peripheral terminals of sensory neurons supports this hypothesis. Furthermore,

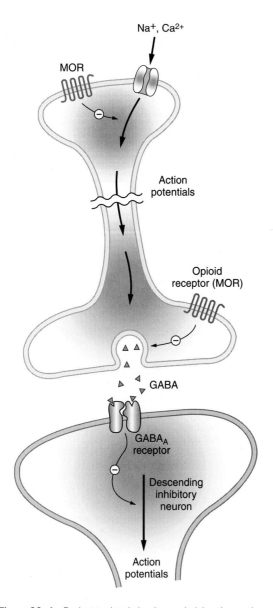

Figure 20–4. Brainstem local circuitry underlying the modulating effect of descending pathways by μ opioid receptor (MOR)–mediated analgesia. The pain inhibitory neuron is indirectly excited by opioids (exogenous or endogenous) that inhibit an inhibitory (GABAergic) interneuron (*GABA*). This results in enhanced inhibition of nociceptive processing in the dorsal horn of the spinal cord.

activation of peripheral μ receptors results in a decrease in sensory neuron activity and transmitter release. For example, administration of opioids into the knees of patients undergoing arthroscopic knee surgery has shown some clinical benefit. With further development, opioids selective for a peripheral site would be useful adjuncts in the treatment of inflammatory pain (Box 20–1). Moreover, new peripherally-acting dynorphins may provide a novel means to treat visceral pain.

Tolerance and Physical Dependence

With frequently repeated administration of therapeutic doses of morphine or its surrogates, there is a gradual loss in effectiveness. This is called tolerance; that is, to reproduce the original response, a larger dose must be administered. Along with tolerance, physical dependence usually develops. Physical dependence is defined as the occurrence of a characteristic **withdrawal** or **abstinence** syndrome when the drug is stopped abruptly. These symptoms include rhinorrhea, lacrimation, chills, gooseflesh, muscle aches, diarrhea, yawning, anxiety, and hostility. A more intense state of precipitated withdrawal results when an opioid antagonist (e.g., naloxone) is administered to a physically dependent individual.

The mechanism of development of tolerance and physical dependence is poorly understood, but persistent activation of μ receptors such as occurs with the treatment of severe chronic pain appears to play a primary role in its induction and maintenance. Recent research suggests that the δ opioid receptor is an important component in the maintenance of tolerance. In addition, the concept of receptor uncoupling has gained prominence. Under this hypothesis, tolerance is due to a dysfunction of structural interactions between the μ receptor and G proteins, second messenger systems, and their target ion channels. Moreover, the NMDA (*N*-methyl-D-aspartate) receptor for glutamate has been shown to play a critical role in tolerance development and maintenance because NMDA receptor antagonists such as ketamine can block tolerance development. In addition to the development of tolerance, persistent administration of opioid analgesics has been observed to sometimes *increase* the sensation of pain (hyperalgesia). Spinally-derived dynorphin is a leading candidate for the mediation of opioid-induced hyperalgesia.

Box 20–1. Ion Channels and Novel Analgesics

Even the most severe acute pain (that lasting hours to days) can usually be well controlled—with significant but tolerable adverse effects—with currently available analgesics, especially the opioids. Chronic pain (lasting weeks to months), however, is not very satisfactorily managed with opioids. It is now known that in chronic pain, presynaptic receptors on sensory nerve terminals in the periphery contribute to increased excitability of sensory nerve endings (peripheral sensitization). The hyperexcitable sensory neuron bombards the spinal cord, leading to increased excitability and synaptic alterations in the dorsal horn (central sensitization). Such changes appear to be important in chronic inflammatory and neuropathic pain states.

In the effort to discover better analgesic drugs for chronic pain, renewed attention is being paid to synaptic transmission in nociception and sensory processing. Potentially important ion channels associated with these processes in the periphery include members of the transient receptor potential family such as the TRPV1 (capsaicin) receptor that is activated by heat and products of inflammation as well as P2X receptors (responsive to purines released from tissue damage). A special type of tetrodotoxin-resistant voltage-gated sodium channel (Nav1.8), also known as the PN3/SNS channel, is apparently uniquely associated with nociceptive neurons in dorsal root ganglia. Mexiletine, which is useful in some chronic pain states, may act by blocking this channel. Certain blockers of voltage-gated N-type calcium channels have shown analgesic effects. A synthetic peptide related to the marine snail toxin ω-conotoxin, which selectively blocks these calcium channels, is in clinical trials as an analgesic. Gabapentin, an anticonvulsant analog of gamma-aminobutyric acid (GABA) (Chapter 14), is an effective treatment for neuropathic (nerve injury) pain. It has recently been shown to block the pain and hyperalgesia associated with inflammation. Potential sites of action of gabapentin include the alpha-2-delta family of calcium channels.

N-methyl-D-aspartate (NMDA) receptors appear to play a very important role in central sensitization at both spinal and supraspinal levels. Although certain NMDA antagonists have demonstrated analgesic activity (e.g., ketamine), it has been difficult to find agents with an acceptably low profile of side effects or neurotoxicity. GABA and acetylcholine (through nicotinic receptors) appear to control the central synaptic release of several transmitters involved in nociception. Nicotine itself and certain nicotine analogs cause analgesia. A nicotinic agonist found in certain frogs (epibatidine) has significant analgesic effect.

Although none of the studies described has yet yielded an approved analgesic drug, they have already provided a better understanding of nociception and analgesia.

ACUTE EFFECTS OF MORPHINE AND ITS SURROGATES

Central Nervous System Effects

The principal effects of opioid analgesics with affinity for μ receptors are in the CNS; the more important effects include analgesia, euphoria, sedation, and respiratory depression. With repeated use, a high degree of tolerance occurs to all of these effects.

Analgesia

The opioids are the most powerful drugs available for the relief of pain. They attenuate both emotional (affective) and sensory aspects of the pain experience. Strong agonists (i.e., those with the highest analgesic efficacy, full agonists) include **morphine, methadone, meperidine, fentanyl, levorphanol,** and **heroin. Codeine, hydrocodone,** and **oxycodone** are partial agonists with mild to moderate analgesic efficacy. **Propoxyphene** is a very weak agonist drug.

Euphoria

Typically, patients or drug users who receive intravenous morphine experience a pleasant floating sensation with lessened anxiety and distress. However, dysphoria, an unpleasant state characterized by restlessness and malaise, may sometimes occur. These effects may occur at doses below those required for maximum analgesia.

Sedation

Drowsiness and clouding of mentation are frequent concomitants of opioid action. There is little or no amnesia. Sleep is induced by opiates more frequently in the elderly than in young, healthy individuals. Ordinarily, the patient can be easily aroused from this sleep. However, the combination of morphine with other CNS-depressant drugs such as the sedative-hypnotics may result in very deep sleep. Marked sedation occurs more frequently with compounds closely related to morphine and its derivatives and less frequently with the synthetic agents such as meperidine and fentanyl.

Respiratory Depression

Opioid actions in the medulla lead to inhibition of the respiratory center, with decreased response to carbon dioxide challenge. With full agonists, respiratory depression may be seen at conventional analgesic doses. The respiratory depression is dose related and is influenced significantly by the degree of sensory input occurring at the time. For example, it is possible to partially overcome opioid-induced respiratory depression by stimulation of various sorts. When strongly painful stimuli that have prevented the depressant action of a large dose of an opioid are relieved, respiratory depression may suddenly become marked. A small to moderate decrease in respiratory function, as measured by $PaCO_2$ elevation, may be well tolerated in the patient without prior respiratory impairment. However, in individuals with asthma, chronic obstructive pulmonary disease, or cor pulmonale, this decrease in respiratory function may not be tolerated. Increased PCO_2 may cause cerebrovascular dilation, resulting in increased cerebral blood flow and increased intracranial pressure.

Antitussive Actions

Suppression of the cough reflex is a well-recognized action of opioids; the exact mechanism, however, is unknown. Codeine in particular has been used to advantage in persons suffering from pathologic cough and in patients in whom it is necessary to maintain ventilation via an endotracheal tube. However, cough suppression by opioids may allow accumulation of secretions and thus lead to airway obstruction and atelectasis.

Miosis

Constriction of the pupils is seen with virtually all opioid agonists except meperidine. Miosis is a pharmacologic action to which little or no tolerance develops; thus, it is valuable in the diagnosis of opioid overdose. Even in highly tolerant addicts, miosis will be seen. This action, which can be blocked by opioid antagonists such as naloxone, is mediated by parasympathetic pathways, which, in turn, can be blocked by atropine. Meperidine has sufficient antimuscarinic action to prevent miosis.

Nausea and Vomiting

The opioid analgesics can activate the brainstem chemoreceptor trigger zone to produce nausea and vomiting. There may also be a vestibular component in this effect because ambulation seems to increase the incidence of nausea and vomiting.

Truncal Rigidity

An intensification of tone in the large trunk muscles has been noted with a number of opioids. Truncal rigidity results from an action of these drugs at supraspinal levels. Truncal rigidity reduces thoracic compliance and thus interferes with ventilation. The effect is most apparent when high doses of the highly lipid-soluble opioids (e.g., fentanyl, sufentanil, alfentanil) are rapidly administered intravenously. Truncal rigidity may be overcome by administration of an opioid antagonist, which of course will also antagonize the analgesic action of the opioid. Preventing truncal rigidity while preserving analgesia requires the concomitant use of neuromuscular-blocking agents.

Peripheral Effects

Cardiovascular System

Most opioids have no significant direct effects on the heart and no major effects on cardiac rhythm (except bradycardia). Meperidine is an exception to this generalization because its antimuscarinic action may result in tachycardia. Blood pressure is usually well maintained in subjects receiving opioids unless the cardiovascular system is stressed, in which case hypotension may occur. This hypotensive effect is probably due to peripheral arterial and venous dilation, which has been attributed to a number of mechanisms including central depression of vasomotor-stabilizing mechanisms and release of histamine. No consistent effect on cardiac output is seen, and the electrocardiogram is not significantly affected. However, caution should be exercised in patients with decreased blood volume, since the above mechanisms make these patients quite susceptible to hypotension. Opioid analgesics affect cerebral circulation minimally except when PCO_2 rises as a consequence of respiratory depression.

Gastrointestinal Tract

Constipation occurs through decreased intestinal peristalsis, which is probably mediated by effects on opioid receptors in the enteric nervous system. In the stomach, motility (rhythmic contraction and relaxation) may decrease but tone (persistent contraction) may increase—particularly in the central portion. In the large intestine, propulsive peristaltic waves are diminished and tone is increased; this delays passage of the fecal mass and allows increased absorption of water, which leads to constipation. This powerful action is the basis for the clinical use of some of these drugs as antidiarrheal agents.

Smooth Muscle

Opioids (with the exception of meperidine) cause contraction of biliary tract smooth muscle, which may cause biliary colic or spasm, increased ureteral and bladder sphincter tone, and a reduction in uterine tone, which may contribute to prolongation of labor.

Renal Effects

Renal function is depressed by opioids. In humans, this is believed to be chiefly due to decreased renal plasma flow. Opioids can decrease systemic blood pressure and glomerular filtration rate. In addition, μ opioids have been found to have an antidiuretic effect in humans. Mechanisms may involve both the CNS and peripheral sites, but the relative contributions of each are unknown. Opioids also enhance renal tubular sodium reabsorption. The role of opioid-induced changes in antidiuretic hormone (ADH) release is controversial. Ureteral and bladder tone are increased by therapeutic doses of the opioid analgesics. Increased sphincter tone may precipitate urinary retention, especially in postoperative patients and older men with prostatic hyperplasia. Occasionally, ureteral colic caused by a renal calculus is made worse by the opioid-induced increase in ureteral tone.

Pruritus

Therapeutic doses of the opioid analgesics (especially morphine) produce flushing and warming of the skin accompanied sometimes by sweating and itching; CNS effects and peripheral histamine release may be responsible for these reactions. Opioid-induced pruritus and, occasionally, urticaria appear more frequently when opioid analgesics are administered parenterally. In addition, when opioids such as morphine are administered by the spinal or epidural route, their usefulness may be limited by intense pruritus over the lips and torso.

■ CLINICAL USES

Successful treatment of pain is a challenging task that begins with careful attempts to assess the source and magnitude of the pain. The amount of pain experienced by the patient is often described by means of a numeric visual analog scale (VAS) with word descriptors ranging from no pain (0) to excruciating pain (10). A similar scale can be used with children and with patients who cannot speak; this scale depicts five faces ranging from smiling (no pain) to crying (maximum pain).

In severe pain, the administration of an opioid analgesic is usually considered a primary part of the overall management plan. Determining the route of administration (oral, parenteral, spinal), duration of drug action, ceiling effect (maximal intrinsic activity), duration of therapy, potential for unwanted side effects, and the patient's past experience with opioids should all be addressed by the prescribing practitioner and monitored by all health-care personnel involved in the patient's care. One of the principal errors made by practitioners in this setting is a failure to assess a patient's pain adequately and to match its severity with an appropriate level of drug therapy. Just as important is the principle that following delivery of the therapeutic plan, its effectiveness must be reevaluated and the plan modified if necessary if the response was excessive or inadequate.

Use of opioid drugs in acute situations may be contrasted with their use in chronic pain management, where a multitude of other factors must be considered, including the development of tolerance to and physical dependence on opioid analgesics.

Analgesia

In the acute setting, strong agonists are usually given parenterally for the treatment of relatively constant moderate to severe pain; whereas sharp, intermittent pain does not appear to be as effectively controlled. The pain associated with cancer and other terminal illnesses must be treated aggressively and often requires a multidisciplinary approach for effective management. Such conditions may require continuous use of potent opioid analgesics and will be associated with some degree of tolerance and dependence. There is, however, incomplete cross-tolerance to the μ-receptor effects between various subclasses of opioids, and this provides the basis for "rotation" of opioids in chronic pain management. If tolerance and dependence occurs, this should not be used as a barrier to providing patients with the best possible care and quality of life. Research in the hospice movement has demonstrated that fixed-interval administration of opioid medication (i.e., a regular dose at a scheduled time) is more effective in achieving pain relief than dosing on demand. New dosage forms of opioids that allow slower release of the drug are now available (e.g., sustained-release forms of morphine and oxycodone).

Their purported advantage is a longer and more stable level of analgesia.

Prolonged analgesia, with some reduction in adverse effects, can be achieved with epidural administration of certain strong agonist drugs (e.g., fentanyl and morphine). If disturbances of gastrointestinal function prevent the use of oral sustained-release morphine, the fentanyl transdermal system (fentanyl patch) can be used over long periods. Administration of strong opioids by nasal insufflation has been shown to be efficacious, but very few are currently available for this route. Opioid analgesics are often used during obstetric labor, but care must be taken to minimize neonatal depression because opioids cross the placental barrier and reach the fetus.

For less severe pain and in the chronic setting, moderate agonists are given by the oral route. In addition, stimulant drugs such as the amphetamines have been shown to enhance the analgesic actions of the opioids and thus may be very useful adjuncts in the patient with chronic pain. Also, other drug groups, such as various anticonvulsants and antidepressants, are useful in the successful management of chronic pain syndrome (Chapters 14 and 19, respectively) and should also be considered.

Cough Suppression

Suppression of cough can be obtained at opioid doses lower than those needed for analgesia. However, in recent years, the use of opioid analgesics to allay cough has diminished largely because a number of effective synthetic compounds have been developed that are neither analgesic nor addictive. See Chapter 35 for additional information. Useful oral antitussive drugs include **codeine** and **dextromethorphan**.

Treatment of Diarrhea

Diarrhea from almost any cause can be controlled with the opioid analgesics, but if diarrhea is associated with infection such use must not substitute for appropriate antimicrobial chemotherapy. Crude opium preparations (e.g., paregoric) were used in the past to control diarrhea, but now synthetic surrogates with more selective gastrointestinal effects and few or no CNS effects are used. Several preparations are available specifically for this purpose (e.g., **diphenoxylate** and **loperamide**). See Chapter 36 for additional information.

Management of Acute Pulmonary Edema

Intravenous morphine has a dramatic ability to reduce dyspnea from pulmonary edema associated with left ventricular failure. The mechanism is not clear but probably involves reduced *perception* of shortness of breath and reduced patient anxiety as well as reduced cardiac preload (reduced venous tone) and afterload (decreased peripheral resistance). Morphine can also be particularly useful when treating the pain associated with myocardial ischemia in patients with acute pulmonary edema. However, other drugs with minimal or no respiratory depressant effects (diuretics) may also be used to manage acute pulmonary edema.

Anesthesia

The opioids are useful as preoperative drugs because of their sedative, anxiolytic, and analgesic properties. The opioids are also used intraoperatively as adjunctive agents in balanced anesthesia protocols (Chapter 15). High-dose intravenous opioids (e.g., morphine, fentanyl) are often a primary component of the anesthetic regimen, most commonly in cardiovascular surgery and other types of high-risk surgery where a primary goal is to minimize cardiovascular depression. In such situations, mechanical respiratory assistance must be provided.

Because of their direct action on the superficial neurons of the spinal cord dorsal horn, opioids can also be used as regional analgesics by administration into the epidural or subarachnoid spaces of the spinal column. Long-lasting analgesia with minimal adverse effects can be achieved by epidural administration of 3 to 5 mg of morphine, followed by slow infusion through a catheter placed in the epidural space. It was initially assumed that the epidural application of opioids might selectively produce analgesia without impairment of motor, autonomic, or sensory functions other than pain. However, respiratory depression may occur after the drug is injected into the epidural space and may require reversal with naloxone. Other effects such as pruritus and nausea and vomiting are common

after epidural and subarachnoid administration of opioids and may also be reversed with naloxone if necessary. Currently, the epidural route is favored because adverse effects are less common. Morphine is the most frequently used agent, but the use of low doses of local anesthetics in combination with fentanyl infused through a thoracic epidural catheter has also become an accepted method of pain control in patients recovering from major upper abdominal surgery. In rare cases of chronic pain management, health-care professionals may elect to implant a programmable infusion pump connected to a spinal catheter for continuous infusion of opioids or other analgesic compounds.

Opioid Dependence

Methadone, one of the longer-acting opioids, is used in the management of opioid withdrawal states and in maintenance programs for addicts. In withdrawal states, methadone permits a slow tapering of the opioid effect that diminishes the intensity of abstinence symptoms. **Buprenorphine** has an even longer duration of action and is sometimes used in withdrawal states. In maintenance programs, the prolonged action of methadone blocks the euphoria-inducing effects of doses of shorter-acting opioids (e.g., heroin, morphine).

ALTERNATIVE ROUTES OF ADMINISTRATION

Rectal suppositories of morphine and hydromorphone have long been used when oral and parenteral routes are undesirable. The transdermal patch provides stable blood levels of drug and better pain control while avoiding the need for repeated parenteral injections. Fentanyl has been the most successful opioid in transdermal application and finds great use in patients experiencing chronic pain. The intranasal route avoids repeated parenteral drug injections and the first-pass metabolism of orally administered drugs. Butorphanol is the mostly widely used opioid currently available in the United States in a nasal formulation. Another alternative to parenteral administration is the buccal transmucosal route, which uses a fentanyl citrate lozenge or a "lollipop" mounted on a stick.

Another type of pain control called patient-controlled analgesia (PCA) is used in many hospitals. PCA permits the patient to control a parenteral (usually intravenous) infusion device by depressing a button to deliver a preprogrammed dose of the desired opioid analgesic. Clinical trials suggest that better pain control is achieved using less opioid, making this approach very useful in postoperative pain control. Overdosage secondary to misuse or improper programming of the PCA device must be guarded against because there is a risk of respiratory depression with hypoxia.

ADVERSE EFFECTS AND TOXICITY

Adverse effects of the opioid analgesics that are extensions of their acute pharmacologic actions include respiratory depression, nausea, vomiting, and constipation (Table 20–3). In addition, tolerance and dependence, diagnosis and treatment of overdosage, and drug interactions must be considered.

Tolerance and Dependence

Tolerance development begins with the first dose of an opioid, but is not usually obvious until after 2 to 3 weeks of frequent exposure to ordinary doses. Tolerance develops most readily when higher doses are given more frequently. Tolerance develops to a different degree for different effects of opioid drugs: marked tolerance is observed for analgesia, euphoria, sedation, respiratory depression, nausea and vomiting, and the

---

Table 20–3.   Adverse effects of the opioid analgesics

Behavioral restlessness, tremulousness, hyperactivity (in dysphoric reactions)
Respiratory depression
Nausea and vomiting
Increased intracranial pressure
Postural hypotension accentuated by hypovolemia
Constipation
Urinary retention
Itching around nose, urticaria (more frequent with parenteral and spinal administration)

---

antitussive effect. Tolerence is minimal for miosis, constipation, and convulsions.

Cross-tolerance is an extremely important characteristic of the opioids; that is, patients tolerant to morphine show a reduction in analgesic response to other agonist opioids. This is particularly true of those agents with primarily μ-receptor agonist activity. Morphine and its congeners exhibit cross-tolerance not only with respect to their analgesic actions but also to their euphoriant, sedative, and respiratory effects. However, the cross-tolerance existing among the μ-receptor agonists can often be partial or incomplete, which supports the rotational use of opioids in managing chronic pain syndrome.

Drug dependence of the opioid type is marked by a relatively specific withdrawal or abstinence syndrome. **Withdrawal syndrome,** because of its severity, is often treated with methadone replacement therapy to remove the drug from the system slowly with less severe withdrawal signs and symptoms (see discussion above). Psychologic dependence, unfortunately, is strongly reinforced by the development of physical dependence. The euphoria, indifference to stimuli, and sedation caused by opioid analgesics tend to promote their compulsive use. The addict experiences abdominal effects much like an intense sexual orgasm; this also contributes to their abuse. However, just as there are pharmacologic differences between the various opioids, there are also differences in psychologic dependence and the severity of withdrawal effects. For example, withdrawal from dependence upon a strong agonist is associated with more severe withdrawal signs and symptoms than withdrawal from a mild or moderate agonist.

Administration of an opioid *antagonist* to an opioid-dependent person is followed by brief but severe withdrawal symptoms. The potential for physical and psychologic dependence of the partial agonist-antagonist opioids appear to be less than that of the agonist drugs.

Overdose

A triad of pupillary constriction, comatose state, and respiratory depression is characteristic of opioid overdose, with the latter being responsible for most fatalities. Diagnosis of overdosage is confirmed if intravenous injection of naloxone, an antagonist drug, results in prompt signs of recovery. Treatment of overdose involves the use of antagonists such as naloxone and other therapeutic measures, especially ventilatory support.

Drug Interactions

The most important drug interactions involving opioid analgesics are additive CNS depression with ethanol, sedative-hypnotics, anesthetics, antipsychotic drugs, tricyclic antidepressants, and antihistamines. Concomitant use of certain opioids (e.g., meperidine) with monoamine oxidase inhibitors increases the incidence of hyperpyrexic coma. Meperidine has also been implicated in the serotonin syndrome when used with selective serotonin reuptake inhibitors (Table 20–4).

Contraindications and Cautions in Therapy

Use of Pure Agonists with Weak Partial Agonists

As described in Chapter 2, a partial agonist behaves like an antagonist when given in the presence of a full agonist. Thus, a weak partial agonist such as pentazocine, if given to a patient also receiving a full agonist (e.g., morphine), may result in diminishing analgesia or even a state of withdrawal; such combinations should be avoided.

Use in Patients with Head Injuries

Respiratory depression caused by opioids causes carbon dioxide retention. This results in cerebral vasodilation. In patients with a head injury, the resulting elevation in intracranial pressure may be lethal.

Use during Pregnancy

Chronic use of opioids during pregnancy may result in physical dependence in the fetus in utero and withdrawal symptoms in the neonate in the early postpartum period. A severe withdrawal syndrome in the infant may result in irritability, shrill crying, diarrhea, or even seizures. When withdrawal symptoms are judged to be relatively mild, treatment is aimed at control of these symptoms with such drugs as diazepam; with more severe withdrawal, small doses of opioids are often necessary.

Use in Patients with Impaired Pulmonary Function

In patients with borderline respiratory reserve, the depressant properties of the opioid analgesics may lead to acute respiratory failure.

Use in Patients with Impaired Hepatic or Renal Function

Most opioids are metabolized primarily in the liver and the metabolites are excreted in the urine. The half-lives of morphine and its congeners are, therefore, prolonged in patients with impaired hepatic or renal function. The parent drug and its metabolites may then accumulate; dosage should therefore be reduced in such patients.

Use in Patients with Endocrine Disease

Patients with adrenal insufficiency (Addison's disease) and those with hypothyroidism (myxedema) may have prolonged and exaggerated responses to opioids.

■ AGONIST-ANTAGONISTS DRUGS

Analgesic Activity

The analgesic activity of mixed agonist-antagonists varies with the individual drug but is less than that of strong agonists like morphine. **Buprenorphine** and

Table 20–4.	Opioid drug interactions
Drug Group	**Interaction with Opioids**
Sedative-hypnotics	Increased central nervous system depression, particularly respiratory depression
Antipsychotic tranquilizers	Increased sedation. Variable effects on respiratory depression. Accentuation of cardiovascular effects (antimuscarinic and α-blocking actions)
MAO inhibitors	Relative contraindication to all opioid analgesics because of the high incidence of hyperpyrexic coma; hypertension has also been reported

MAO = monoamine oxidase.

nalbuphine afford greater analgesia than pentazocine, which is similar to codeine in analgesic efficacy.

Receptors

Nalbuphine and pentazocine are κ agonists, with weak μ-receptor antagonist activity. Buprenorphine is a μ-receptor agonist with weak antagonist effects at κ and δ receptors. These characteristics can lead to unpredictable results if such mixed agonist-antagonist drugs are used together with pure agonists such as morphine. Buprenorphine has a long duration of effect because it binds strongly to μ receptors. Although the prolonged activity of buprenorphine may be clinically useful (e.g., to suppress withdrawal signs in dependency states), this property renders its effects resistant to naloxone reversal.

Effects

The mixed agonist-antagonist drugs usually cause sedation at analgesic doses. Dizziness, sweating, and nausea may also occur, and anxiety, hallucinations, and nightmares are possible adverse effects. Respiratory depression may be less intense than with pure agonists but is not predictably reversed by naloxone. Tolerance develops with chronic use but is less than the tolerance that develops to the pure agonists, and there is minimal cross-tolerance. Physical dependence occurs, but the abuse liability of mixed agonist-antagonist drugs is less than that of the full agonists.

▨ OPIOID ANTAGONISTS

Naloxone, nalmefene, and **naltrexone** are pure opioid receptor antagonists that have few other effects at doses that produce marked antagonism of agonist effects. These drugs have greater affinity for μ receptors than for other opioid receptors. The major clinical use of the opioid antagonists is in the management of acute opioid overdose. Naloxone and nalmefene are given intravenously. Because naloxone has a short duration of action (1 to 2 hours), multiple doses may be required in opioid analgesic overdose. Nalmefene has a duration of action of 8 to 12 hours. Naltrexone has a long elimination half-life, blocking the actions of

strong agonists (e.g., heroin) for at least 24 hours after oral use. Naltrexone also decreases the craving for ethanol and is approved for adjunctive use in alcohol dependency programs.

Miscellaneous

Tramadol is a moderately efficacious central-acting nonopioid, non-NSAID analgesic. Its mechanism of action appears to involve enhanced serotonergic neurotransmission and its analgesic effectiveness can be blocked by coadministration of the serotonin 5-HT_3 receptor antagonist ondansetron. Tramadol also inhibits norepinephrine transporter function and is a weak μ-receptor agonist.

The toxicity of tramadol includes seizures; the drug is relatively contraindicated in patients with a history of epilepsy and for use with other drugs that lower the seizure threshold. Other side effects include nausea and dizziness, but these symptoms typically decrease after several days of therapy. No clinically relevant effects on respiration or the cardiovascular system have been reported thus far.

▨ REHABILITATION FOCUS

Use of opioid analgesics represents one of the most effective methods for treating moderate to severe pain. Physical therapists may encounter patients using these medications when recovering from trauma or following surgery (acute pain relief) and in patients with terminal cancer or chronic pain (chronic pain relief). The common adverse effects of sedation and nausea may be a hindrance to some therapeutic interventions but the pain relief afforded by the drugs may allow for the progression of the rehabilitation program and ultimate achievement of the desired outcomes. The physical therapist should recognize that these drugs can have a profound effect on a patient's respiratory response to exercise due to depression of the medullary chemoreceptors and the potential blunting of the respiratory response to exercise, which can result in hypoxia and hypercapnia.

Another adverse effect of opioid medications is the tendency for these drugs to cause constipation. This could be especially problematic in patients with conditions that decrease gastrointestinal motility (e.g., spinal cord injury, abdominal surgery). For this reason, laxatives or gastrointestinal stimulants are often administered to minimize the risk of fecal impaction caused by the opioid. Physical therapists should be aware of this side effect and educate patients and their caregivers of the potential seriousness of this problem.

Unfortunately, with long-term use of opioids, patients can become physically dependent on their use. When patients are gradually weaned off opioid medications, they may experience withdrawal symptoms including diffuse muscle aches. Although muscle aches caused by opioid withdrawal are not due to actual somatic disorder, many physical agents such as heat and electrotherapy, and manual techniques such as massage and relaxation may provide some relief from these somatic symptoms.

■ CLINICAL RELEVANCE FOR REHABILITATION

Adverse Drug Reactions
- Constipation
- Respiratory depression
- Nausea and vomiting
- Dizziness or mental clouding
- Hypotension
- Development of tolerance and physical dependence

Effects Interfering with Rehabilitation
- Sedation, mental slowing, and drowsiness can affect patient interventions.
- Respiratory depression can lead to hypoxia and hypercapnia.
- Respiratory response to exercise may be blunted.
- Opioid withdrawal may lead to diffuse muscle aches and pains.

Possible Therapy Solutions
- Patients are often not prescribed opioids for long periods of time due to their tolerance and dependence effects. However, therapy interventions should occur at peak levels for maximum analgesic benefit.
- If problems occur, discuss possible alternatives with prescribing practitioner to maximize potential during therapy sessions.
- Be very aware of the abuse potential with this class of medication.

Potentiation of Functional Outcomes Secondary to Drug Therapy
- Opioid analgesics decrease pain levels and allow increased patient participation in rehabilitation.

PROBLEM-ORIENTED PATIENT STUDY

Brief History: The patient is a 58-year-old female with a long history of osteoarthritis of bilateral knees. The patient has been treated conservatively over the past several years for her pain with medication (oral cyclooxygenase-2 [COX-2] inhibitors and intra-articular betamethazone injections) and physical therapy. She stated that she has had progressively more pain and dysfunction over the past year. She and her primary physician determined that it was time for bilateral total knee replacements. The patient subsequently underwent bilateral total knee arthroplasty without complication.

Current Medical Status and Drug Therapy: At 4 days postoperative in the acute care hospital, the patient was using a PCA pump with morphine sulfate for pain control. She also was receiving oral meperidine for breakthrough pain.

Rehabilitation Setting: The patient was referred to physical therapy for active and passive range of motion (ROM) to both lower extremities and

(continued)

PROBLEM-ORIENTED PATIENT STUDY (*Continued*)

upright mobility training prior to admittance to an acute rehabilitation facility.

Problem/Clinical Options: The patient was eager to get started and make progress; however, she stated that she has a low tolerance for pain. Since she has some discomfort associated with active and passive ROM activities, she has asked for her oral drug prior to her therapy visits. On several occasions, the patient has done well with tolerating active and passive ROM exercises with this regimen. However, upon standing and attempting gait training, she experienced rapid onset of fatigue and became very short of breath. On one occasion, the condition was so severe that she experienced syncope. The physical therapist recognized that these signs and symptoms could be due to the amount of opioid analgesic she was taking prior to therapy

sessions. Although the medication had helped her improve active and passive ROM, it was causing adverse effects in her mobility training. The physical therapist spoke with the patient, her nurse, and her primary physician, and it was determined that for optimal outcome the patient would receive gait/mobility training during the first part of her therapy time. She would then be given an oral dose of meperidine prior to active and passive ROM exercises. Although the onset of analgesia might be somewhat delayed, it was felt that this drug regimen would allow her to get the maximal benefit from therapy prior to acute rehabilitation placement. This regimen was carried out for several treatment sessions and proved advantageous as long as the nursing staff was available to provide the oral medication at the time it was needed.

PREPARATIONS AVAILABLE[1]

Analgesic Opioids

Alfentanil (Alfenta)

Buprenorphine (Buprenex, others)
Oral: 2-, 8-mg sublingual tablets
Parenteral: 0.3 mg/mL for injection

Butorphanol (generic, Stadol)
Parenteral: 1, 2 mg/mL for injection
Nasal (generic, Stadol NS): 10 mg/mL nasal spray

Codeine (sulfate or phosphate) (generic)
Oral: 15-, 30-, 60-mg tablets, 15 mg/5 mL solution
Parenteral: 30, 60 mg/mL for injection

Dezocine (Dalgan)
Parenteral: 5, 10, 15 mg/mL for injection

Fentanyl
Parenteral (generic, Sublimaze): 50 mg/mL for injection
Fentanyl Transdermal System (Duragesic): 25-, 50-, 75-, 100-mcg/h delivery
Fentanyl Oralet: 100-, 200-, 300-, 400-mcg oral lozenge
Fentanyl Actiq: 200-, 400-, 600-, 800-, 1200-, 1600-mcg lozenge on a stick

Hydromorphone (generic, Dilaudid)
Oral: 1-, 2-, 3-, 4-, 8-mg tablets; 5 mg/mL liquid
Parenteral: 1, 2, 4, 10 mg/mL for injection
Rectal: 3-mg suppositories

Levomethadyl acetate (Orlaam)
Oral: 10 mg/mL solution. **Note:** Approved only for the treatment of narcotic addiction.

Levorphanol (generic, Levo-Dromoran)
Oral: 2-mg tablets
Parenteral: 2 mg/mL for injection

Meperidine (generic, Demerol)
Oral: 50-, 100-mg tablets; 50 mg/5 mL syrup
Parenteral: 25-, 50-, 75-, 100-mg per dose for injection

Methadone (generic, Dolophine)
Oral: 5-, 10-mg tablets; 40-mg dispersible tablets; 1, 2, 10 mg/mL solutions
Parenteral: 10 mg/mL for injection

Morphine sulfate (generic, others)
Oral: 10-, 15-, 30-mg tablets; 15-, 30-mg capsules; 10, 20, 100 mg/5 mL solution
Oral sustained-release tablets (MS-Contin, others): 15-, 30-, 60-, 100-, 200-mg tablets); Oral sustained-release capsules (Kadian): 20-, 50-, 100-mg capsules
Parenteral: 0.5, 1, 2, 4, 5, 8, 10, 15, 25, 50 mg/mL for injection
Rectal: 5-, 10-, 20-, 30-mg suppositories

Nalbuphine (generic, Nubain)
Parenteral: 10, 20 mg/mL for injection

Oxycodone (generic)
Oral: 5-mg tablets, capsules; 1, 20 mg/mL solutions
Oral sustained-release (OxyContin): 10-, 20-, 40-, 80-, 100-mg tablets

Oxymorphone (Numorphan)
Parenteral: 1, 1.5 mg/mL for injection
Rectal: 5-mg suppositories

Pentazocine (Talwin)
Oral: See analgesic combinations.
Parenteral: 30 mg/mL for injection

Propoxyphene (generic, Darvon Pulvules, others)
Oral: 65-mg capsules, 100-mg tablets. **Note:** This product is not recommended.

Remifentanil (Ultiva)
Parenteral: 3-, 5-, 10-mg powder for reconstitution for injection

Sufentanil (generic, Sufenta)
Parenteral: 50 mcg/mL for injection

Tramadol (Ultram)
Oral: 50-mg tablets

Analgesic Combinations[2]

Codeine/acetaminophen (generic, Tylenol w/Codeine, others)
Oral: 15-, 30-, 60-mg codeine plus 300- or 325-mg acetaminophen tablets or capsules; 12-mg codeine plus 120-mg acetaminophen tablets

Codeine/aspirin (generic, Empirin Compound, others)
Oral: 30-, 60-mg codeine plus 325-mg aspirin tablets

Hydrocodone/acetaminophen (generic, Norco, Vicodin, Lortab, others)
Oral: 2.5-, 5-, 7.5-, 10-mg hydrocodone plus 500- or 650-mg acetaminophen tablets

Hydrocodone/ibuprofen (Vicoprofen)
Oral: 7.5-mg hydrocodone plus 200-mg ibuprofen

Oxycodone/acetaminophen (generic, Percocet, Tylox, others). Note: High-dose acetaminophen has potential for hepatic toxicity with repeated use.
Oral: 5-mg oxycodone plus 325- or 500-mg acetaminophen tablets

Oxycodone/aspirin (generic, Percodan)
Oral: 4.9-mg oxycodone plus 325-mg aspirin

Propoxyphene/aspirin or acetaminophen (Darvon Compound-65, others). Note: This product is not recommended.
Oral: 65-mg propoxyphene plus 389-mg aspirin plus 32.4-mg caffeine; 50-, 65-, 100-mg propoxyphene plus 325- or 650-mg acetaminophen.

Opioid Antagonists

Nalmefene (Revex)
Parenteral: 0.1, 1 mg/mL for injection

Naloxone (Narcan, various)
Parenteral: 0.4, 1 mg/mL; 0.02 mg/mL (for neonatal use) for injection

Naltrexone (ReVia, Depade)
Oral: 50-mg tablets

Antitussives

Codeine (generic, others)
Oral: 15-, 30-, 60-mg tablets; constituent of many proprietary syrups[2]

Dextromethorphan (generic, Benylin DM, Delsym, others)
Oral: 2.5-, 5-, 7.5-, 15-mg lozenges; 3.5, 5, 7.5, 10, 15 mg/5 mL syrup; 30-mg sustained-action liquid; constituent of many proprietary syrups[1]

[1]Antidiarrheal opioid preparations are listed in Chapter 36.

[2]Dozens of combination products are available; only a few of the most commonly prescribed ones are listed here. Codeine combination products available in several strengths are usually denoted No. 2 (15-mg codeine), No. 3 (30-mg codeine), and No. 4 (60-mg codeine). Prescribers should be aware of the possible danger of renal damage with acetaminophen, aspirin, and NSAIDs contained in these analgesic combinations.

REFERENCES

Arcioni R, et al: Ondansetron inhibits the analgesic effects of tramadol: A possible 5-HT(3) spinal receptor involvement in acute pain in humans. *Anesth Analg* 2002;94:1553.

Basbaum AI, Jessel T: The perception of pain. In *Principles of Neural Science*, 4th ed. Kandel ER, et al, eds. New York: McGraw-Hill, 2000.

Benedetti C, Premuda L: The history of opium and its derivatives. In *Advances in Pain Research and Therapy*, Vol 14. Benedetti C, et al, eds. New York: Raven Press, 1990.

Bolan EA, et al: Synergy between mu opioid ligands: Evidence for functional interactions among mu opioid receptor subtypes. *J Pharmacol Exp Ther* 2002; 303:557.

Davis MP, Walsh D: Methadone for relief of cancer pain: A review of pharmacokinetics, pharmacodynamics, drug interactions and protocols of administration. *Support Care Cancer* 2001;9:73.

Laughlin TM, et al: Mechanisms of induction of persistent nociception by dynorphin. *J Pharmacol Exp Ther* 2001;299:6.

Mercadante S: Opioid rotation for cancer pain: Rationale and clinical aspects. *Cancer* 1999;86:1856.

Mitchell JM, et al: A locus and mechanism of action for associative morphine tolerance. *Nat Neurosci* 2000;3:47.

Parris WC, et al: The use of controlled-release oxycodone for the treatment of chronic cancer pain: A randomized, double-blind study. *J Pain Symptom Manage* 1998;16:205.

Shir Y, et al: Methadone is safe for treating hospitalized patients with severe pain. *Can J Anaesth* 2001;48:1109.

Sindrup SH, Jensen TS: Efficacy of pharmacological treatments of neuropathic pain: An update and effect related to mechanism of drug action. *Pain* 1999;83:389.

Tzschentke TM: Behavioral pharmacology of buprenorphine, with a focus on preclinical models of reward and addiction. *Psychopharmacology* (Berl) 2002;161:1.

Vanderah TW, et al: Mechanisms of opioid-induced pain and antinociceptive tolerance: Descending facilitation and spinal dynorphin. *Pain* 2001;92:5.

Von Dossow V, et al: Thoracic epidural anesthesia combined with general anesthesia: The preferred anesthetic technique for thoracic surgery. *Anesth Analg* 2001;92:848.

Wang Z, et al: Pronociceptive actions of dynorphin maintain chronic neuropathic pain. *J Neurosci* 2001;21:1779.

Williams JT, et al: Cellular and synaptic adaptations mediating opioid dependence. *Physiol Rev* 2001;81:299.

Rehabilitation References

Allan L, et al: Transdermal fentanyl versus sustained release oral morphine in strong-opioid naïve patients with chronic low back pain. *Spine* 2005;30:2484.

Bourne MH, et al: Tramadol/acetaminophen tablets in the treatment of postsurgical orthopedic pain. *Am J Orthop* 2005;34:592.

Vogt MT, et al: Analgesic usage for low back pain: Impact on health care costs and service use. *Spine* 2005;30:1075.

Zorowitz RD, et al: Usage of pain medications during stroke rehabilitation: the Post-Stroke Rehabilitation Outcomes Project (PSROP). *Top Stroke Rehab* 2005;12:37.

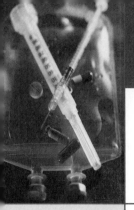

21

DRUGS OF ABUSE

As generally understood, drug abuse includes any illicit use of a drug for nonmedical purposes, usually for altering consciousness, but also for body building. The term also denotes the deliberate use of chemicals that are generally not considered drugs by the lay public, but may be harmful to the user. Often, the motivation for drug abuse appears to be the anticipated feeling of pleasure derived from the central nervous system (CNS) effects of the drug. If physiologic dependence is present, preventing a **withdrawal** or **abstinence syndrome** reinforces continued drug abuse.

The term drug abuse connotes social disapproval and may have different meanings to different people. One may also distinguish drug abuse from drug misuse. To misuse a drug might be to take it for the wrong indication, in the wrong dosage, or for too long a period. In the context of drug abuse, the drug itself is of less importance than the pattern of use. For example, taking 50 mg of diazepam to heighten the effect of a daily dose of methadone is an abuse of diazepam. On the other hand, taking the same excessive daily dose of the drug, but only for its anxiolytic effect, is misusing diazepam.

In this chapter, we discuss the terminology relevant to drugs of abuse, the socioeconomic and cultural considerations of such drug use, and the major classes of these drugs along with some examples from each class. The major classes of drugs that are abused are presented in Figure 21–1, and prototypic agents of each class are presented in Table 21–1.

DEFINITIONS

Dependence refers to the biologic phenomena often associated with drug abuse. **Psychologic dependence** is manifested by compulsive drug-seeking behavior in which the individual uses the drug repetitively for personal satisfaction, often despite known risks to health. Deprivation of the agent for a short period of time typically results in a strong desire or craving for it. Cigarette smoking is one example. **Physiologic dependence** is present when withdrawal of the drug produces symptoms and signs that are frequently the opposite of those sought by the user. A traditional explanation for these manifestations is that the body adjusts to a new homeostasis during the period of drug use and reacts in opposite fashion when this equilibrium is disturbed. Alcohol withdrawal syndrome is perhaps the best-known example, but milder degrees of withdrawal may be observed in people who drink large amounts of coffee. Psychologic dependence almost always precedes physiologic dependence, but does not inevitably lead to physiologic dependence. **Addiction** is usually taken to mean a state of physiologic and psychologic dependence, but the word is too imprecise for scientific usage.

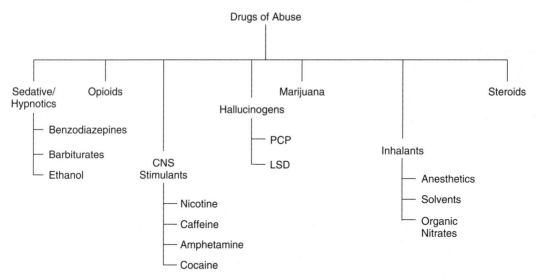

Figure 21–1. Major classes of drugs of abuse. LSD = lysergic acid diethylamide; PCP = phencyclidine.

Tolerance signifies a decreased response to the effects of the drug, necessitating progressively larger doses to achieve the same effect. Tolerance is closely associated with the phenomenon of physiologic dependence. Tolerance is largely due to compensatory responses that mitigate the drug's pharmacodynamic action. *Metabolic tolerance* due to increased disposition of the drug after chronic use is occasionally reported.

Functional tolerance, which may be more common, is due to compensatory changes in receptors, effector enzymes, or membrane actions of the drug.

A number of experimental techniques have been devised to predict the ability of a drug to produce dependence and to assess its likelihood for abuse. Most of these techniques employ self-administration of the drug by animals. The rates of reinforcement can be

Table 21–1. Major classes of drugs of abuse with prototypic substances and additional abused substances

Class	Prototype	Other Significant Agents
Sedative-hypnotics	Ethanol, phenobarbital, chlordiazepoxide	Diazepam, methaqualone, meprobamate, secobarbital, GHB
Opioid analgesics	Heroin	Fentanyl, meperidine, and other strong opioid analgesics
Stimulants	Amphetamine, caffeine, cocaine, nicotine	Methamphetamine, phenmetrazine, DOM, MDA, MDMA
Hallucinogens	LSD, phencyclidine	Mescaline, ketamine, scopolamine
Marijuana	"Grass" or "pot"	Hashish, dronabinol
Inhalants	Nitrous oxide, toluene, amyl nitrite	Chloroform, benzene, ether, isobutyl nitrite
Steroids	Testosterone	Nandrolone, fluoxymesterone, testolactone

DOM = 2,5-dimethoxy-4-methylamphetamine; GHB = gamma-hydroxybutyrate; LSD = lysergic acid diethylamide; MDA = methylenedioxyamphetamine; MDMA = methylenedioxymethamphetamine.

altered to make the animal work harder for each dose of drug, providing a semiquantitative measure as well. Comparisons are made against a standard drug in the class; for example, morphine among the opioids. Withdrawal of dependent animals from drugs assesses the nature of the withdrawal syndrome and can be used to test drugs that might cross-substitute for the standard drug. Most agents with significant potential for psychologic or physiologic dependence can be readily detected by these techniques. However, the actual abuse liability is difficult to predict since many variables enter into the decision to abuse drugs.

■ CULTURAL CONSIDERATIONS

Current attitudes in the United States toward drugs that are claimed to have high abuse potential are reflected in the schedule of controlled drugs (Table 21–2). This schedule is quite similar to those published by international control bodies. Such schedules affect law-abiding manufacturers and ethical prescribers of the drugs, and have little deterrent effect on illicit manufacturers or suppliers. Such schedules have been circumvented by the synthesis of "designer drugs" that make small modifications of the chemical structures of drugs with little or no change in their pharmacodynamic actions. Thus, schedules must constantly be revised to include these attempts to produce compounds not currently listed.

The use of mind-altering drugs is based on a complicated interplay between three factors: the user, the setting in which the drug is taken, and the drug. Thus, the personality of the user and the setting may have a strong influence on what the user experiences. Regardless of these circumstances, it is usually possible to identify a group of effects for a given drug that will be experienced by almost anyone under almost any circumstances if the dosage is adequate.

■ NEUROBIOLOGY OF ABUSED DRUGS

During the last 20 years, substantial progress has been made in elucidating the neurobiology of abused drugs and their effects. Most or all abused drugs act through neurotransmitter systems that involve norepinephrine (NE), dopamine (DA), gamma-aminobutyric acid (GABA), serotonin (5-HT), glutamate, endorphins, or enkephalins. Regardless of the drug and the initial neurotransmitter, a final common pathway in addiction appears to be the dopaminergic mesolimbic system of the brain, with the ventral tegmental area and the nucleus accumbens playing especially important roles. The locus ceruleus appears to play an important role during withdrawal. The latter finding has important

Table 21–2.	Schedules of controlled drugs		
Schedule	**Clinical Value**	**Addiction Potential**	**Examples**
I	No medical use	High	Flunitrazepam, heroin, LSD, marijuana,[1] mescaline, methaqualone, PCP, DOM, MDMA
II	Medical use	High	Strong opioid agonists, cocaine, short half-life barbiturates, amphetamines, cannabinols, methylphenidate
III	Medical use	Moderate	Anabolic steroids, codeine, and moderate opioid agonists, dronabinol, thiopental
IV	Medical use	Low	Benzodiazepines, chloral hydrate, meprobamate, weak opioid agonists, propoxyphene, zaleplon, zolpidem

DOM = 2,5-dimethoxy-4-methylamphetamine; LSD = lysergic acid diethylamide; MDMA = methylenedioxymethamphetamine; PCP = phencyclidine.
[1]Marijuana does not have high addiction potential but is included in this category for historical and political reasons.

treatment implications, such as the use of clonidine (a sympatholytic) for opioid withdrawal.

In the case of stimulants such as amphetamines and cocaine, the connection with dopamine-mediated effects is easily observed, since these drugs directly influence dopaminergic transmission. Other drug classes, such as the benzodiazepines, have specific receptors on chloride channels associated with GABA, whereas other abused drugs, such as phencyclidine, bind to sites on excitatory amino acid receptor–channel complexes. Endogenous ligands have been discovered for the receptors bound by drugs such as opioids and cannabinoids. Examples include β-endorphin (for the μ opioid receptor) and anandamide (for the cannabinoid receptors). These receptors are critical for the acute effects of these abused drugs.

Many neurobiologic findings regarding mechanisms of drug dependence in animal models have been confirmed in human studies. These human studies include administration of drugs while measuring neuroendocrine and behavioral outcomes, assessments of endogenous ligands in cerebrospinal fluid from drug-dependent patients, and neuroimaging studies, particularly neuroreceptor imaging. Available radioligands have permitted examination of dopamine receptors and transporters, opioid receptors, and functional brain activity based on blood flow or glucose utilization. These receptor-neuroimaging studies have demonstrated that chronic abuse of drugs that produces tolerance, dependence, and sensitization may have associated effects on receptor and transporter numbers. These changes are typified by cocaine abuse in which the number of D_2 receptors is decreased, whereas the number of dopamine presynaptic transporters is increased. Blood flow and glucose utilization studies have shown that acute drug use is associated with substantial reductions in cerebral metabolic activity, and that the rate of change is a correlate of the reinforcing effects of abused drugs.

■ MAJOR DRUG GROUPS

Sedative-Hypnotics

Medicinal uses of these drugs, with the exception of ethanol, are discussed in Chapter 13. This group includes barbiturates, benzodiazepines, and ethanol. Benzodiazepines are commonly prescribed drugs for anxiety, and as Schedule IV drugs, are judged to have low abuse liability (Table 21–2). Short-acting barbiturates such as **secobarbital** have high addiction potential and are classified as Schedule II (Table 21–2). In contrast, **flunitrazepam** is considered to have no medicinal value and is classified as Schedule I. Ethanol is not listed in schedules of controlled substances with abuse liability.

Physiologic Effects

Sedative-hypnotics reduce inhibitions, suppress anxiety, and produce relaxation. All of these actions are thought to encourage repetitive use and the development of psychologic dependence. These drugs are CNS depressants, and the depressant effects are enhanced by concomitant use of opioid analgesics, antipsychotic agents, marijuana, and any other drug with sedative properties. Acute overdoses commonly result in death as a result of depression of the medullary respiratory and cardiovascular centers (Table 21–3). Management of overdose includes maintenance of a patent airway plus ventilatory support. **Flumazenil** can be used to reverse the CNS depressant effects of benzodiazepines, but there is no antidote for barbiturates or ethanol. Flunitrazepam (Rohypnol), a potent rapid-onset benzodiazepine with marked amnestic properties, has been used in "date rape." Added to alcoholic beverages, **chloral hydrate** or **gamma-hydroxybutyrate** (**GHB**; sodium oxybate) also renders the victim incapable of resisting rape. However, any sedative-hypnotic, alone or in combination with other CNS depressants, may decrease an individual's ability to resist unwanted sexual advances.

Withdrawal

Physiologic dependence occurs with continued use of sedative-hypnotics. Signs and symptoms of the abstinence syndrome are most pronounced with drugs that have a half-life of less than 24 hours. Examples include **ethanol, secobarbital,** and **methaqualone**. However, physiologic dependence may occur with any sedative-hypnotic, including the longer-acting benzodiazepines. The most important signs of withdrawal derive from excessive CNS stimulation and include anxiety, tremor,

Table 21–3. Manifestations of overdose and withdrawal for selected drugs of abuse

Drug	Overdose Effects	Withdrawal Signs and Symptoms
Barbiturates, benzodiazepines, ethanol[1]	Slurred speech, "drunken" behavior, dilated pupils, weak and rapid pulse, clammy skin, shallow respiration, coma, death	Anxiety, insomnia, delirium, tremors, seizures, death
Heroin; other opioid analgesics	Constricted pupils, clammy skin, nausea, drowsiness, respiratory depression, coma, death	Nausea, chills, sweats, cramps, lacrimation, rhinorrhea, yawning, hyperpnea, tremor
Amphetamines; methylphenidate; cocaine[2]	Agitation, hypertension, tachycardia, delusions, hallucinations, hyperthermia, seizures, death	Apathy, irritability, increased sleep time, disorientation, depression

[1]Ethanol withdrawal includes the excited hallucinatory state of delirium tremens.

[2]Cardiac arrhythmias, myocardial infarction, and stroke occur more frequently in cocaine overdose than with other CNS stimulants.

nausea and vomiting, delirium, and hallucinations (Table 21–3). Seizures are not uncommon, occur later in the withdrawal process, and may be life-threatening.

Treatment of sedative-hypnotic withdrawal involves administration of long-acting sedative-hypnotics, such as **diazepam,** to suppress the acute withdrawal syndrome, followed by gradual dose reduction. **Clonidine** or **propranolol** may also be of value to suppress sympathetic overactivity.

A syndrome of therapeutic withdrawal has occurred upon discontinuance of sedative-hypnotics after long-term therapeutic administration. In addition to the symptoms of classic withdrawal presented in Table 21–3, this syndrome includes weight loss, paresthesias, and headache.

Ethanol

Ethanol is a sedative-hypnotic drug with few medical applications, but its abuse as a recreational drug is responsible for major medical and socioeconomic problems.

Pharmacokinetics

After ingestion, ethanol is rapidly and completely absorbed; the drug is then distributed to most body tissues, and its volume of distribution is equivalent to that of total body water (0.5 to 0.7 L/kg).

Two enzyme systems metabolize ethanol to acetaldehyde (Figure 21–2). The first, alcohol dehydrogenase

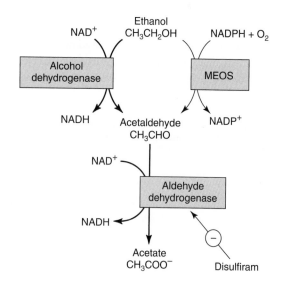

Figure 21–2. Metabolism of ethanol to acetaldehyde by alcohol dehydrogenase and microsomal ethanol-oxidizing system (MEOS). Aldehyde dehydrogenase metabolizes acetaldehyde to acetic acid, and is inhibited by disulfiram.

(ADH), is a cytosolic nicotinamide adenine dinucleotide (NAD)–dependent enzyme, found mainly in the liver and gut, and accounts for the metabolism of low to moderate doses of ethanol. Because of the limited supply of the coenzyme NAD, the reaction has zero-order kinetics that results in a fixed capacity for ethanol metabolism of 7 to 10 g/hour. Gastrointestinal metabolism of ethanol is lower in women than in men, probably accounting for the greater sensitivity of women to equal intake of alcoholic drinks. The second system, the microsomal ethanol-oxidizing system (MEOS), is a liver microsomal mixed-function oxidase system that contributes little to ethanol metabolism at blood ethanol levels below 100 mg/dL. However, the MEOS increases in activity with chronic exposure to ethanol or to inducing agents such as barbiturates. This increase may be partially responsible for the development of tolerance to ethanol. As previously discussed (Chapter 3), one isoform of cytochrome P450 induced by ethanol converts acetaminophen to a hepatotoxic metabolite.

Acetaldehyde formed from the oxidation of ethanol by either system is rapidly metabolized to acetate by aldehyde dehydrogenase, a mitochondrial enzyme found in the liver and many other tissues. Aldehyde dehydrogenase is inhibited by **disulfiram** (Figure 21-2) and other drugs, including metronidazole, oral hypoglycemics, and some cephalosporins. In addition, certain persons of Asian descent with a genetic deficiency of aldehyde dehydrogenase may experience nausea and a flushing reaction from accumulation of acetaldehyde after consumption of small quantities of ethanol.

Acute Physiologic Effects

CNS. The major acute effects of ethanol on the CNS include sedation, loss of inhibition, impaired judgment, slurred speech, and ataxia (Table 21–4). Impairment of driving ability is thought to occur at ethanol blood levels between 60 and 80 mg/dL. Blood levels of 120 to 160 mg/dL are usually associated with gross drunkenness. Levels greater than 300 mg/dL may lead to loss of consciousness, anesthesia, and coma with occasional fatal respiratory and cardiovascular depression. Blood levels greater than 500 mg/dL are usually lethal. Although chronic alcoholics tolerant to the effects of ethanol can function almost normally at much higher blood levels than occasional drinkers, the lethal blood level is little changed. Additive CNS depression occurs with concomitant ingestion of a wide variety of CNS depressants, including sedative-hypnotics, opioid agonists, and many drugs that block muscarinic and H_1 histamine receptors.

The molecular mechanisms underlying the complex CNS effects of ethanol are not fully understood. Specific receptors for ethanol have not been identified. Instead, ethanol appears to modulate the function of a number of signaling proteins. Ethanol facilitates the action of GABA at $GABA_A$ receptors, inhibits the ability of glutamate to activate N-methyl-D-aspartate (NMDA) receptors, and modifies the activities of

Table 21–4.	Blood alcohol concentration (BAC) and clinical effects in nontolerant individuals
BAC (mg/dL)[1]	**Clinical Effect**
50–100	Sedation, subjective "high", increased reaction times
100–200	Impaired motor function, slurred speech, ataxia
200–300	Emesis, stupor
300–400	Coma
>500	Respiratory depression, death

[1]In many parts of the United States, a blood level above 80–100 mg/dL for adults or 10 mg/dL for persons under age 21 is sufficient for conviction of "driving while under the influence."

adenylyl cyclase, phospholipase C, and ion channels. Ethanol "blackouts" may result from interference with NMDA receptors.

OTHER ORGAN SYSTEMS. Ethanol, even at relatively low blood concentrations, significantly depresses cardiac contractility. Vascular smooth muscle is relaxed, which leads to vasodilation, sometimes with marked hypothermia.

Treatment of Alcoholism

CNS DEPRESSION. Intoxication resulting from acute ingestion of ethanol is managed by maintenance of vital signs and prevention of aspiration after vomiting. Correction of electrolyte imbalance may be required in these patients as well. Thiamine is also administered to protect against the Wernicke-Korsakoff syndrome. This syndrome is a relatively uncommon but important entity characterized by paralysis of external eye muscles, ataxia, and a confused state that can progress to coma and death. The syndrome is associated with thiamine deficiency but is rarely seen in the absence of alcoholism. Often, the ocular signs, ataxia, and confusion improve upon prompt administration of thiamine. However, most patients are left with a chronic disabling memory disorder known as Korsakoff's psychosis.

ALCOHOL WITHDRAWAL SYNDROME. In the chronic user of ethanol, discontinuance can lead to a withdrawal syndrome characterized by insomnia, tremor, anxiety, and, in severe cases, life-threatening seizures and delirium tremens (DTs). Peripheral effects include nausea, vomiting, diarrhea, and arrhythmias. The withdrawal syndrome is usually managed by administration of thiamine, correction of electrolyte imbalance, and administration of sedative-hypnotics such as **lorazepam** or **diazepam**. The sedative-hypnotics dosage is then gradually tapered. The intensity of the withdrawal syndrome may also be reduced by clonidine or propranolol.

ABSTINENCE. Alcoholism is a complex sociomedical problem characterized by a high relapse rate. The aldehyde dehydrogenase inhibitor disulfiram is used adjunctively in some treatment programs. If ethanol is consumed by a patient who has taken disulfiram, acetaldehyde accumulation leads to nausea, headache, flushing, and hypotension. Because of its highly aversive effects, it is rarely used. Several CNS neurotransmitter systems appear to be targets for drugs that may reduce the craving for alcohol. The opioid receptor antagonist **naltrexone** has been useful in this context, presumably through its ability to decrease the effects of endogenous opioid peptides in the brain. Other agents under investigation for treatment of alcoholism include **acamprosate**, an NMDA receptor antagonist, **ondansetron**, a 5-HT$_3$ receptor antagonist, and **topiramate**, a presynaptic inhibitor of GABA reuptake.

Opioid Analgesics

The medicinal uses of these drugs are discussed in Chapter 20. The opioid analgesics (Table 21–1) are responsible for many cases of drug abuse. The group includes a wide spectrum of scheduled drugs from **heroin** to **propoxyphene**. Heroin is a Schedule I drug, and propoxyphene is a Schedule IV drug (Table 21–2), reflecting the differences in addiction liability.

Physiologic Effects

The most commonly abused drugs in this group are **heroin**, **morphine**, **oxycodone**, and, among health professionals, **meperidine** and **fentanyl**. The effects of intravenous heroin are described by abusers as a "rush" or orgasmic feeling, followed by euphoria and then sedation. Intravenous administration of opioids is associated with rapid development of tolerance and psychologic and physiologic dependence. Oral administration or smoking of opioids causes milder effects, with a slower onset of tolerance and dependence. Overdose of opioids leads to respiratory depression progressing to coma and death (Table 21–3). Overdose is managed with intravenous **naloxone** or **nalmefene** and ventilatory support.

Withdrawal

Deprivation of opioids in physiologically dependent individuals leads to an abstinence syndrome that includes lacrimation, rhinorrhea, yawning, sweating, weakness, gooseflesh ("cold turkey"), nausea and vomiting, tremor, muscle jerks ("kicking the habit"), and hyperpnea (Table 21–3). Although extremely unpleasant, withdrawal from opioids is rarely fatal, unlike withdrawal from sedative-hypnotics. Treatment involves replacement of the illicit drug with a pharmacologically equivalent agent, such as methadone, followed by slow dose reduction of the medication. Clonidine and buprenorphine, a longer-acting opioid, have also been used to suppress withdrawal symptoms. The administration of naloxone to someone who is using strong opioids may cause more rapid and more intense symptoms of withdrawal. Neonates born to mothers physiologically dependent on opioids require special management of withdrawal symptoms.

Stimulants

Caffeine and nicotine are commonly used licit stimulant drugs, whereas greater euphoria-producing stimulants, such as cocaine and amphetamines, are commonly used illicit drugs. Nicotine is also discussed briefly in Chapter 5. Despite their similar behavioral effects, caffeine, nicotine, cocaine, and amphetamine have very different structures and sites of action in the brain.

Caffeine and Nicotine

Caffeine, a methylxanthine compound, appears to exert its central and at least some of its peripheral actions by blocking adenosine receptors. Some effects at higher concentrations may be due to blockade of phosphodiesterase, the enzyme responsible for metabolizing cyclic adenosine monophosphate (cAMP) and cyclic guanosine monophosphate (cGMP). Because caffeine does not act on dopaminergic brain structures related to reward and addiction, its abuse and dependence potential are quite small. Nicotine is one of the most widely used licit drugs because it is heavily promoted and produces powerful psychologic and physiologic dependence. About 28% of adults in the United States smoke cigarettes because they have become dependent on nicotine. Additionally, the use of smokeless tobacco products, such as snuff and chewing tobacco, has increased in adolescents. In the United States, deaths directly attributable to smoking account for 20% of all deaths and 30% of cancer deaths. About 90% of cases of chronic obstructive pulmonary disease in the United States are due to smoking.

PHYSIOLOGIC EFFECTS. Caffeine in beverages and nicotine in tobacco products are legal in most Western cultures even though they have adverse medical effects. Psychologic dependence on caffeine and nicotine has been recognized for some time. More recently, demonstration of abstinence signs and symptoms has provided evidence for physiologic dependence to both compounds.

WITHDRAWAL. The anxiety and mental discomfort experienced from discontinuing nicotine are major impediments to quitting the habit. Withdrawal from caffeine is accompanied by lethargy, irritability, and headaches. Perhaps surprisingly, withdrawal symptoms appear to occur in fewer than 3% of regular coffee drinkers.

TOXICITY. Acute toxicity from overdosage of caffeine or nicotine includes excessive CNS stimulation with tremor, insomnia, and nervousness; cardiac stimulation and arrhythmias; and, in the case of nicotine, respiratory paralysis. Severe toxicity has been reported in small children who ingest discarded nicotine gum or nicotine patches, which are used as substitutes for tobacco products. The morbidity associated with caffeine overdose, which can include disturbing effects on sleep and heart rhythm, is much less than the morbidity associated with other stimulants.

Amphetamines and Cocaine

Cocaine is a plant product that has been used for at least 1,200 years in the custom of chewing coca leaves by natives of the South American Andes. In contrast, amphetamine was synthesized in the late 1920s and has a large number of analogs. A closely related natural alkaloid, **cathinone**, produces effects indistinguishable from those of the amphetamines, and is found in the plant khat. Amphetamines probably act mainly by increasing release of catecholaminergic neurotransmitters such as dopamine. These drugs cause intracellular dopamine release from synaptic vesicles within the nerve terminal. Increased dopamine within the synaptic terminal results in dopamine transporters releasing dopamine into the synapse. This release contrasts with traditional exocytosis of dopamine

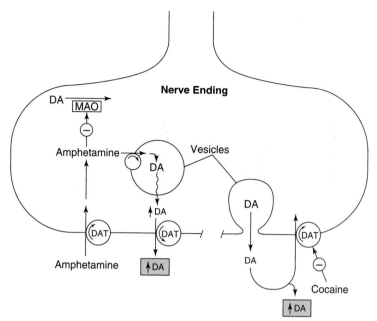

Figure 21–3. A model for the action of cocaine and amphetamine at a dopaminergic synapse in the central nervous system. Cocaine (*right side*) blocks the dopamine reuptake transporter (DAT). Amphetamine (*left side*) has several effects. It enters the nerve ending via transport by the DAT and displaces dopamine (DA) from vesicles by altering their pH. It also inhibits dopamine metabolism by MAO in the nerve ending. The increased intraneuronal dopamine causes reversal of the DAT and dopamine floods into the synapse.

from the presynaptic terminal. Amphetamine and related analogs also inhibit intracellular monoamine oxidase (MAO) metabolism of dopamine (Chapter 4).

Cocaine reduces dopamine and NE reuptake into the neuron by inhibiting the dopamine and NE reuptake transporters. A useful model of the action of these two drugs in the reward centers of the CNS is shown in Figure 21–3. Note that both drugs result in increased dopamine concentration in the synapse.

AMPHETAMINES

Physiologic Effects. Amphetamines cause a feeling of euphoria and self-confidence that contributes to the rapid development of psychologic dependence. Drugs in this class include **dextroamphetamine** and **methamphetamine** ("speed"), a crystal form of which ("ice") can be smoked. Chronic high-dose abuse can lead to a psychotic state, with delusions and paranoia that may

be difficult to differentiate from schizophrenia. Symptoms of overdose include agitation, restlessness, tachycardia, hyperthermia, hyperreflexia, and possibly seizures (Table 21–3). There is no specific antidote, and supportive measures are directed toward control of body temperature and protection against cardiac arrhythmias and seizures. Chronic abuse of amphetamines is also associated with the development of necrotizing arteritis, leading to cerebral hemorrhage and renal failure.

Tolerance and Withdrawal. Tolerance can be marked, and an abstinence syndrome, characterized by increased appetite, sleepiness, exhaustion, and mental depression, can occur on withdrawal. Antidepressant drugs may be indicated.

CONGENERS OF AMPHETAMINES. Several chemical congeners of amphetamines have hallucinogenic properties. These include **2,5-dimethoxy-4-methylam-phetamine** (DOM, STP), **methylene dioxyamphetamine** (MDA), and **methylene dioxymethamphetamine** (MDMA; "ecstasy"). MDMA is purported to facilitate interpersonal communication and act as a sexual enhancer. MDMA and similar substances are sometimes grouped together as "RAVE" drugs. Positron emission tomography studies of the brains of regular users of MDMA show a depletion of neurons in serotonergic tracts. Overdose toxicity includes the clinical features seen with overdose of amphetamine and the potential for hyperthermia.

COCAINE

Physiologic Effects. Cocaine ("super-speed") has marked amphetamine-like effects. Its abuse continues to be widespread in the United States partly because of the availability of a free-base form ("crack") that can be smoked. The euphoria, self-confidence, and mental alertness produced by cocaine are short-lasting and strongly reinforce its continued use.

Overdoses with cocaine commonly result in fatalities from arrhythmias, seizures, or respiratory arrest (Table 21–3). Cardiac toxicity is partly due to blockade of norepinephrine reuptake. Its local anesthetic action also contributes to the production of seizures. In addition, the powerful vasoconstrictor action of cocaine may lead to severe hypertensive episodes, resulting in myocardial infarctions and strokes. No specific antidote is available. Cocaine abuse during pregnancy is associated with increased fetal morbidity and mortality.

Withdrawal. The abstinence syndrome after withdrawal from cocaine is similar to that after amphetamine discontinuance. Severe depression of mood is common and strongly reinforces the compulsion to use the drug. Antidepressant drugs may be indicated. Infants born to mothers who abuse cocaine or amphetamines have possible teratogenic abnormalities, increased morbidity and mortality, and may be cocaine dependent. The signs and symptoms of withdrawal are listed in Table 21–3.

Hallucinogens

These agents modulate several different neurotransmitters. They include modulators of glutamate at NMDA receptors, with **phencyclidine (PCP)** as the prototypic drug. Others, exemplified by **lysergic acid diethylamide (LSD)**, may modulate actions of norepinephrine, dopamine, and serotonin.

Phencyclidine

PCP ("angel dust") is probably the most dangerous of the currently popular hallucinogenic agents. Receptors for PCP have been identified in the brain, and PCP acts as an antagonist at NMDA receptors. Psychotic reactions are common with PCP, and impaired judgment often leads to reckless behavior. This drug should be classified as a *psychotomimetic.* Effects of overdosage with PCP include nystagmus, marked hypertension, hyperthermia, and seizures, which may be fatal. Parenteral benzodiazepines (e.g., diazepam, lorazepam) are used to curb excitation and protect against seizures. Ketamine, a structural congener of PCP, is also abused.

Miscellaneous Hallucinogenic Agents

Several drugs with similar hallucinogenic effects have been classified as having abuse liability, including **LSD**, **mescaline**, and **psilocybin**. These three substances chemically resemble the three major neurotransmitters: NE, DA, and 5-HT. LSD is a partial agonist at 5-HT_{1A} and 5-HT_{1C} receptor subtypes. Agonist interactions may be relevant to the hallucinogenic effects, while 5-HT_2 receptor antagonist interactions may be more important in the peripheral effects.

Hallucinogenic effects may also occur with scopolamine and other antimuscarinic agents. The perceptual and psychologic effects of such drugs are usually accompanied by marked somatic effects, particularly nausea, weakness, and paresthesias. Panic reactions ("bad trips") may also occur. There is little evidence that use of these agents leads to the development of physiologic dependence.

Marijuana

Marijuana ("grass" or "pot") is a collective term for the psychoactive constituents present in crude extracts of the plant *Cannabis sativa* (hemp), the active components of which include the compounds **tetrahydrocannabinol (THC)**, **cannabidiol (CBD)**, and **cannabinol (CBN)**. Hashish is a partially purified material that is more potent. A G protein–coupled *cannabinoid receptor* (CB1) has been identified and is most numerous in the outflow nuclei of the basal ganglia, the substantia nigra, pars reticulata, globus pallidus, hippocampus, and brainstem.

Physiologic Effects

Central effects of marijuana result in feelings of being "high." Effects include euphoria, disinhibition, uncontrollable laughter, changes in perception, and achievement of a dream-like state. Mental concentration may be difficult. Vasodilation occurs, and the pulse rate is characteristically increased. Habitual users show reddened conjunctivae. A mild withdrawal state has been noted only in long-term heavy users of marijuana. The dangers of marijuana use are its impairment of judgment and reflexes, effects that are potentiated by concomitant use of sedative-hypnotics, including ethanol. Therapeutic effects of marijuana include its ability to decrease intraocular pressure and its antiemetic actions. **Dronabinol** is a controlled-substance formulation (Schedule III) of THC that is used to combat nausea in cancer chemotherapy.

Inhalants

Certain gases or volatile liquids are abused because they provide a feeling of euphoria or disinhibition. These substances may be divided into three major groups: anesthetics, industrial solvents, and organic nitrites.

Anesthetics

This group includes **nitrous oxide, chloroform**, and **diethyl ether**. The general anesthetics are discussed in Chapter 15. These agents are hazardous because they affect judgment and induce loss of consciousness. Inhalation of nitrous oxide as the pure gas with no oxygen has caused asphyxia and death. Ether and chloroform sensitize the heart to arrhythmias. Also, ether is highly flammable.

Industrial Solvents

Solvents and a wide range of volatile compounds are present in commercial products such as gasoline, paint thinners, aerosol propellants, glues, rubber cement, and shoe polish. Because of their ready availability, these substances are most frequently abused by children in early adolescence. Active ingredients that have been identified include benzene, hexane, methylethylketone, toluene, and trichloroethylene. Many of these are toxic to the liver, kidneys, lungs, bone marrow, and peripheral nerves and cause brain damage in animals.

Organic Nitrites

Amyl nitrite, isobutyl nitrite, and other organic nitrites are referred to as "poppers" and are mainly used as sexual intercourse "enhancers." Inhalation of the nitrites causes dizziness, tachycardia, hypotension, and flushing. With the exception of methemoglobinemia, few serious adverse effects have been reported.

Steroids

In many countries, including the United States, anabolic steroids are controlled substances (Schedule III) based on their potential for abuse (Table 21–2). Effects sought by abusers are increases in muscle mass and strength rather than euphoria. However, excessive use can have adverse behavioral, cardiovascular, endocrine, and musculoskeletal effects. Premature closure of the epiphyses, masculinization in females, and acne, which is sometimes severe, are predictable androgenic adverse effects. Hepatic dysfunction has been reported, and the abuse of anabolic steroids may pose an increased risk of myocardial infarction. Behavioral manifestations include increases in libido and aggression ("roid rage"). A withdrawal syndrome has been described as fatigue and depression of mood.

■ REHABILITATION FOCUS

The comorbidities associated with drugs of abuse are some of the most difficult problems facing health-care professionals. These compounds are self-administered by patients, often without divulging their use to health-care professionals. The problem is further complicated by the fact that the clinical manifestations and complications vary depending on which drugs are being abused. The most significant adverse effects that may affect rehabilitation treatments are those associated with the cardiovascular and the central nervous systems.

Among licit agents, both caffeine and nicotine have some sympathomimetic effects, and may increase the incidence of adverse events during therapy due to increasing blood pressure and heart rate and sensitization of the heart to arrhythmias. Additionally, smoking tobacco results in an increase in carbon monoxide (CO) and carboxyhemoglobin in the blood. Carboxyhemoglobin is the result of CO binding to hemoglobin. Carbon monoxide binds to hemoglobin with an affinity 200 times greater than that of oxygen, and the bound CO prevents the binding of oxygen to hemoglobin. Heavy smokers may have up to 9% of their hemoglobin as carboxyhemoglobin, and a significant decrease in their exercise capacity resulting from the reduced capacity of their blood to deliver oxygen to the tissues. Regular smoking of marijuana carries a similar reduction in exercise capacity resulting from carboxyhemoglobin.

The use of illicit agents may be complicated by patient denial of their use. Therefore, health-care professionals need to recognize both the manifestations of the abuse of these illicit agents and the manifestations of withdrawal from such use. For CNS stimulants such as amphetamines and cocaine, the potential for adverse cardiovascular, thermoregulatory, or CNS adverse events occurs during the abuse stage, with a higher incidence for cocaine compared to amphetamines. Patients in abstinence treatment programs for CNS stimulants will often have the opposite clinical presentation. Patients will be depressed and fatigued, have delayed psychomotor responses, and possibly complain of myalgia and arthralgia.

Patients abusing CNS depressants and opioids will present with manifestations opposite to those of abusers of CNS stimulants. The depression and fatigue with delayed psychomotor responses will occur during the abuse period, whereas the risk for CNS adverse events, such as seizures may occur during periods of abstinence.

For the hallucinogens, the incidence of morbidity and mortality is higher for PCP and ketamine compared to LSD and the other agents. The clinician should recognize the potential cardiovascular manifestations of PCP (hypertension and tachycardia) that interfere with therapy. Aggressive behavior may be associated with PCP intoxication. The manifestations of marijuana abuse are delayed psychomotor activity

and decreased exercise capacity as a result of elevated carboxyhemoglobin.

Chronic abuse of steroids results in elevated low-density lipoproteins (LDLs) and the associated pathophysiologies associated with elevated LDL and atherosclerosis. Patients taking very high doses of androgenic steroids may manifest hostility and aggressiveness.

■ CLINICAL RELEVANCE FOR REHABILITATION

Adverse Drug Reactions

A major problem with drugs of abuse is the reservations that patients have in telling health-care professionals of their use.

- CNS stimulants (cocaine, amphetamines) and hallucinogens (phencyclidine, ketamine) are cardiovascular stimulants.
- Opioid analgesics, alcohol, and other CNS depressants are respiratory depressants.
- Hallucinogens (LSD, phencyclidine, ketamine, others), opioid analgesics, alcohol, marijuana, and CNS depressants can cause cognitive changes.
- Anabolic steroids can cause behavioral changes.
- Alcohol, CNS depressants, marijuana, and opioid analgesics decrease psychomotor skills.
- Marijuana and organic nitrites can cause orthostatic hypotension.
- During withdrawal from CNS stimulants, the patient may demonstrate decreased cognitive and psychomotor function.
- Withdrawal from alcohol and CNS depressants can result in increased CNS and autonomic (sympathetic) activity.

Effects Interfering with Rehabilitation

- Central nervous system stimulants (cocaine, amphetamines) and hallucinogens (phencyclidine, ketamine) predispose the patient to increased risk of hyperthermia, severe hypertension, seizures, cardiac arrhythmias, angina pectoris, and myocardial infarction.

- Opioid analgesics, alcohol, and other CNS depressants decrease respiratory drive with hypoxia as the clinical manifestation.
- Cognitive and behavioral changes can result from many drugs of abuse.
    - Psychotomimetics (phencyclidine, ketamine) can make the patient combative.
    - Hallucinogens (LSD, marijuana, others) can cause hallucinations.
    - Alcohol, opioid analgesics, and other CNS depressants can decrease inhibitions, resulting in abnormal behavior.
    - Anabolic steroids can increase aggressive behavior ("roid rage").
- Current use of alcohol, other CNS depressants, marijuana, and opioid analgesics increases the risk of falls and injury.
- Orthostatic hypotension may cause patients to faint when transferring from a sitting or supine position to standing, exiting from warm aquatherapy area, or if aerobic exercise is terminated without an appropriate cool-down period.
- Withdrawal from CNS stimulants (cocaine, amphetamines) can result in sleepiness, mental depression, and exhaustion.
- Withdrawal from CNS depressants and alcohol can result in seizures, arrhythmias, increased anxiety, and agitation.

Possible Therapy Solutions

- Recommend that patients discuss use of these drugs with their referring health-care provider or appropriate therapeutic groups (e.g., Alcoholics Anonymous, Narcotics Anonymous).

Potentiation of Functional Outcomes Secondary to Drug Therapy

- None of the drugs of abuse potentiate functional outcomes in rehabilitation.

PROBLEM-ORIENTED PATIENT STUDY

Brief History: The patient is a 54-year-old male who is employed at an automotive assembly plant. Two weeks ago, he injured his low back while on the assembly line. The patient states that he was rotating and bending when he felt a sudden pain in the left side of his low back. The patient was immediately taken to the emergency room where he was evaluated and given a diagnosis of low back musculoskeletal strain. The patient was provided with Tylenol III (codeine and acetaminophen) for pain relief on an as-needed basis. The patient was scheduled for evaluation and enrollment in a work-hardening program prior to return to full-time employment at the plant.

Current Medical Status and Drug Therapy: The patient was evaluated 1 week ago at the rehabilitation clinic. At evaluation, the patient stated that he occasionally has chest pains related to exertion and was diagnosed with exertional angina. He states that the problem does not occur often and he has refused drugs other than an aspirin a day. The patient also stated that he has smoked half a pack of cigarettes a day for 30-plus years.

Rehabilitation Setting: The initial rehabilitation treatments were designed to decrease complaints of low back pain. During the past week, the patient states that he continues to take Tylenol III on a daily basis. The patient arrives today at 8:30 to begin the work-hardening component of rehabilitation. The patient states that he has taken Tylenol III and eaten breakfast consisting of "coffee and a couple of cigarettes" about 60 minutes ago. The work-hardening program is a set of aerobic activities designed to mimic the activities of the patient at the plant in order to improve biomechanical function and reduce the incidence of

(continued)

PROBLEM-ORIENTED PATIENT STUDY (*Continued*)

workplace injuries. The patient begins activities and continues for about 10 minutes. At that time, he complains of shortness of breath and pain along the left arm. His blood pressure and heart rate are subsequently measured at 155/92 mm Hg and 99 bpm and regular. The patient is monitored and the angina and dyspnea dissipate during the next 20 minutes. Blood pressure and heart rate at this time are 131/84 mm Hg and 83 bpm.

Problem/Clinical Options: The morning of the work-hardening program the patient took two cardiovascular stimulants—nicotine and caffeine—at breakfast. Smoking also increased his carboxyhemoglobin and decreased both the oxygen-carrying capacity of the blood and exercise tolerance. The Tylenol III, containing an opioid (codeine),

inhibited central respiratory drive. This combination of licit and prescribed drugs predisposed the patient to exertional cardiac hypoxia, especially since the patient has a documented history of exertional angina. The therapist should contact the referring physician for approval of additional work-hardening participation prior to the next scheduled appointment. The therapist should also recommend that the patient avoid smoking and drinking coffee prior to participating in the work-hardening program because of the potential of these agents to increase the chance of exertional angina during aerobic activity. Administration of Tylenol III prior to the work-hardening program should be discussed with the referring health-care provider.

PREPARATIONS AVAILABLE

Drugs for the Treatment of Acute Alcohol Withdrawal Syndrome

Acamprosate (Campral)
Oral: 333 mg delayed release

Diazepam (generic, Valium, others)
Oral: 2-, 3-, 10-mg tablets; 5 mg/5 mL solutions
Parenteral: 5 mg/mL for injection

Lorazepam (generic, Alzapam, Ativan)
Oral: 0.5-, 1-, 2-mg tablets
Parenteral: 2, 4 mg/mL for injection

Oxazepam (generic, Serax)
Oral: 10-, 15-, 30-mg capsules; 15-mg tablets

Thiamine (generic)
Parenteral: 100 mg/mL for IV injection

Drugs for the Prevention of Alcohol Abuse

Disulfiram (generic, Antabuse)
Oral: 250-, 500-mg tablets

Naltrexone (ReVia)
Oral: 50-mg tablets

REFERENCES

Everitt BJ, et al: The neuropsychological basis of addictive behaviour. *Brain Res Brain Res Rev* 2001; 36:129.

Lüscher C: Drugs of abuse. *Basic & Clinical Pharmacology*, 10th ed. Katzung BK, ed. New York: McGraw-Hill, 2007.

Melichar JK, et al: Addiction and withdrawal–current views. *Curr Opin Pharmacol* 2001;1:84.

Nestler EJ: Molecular basis of long-term plasticity underlying addiction. *Nat Rev Neurosci* 2001; 2:119.

Weiss F, et al: Compulsive drug-seeking behavior and relapse. Neuroadaptation, stress, and conditioning factors. *Ann N Y Acad Sci* 2001;937:1.

Websites: www.health.org and www.drugabuse.gov

Sedatives, Ethanol, and Gamma-Hydroxybutyrate

Brent J, et al: Fomepizole for the treatment of ethylene glycol poisoning. Methylpyrazole for Toxic Alcohols Study Group. *N Engl J Med* 1999;340,832.

CDC Fetal Alcohol Syndrome ebsite:http://www.cdc.gov/ncbddd/fas/

Hoffman PL, et al: Transgenic and gene "knockout" models in alcohol research. *Alcohol Clin Exp Res* 2001; 25(Suppl):606.

Jacobsen D: New treatment for ethylene glycol poisoning. *N Engl J Med* 1999;340:879.

Li TK: Pharmacogenetics of responses to alcohol and genes that influence alcohol drinking. *J Stud Alcohol* 2000;61:5.

Longo LP, Johnson B: Addiction: Part I. Benzodiazepines—side effects, abuse risk, and alternatives. *Am Fam Physician* 2000;61:2121.

National Institute on Drug Abuse (NIDA). Website on Alcohol: http://www.nida.nih.gov/DrugPages/Alcohol.html

Nelson S, Knolls JK: Alcohol, host defence and society. *Nat Rev Immunol* 2002;2:205.

Okun MS, et al: GHB: An important pharmacologic and clinical update. *J Pharm Pharm Sci* 2001;4:167.

Olney JW, et al: The enigma of fetal alcohol neurotoxicity. *Ann Med* 2002;34:109.

Spies CD, et al: Effects of alcohol on the heart. *Curr Opin Crit Care* 2001;7:337.

Opioids

Gonzalez G, et al: Treatment of heroin (Diamorphine) addiction: Current approaches and future prospects. *Drugs* 2002;62:1331.

Stimulants

Balfour D, Le Houezec J: Advances in neuroscience and pharmacology of nicotine. 3rd SRNT Europe Conference. *Nicotine Tob Res* 2002;4:229.

Davidson C, et al: Methamphetamine neurotoxicity: Necrotic and apoptotic mechanisms and relevance to human abuse and treatment. *Brain Res Brain Res Rev* 2001;36:1.

Feinstein AR, et al: Do caffeine-containing analgesics promote dependence? A review and evaluation. *Clin Pharmacol Ther* 2000;68:457.

Kosten TR, et al: The potential of dopamine agonists in drug addiction. *Exp Opin Investig Drugs* 2002;11:491.

Reneman L, et al: Cortical serotonin transporter density and verbal memory in individuals who stopped using 3,4-methylenedioxymethamphetamine (MDMA or "ecstasy"): Preliminary findings. *Arch Gen Psychiatry* 2001;58:901.

Hallucinogens

Halpern JH, Pope HG Jr: Hallucinogens on the Internet: A vast new source of underground drug information. *Am J Psychiatry* 2001;158:481.

Koesters SC, et al: MDMA ("ecstasy") and other "club drugs." The new epidemic. *Pediatr Clin North Am* 2002;49:415.

Website: www.clubdrugs.org

Marijuana

Ashton CH: Pharmacology and effects of cannabis: A brief review. *Br J Psychiatry* 2001;178:101.

Gruber AJ, Pope HG Jr: Marijuana use among adolescents. *Pediatr Clin North Am* 2002;49:389.

Maldonado R, Rodríguez de Fonseca F: Cannabinoid addiction: Behavioral models and neural correlates. *J Neurosci* 2002;22:3326.

Pope HG Jr, et al: Neuropsychological performance in long-term cannabis users. *Arch Gen Psychiatry* 2001;58:909.

Inhalants

Neumark YD, et al: The epidemiology of adolescent inhalant drug involvement. *Arch Pediatr Adolesc Med* 1998;152:781.

Riegel AC, French ED: Abused inhalants and central reward pathways: Electrophysiological and behavioral studies in the rat. *Ann N Y Acad Sci* 2002;965:281.

Rosenberg NL, et al: Neuropsychologic impairment and MRI abnormalities associated with chronic solvent abuse. *J Toxicol Clin Toxicol* 2002;40:21.

Steroids

Bahrke MS, et al: Risk factors associated with anabolic-androgenic steroid use among adolescents. *Sports Med* 2000;29:397.

Pope HG, et al: Effects of supraphysiological doses of testosterone on mood and aggression in normal men. *Arch Gen Psychiatry* 2000;57:133.

Website: www.steroidabuse.org

Rehabilitation

Benzaquen BS, et al: Effects of cocaine on the coronary arteries. *Am Heart J* 2001;142:402.

Boissonnault WG, Koopmeiners MB: Medical history profile: orthopaedic physical therapy outpatients. *J Orthop Sports Phys Ther* 1994;20:2.

Daher Ede F, et al: Rhabdomyolysis and acute renal failure after strenuous exercise and alcohol abuse: case report and literature review. *Sao Paulo Med J* 2005; 123:33.

Das G. Cardiovascular effects of cocaine abuse. *Int J Clin Pharmacol Ther Toxicol* 1993;31:521.

Duarte JA, et al: Strenuous exercise aggravates MDMA-induced skeletal muscle damage in mice. *Toxicology* 2005;206:349.

Foltin RW, et al: Cardiovascular effects of cocaine in humans: Laboratory studies. *Drug Alcohol Depend* 1995; 37:193.

George AJ: Central nervous system stimulants. Baillieres Best *Pract Res Clin Endocrinol Metab* 2000;14:79.

Maki T, et al: Effect of ethanol drinking, hangover, and exercise on adrenergic activity and heart rate variability in patients with a history of alcohol-induced atrial fibrillation. *Am J Cardiol* 1998;82:317.

Marques-Magallanes JA, et al: Impact of habitual cocaine smoking on the physiologic response to maximum exercise. *Chest* 1997;112:1008.

Millis RM: Effects of recreational drugs on physical activity. *J Natl Med Assoc* 1987;79:59.

Nademanee K: Prevalence of myocardial ischemia in cocaine addicts. *NIDA Res Monogr* 1991;108:116.

Parrott AC: MDMA (3,4-methylenedioxymethamphetamine) or ecstasy: The neuropsychobiological implications of taking it at dances and raves. *Neuropsychobiology* 2004;50:329.

Pradhan SN: Phencyclidine (PCP): Some human studies. *Neurosci Biobehav Rev* 1984;8:493.

Seymour HR, et al: Severe ketoacidosis complicated by "ecstasy" ingestion and prolonged exercise. *Diabet Med* 1996;13:908.

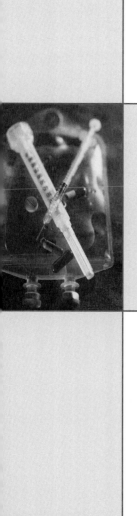

SELECTED TOPICS IN ENDOCRINE FUNCTION

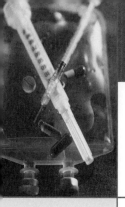

22

GROWTH, THYROID, AND GONADAL PHARMACOLOGY

The endocrine system integrates major organ systems with each other and with the nervous system. The endogenous ligands that the endocrine system uses to perform this integrative task are called **hormones**. Hormones are released from specialized cells, circulate in the blood, and regulate physiologic processes in one or more target organs. In many endocrine systems, several hormones act in series to regulate organ function. The release of one hormone in the series regulates the release of the next hormone. A series of this type provides multiple levels of regulation and integration and also provides the opportunity for *negative feedback*, in which the last hormone in the series can reduce the production of earlier hormones in the series and thereby regulate its own production (Figure 22–1). The endocrine system provides many useful therapeutic targets and many drugs either mimic or block the effects of naturally occurring hormones.

This chapter will focus on drugs that regulate three related endocrine systems. These are (1) the hypothalamic-pituitary endocrine system, which exerts control over many integrative functions and other endocrine tissues and interacts directly with the nervous system; (2) the thyroid gland, an essential regulator of growth, development, and normal function of many organ systems; and (3) the gonadal system, which regulates the development and function of reproductive tissues. Separate chapters will cover the pharmacology of drugs that influence the function of hormones produced by the adrenal gland (Chapter 23), hormones that regulate blood glucose (Chapter 24), and those involved with bone mineralization (Chapter 25).

HYPOTHALAMIC HORMONES

The overall control of metabolism, growth, and reproduction is mediated by a combination of neural and endocrine systems located in the hypothalamus and pituitary gland. The pituitary consists of an anterior lobe (*adenohypophysis*) and a posterior lobe (*neurohypophysis*). The pituitary is connected to the hypothalamus by a stalk of neurosecretory fibers and blood vessels, including a portal venous system that drains the hypothalamus and perfuses the anterior pituitary. The portal venous system carries small regulatory peptide releasing hormones from the hypothalamus to the anterior pituitary. These releasing hormones regulate release of anterior pituitary hormones, which subsequently regulate target tissues throughout the body (Table 22–1). The hormones released from the posterior lobe of the pituitary (oxytocin and vasopressin) are synthesized in the hypothalamus and transported via neurosecretory fibers in the pituitary stalk to the

299

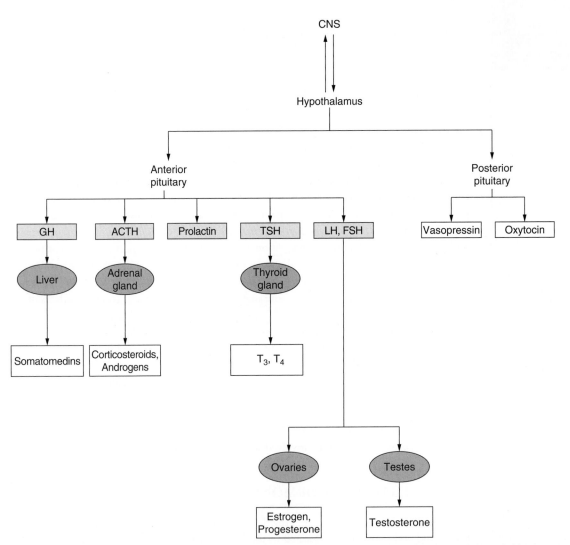

Figure 22–1. Multistep hormonal control of the hypothalamic-pituitary-terminal organ cascade with feedback control. Hormones from the terminal (target) organ regulate release of hormones higher up in the cascade. In most cases, the terminal hormone exerts negative feedback effects, although positive feedback systems also occur. Hormones of the adrenal gland depicted are discussed in Chapter 23. ACTH = adrenocorticotropic hormone; ADH = antidiuretic hormone; CNS = central nervous system; FSH = follicle stimulating hormone ; LH = luteinizing hormone; TSH = thyroid-stimulating hormone.

Table 22–1.	Links among hypothalamic, pituitary, and target gland hormones		
Hypothalamic Hormone	**Pituitary Hormone**	**Target Organ**	**Target Organ Hormone**
Growth hormone–releasing hormone (GHRH)	Growth hormone (GH)	Liver	Somatomedins
Somatostatin[1]	Growth hormone (GH)	Liver	Somatomedins
Thyrotropin-releasing hormone (TRH)	Thyroid-stimulating hormone (TSH)	Thyroid	Thyroxine, triiodothyronine
Corticotropin-releasing hormone (CRH)	Adrenocorticotropic hormone (ACTH)	Adrenal cortex	Glucocorticoids, mineralo-corticoids, androgens
Gonadotropin-releasing hormone (GnRH)	Follicle-stimulating hormone (FSH), luteinizing hormone (LH)	Gonads	Estrogen, progesterone, testosterone
Prolactin-inhibiting hormone (PIH; dopamine)	Prolactin (PRL)	Anterior pituitary	
Oxytocin	None	Smooth muscles, especially uterus	
Vasopressin	None	Renal tubule, smooth muscle	

[1]Inhibits GH and TSH release. Also found in gastrointestinal tissues; inhibits release of gastrin, glucagon, and insulin.

posterior lobe from which they are released into the circulation (Table 22–1).

Hypothalamic and pituitary hormones, and their synthetic analogs, have pharmacologic applications in three areas: (1) replacement therapy for hormone deficiency states, (2) antagonist therapy for diseases resulting from excessive production of, or response to, pituitary hormones, and (3) diagnostic tools for performing stimulation tests.

Growth Hormone–Releasing Hormone

Growth hormone–releasing hormone (GHRH) is a hypothalamic hormone that stimulates the release of growth hormone (GH) from the anterior pituitary. GH (also known as somatotropin) is an important regulator of growth in children and tissue maintenance

in adults. Two short synthetic peptides with activity similar to GHRH are available for clinical use. In normal individuals, these peptides produce a rapid increase in plasma GH concentrations. They are occasionally used as a diagnostic tool in patients with GH deficiency to determine whether the cause of GH deficiency is due to a problem in the hypothalamus, pituitary, or tissues targeted by GH.

Somatostatin

Somatostatin (somatotropin release-inhibiting hormone, SRIF), a 14-amino-acid peptide, is found in the pancreas and other parts of the gastrointestinal system as well as in the central nervous system. This hormone inhibits the release of a number of hormones including GH, glucagon, insulin, and gastrin. Because of its short duration of action, somatostatin itself is of no clinical value. **Octreotide,** a synthetic somatostatin analog with a longer duration of action, is used to reduce symptoms caused by certain tumors that produce excessive concentrations of hormones. Tumors that are partially responsive to octreotide's inhibitory effects include GH-secreting tumors that cause acromegaly, carcinoid tumors, gastrinoma, and glucagonoma. Regular octreotide must be administered subcutaneously two to four times daily. Once a brief course of regular octreotide has been demonstrated to be effective and tolerated, a slow-release intramuscular (IM) formulation is administered every 4 weeks for long-term therapy. Adverse effects associated with octreotide primarily involve the gastrointestinal system and the heart.

Thyrotropin-Releasing Hormone

Thyrotropin-releasing hormone (TRH), or **protirelin,** is a tripeptide that stimulates **thyrotropin** (thyroid-stimulating hormone, TSH) release from the anterior pituitary. TRH also increases prolactin production by the anterior pituitary, but has no effect on the release of GH or adrenocorticotropin (ACTH). TRH has been used in diagnostic testing of thyroid dysfunction.

Corticotropin-Releasing Hormone

Corticotropin-releasing hormone (CRH) is a 41-amino-acid peptide that stimulates secretion of both ACTH and the closely related peptide β-endorphin from the anterior pituitary. CRH is used to diagnose the source of ACTH secretion abnormalities. ACTH-secreting tumors located within the pituitary usually respond to exogenous CRH with an increase in ACTH secretion. In contrast, ACTH secretion by tumors located outside the pituitary rarely responds to exogenous CRH.

Gonadotropin-Releasing Hormone

Gonadotropin-releasing hormone (GnRH), a decapeptide, coordinates reproductive function in males and females by regulating release of two gonadotropins—luteinizing hormone (LH) and follicle-stimulating hormone (FSH)—from the anterior pituitary. When administered in a pulsatile fashion that mimics the endogenous pattern of secretion, recombinant GnRH stimulates gonadotropin release. Pulsatile GnRH

administration is used to determine the basis of delayed puberty in adolescents and, rarely, to treat infertility caused by hypothalamic dysfunction in both sexes.

Leuprolide was the first of several synthetic peptides with GnRH agonist activity. When given in pulsatile doses, these synthetic peptides, like GnRH, stimulate gonadotropin release. In contrast, steady dosing *inhibits* gonadotropin release by causing down-regulation of GnRH receptors in pituitary cells that normally release gonadotropins. Steady dosage of GnRH agonists is used to suppress gonadotropin secretion in patients with prostatic carcinoma or other gonadal steroid-sensitive tumors, endometriosis, or precocious puberty. GnRH agonists are also used to suppress endogenous gonadotropin release in women undergoing controlled ovarian hyperstimulation and in assisted reproduction technology such as in vitro fertilization.

Ganirelix and **cetrorelix** are new GnRH *antagonists* that can be used to prevent premature surges of LH during controlled ovarian hyperstimulation. These GnRH antagonists may also be effective in disorders that are currently treated with GnRH agonists, including endometriosis, uterine fibroids, and prostatic cancer.

Prolactin-Inhibiting Hormone

Dopamine (also called prolactin-inhibiting hormone, PIH) is the primary physiologic regulator of prolactin release. Acting through D2 dopamine receptors, dopamine *inhibits* prolactin release. Dopamine itself is not used to treat hyperprolactinemia. Instead, **bromocriptine** and other orally active ergot derivatives such as **pergolide** are used to reduce prolactin secretion from normal glands as well as from prolactinomas.

■ ANTERIOR PITUITARY HORMONES

Growth Hormone (Somatotropin)

Recombinant forms of human GH are **somatropin** and **somatrem;** the latter is somatotropin with an extra methionine added to the protein. Recombinant growth hormone is used to treat GH deficiency in children and adults. Girls with Turner's syndrome treated with GH frequently achieve increased final adult height. GH treatment also improves growth in children with failure to thrive secondary to chronic renal failure or HIV infection. Growth hormone is also helpful in treating adults with acquired immune deficiency syndrome (AIDS)–associated wasting.

Thyroid-Stimulating Hormone

In thyroid cells, thyroid-stimulating hormone (TSH) increases iodine uptake and production of thyroid hormones. TSH has been used as a diagnostic tool to distinguish primary from secondary hypothyroidism.

Adrenocorticotropin Hormone

Adrenocorticotropin (ACTH) is a large peptide formed from a larger precursor peptide, pro-opiomelanocortin. This precursor is also the source of α-melanocyte-stimulating hormone, β-endorphin, and met-enkephalin. **Cosyntropin,** a synthetic ACTH analog, is used for diagnostic purposes in patients with abnormal corticosteroid production.

Follicle-Stimulating Hormone

Follicle-stimulating hormone (FSH) is a glycoprotein that stimulates gametogenesis and follicle development in women and spermatogenesis in men. Two preparations are available for clinical use. Urofollitropin can be purified from the urine of postmenopausal women and is available in a recombinant form, follitropin-α (rFSH). These products are used in combination with other drugs to treat infertility in both sexes.

Luteinizing Hormone

In women, luteinizing hormone (LH) acts in concert with FSH to regulate gonadal steroid production, follicular development, and ovulation. In men, LH regulates testosterone production. A recombinant form of LH is available for clinical use. Human chorionic gonadotropin (hCG), which is almost identical to LH in structure, is used for treatment of hypogonadism in men and women and as part of controlled ovarian hyperstimulation and assisted reproductive technology programs.

Menotropins

Menotropins are human menopausal gonadotropins that consist of a mixture of FSH and LH purified from the urine of postmenopausal women. The product is used in combination with hCG in the treatment of hypogonadal states and as part of controlled ovarian hyperstimulation and assisted reproductive technology programs.

■ THYROID AND ANTITHYROID DRUGS

The thyroid gland secretes two types of hormones. The first is calcitonin, a peptide that is important in calcium metabolism and bone mineralization; calcitonin is discussed in Chapter 25. The second type of thyroid hormone consists of two iodine-containing hormones, thyroxine (T_4) and triiodothyronine (T_3), which have broad effects on growth, development, and metabolism (Figure 22–2).

Thyroid Hormones

Control, Synthesis, Transport, and Mechanism of Action

Thyroid function is controlled by TSH release from the anterior pituitary and by iodine availability. High levels of thyroid hormones inhibit TSH release, providing an effective negative feedback control mechanism.

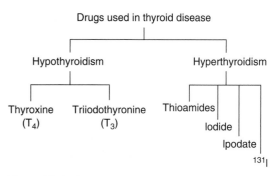

Figure 22–2. Treatment of thyroid disease. Pharmacologic treatment may be divided into supplementation with exogenous hormones when thyroid function is insufficient (hypothyroidism), or inhibition of thyroid function when thyroid hormones are in excess (hyperthyroidism).

Iodine, derived from food or iodine supplements, is necessary for the synthesis of thyroid hormones. Iodine uptake is an active process, and the iodide ion is highly concentrated in the thyroid gland (Figure 22–3). The tyrosine residues of the protein thyroglobulin are iodinated in the gland to form monoiodotyrosine (MIT) or diiodotyrosine (DIT). Whereas T_4 is formed from the combination of 2 molecules of DIT, T_3 is formed from the combination of one molecule each of MIT and DIT. Inadequate iodine intake results in a diffuse enlargement of the thyroid gland called **goiter**. Higher than normal iodide concentrations inhibit iodination of tyrosine, an effect that is useful in the treatment of thyroid disease. In Graves' disease, lymphocytes release a thyroid-stimulating immunoglobulin that causes thyrotoxicosis. Because these lymphocytes are not susceptible to negative feedback, blood concentrations of thyroid hormone may become very high.

The thyroid gland secretes both T_3 and T_4. Although the T_3 released from the thyroid is active, most circulating T_3 is formed by the deiodination of T_4 in the tissues. Both T_3 and T_4 are transported in the blood by thyroxine-binding globulin (TBG), a protein synthesized by the liver. T_3 is about 10 times more potent than T_4. Because T_4 is converted to T_3 in target cells, the liver, and the kidneys, most of the effect of circulating T_3 is probably due to deiodination of T_4 in the tissues.

Thyroid hormone binds to intracellular receptors that control expression of genes responsible for many metabolic processes. Proteins synthesized under T_3 control differ depending on the tissue involved. These

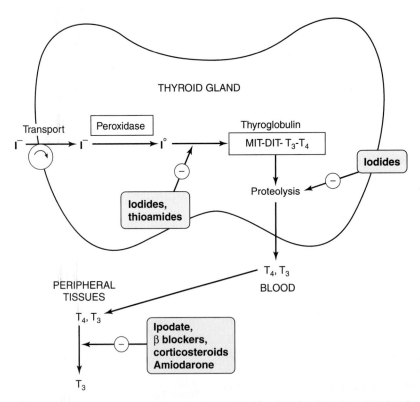

Figure 22–3. Biosynthesis of thyroid hormones and the sites of action of various drugs that interfere with thyroid hormone biosynthesis. DIT = diiodotyrosine; MIT = monoiodotyrosine; T_3 = triiodothyronine; T_4 = thyroxine.

proteins include Na+/K+ ATPase, specific contractile proteins in smooth muscle and the heart, enzymes involved in lipid metabolism, and important developmental components in the brain. In addition, T_3 may also have a separate membrane receptor-mediated effect in some tissues.

Physiologic Effects

The actions of thyroid hormones include normal growth and development of the nervous, skeletal, and reproductive systems and regulation of metabolism of fats, carbohydrates, proteins, and vitamins. The key features of excess thyroid activity (hyperthyroidism) and insufficient thyroid function (hypothyroidism) are listed in Table 22–2.

Clinical Use

Thyroid hormone therapy can be accomplished with either T_4 or T_3. Synthetic T_4 (**levothyroxine**) is usually the first choice. T_3 acts more quickly, but has a shorter half-life and is more expensive.

Adverse Effects

Toxicity due to excessive supplementation of thyroid hormones is expressed as hyperthyroidism (Table 22–2). Older patients, those with cardiovascular disease, and those with long-standing hypothyroidism are highly sensitive to the stimulatory effects of T_4 on the heart, and this sensitivity should be considered in the rehabilitation process associated with these patients.

Antithyroid Drugs

Thioamides

Propylthiouracil (PTU) and **methimazole** are small sulfur-containing molecules that inhibit thyroid hormone production by several mechanisms. The most important mechanism is blocking iodination of the tyrosine residues of thyroglobulin (Figure 22–3). In addition, these drugs may block coupling of DIT and MIT. The thioamides can be taken orally and are effective in most patients with uncomplicated hyperthyroidism. Because synthesis (rather than release) of thyroid hormone is inhibited, the onset of activity of these drugs is usually slow, often requiring 3 to 4 weeks for full effect. However, high-dose PTU also inhibits the conversion of T_4 to T_3. PTU is less likely than

methimazole to cross the placenta and enter breast milk, but it should be used cautiously in pregnant and nursing women. The most common toxic effect is skin rash. Rarely, severe immune reactions occur, but these are usually reversible. These include vasculitis, hypoprothrombinemia, and agranulocytosis.

Iodide Salts and Iodine

Iodide salts inhibit thyroid hormone release; possibly by inhibiting thyroglobulin proteolysis (Figure 22–3). These salts also decrease the size and vascularity of the hyperplastic thyroid gland. Because iodide salts inhibit release as well as synthesis of thyroid hormones, their onset of action occurs relatively rapidly—within 2 to 7 days. However, their effects are transient; the thyroid gland "escapes" from the iodide block after several weeks of treatment. Iodide salts are used to manage severe hyperthyroidism, a "thyroid storm" (life-threatening sudden acute exacerbation of all of the symptoms of hyperthyroidism), and to prepare patients for surgical resection of a hyperactive thyroid. The usual forms of this drug are oral solutions such as Lugol's solution (iodine and potassium iodide) or saturated solution of potassium iodide.

Radioactive Iodine and Iodinated Radiocontrast Media

Radioactive iodine (^{131}I) is taken up and concentrated in the thyroid gland so avidly that a dose large enough to damage the gland severely can be given without endangering other tissues. Unlike the thioamides and iodide salts, an effective dose of ^{131}I can produce a permanent cure of hyperthyroidism without surgery. ^{131}I should not be used in pregnant or nursing women.

Certain iodinated radiocontrast media, such as **ipodate**, effectively suppress the conversion of T_4 to T_3 in the liver, kidney, and other peripheral tissues (Figure 22–3). Inhibition of hormone release from the thyroid may also play a part. Ipodate is useful for rapidly reducing T_3 concentrations in hyperthyroidism.

Other Drugs

Other agents used in the treatment of hyperthyroidism include the β-adrenergic receptor antagonists (Chapter 6). These agents are particularly useful in controlling the

Table 22–2.   Manifestations of hyperthyroidism and hypothyroidism

System	Hyperthyroidism	Hypothyroidism
Skin and appendages	Warm, moist skin; sweating; heat intolerance; fine, thin hair; Plummer nails; pretibial dermopathy (Graves' disease)	Pale, cool, puffy; dry and brittle hair; brittle nails
Eyes, face	Retraction of upper lid with wide stare; periorbital edema; exophthalmos; diplopia (Graves' disease)	Drooping of eyelids; periorbital edema, loss of temporal aspects of eyebrows; puffy, nonpitting facies; large tongue
Cardiovascular system	Decreased peripheral vascular resistance; increased heart rate, stroke volume, cardiac output, pulse pressure; high-output heart failure; increased inotropic and chronotropic effects; arrhythmias; angina	Increased peripheral vascular resistance; decreased heart rate, stroke volume, cardiac output, pulse pressure; low-output heart failure; ECG: bradycardia, prolonged PR interval, flat T wave, low voltage; pericardial effusion
Respiratory system	Dyspnea; decreased vital capacity	Pleural effusions; hypoventilation and CO_2 retention
Gastrointestinal system	Increased appetite; increased frequency of bowel movements; hypoproteinemia	Decreased appetite; decreased frequency of bowel movements; ascites
Central nervous system	Nervousness; hyperkinesia; emotional lability	Lethargy; general slowing of mental processes; neuropathies
Musculoskeletal system	Weakness and muscle fatigue; increased deep tendon reflexes; hypercalcemia; osteoporosis	Stiffness and muscle fatigue; decreased deep tendon reflexes; increased alkaline phosphatase, LDH, AST
Renal system	Mild polyuria; increased renal blood flow; increased glomerular filtration rate	Impaired water excretion; decreased renal blood flow; decreased glomerular filtration rate
Hematopoietic system	Increased erythropoiesis; anemia[1]	Decreased erythropoiesis; anemia[1]
Reproductive system	Menstrual irregularities; decreased fertility; increased gonadal steroid metabolism	Hypermenorrhea; infertility; decreased libido; impotence; oligospermia; decreased gonadal steroid metabolism
Metabolic system	Increased basal metabolic rate; negative nitrogen balance; hyperglycemia; increased free fatty acids; decreased cholesterol and triglycerides; increased hormone degradation; increased requirements for fat- and water-soluble vitamins; increased drug metabolism	Decreased basal metabolic rate; slight positive nitrogen balance; delayed degradation of insulin, with increased sensitivity; increased cholesterol and triglycerides; decreased hormone degradation; decreased requirements for fat- and water-soluble vitamins; decreased drug metabolism

AST = aspartate aminotransferase; ECG = electrocardiograph; LDH = lactate dehydrogenase.

[1]The anemia of hyperthyroidism is usually normochromic and caused by increased red blood cell turnover. The anemia of hypothyroidism may be normochromic, hyperchromic, or hypochromic and may be due to decreased production rate, decreased iron absorption, decreased folic acid absorption, or to autoimmune pernicious anemia.

Table 22–3. Drug effects and thyroid function

Drug Effect	Drugs
Change in Thyroid Hormone Synthesis	
Inhibition of TRH or TSH secretion without induction of hypothyroidism	Dopamine, levodopa, corticosteroids, somatostatin
Inhibition of thyroid hormone synthesis or release with the induction of hypothyroidism (or occasionally hyperthyroidism)	Iodides (including amiodarone), lithium, aminoglutethimide, thioamides, ethionamide
Alteration of Thyroid Hormone Transport and Serum Total T_3 and T_4 Levels, but Usually No Modification of FT_4[1] or TSH	
Increased TBG	Estrogens, tamoxifen, heroin, methadone, mitotane, fluorouracil
Decreased TBG	Androgens, glucocorticoids
Displacement of T_3 and T_4 from TBG with transient hyperthyroxinemia	Salicylates, fenclofenac, mefenamic acid, furosemide
Alteration of T_4 and T_3 Metabolism with Modified Serum T_3 and T_4 Levels but Not FT_4 or TSH Levels	
Induction of increased hepatic enzyme activity	Phenytoin, carbamazepine, phenobarbital, rifampin, rifabutin, nicardipine, imatinib, protease inhibitors
Inhibition of 5′-deiodinase with decreased T_3, increased rT_3[2]	Iopanoic acid, ipodate, amiodarone, β blockers, corticosteroids, propylthiouracil, flavonoids
Other interactions	
Interference with T_4 absorption	Cholestyramine, colestipol, aluminum hydroxide, sucralfate, raloxifene, ferrous sulfate, some calcium preparations, bran, soy, ciprofloxacin, sodium polystyrene sulfonate
Induction of autoimmune thyroid disease with hypothyroidism or hyperthyroidism	Interferon-α, interleukin-2

TBG = thyroxine-binding globulin; TRH = thyroxine-releasing hormone; TSH = thyroid-stimulating hormone.

[1] FT_4 is free thyroxine not bound to TBG.

[2] rT_3 is an inactive deiodinated metabolite of T_4.

tachycardia and other cardiac abnormalities of severe hyperthyroidism. Propranolol also inhibits the conversion of T_4 to T_3 (Figure 22–3). Finally, a number of other drugs not used in the treatment of thyroid dysfunction may affect thyroid hormone levels by altering thyroid hormone synthesis, transport, or metabolism (Table 22–3).

GONADAL HORMONES AND INHIBITORS

The gonadal hormones include the steroids of the ovary (estrogens and progesterone) and testis (chiefly testosterone) (Figure 22–4). Because of their use as contraceptives, many synthetic estrogens and progesterone

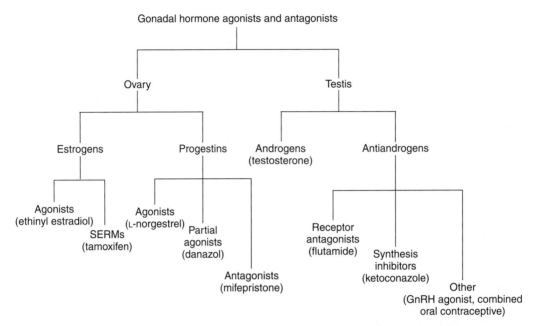

Figure 22–4. Drug classes used for contraception and treatment of gonadal dysfunction. Gonadal hormones are divided into steroids of the ovary (i.e., estrogens and progesterone receptor agonists) and those of the testis (chiefly testosterone). Subsequent divisions include drugs that inhibit synthesis of steroid hormones, partial receptor agonists, receptor antagonists, and those that act as agonists in some tissues and antagonists in other tissues. This last division of mixed agonists is called selective estrogen receptor modulators (SERMs).

receptor agonists have been produced. These include receptor agonists, partial agonists, antagonists, and some drugs with mixed effects. Drugs with mixed effects demonstrate agonist effects in some tissues and antagonist effects in other tissues. Mixed agonists with estrogenic effects are called **selective estrogen receptor modulators** (SERMs). Synthetic androgens, all of which have anabolic activity, are also available for clinical use. A diverse group of drugs with antiandrogenic effects are also used in the treatment of prostatic cancer, benign prostatic hyperplasia, and hirsutism in women.

Ovarian Hormones

The ovary is the primary source of sex hormones in women during the childbearing years (i.e., between puberty and menopause). During each menstrual cycle, in response to FSH and LH from the anterior pituitary, a follicle in the ovary matures, secretes

increasing amounts of estrogen, releases an ovum, and finally transforms into a progesterone-secreting corpus luteum. If the ovum is not fertilized and implanted, the corpus luteum degenerates. The uterine endometrium, which proliferated as a result of stimulation by estrogen, is shed as part of the menstrual flow, and the cycle repeats. Both estrogen and progesterone enter into cells and bind to cytosolic receptors. The receptor–hormone complex translocates into the nucleus, where it modulates gene expression.

Estrogens

The major ovarian estrogen in women is estradiol. Although estradiol has low oral bioavailability, its bioavailability is increased in a micronized form. The drug can also be administered via transdermal patch or vaginal cream. Long-acting esters of estradiol that are converted in the body to estradiol, such as estradiol cypionate, can be administered by IM injection. Mixtures of conjugated estrogens from biologic sources (e.g., Premarin) are used orally for hormone replacement therapy (HRT). **Ethinyl estradiol** and **mestranol** are synthetic estrogens with high bioavailability that are used in hormonal contraceptives.

PHYSIOLOGIC EFFECTS. Estrogen is essential for normal female sexual development. The hormone is responsible for growth of the vagina, uterus, and uterine tubes during childhood, appearance of secondary sexual characteristics, and the growth spurt associated with puberty. Estrogen also has multiple metabolic effects. The hormone modifies serum protein levels and reduces bone resorption. Estrogen also enhances blood coagulability and increases plasma triglyceride and high-density lipoprotein (HDL) cholesterol levels while reducing low-density lipoprotein (LDL) cholesterol. Continuous administration of estrogen, especially in combination with a progestin, inhibits the secretion of gonadotropins from the anterior pituitary (Figure 22–5).

CLINICAL USE. Estrogens are used in the treatment of hypogonadism in young females (Table 22–4). Another use is as HRT in women with estrogen deficiency resulting from premature ovarian failure, menopause, or surgical removal of the ovaries. HRT ameliorates hot flushes and atrophic changes in the urogenital tract. Estrogen is also effective in preventing bone loss and osteoporosis; however, there is an increased risk of adverse cardiovascular events and breast cancer when estrogen is used by postmenopausal women for this pharmacologic effect. Finally, the estrogens are components of hormonal contraceptives (see discussion below).

ADVERSE EFFECTS. In hypogonadal girls, the dose of estrogen must be adjusted carefully to prevent premature closure of the epiphyses of the long bones, resulting in short stature. The relationship between long-term estrogen therapy and cancer continues to be actively investigated. When used alone for HRT in women with a uterus, estrogen increases the risk of endometrial cancer. However, this effect can be prevented by combining estrogen with a progestin. Estrogen use by postmenopausal women is also associated with a small increase in the risk of breast cancer, myocardial infarction, and stroke. These increased risks are not ameliorated by concurrent progestin therapy. Dose-dependent toxicities include nausea, breast tenderness, increased risk of migraine headache, thromboembolic events (e.g., deep vein thrombosis), gallbladder disease, hypertriglyceridemia, and hypertension.

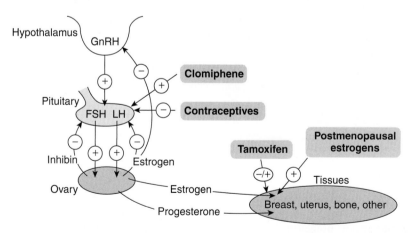

Figure 22–5. Sites of action of several ovarian hormones and their analogs. Clomiphene, a mixed agonist-antagonist, is an antagonist at pituitary and hypothalamic estrogen receptors; this prevents negative feedback and increases the output of pituitary gonadotropins. Tamoxifen, a SERM, is an antagonist at estrogen receptors in the breast, but acts as an agonist in other tissues. Hormonal contraceptives reduce FSH and LH output from the pituitary by activating receptors that mediate feedback inhibition, and have important effects in the genital tract (not shown).

Table 22–4. Representative applications for the gonadal hormones and hormone antagonists

Clinical Application	Drugs
Hypogonadism in girls, women	Conjugated estrogens ethinyl estradiol, estradiol esters
Hormone replacement therapy	Estrogen component: conjugated estrogens, estradiol, estrone, estriol
	Progestin component: progesterone, medroxyprogesterone acetate
Oral hormonal contraceptive	Combined: ethinyl estradiol or mestranol plus a progestin
	Progestin only: norethindrone or norgestrel
Parenteral contraceptive	Medroxyprogesterone as a depot IM injection
	Ethinyl estradiol and L-noregestromin as a weekly patch
	Ethinyl estradiol and etonogestrel as a monthly vaginal ring
	Etonogestrel as a subcutaneous implant
	L-norgestrel as an intrauterine device (IUD)
Postcoital (emergency) contraceptive	L-norgestrel, combined oral contraceptives
Intractable dysmenorrhea or uterine bleeding	Conjugated estrogens, ethinyl estradiol, oral contraceptive, GnRH agonist, depot injection of medroxyprogesterone acetate
Infertility	Clomiphene; hMG and hCG; GnRH analogs; progesterone; bromocriptine
Abortifacient	Mifepristone (RU 486) and prostaglandin
Endometriosis	Oral contraceptive, depot injection of medroxyprogesterone acetate, GnRH agonist, danazol
Breast cancer	Tamoxifen, aromatase inhibitors (e.g., anastrozole)
Osteoporosis in postmenopausal women	Conjugated estrogens, estradiol, raloxifene
Hypogonadism in boys, men; replacement therapy	Testosterone enanthate or cypionate; methyltestosterone; fluoxymesterone, testosterone (patch)
Anabolic protein synthesis	Oxandrolone, stanozolol
Prostate hyperplasia (benign)	Finasteride
Prostate carcinoma	GnRH agonist, androgen receptor antagonist (e.g., flutamide)
Hirsutism	Combined oral contraceptive, spironolactone, flutamide, GnRH agonist

IM = intramuscular; GnRH = gonadotropin-releasing hormone; hCG = human chorionic gonadotropin; hMG = menotropins.

Progestins

Progesterone is the major progestin in humans. Micronized form is used orally for HRT and progesterone-containing vaginal creams are also available. Synthetic progestins (e.g., **medroxyprogesterone**) have improved oral bioavailability. The 19-nortestosterone compounds differ primarily in their degree of androgenic effects. Older drugs such as L-**norgestrel** and **norethindrone** are more androgenic than the newer progestins such as **norgestimate** and **desogestrel**.

PHYSIOLOGIC EFFECTS. Progesterone induces secretory changes in the endometrium and is required for the maintenance of pregnancy. Other progestins also stabilize the endometrium but do not support pregnancy. Progestins do not significantly affect plasma proteins, but they affect carbohydrate metabolism and stimulate fat deposition. High doses suppress gonadotropin secretion and often prevent ovulation.

CLINICAL USE. Progestins are used as contraceptives, either alone or in combination with an estrogen. As previously discussed, they are used in combination with an estrogen in HRT to prevent estrogen-induced endometrial cancer. Progesterone is used in assisted reproductive technology programs to promote and maintain pregnancy.

ADVERSE EFFECTS. The toxicity of progestins is low. However, they may increase blood pressure and decrease high-density plasma lipoprotein (HDL) cholesterol. Long-term use of high doses in premenopausal women is associated with a reversible decrease in bone density and delayed resumption of ovulation after termination of therapy.

Hormonal Contraceptives

Hormonal contraceptives contain either a combination of an estrogen and a progestin or a progestin alone. Hormonal contraceptives are available in a variety of preparations, including oral pills, long-acting injections, transdermal patches, vaginal rings, and intrauterine devices (IUDs) (Table 22–4). Three different types of oral contraceptives for women are available in the United States. Monophasic preparations are a combination of estrogen-progestin tablets that are taken in constant dosage throughout the menstrual cycle. Biphasic and triphasic preparations are combination preparations in which the progestin or estrogen dosage, or both, changes during the month to more closely mimic hormonal changes in a menstrual cycle. The third type of preparation contains only progestin.

The postcoital contraceptives (also known as "emergency contraception") will prevent pregnancy if administered within 72 hours after unprotected sexual intercourse. Several types of oral preparations are effective: estrogens alone, L-norgestrel (progestin alone), combination pills containing an estrogen and a progestin, and **mifepristone** (RU 486), a progesterone antagonist.

Mechanism of Action

The combination hormonal contraceptives have several actions. The primary action is inhibition of ovulation. Additional changes in the cervical mucus glands, uterine tubes, and endometrium also decrease the likelihood of fertilization and implantation. Progestin-only agents do not always inhibit ovulation and instead act through the other mechanisms listed. The mechanisms of action of postcoital contraceptives are not well understood. When administered before the LH surge, they inhibit ovulation. They also affect cervical mucus, tubal function, and endometrial lining.

Other Clinical Uses and Beneficial Effects

Additional clinical uses of combination hormonal contraceptives are presented in Table 22–4. Combination hormonal contraceptives are used to prevent estrogen deficiency in young women with primary hypogonadism after their growth has been achieved. Combinations of hormonal contraceptives and progestins are used to treat acne, hirsutism, dysmenorrhea, and endometriosis. Users of combination hormonal contraceptives have reduced risks of ovarian cysts, ovarian and endometrial cancer, benign breast disease, and pelvic inflammatory disease as well as a lower incidence of ectopic pregnancy, iron deficiency anemia, and rheumatoid arthritis.

Adverse Effects

The incidence of dose-dependent toxicity has fallen since the introduction of the low-dose combined oral contraceptives. The most notable adverse effects include thromboembolism and a potentially increased risk of developing breast cancer at a younger age.

Increased risk of thromboembolism results from the effect of the combined hormonal contraceptives' estrogenic component on liver synthesis of blood coagulation factors. There is a well-documented increase in the risk of thromboembolic events in older women, smokers, women with a personal or family history of such problems, and women with genetic defects that affect the production or function of clotting factors. This increased risk results in an elevated potential for myocardial infarction, stroke, deep vein thrombosis, and pulmonary embolism. However, risk of thromboembolism incurred by the use of combined hormonal contraceptives is usually less than that imposed by pregnancy.

Evidence also suggests that the lifetime risk of breast cancer in women who are current or past users of hormonal contraceptives is not affected by oral contraceptive use, but there may be an earlier onset of breast cancer.

The potential for other toxicities also exists. The low-dose combined oral and progestin-only contraceptives cause significant breakthrough bleeding, especially during the first few months of therapy. Other toxicities of the hormonal contraceptives include nausea, breast tenderness, headache, skin pigmentation, and depression. Preparations containing older, more androgenic progestins can cause weight gain, acne, and hirsutism. The high dose of estrogen in the estrogen-containing postcoital contraceptives is associated with significant nausea.

Selective Estrogen Receptor Modulators

Selective estrogen receptor modulators (SERMs) are mixed estrogen receptor ligands that act as agonists in some tissues and as partial agonists or antagonists in other tissues.

Tamoxifen is a SERM effective in the treatment of hormone-responsive breast cancer, where it acts as an antagonist to prevent receptor activation by endogenous estrogens (Figure 22–5). Prophylactic use of tamoxifen reduces the incidence of breast cancer in women who are at very high risk. However, tamoxifen acts as an agonist at endometrial estrogen receptors, causing hyperplasia and increasing the risk of endometrial cancer. Tamoxifen can cause hot flushes, reflecting an antagonist effect, whereas it also increases risk of venous thrombosis, an agonist effect. In bone, tamoxifen has more agonist than antagonist estrogenic actions, thus preventing osteoporosis in women who are taking the drug for breast cancer. **Toremifene** is structurally related to tamoxifen and has similar properties, indications, and toxicities.

Raloxifene, which is approved for prevention of osteoporosis in postmenopausal women and the prevention of breast cancer in high-risk women, has a partial agonist effect on bone. Like tamoxifen, raloxifene has antagonist effects in breast tissue and reduces the incidence of breast cancer in women who are at very high risk. Unlike tamoxifen, the drug has no estrogenic effects on endometrial tissue. Adverse effects also include hot flushes and increased risk of venous thrombosis.

Other Estrogen and Progesterone Agonists, Antagonists, and Synthesis Inhibitors

Clomiphene is used to induce ovulation in anovulatory women who wish to become pregnant. The drug is a nonsteroidal compound with tissue-selective actions. By selectively blocking estrogen receptors in the anterior pituitary, clomiphene reduces negative feedback and increases FSH and LH secretion. This increase in gonadotropins stimulates ovulation.

Mifepristone (RU 486) is an orally active steroid antagonist of progesterone and glucocorticoid receptors. Mifepristone is primarily used as an abortifacient in early pregnancy, up to 49 days after the last menstrual period. When given as a single oral dose followed by administration of a prostaglandin E or prostaglandin F analog, a very high percentage of complete abortion is achieved with a low incidence of serious toxicity.

Danazol is a weak partial agonist that binds to progestin, androgen, and glucocorticoid receptors. Danazol also inhibits several P450 enzymes involved in gonadal steroid synthesis. The drug is sometimes used in the treatment of endometriosis and fibrocystic breast disease.

Aromatase inhibitors such as **anastrozole** and related compounds are nonsteroidal inhibitors of aromatase, the enzyme required for estrogen synthesis. These drugs are used in the treatment of breast cancer (Chapter 31).

Androgens

The hypothalamic-pituitary control of the secretion of testosterone and related androgens is presented in Figure 22–6. Testosterone and related androgens are produced in the testis, the adrenal gland, and, to a small extent, the ovary. Testosterone is synthesized from progesterone and dehydroepiandrosterone (DHEA). The latter also has a sulfated form (DHEAS). In the plasma, testosterone is partly bound to a transport protein, sex hormone–binding globulin (SHBG). Testosterone itself is active in some tissues,

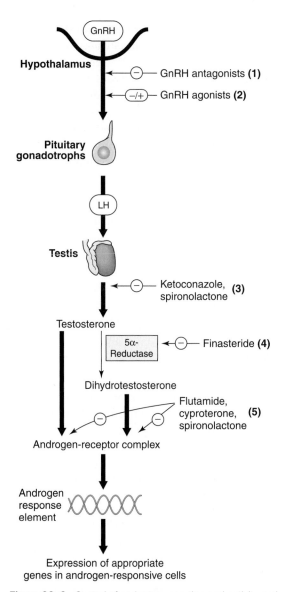

Figure 22–6. Control of androgen secretion and activity and some sites of action of antiandrogens: **(1)** competitive inhibition of gonadotropin-releasing hormone (GnRH) receptors; **(2)** stimulation (+) or inhibition (-) by GnRH agonists; **(3)** inhibition of testosterone synthesis by ketoconazole and possibly spironolactone; **(4)** inhibition of dihydrotestosterone production by finasteride; **(5)** inhibition of androgen binding at its receptor by flutamide and other drugs.

but it is converted in several organs (such as the prostate gland) to **dihydrotestosterone** (DHT), which is the active hormone in those tissues. Because of rapid hepatic metabolism, orally administered testosterone has little effect. The drug may be given by injection of long-acting esters or as a transdermal patch. Orally active variants are also available (Table 22–4).

Many androgens have been synthesized in an effort to increase anabolic effects (increasing muscle mass) without increasing androgenic actions (producing masculine characteristics). **Oxandrolone** and **stanozolol** are examples of drugs that, in laboratory testing, have an increased ratio of anabolic:androgenic action. However, all of the so-called anabolic steroids have androgenic agonist effects when used in humans.

Physiologic Effects

Like the steroid hormones discussed previously, androgens enter cells and bind to cytosolic receptors (Figure 22–6). The hormone–receptor complex enters the nucleus and modulates the expression of target genes. Testosterone is necessary for normal development of the male fetus and infant and is responsible for major changes in the male at puberty. These changes include growth of the penis, larynx, and skeleton; development of facial, pubic, and axillary hair; darkening of skin; and enlargement of muscle mass. After puberty, testosterone maintains secondary sex characteristics, fertility, and libido. Finally, testosterone (as dihydrotestosterone) acts on hair cells to cause male-pattern baldness.

The major effect of androgens, in addition to development and maintenance of normal male characteristics, is an anabolic action that involves increased muscle size and strength and increased red blood cell production. Urea excretion is reduced, and nitrogen balance becomes more positive. Testosterone also helps maintain normal bone density.

Clinical Use

The primary clinical use of the androgens is for replacement therapy in hypogonadism (Table 22–4). They have also been used to stimulate red blood cell production in certain anemias and to promote weight gain in patients with wasting syndromes (e.g., AIDS-associated wasting). The anabolic effects have been exploited illicitly by athletes in attempts to increase muscle mass and strength and enhance athletic performance. Therefore, they are banned by amateur and professional athletic organizations.

Adverse Effects

Use of androgens by females results in menstrual irregularity and virilization, which includes hirsutism, enlarged clitoris, and deepening of the voice. In women who are pregnant with a female fetus, exogenous androgens can cause virilization of the fetus' external genitalia. Paradoxically, excessive doses of androgens in men can result in feminization, which is characterized by gynecomastia, testicular shrinkage, and infertility. This feminization results from feedback inhibition of the anterior pituitary and conversion of exogenous androgens to estrogens. High doses in males also cause behavioral changes including hostility and aggression ("roid rage") (Chapter 21). In both sexes, high doses of anabolic steroids can cause cholestatic jaundice, elevation of liver enzyme levels, possibly hepatocellular carcinoma, increased lipid levels (resulting in atherosclerosis), and sodium retention (resulting in hypertension).

Antiandrogens

Decreasing the effects of androgens is an important mode of therapy for both benign and malignant prostate disease, precocious puberty, hair loss, and hirsutism. Several drugs are available that act at different sites in the androgen pathway (Figure 22–6).

Gonadotropin-Releasing Hormone Analogs

A reduction in gonadotropin secretion, especially LH secretion, lowers the production of testosterone. As described earlier, this can be effectively accomplished with long-acting depot preparations of **leuprolide** or similar GnRH agonists. These analogs are used in prostatic carcinoma. During the first week of therapy, an androgen receptor antagonist such as **flutamide** is added to prevent the tumor flare that can result from the surge in testosterone synthesis caused by the initial agonist action of the GnRH analog. Within several weeks, testosterone production falls to normal and then far below normal.

Inhibitors of Steroid Synthesis

All steroid hormones are derivatives of cholesterol. Steroid hormones include the gonadal hormones

discussed here and the corticosteroids discussed in Chapter 23. **Ketoconazole**, an antifungal agent (Chapter 29), inhibits cytochrome P450 enzymes necessary for the synthesis of gonadal and adrenal steroids. Ketoconazole has been used to suppress adrenal steroid synthesis in patients with steroid-responsive metastatic tumors. Part of the antiandrogen effect of **spironolactone**, a drug used principally as a potassium-sparing diuretic (Chapter 7), is due to its inhibition of 17α-reductase, an enzyme involved in androgen synthesis.

5α-Reductase Inhibitors

Testosterone is converted to DHT by the enzyme 5α-reductase. Some tissues, most notably the prostate and hair follicles, depend on DHT rather than testosterone for androgenic stimulation. 5α-Reductase is inhibited by **finasteride**, a drug used to treat benign prostatic hyperplasia and, at a lower dose, to prevent hair loss in men. Because the drug does not interfere with the action of testosterone, it is less likely than other antiandrogens to cause impotence, infertility, and loss of libido.

Receptor Inhibitors

Flutamide and related drugs are nonsteroidal compounds that act as competitive antagonists at androgen receptors. These drugs are used to decrease the action of endogenous androgens in patients with prostate carcinoma. The diuretic spironolactone also inhibits androgen receptors, and is used in the treatment of hirsutism.

Combined Hormonal Contraceptives

Combined hormonal contraceptives exert an antiandrogenic effect when they are used in women with hirsutism, which is caused by excess production of androgenic steroids. The estrogen in the contraceptive causes the liver to increase production of sex hormone–binding globulin, which in turn acts to reduce the concentration of free androgen in the blood.

■ REHABILITATION FOCUS

Many endocrine drugs directly influence the practice of the physical therapist, while others directly influence patients' responses to the rehabilitation process.

Many postmenopausal women use estrogens and progestins for HRT. A small number of these women experience breast or endometrial cancers, or cardiovascular events to which the HRT contributed. Subsequent rehabilitation may be required by these patients. Androgen supplementation in geriatric males with hypogonadism or decreased testosterone levels improves bone mineral density and exercise tolerance. However, abuse of these drugs by athletes promotes abnormal distribution of cholesterol in serum lipoproteins and increases the risk of atherosclerosis and cardiovascular morbidities. Physical therapists should be aware of these adverse effects and counsel athletes appropriately.

Drugs that affect endocrine function may also directly influence the response of the patient to rehabilitation. For example, excessive supplementation with thyroxine (T_4) presents as hyperthyroidism. The cardiovascular and respiratory dysfunction caused by hyperthyroidism may not appear at rest, but can be precipitated with exercise.

▇ CLINICAL RELEVANCE FOR REHABILITATION

Adverse Drug Reactions

Thyroid hormones
- Exercise intolerance associated with both hyperthyroidism and hypothyroidism

- Intolerance to temperature changes
- Hypothyroidism: cold intolerance
- Hyperthyroidism: heat intolerance

Estrogens and progesterone receptors agonists
- Deep vein thrombosis
- Myocardial infarction
- Hypertension

Effects Interfering with Rehabilitation
- Decreased capacity to participate in aerobic conditioning due to thyroid dysfunction
- Increased risk for embolic event during therapy
- Increased risk of myocardial infarction during therapy

Possible Therapy Solutions
- Examine for potential deep vein thrombosis prior to therapy.
- Check heart rate and blood pressure prior to and following therapy.

Potentiation of Functional Outcomes Secondary to Drug Therapy
- Progressive resistance training has been shown to augment increases in strength and lean body mass by testosterone analogs in certain patient populations with cachexia (i.e., wasting).

PROBLEM-ORIENTED PATIENT STUDY

Brief History: The patient is a 53-year-old female with a 10-year history of mild hypertension that is stabilized with current medications. She also has a 1-year history of bipolar disorder that is being pharmacologically treated. The patient was diagnosed 3 weeks ago with fibromyalgia. She is working with a physical therapist at an outpatient clinic and wellness center to develop an exercise program to assist in pain relief prior to an alternative treatment option of strong analgesics. The patient has been actively participating in the exercise program at the wellness center. She has an appointment with the therapist on a weekly basis for review of the exercise program and assessment of her fibromyalgia symptoms.

Current Medical Status and Drug Therapy: Recent blood pressure measurements were 130/82 mm Hg with a heart rate of 80 beats per minute. Medications include enalapril and hydrochlorothiazide/amiloride combination for hypertension. Bipolar disorder is being treated with lithium carbonate. One week ago, the patient was also diagnosed with functional hypothyroidism that probably resulted from

(continued)

PROBLEM-ORIENTED PATIENT STUDY (*Continued*)

the lithium treatment. The patient was prescribed levothyroxine and started the medication that day.

Rehabilitation Setting: The patient arrived for the weekly assessment with the physical therapist. She complained that within the past week her muscle weakness increased and her ability to perform the exercise program decreased significantly. Specifically, she was short of breath during her work on the stationary bicycle. Additionally, pain complaints associated with her fibromyalgia increased. The therapist measured her blood pressure and heart rate at 142/86 mm Hg and 96 beats per minute and irregular.

Problem/Clinical Options: The exogenous thyroid medication the patient recently started has resulted in hyperthyroidism. The adverse effects of the medication did not manifest until the patient was exercising. Hyperthyroidism decreased the patient's exercise tolerance directly through an effect on skeletal muscles and indirectly through decreased cardiac and pulmonary function. Finally, the chronic pain associated with the fibromyalgia was heightened. The therapist should recommend that the patient discontinue her exercise program until she is reevaluated by her physician. Because atrial fibrillation is likely, the therapist should immediately inform the physician of these signs and symptoms of hyperthyroidism.

PREPARATIONS AVAILABLE

Hypothalamic and Pituitary Agents

Bromocriptine (Parlodel)
Oral: 2.5-mg tablets, 5-mg capsules

Cabergoline (Dostinex)
Oral: 0.5-mg scored tablets

Cetrorelix (Cetrotide)
Parenteral 0.25, 3 mg/vial with diluent for subcutaneous injection

Chorionic gonadotropin (hCG) (generic, Profasi, A.P.L., Pregnyl, others)
Parenteral powder to reconstitute 500, 1000, 2000 units/mL for injection

Corticorelin ovine (Acthrel)
Parenteral 0.1 mg for IV injection

Corticotropin (H.P. Acthar Gel)
Parenteral 80 units/mL

Cosyntropin (Cortrosyn)
Parenteral 0.25 mg/vial with diluent for IV or IM injection

Follitropin alfa (Gonal-F)
Parenteral 37.5, 150 IU powder for injection

Follitropin beta (FSH) (Follistim)
Parenteral 75 IU powder for injection

Ganirelix (Antagon)
Parenteral 500 mcg/mL for injection

Gonadorelin acetate (GnRH) (Lutrepulse)
Parenteral powder to reconstitute for injection via Lutrepulse pump (0.8, 3.2 mg/vial)

Gonadorelin hydrochloride (GnRH) (Factrel)
Parenteral 100, 500 mg for injection

Goserelin acetate (Zoladex)
Parenteral 3.6-, 10.8-mg subcutaneous implant

Histrelin (Supprelin)
Parenteral 120, 300, 600 mg for subcutaneous injection

Leuprolide (generic, Lupron)
Parenteral 5 mg/mL for subcutaneous injection

Parenteral depot suspension (Lupron Depot, Depot-Ped, Depot-3, Depot-4): lyophilized microspheres to reconstitute for IM injection (3.75, 7.5, 11.25, 15, 22.5, 30 mg/vial)
Parenteral implant: 72 mg

Menotropins (hMG) (Pergonal, Repronex)
Parenteral 75 IU FSH and 75 IU LH activity, 150 IU FSH and 150 IU LH activity, each with diluent

Nafarelin (Synarel)
Nasal: 2 mg/mL (200 mcg/spray)

Octreotide (Sandostatin)
Parenteral 0.05, 0.1, 0.2, 0.5, 1 mg/mL for subcutaneous or IV administration
Parenteral depot injection (Sandostatin LAR Depot): 10, 20, 30 mg for IM injection only

Pergolide (Permax)
Oral: 0.05-, 0.25-, 1-mg tablets

Protirelin (Thypinone, Relefact TRH, Thyrel TRH)
Parenteral 500 mg/mL for injection

Sermorelin (Geref)
Parenteral 0.5, 1 mg for subcutaneous injection; 50-mcg powder to reconstitute for intravenous injection

Somatrem (Protropin)
Parenteral 5, 10 mg/vial with diluent for subcutaneous or IM injection

Somatropin (Genotropin, Humatrope, Nutropin, Nutropin AQ, Norditropin, Serostim, Saizen)
Parenteral 0.2, 0.4, 0.6, 0.8, 1.0, 1.2, 1.4, 1.5, 1.6, 1.8, 2, 4, 5, 5.8, 6, 8, 10, 12, 13.5, 13.8, 15, 18, 22.5, 24 mg/vial with diluent for subcutaneous or IM injection

Thyrotropin alpha (Thyrogen)
Parenteral 1.1 mg (4 IU)/vial with diluent for IM injection

Triptorelin (Trelstar)
Parenteral 3.75, 11.25 mg for IM injection

Urofollitropin (Fertinex, Bravelle)
Parenteral powder to reconstitute for injection, 75, 150 IU FSH activity per ampule

Thyroid Agents

Levothyroxine (T_4) (generic, Levoxyl, Levo-T, Synthroid, Unithroid)
Oral: 0.025-, 0.05-, 0.075-, 0.088-, 0.1-, 0.112-, 0.125-, 0.137-, 0.15-, 0.175-, 0.2-, 0.3-mg tablets
Parenteral 200, 500 mcg per vial (100 mcg/mL when reconstituted) for injection

Liothyronine (T_3) (generic, Cytomel, Triostat)
Oral: 5-, 25-, 50-mcg tablets
Parenteral 10 mcg/mL

Liotrix (a 4:1 ratio of T_4:T_3) (Thyrolar)
Oral: tablets containing 12.5, 25, 30, 50, 60, 100, 120, 150, 180 mcg T_4 and one-fourth as much T_3

Thyroid desiccated (USP) (generic, Armour Thyroid, Thyroid Strong, Thyrar, S-P-T)
Oral: tablets containing 15, 30, 60, 90, 120, 180, 240, 300 mg; capsules (S-P-T) containing 120, 180, 300 mg

Antithyroid Agents

Diatrizoate sodium (Hypaque)
Parenteral 25% (150 mg iodine/mL); 50% (300 mg iodine/mL) (unlabeled use)

Iodide (^{131}I) sodium (Iodotope, Sodium Iodide I^{131} Therapeutic)
Oral: available as capsules and solution

Iopanoic acid (Telepaque)
Oral: 500-mg tablets (unlabeled use)

Ipodate sodium (Oragrafin Sodium, Bilivist)
Oral: 500-mg capsules (unlabeled use)

Methimazole (Tapazole)
Oral: 5-, 10-mg tablets

Potassium iodide
Oral solution (generic, SSKI): 1 g/mL
Oral solution (Lugol solution): 100 mg/mL potassium iodide plus 50 mg/mL iodine
Oral syrup (Pima): 325 mg/5 mL

Oral controlled-action tablets (Iodo-Niacin): 135 mg potassium iodide plus 25 mg niacinamide hydroiodide
Oral potassium iodide tablets (generic, IOSAT, RAD-Block, Thyro-Block): 65, 130 mg

Propylthiouracil (PTU) (generic)
Oral: 50-mg tablets

Thyrotropin; recombinant human TSH (Thyrogen)
Parenteral 0.9 mg per vial

Estrogens

Conjugated estrogens (Premarin)
Oral: 0.3-, 0.625-, 0.9-, 1.25- 2.5-mg tablets
Parenteral 25 mg/5 mL for IM, IV injection
Vaginal: 0.625 mg/g cream base

Dienestrol (Ortho Dienestrol, DV)
Vaginal: 10 mg/g cream

Diethylstilbestrol diphosphate (Stilphostrol)
Oral: 50-mg tablets
Parenteral 50 mg/mL injection

Esterified estrogens (Menest, Estratab)
Oral: 0.3-, 0.625-, 1.25-, 2.5-mg tablets

Estradiol cypionate in oil (generic, Depo-Estradiol cypionate)
Parenteral 5 mg/mL for IM injection

Estradiol (generic, Estrace)
Oral: 0.5-, 1-, 2-mg tablets
Vaginal: 0.1 mg/g cream

Estradiol transdermal (Estraderm, others)
Transdermal: patches with 0.025, 0.0375, 0.05, 0.075, 0.1 mg/d release rates

Estradiol valerate in oil (generic)
Parenteral 10, 20, 40 mg/mL for IM injection
Oral contraceptives are listed in Table 40–3.

Estrone aqueous suspension (generic, Kestrone 5)
Parenteral 5 mg/mL for injection

Estropipate (generic, Ogen)
Oral: 0.625-, 1.25-, 2.5-, 5-mg tablets
Vaginal: 1.5 mg/g cream base

Ethinyl estradiol (Estinyl)
Oral: 0.02-, 0.05-, 0.5-mg tablets

Progestins

Etonogestrel (Implanon)
Kit for subcutaneous implant; 1 rod of 68 mg

Hydroxyprogesterone caproate (generic, Hylutin)
Parenteral 125, 250 mg/mL for IM injection

Medroxyprogesterone acetate (generic, Provera)
Oral: 2.5-, 5-, 10-mg tablets
Parenteral (Depo-Provera): 150, 400 mg/mL for IM injection

Megestrol acetate (generic, Megace)
Oral: 20-, 40-mg tablets; 40 mg/mL suspension

Norethindrone acetate (generic, Aygestin)
Oral: 5-mg tablets

Norgestrel (Ovrette) (Also Table 40–3)
Oral: 0.075-mg tablets

Progesterone (generic)
Oral: 100-mg capsules
Topical: 8% vaginal gel
Parenteral 50 mg/mL in oil for IM injection

Androgens and Anabolic Steroids

Fluoxymesterone (generic, Halotestin)
Oral: 2-, 5-, 10-mg tablets

Methyltestosterone (generic)
Oral: 10-, 25-mg tablets; 10-mg capsules; 10-mg buccal tablets
Parenteral 200 mg/mL injection

Nandrolone decanoate (Deca-Durabolin, others)
Parenteral 100, 200 mg/mL in oil for injection

Oxandrolone (Oxandrin)
Oral: 2.5-mg tablets

Oxymetholone (Androl-50)
Oral: 50-mg tablets

Stanozolol (Winstrol)
Oral: 2-mg tablets

Testolactone (Teslac)
Oral: 50-mg tablets

Testosterone aqueous (generic, others)
Parenteral 25, 50, 100 mg/mL suspension for IM

Testosterone cypionate in oil (generic, others)
Parenteral 100, 200 mg/mL for IM injection

Testosterone enanthate in oil (generic)
Parenteral 200 mg/mL for IM injection

Testosterone propionate in oil (generic, Testex)
Parenteral 100 mg/mL for IM injection
Testosterone transdermal system
Patch (Testoderm): 4, 5, 6 mg/24 h release rate
Patch (Androderm): 2.5, 5 mg/24 h release rate
Gel (Androgel): 25, 50 mg total
Testosterone pellets (Testopel)
Parenteral 75 mg/pellet for parenteral injection (not IV)

SERMs, Antagonists, and Inhibitors

Anastrozole (Arimidex)
Oral: 1-mg tablets

Bicalutamide (Casodex)
Oral: 50-mg tablets

Clomiphene (generic, Clomid, Serophene, Milophene)
Oral: 50-mg tablets

Danazol (generic, Danocrine)
Oral: 50-, 100-, 200-mg capsules

Dutasteride (Avodart)
Oral: 0.5-mg tablets

Exemestane (Aromasin)
Oral: 25-mg tablets

Finasteride
Oral: 1-mg tablets (Propecia); 5-mg tablets (Proscar)

Flutamide (Eulexin)
Oral: 125-mg capsules

Fulvestrant (Faslodex)
Parenteral 50 mg/mL for IM injection

Letrozole (Femara)
Oral: 2.5-mg tablets

Mifepristone (Mifeprex)
Oral: 200-mg tablets

Nilutamide (Nilandron)
Oral: 50-, 150-mg tablets

Raloxifene (Evista)
Oral: 60-mg tablets

Tamoxifen (generic, Nolvadex)
Oral: 10-, 20-mg tablets

Toremifene (Fareston)
Oral: 60-mg tablets

REFERENCES

Agarwal SK: Comparative effects of GnRH agonist therapy. Review of clinical studies and their implications. *J Reprod Med* 1998;43(Suppl):293. American Thyroid Association (http://thyroid.org/)

Anderson GL, et al: Women's Health Initiative Steering Committee. Effects of conjugated equine estrogen in postmenopausal women with hysterectomy: The Women's Health Initiative randomized controlled trial. *JAMA* 2004;291:1701.

Atkins P, et al: Drug therapy for hyperthyroidism in pregnancy: Safety issues for mother and fetus. Drug Saf 2000;23:229.

Bagatell CJ, Bremmer WJ: Androgens in men—uses and abuses. *N Engl J Med* 1996;334:707.

Bevan JS, et al: Primary medical therapy for acromegaly: An open, prospective, multicenter study of the effects of subcutaneous and intramuscular slow-release octreotide on growth hormone, insulin-like growth factor-I, and tumor size. *J Clin Endocrinol Metab* 2002; 87:4554.

Cook DM, et al: The pharmacokinetic and pharmacodynamic characteristics of a long-acting growth hormone (GH) preparation (Nutropin Depot) in GH-deficient adults. *J Clin Endocrinol Metab* 2002;87:4508.

Cooper DS: Clinical practice: Subclinical hypothyroidism. *N Engl J Med* 2001;345:260.

Daya S: Updated meta-analysis of recombinant follicle-stimulating hormone (FSH) versus urinary FSH for ovarian stimulation in assisted reproduction. *Fertil Steril* 2002;77:711.

Dong BJ: How medications affect thyroid function. *West J Med* 2000;172:102.

Edwards DP, Boonyaratanakornkit V: Rapid extranuclear signaling by the estrogen receptor (ER): MNAR couples ER and Src to the MAP Kinase signaling pathway. *Mol Interv* 2002;3:12.

Fontanilla JC, et al: The use of oral radiographic contrast agents in the management of hyperthyroidism. *Thyroid* 2001;11:561.

Gardner DG, Shoback D: *Greenspan's Basic & Clinical Endocrinology*, 8th ed. New York: McGraw-Hill, 2007.

Glasier A, et al: Mifepristone (RU 486) compared with high-dose estrogen and progestogen for emergency postcoital contraception. *N Engl J Med* 1992;327:1041.

Golditz GA, et al: Hormone replacement therapy and the risk of breast cancer: Results from epidemiologic studies. *Am J Obstet Gynecol* 1993;168: 1473.

Grey AB, et al: The effect of the anti-estrogen tamoxifen on cardiovascular risk factors in normal postmenopausal women. *J Clin Endocrinol Metab* 1995;80:8192.

Grodstein F, et al: Postmenopausal estrogen and progestin use and the risk of cardiovascular disease. *N Engl J Med* 1996;335:453.

Gruters A, et al: Long-term consequences of congenital hypothyroidism in the era of screening programs. *Endocrinol Metab* 2002;16:369.

Lacey JV Jr, et al: Oral contraceptives as risk factors for cervical adenocarcinomas and squamous cell carcinomas. *Cancer Epidemiol Biomarkers Prev* 1999;8:1079.

Leschek EW, et al: Effect of growth hormone treatment on adult height in peripubertal children with idiopathic short stature: A randomized, double-blind, placebo-controlled trial. *J Clin Endocrinol Metab* 2004;89:3140.

Love RR, et al: Effects of tamoxifen on bone mineral density in postmenopausal women with breast cancer. *N Engl J Med* 1992;326:852.

Manson JE, et al: Estrogen plus progestin and the risk of coronary heart disease. *N Engl J Med* 2003;349:523.

Markou K, et al: Iodine-induced hyperthyroidism. *Thyroid* 2001;11:501.

Papadakis MA, et al: Growth hormone replacement in healthy older men improves body composition but not functional ability. *Ann Intern Med* 1996;124:708.

Price VH: Treatment of hair loss. *N Engl J Med* 1999;341:964.

Rhoden EL, Morgenthaler A: Risks of testosterone-replacement therapy and recommendations for monitoring. *N Engl J Med* 2004;350:482.

Rittmaster RS: Medical treatment of androgen-dependent hirsutism. *J Clin Endocrinol Metab* 1995;80:2559.

Rossouw JE, et al: Risks and benefits of estrogen plus progestin in healthy postmenopausal women: Principal results from the Women's Health Initiative randomized controlled trial. *JAMA* 2002;288:321.

Smallridge RC, Ladenson PW: Hypothyroidism in pregnancy: Consequences to neonatal health. *J Clin Endocrinol Metab* 2001;86:2349.

Tang XT, et al: Cellular mechanisms of growth inhibition of human epithelial ovarian cancer cell line by LH-releasing hormone antagonist cetrorelix. *J Clin Endocrinol Metab* 2002;87:3721.

Toft AD: Clinical practice: Subclinical hyperthyroidism. *N Engl J Med* 2001;345:512.

Van Wely M, et al: Human menopausal gonadotropin versus recombinant follicle stimulation hormone for ovarian stimulation in assisted reproductive cycles (Cochrane Review). *Cochrane Database Syst Rev* 2003;(1):CD003973.

Weisberg E: Interactions between oral contraceptives and antifungals/antibacterials. Is contraceptive failure the result? *Clin Pharmacokinet* 1999;36:309.

Wiersinga QM: Thyroid hormone replacement therapy. *Horm Res* 2001;56(Suppl 1):74.

Windisch PA, et al: Recombinant human growth hormone for AIDS-associated wasting. *Ann Pharmacother* 1998;32:437.

Woeber KA: Update on the management of hyperthyroidism and hypothyroidism. *Arch Intern Med* 2000;160:1067.

Women's Health Initiative Investigators: Risk and benefits of estrogen plus progestin in healthy postmenopausal women. Principal results from the Women's Health Initiative randomized controlled trial. *JAMA* 2002;288:321.

Rehabilitation

Burmeister LA, Flores A: Subclinical thyrotoxicosis and the heart. *Thyroid* 2002;12:495.

Dudgeon WD, et al: Counteracting muscle wasting in HIV-infected individuals. *HIV Med* 2006;7:200.

Florakis D, et al: Sustained reduction in circulating cholesterol in adult hypopituitary patients given low dose titrated growth hormone replacement therapy: A two year study. *Clin Endocrinol* (Oxf) 2000;53:453.

Gruenewald DA, Matsumoto AM: Testosterone supplementation therapy for older men: Potential benefits and risks. *J Am Geriatr Soc* 2003;51:101; discussion 115.

Kahaly GJ, et al: Cardiovascular hemodynamics and exercise tolerance in thyroid disease. *Thyroid* 2002;12:473.

Kahaly GJ, et al: Cardiac risks of hyperthyroidism in the elderly. *Thyroid* 1998;8:1165.

Raza JA, et al: Ischemic heart disease in women and the role of hormone therapy. *Int J Cardiol* 2004;96:7.

Roffi M, et al: Thyrotoxicosis and the cardiovascular system: Subtle but serious effects. *Cleve Clin J Med* 2003;70:57.

Sattler FR, et al: Effects of pharmacological doses of nandrolone decanoate and progressive resistance training in immunodeficient patients infected with human immunodeficiency virus. *J Clin Endocrinol Metab* 1999;84:1268.

23

CORTICOSTEROIDS AND CORTICOSTEROID ANTAGONISTS

The endogenous corticosteroids are produced by the adrenal cortex and are essential for life. As with the gonadal steroid hormones discussed in Chapter 22, corticosteroids are synthesized from cholesterol. They comprise two major physiologic and pharmacologic groups, **glucocorticoids** and mineralocorticoids (Figure 23–1). Glucocorticoids have important effects on intermediary metabolism, catabolism, immune responses, and inflammation. Mineralocorticoids regulate sodium and potassium transport in the collecting tubules of the kidney. A third group, the adrenal androgens (dehydroepiandrosterone [DHEA] and androstenedione) constitute the major endogenous precursors of estrogen in females in whom ovarian function is deficient or absent (e.g., postmenopausal) and in preadolescent males. Drugs that modulate the physiologic effects of endogenous corticosteroids either mimic the corticosteroids or inhibit corticosteroid synthesis or receptor interactions.

Like other hormones under the control of the hypothalamic and pituitary endocrine system, glucocorticoids provide feedback inhibition of their own production by acting in the hypothalamus and pituitary. Glucocorticoids inhibit the production of **corticotropin-releasing factor** (CRF) within the hypothalamus and **adrenocorticotropic hormone** (ACTH) within the pituitary. CRF controls the release of ACTH, which in turn regulates corticosteroid production within the adrenal cortex. A key action of *exogenous* glucocorticoids is activation of this feedback inhibition system with subsequent suppression of endogenous adrenal steroid production. After chronic treatment with exogenous glucocorticoids, recovery of the endogenous system takes weeks to months.

A large number of synthetic glucocorticoids are available. They can be delivered by a variety of routes, including oral, intravenous, intra-articular, and topical.

GLUCOCORTICOIDS

Mechanism of Action

Steroid hormones enter the cell and bind to cytosolic receptors. The complex of the receptor and its bound steroid translocates to the nucleus where it alters gene expression by binding to **glucocorticoid response elements** (GREs) (Figure 23–2). Tissue-specific responses to steroids are made possible by the presence of different protein regulators in each tissue that control the interaction between the hormone-receptor complex, other transcription factors, and particular response elements.

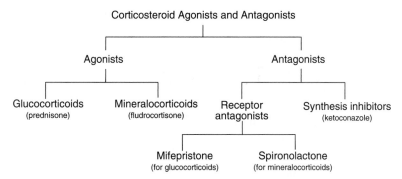

Figure 23–1. Classification of drugs that mimic or block the effects of endogenous corticosteroids.

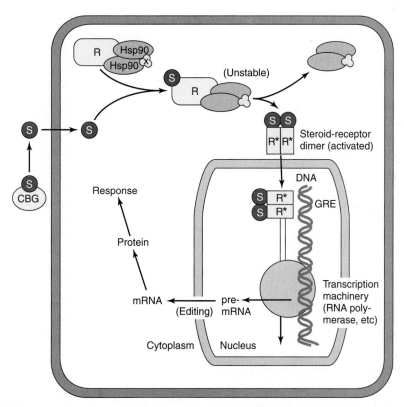

Figure 23–2. Mechanism of glucocorticoid action. This figure models the interaction of a steroid (S), with its receptor (R) and the subsequent events in a target cell. The steroid is present in the blood—bound to the corticosteroid-binding globulin (CBG)—but it enters the cell as the free form. The intracellular receptor (R) is bound to stabilizing proteins, including heat shock protein 90 (Hsp90) and several others. When the complex binds a molecule of steroid, the Hsp90 and associated molecules are released. The steroid-receptor complex enters the nucleus as a dimer, binds to the glucocorticoid response element (GRE), and thereby regulates gene transcription by RNA polymerase II and associated transcription factors. The resulting mRNA is edited and exported to the cytoplasm for the production of protein that contributes to the final hormone response.

Organ and Tissue Effects

Glucocorticoids have multiple effects within the body. They are important regulators of intermediary metabolism of carbohydrates, lipids, and proteins, and cause a general catabolic effect. Glucocorticoids also stimulate **gluconeogenesis.** As a result, blood glucose level rises, and insulin secretion is stimulated. Both **lipolysis** and **lipogenesis** are stimulated, with a net increase of fat deposition in certain areas, particularly the face, shoulders, and back. Chronic use of high doses of corticosteroids results in a characteristic appearance described as "cushingoid," which is named after the adrenal hypercortisolism associated with excessive pituitary production of ACTH (Cushing's syndrome). The cushingoid appearance includes a "moon face" and "buffalo hump" on the posterior base of the neck. Glucocorticoids stimulate muscle protein breakdown and amino acid release, which results in skeletal muscle wasting and deconditioning with chronic corticosteroid use. In addition, lymphoid and connective tissue, fat, and skin undergo wasting under the influence of high concentrations of these steroids. Catabolic effects on bone can lead to osteoporosis. In children, growth is inhibited.

Glucocorticoids have very important anti-inflammatory and immunosuppressive effects (Chapters 32 and 34). These drugs have a dramatic effect on the distribution and function of leukocytes. They increase neutrophils and decrease lymphocytes, eosinophils, basophils, and monocytes. The migration of leukocytes is also inhibited. The mechanisms underlying these anti-inflammatory effects include decreases in eicosanoid metabolism and decreases in the production of cytokines that participate in inflammatory reactions (e.g., interleukin-2, interleukin-3, and **platelet-activating factor**). The immunosuppressive effects of glucocorticoids include inhibition of mechanisms involved in cell-mediated immunologic functions, especially those dependent on lymphocytes. Glucocorticoids are actively lymphotoxic and, for this reason, are important in the treatment of hematologic cancers. The drugs do not interfere with the development of normal acquired immunity, but delay rejection reactions in patients with organ transplants.

Endogenous glucocorticoids, such as cortisol, are required for normal renal excretion of water loads. The glucocorticoids also have effects on the central nervous system (CNS). When given in large doses, especially for long periods of time, these drugs can cause profound behavioral changes. Large doses stimulate gastric acid secretion and decrease resistance to ulcer formation.

Clinical Uses

Glucocorticoids are used in a wide variety of conditions including both adrenal and nonadrenal disorders. Some common therapeutic uses are presented in Table 23–1. Glucocorticoids are essential to preserving life in patients with chronic adrenal cortical insufficiency (Addison's disease), and high doses are necessary in acute adrenal insufficiency (addisonian crisis), which can be precipitated in patients with Addison's disease by infection, surgery, or trauma. Glucocorticoids are also used in certain types of congenital adrenal hyperplasia, in which synthesis of abnormal forms of corticosteroids are stimulated by ACTH. In these conditions, administration of a potent synthetic glucocorticoid suppresses ACTH secretion sufficiently to reduce synthesis of the abnormal steroids.

Many nonadrenal disorders respond to corticosteroid therapy. Some of these are inflammatory or immunologic in nature. Examples include asthma, organ transplant rejection, arthritis and other diseases of connective tissue, and exophthalmos (an ocular disorder associated with Graves' disease). Other applications include the treatment of hematopoietic cancers, neurologic disorders, chemotherapy-induced vomiting, hypercalcemia, and high-altitude sickness. **Betamethasone,** a synthetic glucocorticoid with a low degree of protein binding, is given to women in premature labor to hasten maturation of the fetal lungs. The degree of benefit conferred by exogenous corticosteroids differs considerably in various disorders, but toxicity often limits their long-term use.

▉ IMPORTANT GLUCOCORTICOIDS

Properties of some important glucocorticoid drugs are presented in Table 23–2. The major endogenous glucocorticoid is **cortisol (hydrocortisone).** Endogenous cortisol secretion is regulated by ACTH and varies with the circadian rhythm. Peak plasma cortisol levels occur in the morning and the trough occurs about midnight. In the plasma, cortisol is 95% bound to corticosteroid-binding

Table 23–1. Examples of therapeutic indications for glucocorticoids in nonadrenal disorders

Disorder	Examples
Allergic reactions	Angioneurotic edema, asthma, bee stings, contact dermatitis, drug reactions, allergic rhinitis, serum sickness, urticaria
Collagen-vascular disorders	Giant cell arteritis, lupus erythematosus, mixed connective tissue syndromes, polymyositis, polymyalgia rheumatica, rheumatoid arthritis, temporal arteritis
Eye diseases	Acute uveitis, allergic conjunctivitis, choroiditis, optic neuritis
Gastrointestinal diseases	Inflammatory bowel disease, nontropical sprue, subacute hepatic necrosis
Hematologic disorders	Acquired hemolytic anemia, acute allergic purpura, leukemia, autoimmune hemolytic anemia, idiopathic thrombocytopenic purpura, multiple myeloma
Systemic inflammation	Acute respiratory distress syndrome (sustained therapy with moderate dosage accelerates recovery and decreases mortality)
Infections	Gram-negative septicemia (occasionally helpful to suppress excessive inflammation)
Inflammatory conditions of bones and joints	Arthritis, bursitis, tenosynovitis
Neurologic disorders	Cerebral edema (large doses of dexamethasone are given to patients following brain surgery to minimize cerebral edema in the postoperative period), multiple sclerosis
Organ transplants	Prevention and treatment of rejection
Pulmonary diseases	Aspiration pneumonia, bronchial asthma, prevention of infant respiratory distress syndrome, sarcoidosis
Renal disorders	Nephrotic syndrome
Skin diseases	Atopic dermatitis, dermatoses, lichen simplex chronicus (localized neurodermatitis), mycosis fungoides, pemphigus, seborrheic dermatitis, xerosis
Thyroid diseases	Malignant exophthalmos, subacute thyroiditis
Miscellaneous	Hypercalcemia, mountain sickness, chemotherapy-induced nausea and vomiting

Table 23–2. Properties of representative corticosteroids

Agent	Duration of Action (hours)	Anti-inflammatory Potency[1]	Salt-retaining Potency[1]	Topical Activity
Primarily glucocorticoid				
Cortisol	8–12	1	1	0
Prednisone	12–24	4	0.3	(+)
Triamcinolone	15–24	5	0	+++
Dexamethasone	24–36	30	0	+++++
Primarily mineralocorticoid				
Aldosterone	1–2	0.3	3000	0
Fludrocortisone	8–12	10	125–250	0

[1]Relative to cortisol

globulin. Exogenously administered cortisol is well absorbed from the gastrointestinal tract and is cleared by the liver. Compared with its synthetic congeners, it has a short duration of action. Although it diffuses poorly across normal skin, topical cortisol preparations are readily absorbed across inflamed skin and mucous membranes. Cortisol also has a small, but significant, salt-retaining mineralocorticoid effect. This is an important cause of hypertension in patients with a cortisol-secreting adrenal tumor or a pituitary ACTH-secreting tumor (Cushing's syndrome).

The mechanism of action of the synthetic glucocorticoids is identical to that of endogenous cortisol. A large number of glucocorticoid preparations are available for use. **Prednisone** and its active metabolite—**prednisolone, dexamethasone,** and **triamcinolone** are representatives. Compared with cortisol, their properties include longer half-life and duration of action, reduced salt-retaining effect, and better penetration of lipid barriers for topical activity. Special glucocorticoids have been developed for use in asthma and other conditions in which activity on mucous membranes or skin is required, but systemic effects need to be avoided. For example, **beclomethasone** and **budesonide** readily penetrate airway mucosa, but have very short half-lives after they enter the blood, so that systemic effects and toxicity are greatly reduced.

Toxicity

Most of the toxic effects of the glucocorticoids are predictable from the effects already described. Metabolic effects include skeletal growth inhibition, insulin-resistant diabetes mellitus, muscle wasting, and osteoporosis. Chronic salt and water retention can lead to hypertension. Hyperlipidemia and subsequent atherosclerosis increase the risk of adverse cardiovascular events. Peptic ulcers may also occur. Affective changes initially include insomnia and **euphoria** ("steroid high") followed by depression and occasionally psychosis. An important consequence of chronic corticosteroid therapy is adrenal suppression secondary to suppression of ACTH secretion by the pituitary. Abrupt discontinuation of corticosteroid in someone who has been treated chronically will result in a potentially life-threatening **addisonian crisis**.

Methods for minimizing corticosteroid toxicity include local administration such as aerosols for asthma, alternate-day therapy to reduce pituitary suppression, and dose tapering soon after achieving a therapeutic response. To avoid adrenal insufficiency in patients who have had long-term therapy, additional "stress doses" may need to be given during serious illness or before major surgery. Patients who are being withdrawn from glucocorticoids after protracted use should have their doses tapered slowly over the course of several months to allow recovery of normal adrenal function.

■ MINERALOCORTICOIDS

The major endogenous mineralocorticoid in humans is **aldosterone**, which has previously been discussed in connection with hypertension and control of its secretion by angiotensin II (Chapters 4 and 7). Secretion of aldosterone is regulated by both ACTH and the renin-angiotensin system and is important in the regulation of blood volume and blood pressure (Figure 4-5). Aldosterone has a short half-life and little glucocorticoid activity (Table 23–2). The mechanism of aldosterone action is similar to that of glucocorticoids. The mineralocorticoid receptor shares similar homology with the glucocorticoid receptor. Other mineralocorticoids include **deoxycorticosterone** (the naturally occurring precursor of aldosterone) and a synthetic analog, **fludrocortisone**. The latter has significant glucocorticoid activity (Table 23–2). Because of its long duration of action, fludrocortisone is favored for replacement therapy after surgical removal of the adrenal gland; chronic, stable Addison's disease; and in other conditions in which mineralocorticoid therapy is needed.

■ CORTICOSTEROID ANTAGONISTS

Corticosteroid receptor antagonists or inhibitors of corticosteroid synthesis are used to antagonize the effects of endogenous corticosteroids. The mineralocorticoid receptor antagonists, **spironolactone** and **eplerenone**, were discussed in connection with the diuretics (Chapter 7) and heart failure (Chapter 9). **Mifepristone** (RU 486), an antagonist of glucocorticoid and progesterone receptors, was previously discussed (Chapter 22) and has been used in the treatment of Cushing's syndrome.

Corticosteroids and the gonadal hormones are synthesized from cholesterol. **Ketoconazole,** an antifungal drug, inhibits this process (Figure 22–6) and has been used in several conditions in which reduced steroid levels are desirable. These include adrenal carcinoma, hirsutism, and breast and prostate cancers. **Aminoglutethimide** blocks the conversion of cholesterol to pregnenolone and also inhibits synthesis of all hormonally active steroids. Aminoglutethimide can be used in conjunction with other drugs for treatment of steroid-producing adrenocortical cancer. These drugs are used in the treatment of adrenal cancer when surgical therapy is impractical or unsuccessful because of metastases.

REHABILITATION FOCUS

The glucocorticoid class of pharmacologic agents significantly influences the clinical practice of physical therapists for several reasons. First, many patients with orthopedic dysfunction referred for rehabilitation have previously taken or are currently receiving glucocorticoids. Local glucocorticoid injections are commonly used in patients with orthopedic dysfunctions ranging from carpal tunnel syndrome to ankylosing spondylitis. These injections decrease pain and inflammation at the site of tissue injury. Rehabilitation services are often a necessary adjunct to pharmacotherapy if optimal outcome with minimal recurrence is to be achieved. Second, long-term use of glucocorticoids often results in adverse effects that require the expertise of the physical therapist. For example, long-term glucocorticoid use increases the incidence of hyperglycemia and type 2 diabetes mellitus. Thus, the therapist may see these patients for complications resulting from diabetes, as discussed in Chapter 24. Myopathy is also a consequence of prolonged glucocorticoid use. Depending upon the severity, myopathy may require rehabilitation because of significant type 2 muscle fiber atrophy. Aseptic necrosis of the hip is a well-documented toxicity of long-term systemic glucocorticoid use, which can result in fractures and other hip dysfunction. Physical therapists also use glucocorticoids to treat their patients. Therapists deliver glucocorticoids transcutaneously by iontophoresis or phonophoresis. For drug delivery, iontophoresis uses electromotive charge-charge repulsion, whereas phonophoresis uses the mechanical energy of ultrasound. These modalities increase glucocorticoid transcutaneous flux and improve clinical outcomes in conditions ranging from plantar fasciitis to epithelioid granulomas in patients with sarcoidosis. Critical issues currently debated in the literature for these drug delivery modalities include the depth of tissue penetration of drugs and parameters that optimize transcutaneous delivery. The reader should note that localized drug delivery does not prevent systemic absorption. Because phonophoretic or iontophoretic administration of glucocorticoids may require a prescription, therapists should consult appropriate state authorities prior to administering these drugs.

CLINICAL RELEVANCE FOR REHABILITATION

Adverse Drug Reactions
Glucocorticoids
- Type 2 diabetes mellitus
- Muscle wasting
- Hypertension
- Behavioral changes
- Immunosuppression
- Gastrointestinal distress

Effects Interfering with Rehabilitation
- Increased risk of infection
- Decreased endurance
- Increased risk for cardiovascular dysfunction such as angina pectoris or dysrhythmias
- Exacerbation of exercise-induced hyperglycemia

Possible Therapy Solutions
- Monitor blood glucose levels in hyperglycemic patients
- Check blood pressure and heart rate in all patients
- Look for manifestations of dependent edema
- Educate patient about increased risk of infection

Potentiation of Functional Outcomes Secondary to Drug Therapy
- Iontophoretic and phonophoretic delivery of glucocorticoids may decrease pain and associated inflammation and increase function during the rehabilitation process.

PROBLEM-ORIENTED PATIENT STUDY

Brief History: The patient is a 20-year-old cross-country runner in her junior year of college. She was diagnosed with plantar fasciitis related to her collegiate sport. The team physician referred her to rehabilitation for conservative treatment in an attempt to allow her continued participation on the cross-country team. The patient has no other significant medical problems.

Current Medical Status and Drug Therapy: The patient was given a prescription for meloxicam, a nonsteroidal anti-inflammatory drug (Chapter 34) to take on an "as needed" basis to decrease plantar pain and inflammation.

Rehabilitation Setting: When the patient arrived at the outpatient clinic, her primary symptom was heel pain at the calcaneal origin of the plantar fascia. She was evaluated for active and passive range of motion at the ankle and foot. The patient was examined standing with and without her running shoes, and she was filmed while running on a treadmill. Finally, her running shoes were examined for construction and usage.

Problem/Clinical Options: Plantar fasciitis is a common cause of heel pain in adults, in both athletes and nonathletes. Multiple causes can produce this musculoskeletal dysfunction. Poorly designed athletic shoes and athletic shoes worn beyond their functional life span are significant contributing causes.

A treatment regimen was developed for this patient. To decrease the pain and inflammation, the patient was instructed to ice the plantar surface of the mid-foot following daily training to decrease pain and inflammation. Treatment sessions with the physical therapist consisted of stretching the plantar fascia and gastrocnemius-soleus muscle complex and strengthening exercises for the extrinsic muscles. At the end of each session, dexamethasone-phosphate was iontophoresed from the cathode (mA.minutes) into the plantar region. Addition of dexamethasone-phosphate iontophoresis to a treatment plan for plantar fasciitis has been demonstrated to shorten recovery time. The patient was advised to consider additional consultation for different running shoes or to replace her current shoes more frequently to help prevent recurrent bouts of plantar fasciitis. Failure of conservative rehabilitation treatment for plantar fasciitis may require glucocorticoid injection into the plantar fascia or, as a last resort, surgical procedures.

PREPARATIONS AVAILABLE[1]

Glucocorticoids for Oral and Parenteral Use[1]

Betamethasone (Celestone)
Oral: 0.6-mg tablets; 0.6 mg/5 mL syrup

Betamethasone sodium phosphate (Celestone Phosphate)
Parenteral: 4 mg/mL for IV, IM, intralesional, or intra-articular injection

Cortisone (generic, Cortone Acetate)
Oral: 5-, 10-, 25-mg tablets
Parenteral: 50 mg/mL solution

Dexamethasone (generic, Decadron, others)
Oral: 0.25-, 0.5-, 0.75-, 1-, 1.5-, 2-, 4-, 6-mg tablets; 0.5 mg/5 mL elixir; 0.5 mg/5 mL, 0.5 mg/0.5 mL solution

Dexamethasone acetate (generic, Decadron-LA, others)
Parenteral: 8 mg/mL suspension for IM, intralesional, or intra-articular injection; 16 mg/mL suspension for intralesional injection

Dexamethasone sodium phosphate (generic, Decadron Phosphate, others)
Parenteral: 4, 10, 20 mg/mL for IV, IM, intralesional, or intra-articular injection; 24 mg/mL for IV use only

Hydrocortisone (cortisol) (generic, Cortef)
Oral: 5-, 10-, 20-mg tablets

Hydrocortisone acetate (generic)
Parenteral: 25, 50 mg/mL suspension for intralesional, soft tissue, or intra-articular injection

Hydrocortisone cypionate (Cortef)
Oral: 10 mg/5 mL suspension

Hydrocortisone sodium phosphate (Hydrocortone)
Parenteral: 50 mg/mL for IV, IM, or SC injection

Hydrocortisone sodium succinate (generic, SoluCortef)
Parenteral: 100, 250, 500, 1000 mg/vial for IV, IM injection

Methylprednisolone (generic, Medrol)
Oral: 2-, 4-, 8-, 16-, 24-, 32-mg tablets

Methylprednisolone acetate (generic, DepoMedrol)
Parenteral: 20, 40, 80 mg/mL for IM, intralesional, or intra-articular injection

Methylprednisolone sodium succinate (generic, Solu-Medrol)
Parenteral: 40, 125, 500, 1000, 2000 mg/vial for injection

Prednisolone (generic, Delta-Cortef, Prelone)
Oral: 5-mg tablets; 5, 15 mg/5 mL syrup

Prednisolone acetate (generic)
Parenteral: 25, 50 mg/mL for soft tissue or intra-articular injection

Prednisolone sodium phosphate (Hydeltrasol, others)
Oral: 5 mg/5 mL solution
Parenteral: 20 mg/mL for IV, IM, intra-articular, or intralesional injection

Prednisolone tebutate (generic)
Oral: 5 mg/5 mL liquid
Parenteral: 20 mg/mL for intra-articular or intralesional injection

Prednisone (generic, Meticorten)
Oral: 1-, 2.5-, 5-, 10-, 20-, 50-mg tablets; 1, 5 mg/mL solution and syrup

Triamcinolone (generic, Aristocort, Kenacort)
Oral: 4-, 8-mg tablets; 4 mg/5 mL syrup

Triamcinolone acetonide (generic, Kenalog)
Parenteral: 3, 10, 40 mg/mL for IM, intra-articular, or intralesional injection

Triamcinolone diacetate (generic)
Parenteral: 25, 40 mg/mL for IM, intra-articular, or intralesional injection

Triamcinolone hexacetonide (Aristospan)
Parenteral: 5, 20 mg/mL for intra-articular, intralesional, or sublesional injection

---

[1]For Glucocorticoids for Aerosol Use, see Chapter 35; for Glucocorticoids for Gastrointestinal Use, see Chapter 36.

Mineralocorticoids

Fludrocortisone acetate (generic, Florinef Acetate)
Oral: 0.1-mg tablets

Adrenal Steroid Inhibitors

Aminoglutethimide (Cytadren)
Oral: 250-mg tablets

Ketoconazole (generic, Nizoral)
Oral: 200-mg tablets (unlabeled use)

Mifepristone (Mifeprex)
Oral: 200-mg tablets

REFERENCES

Alesci S, et al: Glucocorticoid-induced osteoporosis: From basic mechanisms to clinical aspects. *Neuroimmunomodulation* 2005;12:1.

Bamberger CM, et al: Molecular determinants of glucocorticoid receptor function and tissue sensitivity to glucocorticoids. *Endocr Rev* 1996; 17:245.

Barnes PJ, Adcock I: Anti-inflammatory actions of steroids: Molecular mechanisms. *Trends Pharmacol Sci* 1993; 14:436.

Chrousos GP: Glucocorticoid therapy and withdrawal. *Curr Pract Med* 1999;1:291.

Czock, D et al: Pharmacokinetics and pharmacodynamics of systemically administered glucocorticoids. *Clin Pharmacokinet* 2005;44:61.

Franchimont D, et al: Glucocorticoids and inflammation revisited: The state of the art. *Neuroimmunomodulation* 2002–03;10:247.

Hochberg Z, et al: Endocrine withdrawal syndromes. *Endocrine Rev* 2003;24:523.

Tuckermann JP, et al: Molecular mechanisms of glucocorticoids in the control of inflammation and lymphocyte apoptosis. *Crit Rev Clin Lab Sci* 2005;42:71.

Tyrell JB, et al: Adrenal cortex. In *Basic & Clinical Endocrinology*, 7th ed. Greenspan FS, Gardner DG, eds. New York: McGraw-Hill, 2003.

Rehabilitation

Banga AK, Panus PC: Clinical applications of iontophoretic devices in rehabilitation medicine. *Crit Rev Phys Rehab Med* 1998;10:147.

Blackford J, et al: Iontophoresis of dexamethasone-phosphate into the equine tibiotarsal joint. *J Vet Pharmacol Ther* 2000;23:229.

Byl NN: The use of ultrasound as an enhancer for transcutaneous drug delivery: Phonophoresis. *Phys Ther* 1995;75:539.

Byl NN, et al: The effects of phonophoresis with corticosteroids: a controlled pilot study. *J. Orthop. Sports Phys Ther* 1993;18:590.

Cobiella CE: Shoulder pain in sports. *Hosp Med* 2004; 65:652.

Crosby W, Humble RN: Rehabilitation of plantar fasciitis. *Clin Podiatr Med Surg* 2001;18:225.

Dougados M, et al: Conventional treatments for ankylosing spondylitis. *Ann Rheum Dis* 2002;61(Suppl 3):iii40.

Gogstetter DS, Goldsmith LA: Treatment of cutaneous sarcoidosis using phonophoresis. *J Am Acad Dermatol* 1999;40:767.

Gudeman SD, et al: Treatment of plantar fasciitis by iontophoresis of 0.4% dexamethasone. A randomized, double-blind, placebo-controlled study. *Am J Sports Med* 1997;25:312.

Harris PR: Iontophoresis: Clinical research in musculoskeletal inflammatory conditions. *J Orthop Sports Phys Ther* 1982;4:109.

Hart LE: Corticosteroid injections, physiotherapy, or a wait-and-see policy for lateral epicondylitis? *Clin J Sport Med* 2002;12:403.

Hawkins RJ, Hobeika PE; Impingement syndrome in the athletic shoulder. *Clin Sports Med* 1983;2:391.

Newcomer KL, et al: Corticosteroid injection in early treatment of lateral epicondylitis. *Clin J Sport Med* 2001;11:214.

Panus PC: Physical agents for transdermal drug delivery: Iontophoresis and phonophoresis. In *Physical Agents: Theory and Practice*, 2nd ed. Behrens B, Michlovitz SL, eds. Philadelphia: F.A. Davis, 2006:233.

Polsonetti BW, et al: Steroid-induced myopathy in the ICU. *Ann Pharmacother* 2002;36:1741.

Schepsis AA, et al: Plantar fasciitis. Etiology, treatment, surgical results, and review of the literature. *Clin Orthop Relat Res* 1991;185.

Smidt N, et al: Corticosteroid injections, physiotherapy, or a wait-and-see policy for lateral epicondylitis: a randomised controlled trial. *Lancet* 2002;359:657.

Smutok MA, et al: Failure to detect dexamethasone phosphate in the local venous blood postcathodic iontophoresis in humans. *J Orthop Sports Phys Ther* 2002;32:461.

Tisdel CL, et al: Diagnosing and treating plantar fasciitis: A conservative approach to plantar heel pain. *Cleve Clin J Med* 1999;66:231.

Vad V, et al: Exercise recommendations in athletes with early osteoarthritis of the knee. *Sports Med* 2002;32:729.

Wilk BR, et al: Defective running shoes as a contributing factor in plantar fasciitis in a triathlete. *J Orthop Sports Phys Ther* 2000;30:21.

Young CC, et al: Treatment of plantar fasciitis. *Am Fam Physician* 2001;63:467, 477.

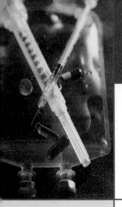

24

PANCREATIC HORMONES AND ANTIDIABETIC DRUGS

The islets of Langerhans in the pancreas contain four main types of endocrine cells (Table 24–1). These cells include **glucagon**-producing alpha cells (A or α), **insulin**- and **amylin**-producing beta cells (B or β), **somatostatin**-producing delta cells (D or δ), and **pancreatic polypeptide**-producing cells (F). Of these, the insulin-producing B cells are the most numerous. The most common disease related to pancreatic function is **diabetes mellitus** (DM), a deficiency of insulin production or effect.

Knowledge of the mechanism of action and physiologic function of insulin is critical in understanding the clinical use of insulin and oral hypoglycemic drugs as the pharmacologic treatments of DM.

Insulin is required in type 1 DM, and several parenteral formulations of insulin are available (Figure 24–1). Type 2 DM can be treated with drug classes that include four types of oral antidiabetic drugs, incretin mimetics, and an amylinomimetic (Figure 24–1), as well as insulin, if required. Glucagon, a hormone that affects the liver, cardiovascular system, and gastrointestinal tract, can be used to treat severe hypoglycemia in patients with DM.

■ INSULIN

Insulin is synthesized as proinsulin, an 86–amino acid single-chain polypeptide. Proinsulin is processed in the Golgi apparatus of pancreatic B cells and then packaged into granules in the form of crystals consisting of two atoms of zinc and six molecules of insulin. In the Golgi apparatus, cleavage of proinsulin removes a 31–amino acid C peptide and leaves two peptide chains that are then cross-linked by two disulfide bonds. Neither proinsulin nor C peptide appears to have important physiologic actions.

Insulin release from pancreatic B cells occurs at a low basal rate, and at a much higher rate in response to a variety of stimuli, especially glucose. The mechanism by which glucose regulates insulin release is well understood. In B cells, glucose metabolism increases intracellular adenosine triphosphate (ATP) levels. ATP-regulated potassium channels respond to increased ATP concentrations by closing, thus reducing potassium conductance (Figure 24–2). Closure of potassium channels results in membrane depolarization (fewer positive ions leaving the cell), which in turn promotes opening of voltage-gated calcium channels. The resulting increase in intracellular free calcium triggers insulin secretion.

Insulin circulates in the blood and exerts its effects by activating insulin receptors located on almost all cells. The insulin receptor is a transmembrane tyrosine kinase receptor. When activated by insulin binding, the insulin receptor phosphorylates itself and a set of intracellular

Table 24–1.	Pancreatic islet cells and their secretory products	
Cell Types	Approximate Percentage of Islet Mass	Secretory Products
A cell (alpha)	20	Glucagon, proglucagon
B cell (beta)	75	Insulin, C peptide, proinsulin, amylin
D cell (delta)	3–5	Somatostatin
F cell (PP cell)[1]	<2	Pancreatic polypeptide

[1]Within pancreatic polypeptide-rich lobules of adult islets, located only in the posterior portion of the head of the human pancreas, glucagon cells are scarce (<0.5%) and F cells make up as much as 80% of the cells.

proteins that comprise intracellular signaling pathways. This series of phosphorylations within the cell results in multiple effects including translocation of **glucose transporters** (GLUTs) to the plasma membrane, changes in activity of enzymes involved in carbohydrate, protein, and lipid metabolism, and complex effects on cell growth and division.

Physiologic Effects

While insulin has important effects in almost every tissue of the body, the principal targets are liver, muscle, and adipose tissue (Figure 24–3). The cellular functions regulated by insulin in these tissues are outlined in Table 24–2. In the liver, insulin increases glycogen synthesis by increasing the activity of enzymes that convert glucose to glycogen (e.g., glucokinase, glycogen synthase) and by inhibiting enzymes involved in glycogenolysis and gluconeogenesis (e.g., glycogen phosphorylase, glucose-6-phosphate, phosphoenolpyruvate carboxykinase, and fructose-1,6-bisphosphatase). Insulin also promotes glycolysis and carbohydrate oxidation by increasing the activity of enzymes that convert glucose to pyruvate (e.g., phosphofructokinase and pyruvate kinase) and the enzyme that accomplishes oxidation of pyruvate (pyruvate dehydrogenase). Finally, insulin increases the synthesis and storage of triglycerides and the formation of very low-density lipoprotein (VLDL) and decreases protein catabolism. In muscle, insulin stimulates glucose uptake by recruiting GLUT4 transporters to the plasma membrane. Through effects on enzymes in metabolic pathways, insulin promotes glycogen synthesis, glycolysis, and carbohydrate oxidation. Insulin also promotes protein synthesis and

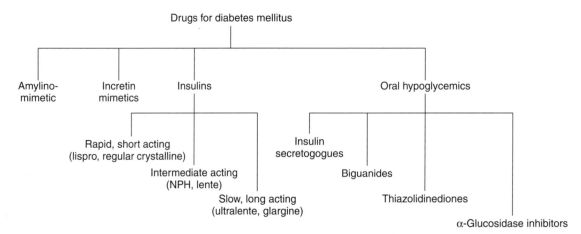

Figure 24–1. Drug classes used in the treatment of diabetes mellitus. Drug classes may be initially divided into insulin, amylinomimetics, incretin mimetics, and oral hypoglycemics. The oral hypoglycemics are subsequently divided into four classes based on mechanism of action.

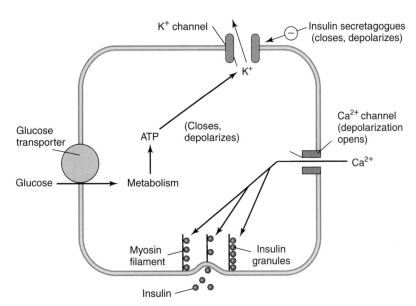

Figure 24–2. Model of insulin release from pancreatic B cell by glucose and insulin secretagogues. In the resting cell with normal (low) ATP levels, potassium moves out of the cell down its concentration gradient through ATP-gated potassium channels. This conductance helps maintain a relatively hyperpolarized potential. In this state, insulin release is minimal. When extracellular and, consequently, intracellular glucose concentration rises, ATP production increases. ATP binds to and closes these potassium channels and the cell depolarizes (positive charges stay inside the cell). Voltage-gated calcium channels open in response to depolarization, allowing calcium to enter the cell. Increased intracellular calcium results in increased insulin secretion. Insulin secretagogues close ATP-dependent potassium channels, thereby depolarizing the membrane and increasing insulin release. (Modified and reproduced, with permission, from Greenspan F, Baxter JD, eds. *Basic & Clinical Endocrinology*, 4th ed. Norwalk, CT, 1994. Now published by McGraw-Hill, New York.)

inhibits protein breakdown. Finally, insulin promotes glucose uptake in adipose tissue through GLUT4 transporters. Through effects on enzymes involved in glycolysis and lipid synthesis, glucose is used to fuel synthesis of triglycerides. Simultaneously, insulin inhibits the breakdown of triglycerides to glycerol and free fatty acids. In addition, insulin stimulates synthesis of lipoprotein lipase, which liberates fatty acids from circulating chylomicrons and VLDL so they can enter adipocytes and be converted into triglycerides. Insulin's net effect in liver, muscle, and adipose tissue is to move glucose from blood into cells, which boosts supplies of glycogen and lipids that can later be used to supply energy during fasting.

■ DIABETES MELLITUS

DM is diagnosed on the basis of more than one fasting blood glucose concentration in excess of 126 mg/dL, a 2-hour oral glucose tolerance test equal to or greater than 200 mg/dL, or a "casual" blood glucose level of greater than 200 mg/dL. Casual is defined as any time during a 24-hour period without regard to the time of the last meal. The serum concentration of hemoglobin $(Hb)A_{1c}$, a glycosylated hemoglobin, is another important index of the recent glycemic state of a patient. Thus, HbA_{1c} serves as an index of glucose levels over the previous 6 to 12 weeks (although it is heavily weighted toward the most recent 2 weeks), whereas

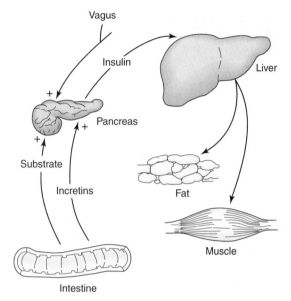

Figure 24–3. Insulin release from the pancreas is stimulated by increased blood glucose, vagal nerve stimulation, incretins (peptide hormones produced in the intestinal epithelium in response to food), and other factors. Insulin promotes synthesis (from circulating nutrients) and storage of glycogen, triglycerides, and protein in its major target tissues: liver, fat, and muscle.

Table 24–2.	Endocrine effects of insulin

Effect on liver:
  Reversal of catabolic features of insulin deficiency
    Inhibits glycogenolysis
    Inhibits conversion of fatty acids and amino acids to keto acids
    Inhibits conversion of amino acids to glucose
  Anabolic action
    Promotes glucose storage as glycogen (induces glucokinase and glycogen synthase, inhibits phosphorylase)
    Increases triglyceride synthesis and very low-density lipoprotein formation
Effect on muscle:
  Increased protein synthesis
    Increases amino acid transport
    Increases ribosomal protein synthesis
  Increased glycogen synthesis
    Increases glucose transport
    Induces glycogen synthase and inhibits phosphorylase
Effect on adipose tissue:
  Increased triglyceride storage
    Lipoprotein lipase is induced and activated by insulin to hydrolyze triglycerides from lipoproteins
    Glucose transport into cell provides glycerol phosphate to permit esterification of fatty acids supplied by lipoprotein transport
  Intracellular lipase is inhibited

blood or urine glucose concentration reflects glucose control near the time of sample collection. The normal range for HbA_{1c} in nondiabetic individuals is 4 to 6%, and the recommended level for diabetics is 7% or less.

The disease states that are included in the diagnosis of DM fall into three major categories: type 1 (insulin-dependent DM), type 2 (non-insulin-dependent DM), and gestational DM (diabetes of pregnancy). Other forms of DM are uncommon. Regardless of the cause of DM, the treatment of DM requires careful attention to blood glucose and HbA_{1c} concentrations.

Type 1 Diabetes Mellitus

The hallmarks of type 1 DM are selective B-cell destruction in the islets of Langerhans, severe or absolute insulin deficiency, and a high risk of ketoacidosis. This latter dangerous condition results from excessive metabolism of fat when glucose utilization is impaired. Administration of insulin is required in patients with type 1 DM. Type 1 DM is further subdivided into immune and idiopathic causes. The immune form, in which a patient's immune system mounts a destructive immunologic response to the pancreatic B cells, is the most common form of type 1 DM. Although most patients are younger than 30 years of age at the time of diagnosis of type 1 DM, the onset can occur at any age. Type 1 DM is found in all ethnic groups, but the highest incidence is in people from northern Europe and Sardinia. Susceptibility appears to involve a multifactorial genetic linkage, but only 15 to 20% of patients have a positive family history.

Type 2 Diabetes Mellitus

Type 2 DM is characterized by tissue resistance to the action of insulin combined with a *relative* deficiency in insulin secretion. A given individual may have more resistance or more B-cell deficiency, and the abnormalities may be mild or severe. Although insulin is produced by B cells in patients with type 2 DM, the amount secreted (which may be quite high) is inadequate to overcome the resistance, and blood glucose levels rise. The impaired insulin action also affects fat metabolism, resulting in increased free fatty acid flux and triglyceride levels, and a low serum concentration of high-density lipoprotein (HDL), the lipoprotein that has a protective effect against atherosclerosis. Individuals with type 2 DM may not require insulin to survive, but 30% or more will benefit from insulin therapy at some time during their lives to control high blood glucose levels. Ten to twenty percent of individuals in whom type 2 DM was initially diagnosed may actually have both type 1 and type 2 DM, or have a slowly progressing type 1, and ultimately will require full insulin replacement. Dehydration in untreated and poorly controlled individuals with type 2 DM can lead to a life-threatening condition called "non-ketotic hyperosmolar coma." In this condition, blood glucose may rise to six to twenty times the normal range, and an altered mental state develops that may progress to loss of consciousness. Urgent medical care and rehydration is required. Although people with type 2 DM ordinarily do not develop ketosis, ketoacidosis may occur as the result of a stressor such as infection or the use of a medication that enhances insulin resistance such as a glucocorticoid (Chapter 23).

Gestational Diabetes Mellitus

Gestational DM is defined as any abnormality in glucose levels noted for the first time during pregnancy, and is diagnosed in approximately 4% of pregnancies in the United States. During pregnancy, a hormone produced by the placenta (human placental lactogen) with homology to growth hormone and prolactin exerts an anti-insulin effect. This causes insulin resistance and DM in some women, particularly in the last trimester. Because gestational DM carries risks for maternal and fetal outcomes, pregnant women are routinely screened for gestational diabetes with glucose challenge tests in the second trimester. The standard therapy for gestational diabetes is insulin. However, recent clinical trials suggest that some oral antidiabetic drugs are safe in pregnancy.

DRUGS FOR TYPE 1 AND 2 DIABETES MELLITUS

Insulin Preparations

Insulins derived from animals (pork or beef) are no longer available in the United States. Pharmaceutical human insulin is manufactured by recombinant DNA technology. Because the native insulin molecule has a half-life of only a few minutes in the circulation, many preparations are formulated to release the hormone slowly into the circulation. The available insulin formulations provide five rates of onset and durations of effect: ultra-rapid onset, rapid onset with short action, intermediate onset and action, slow onset with peak action, and ultra-slow onset with no peak (i.e., plateau only) action (Table 24–3). All insulin preparations contain zinc. The ratio of zinc and other substances to insulin influences the rate of release of active hormone from the site of administration and the duration of action (Figure 24-4).

Ultra-rapid action insulins are represented by **insulin lispro, insulin aspart,** and **insulin glulisine.** These preparations are recombinant human insulins that contain transpositions of two amino acids or replacement of one or more native amino acids. These changes alter physical properties of the peptides so that they dissolve more rapidly at the site of administration and enter the circulation approximately twice as fast as regular crystalline insulin. These insulins are suitable for use immediately before meals. Unlike other insulin preparations, increasing the dose only increases the maximum effect, not the duration of effect.

Regular crystalline-zinc insulin is a rapid-onset and short-action formulation. The insulin is used intravenously in emergencies or administered subcutaneously in maintenance regimens, alone or mixed with intermediate- or long-acting preparations. Before the

Table 24–3. Insulin: types and activity[1]

Pharmacokinetic Type	Form	Activity (hours) Peak	Activity (hours) Duration
Ultra–rapid-onset			
Insulin lispro, insulin aspart, insulin glulisine[1]	Human, analog	0.25–0.5	3–4
Rapid-onset with short action			
Insulin injection USP (regular, crystalline zinc)[2]	Human	0.5–3	5–7
Intermediate-onset and action			
NPH insulin (isophane insulin suspension USP)[1]	Human	8–12	18–24
Lente insulin (insulin zinc suspension USP)[1]	Human	8–12	18–24
Slow-onset with peak action			
Ultralente insulin (insulin zinc suspension extended USP)[1]	Human	8–16	18–28
Ultra–long-onset with no peak action			
Insulin glargine, insulin detemir[1]	Human, analog	No peak	>24

USP = *United States Pharmacopeia.*
[1]Preparations available include 100 U/mL.
[2]Preparations available include 100 U/mL and one 500 U/mL.

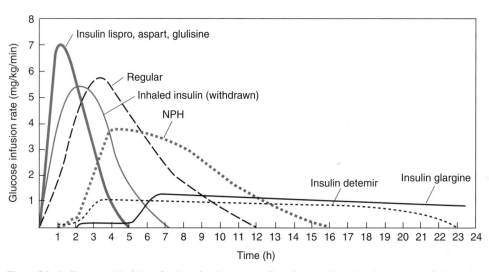

Figure 24–4. Extent and duration of action of various types of insulin as indicated by the glucose infusion rates (mg/kg/min) required to maintain a constant glucose concentration. The durations of action shown are typical of an average dose of 0.2 to 0.3 units/kg; except for insulin lispro and insulin aspart, duration increases when dosage is increased.

development of the ultra-rapid insulins, regular insulin was the primary rapid-onset agent. However, regular insulin requires administration 1 hour or more before each meal.

A special formulation of regular insulin was approved for inhalation (Exubera) in 2007. This was the first insulin formulation that did not require injection, but interest was too low to support continued production and the drug was discontinued.

The major intermediate-onset and intermediate-action preparation currently available is **isophane insulin suspension (NPH insulin)**. This preparation is given by subcutaneous injection; it is not suitable for intravenous use. Intermediate-onset NPH insulin can be mixed in the syringe or purchased premixed with regular insulin for convenience of administration.

Insulins with very slow onset and prolonged action are represented by **ultralente insulin, insulin glargine**, and **insulin detemir**. Ultralente insulin has a very delayed peak at 12 hours after injection and has fallen out of favor. Insulins glargine and detemir achieve a plateau within 3 to 6 hours and maintain a relatively constant blood level for up to 24 hours. These formulations are usually given in the morning only or in the morning and evening to provide maintenance or basal levels for 12 to 24 hours. This basal insulin level may be supplemented (especially in the case of insulins glargine and detemir) with injections of insulin lispro or regular insulin during the day to meet the requirements of carbohydrate intake.

Insulin Delivery Systems

The standard mode of insulin therapy is subcutaneous injection with conventional disposable needles and syringes. More convenient means of administration are also available. Portable pen-sized injectors are used to facilitate subcutaneous injection. Some contain replaceable cartridges, whereas others are disposable. Continuous subcutaneous insulin infusion pumps avoid the need for multiple daily injections and provide flexibility in the scheduling of patients' daily activities. These programmable pumps deliver a constant 24-hour basal rate, and manual adjustments in the rate of delivery can be made to accommodate changes in insulin requirements. Dosage changes may be required prior to meals or exercise. While insulin pumps have many advantages over subcutaneous injections, the pump and its disposable accessories (e.g., tubing) are expensive. The inhaled formulation of insulin had pharmacokinetic properties that made it useful for covering mealtime insulin requirements. This insulin formulation was administered within 10 minutes prior to a meal.

Adverse Effects

Diabetic patients who use insulin are subject to two types of complications: hypoglycemia, from excessive insulin effect, and immunologic toxic effects, from the development of antibodies. Hypoglycemia is very dangerous because brain damage may result. Rapid development of hypoglycemia in individuals with intact hypoglycemic awareness causes autonomic hyperactivity, with both sympathetic and parasympathetic manifestations. The sympathetic manifestations include tachycardia, palpitations, sweating, and tremulousness. The parasympathetic manifestations include nausea and hunger. Hypoglycemia may progress to convulsions and coma if untreated. In diabetic patients who experience frequent hypoglycemic episodes, autonomic warning signs can be less frequent or even absent. These patients can develop severe manifestations of hypoglycemia, including confusion, weakness, bizarre behavior, coma, or seizures without warning. Every patient with DM who is receiving hypoglycemic drug therapy should have an identification bracelet, necklace, or card in the wallet or purse, as well as some form of rapidly absorbed glucose. In patients with hypoglycemia, prompt administration of glucose or simple sugars is essential. The glucose may be given either as sugar or candy by mouth or as intravenous glucose. Alternatively, an intramuscular injection of glucagon can be used to raise serum glucose concentrations. Patients with advanced renal disease, the elderly, and children younger than 7 years are most susceptible to hypoglycemia and its detrimental effects.

The most common form of insulin-induced immunologic complication is the formation of antibodies to insulin or noninsulin protein contaminants, which results in resistance to insulin's action or allergic reactions. With the current use of highly purified human insulins, immunologic complications are very uncommon. Insulin may also cause weight gain, which is particularly undesirable in patients with type 2 DM, who are frequently overweight.

Amylinomimetic

Amylin, a 37–amino acid protein that activates G protein–coupled receptors, is co-secreted with insulin from the B cells. **Pramlintide** is a synthetic analog of amylin. Administration of pramlintide has multiple effects on glucose regulation. The drug reduces post-prandial glucose elevation by prolonging gastric emptying and reducing glucagon secretion following a meal. Through centrally mediated appetite suppression, it reduces caloric intake and causes weight loss, an important benefit for overweight patients. Administration is by subcutaneous injection, with a time to peak plasma concentration of 20 minutes and a half-life of 48 minutes (Table 24–4). Pramlintide is used in both types 1 and 2 DM.

Adverse Effects

Headaches, nausea, vomiting, and loss of appetite occur. Severe hypoglycemia also occurs and is more common in patients with type 1 DM compared to patients with type 2 DM. Arthralgia has been reported in some patients, and allergic reactions are possible.

Incretin Mimetic

Exenatide, a newer drug for treating type 2 diabetes, is a long-acting peptide with a high degree of homology to a hormone called **glucagon-like peptide-1** (GLP-1). A finding that long puzzled endocrinologists was the ability of oral glucose to induce more insulin release than an equivalent amount of intravenous glucose. This finding suggested the existence of a gastrointestinal tract–derived substance that stimulates insulin release. Further research led to discovery of two hormones, called **incretins**, that are released from endocrine cells in the bowel epithelium in response to food. One of these is GLP-1. GLP-1 and exenatide have multiple effects. In addition to augmentation of glucose-stimulated insulin release from pancreatic B cells, they retard gastric emptying, inhibit glucagon secretion, and produce a sense of satiety. Exenatide

Table 24–4.	Representative drugs used to treat type 2 diabetes mellitus
Drug	**Duration of Action (hours)**
Insulin secretagogues	
Sulfonylureas	
Chlorpropamide	Up to 60
Tolbutamide	6–12
Glimepiride	12–24
Glipizide	10–24
Glyburide	10–24
Meglitinides	
Repaglinide	1–3
D-Phenylalanine derivative	
Nateglinide	4
Biguanides	
Metformin	10–12
Thiazolidinediones	
Pioglitazone	15–24
Rosiglitazone	>24
α-Glucosidase inhibitors	
Acarbose	3–4
Miglitol	3–4
Amylinomimetic[1]	
Pramlintide	3
Incretin mimetic	
Exenatide	5–10

[1]Pramlintide is also used to treat type 1 DM.

must be injected subcutaneously twice daily, has a time to peak plasma concentration of approximately 2 hours, and has an elimination half-life of 2.5 hours; the duration is given in Table 24–4. Exenatide has modest therapeutic utility, and is always used in combination with metformin or a secretagogue.

Adverse Effects

Nausea, especially early in the course of treatment, is a problem and can be accompanied by vomiting and diarrhea. Hypoglycemia has occurred when exenatide is combined with an insulin secretagogue but has not been seen when exenatide is combined with metformin.

Oral Antidiabetic Drugs

Five groups of drugs are used for the oral treatment of type 2 DM: insulin secretagogues, biguanides, thiazolidinediones, gliptins, and α-glucosidase inhibitors. Important members of these groups are listed in Table 24–4.

Insulin Secretagogues

The primary action of the insulin secretagogues is to stimulate the release of endogenous insulin. Most of the insulin secretagogues are in the chemical class known as **sulfonylureas**. The sulfonylureas close the ATP-regulated potassium channels in the pancreatic B cell membranes; channel closure depolarizes the cells, which triggers insulin release (Figure 24–2). Insulin secretagogues are not effective in patients who lack functional B cells. These drugs may also reduce glucagon release and increase the number of functional insulin receptors in peripheral tissues. The second-generation sulfonylureas such as **glyburide, glipizide,** or **glimepiride** are considerably more potent and much more commonly used than the older agents such as **tolbutamide** or **chlorpropamide**.

Repaglinide and **nateglinide** are newer insulin secretagogues. Repaglinide is from a chemical class called meglitinides, whereas nateglinide is a D-phenylalanine derivative. Both of these drugs also promote insulin release by closing ATP-regulated potassium channels in pancreatic B cell membranes. The most notable difference between the newer drugs and sulfonylureas is the rapid onset and short duration of action of the newer agents (Table 24–4). They can be taken just before meals to control postprandial glucose concentrations.

ADVERSE EFFECTS. Hypoglycemia is the most common adverse effect of the secretagogues. Occasionally, rash and allergy are reported. The older sulfonylureas, which include tolbutamide and chlorpropamide, are extensively bound to serum proteins, and drugs that compete for protein binding may enhance their hypoglycemic effects. Chlorpropamide has a long duration of action, and liver and kidney disease may greatly increase blood levels of the drug. Like insulin, insulin secretagogues cause weight gain, which is undesirable in the large number of patients with type 2 DM who are overweight.

Biguanides

The biguanides act by a poorly understood mechanism to reduce postprandial and fasting glucose levels in patients with type 2 DM. Their effects do not depend on functional B islet cells. Proposed mechanisms for their action include reduced hepatic gluconeogenesis, stimulation of glycolysis in peripheral tissues, reduction of glucose absorption from the gastrointestinal tract, and reduction of plasma glucagon levels. Several biguanides are in use overseas. **Metformin** is the only member of this group available in the United States. Unlike the sulfonylureas, the biguanides do not cause hypoglycemia. Unlike all other oral antidiabetic drugs and insulin, metformin does not cause weight gain. The duration of action of metformin is intermediate when compared to most other oral antidiabetic drugs (Table 24–4).

ADVERSE EFFECTS. The most common toxicity associated with metformin is nausea and diarrhea, and the most serious toxicity is lactic acidosis. The increased risk of lactic acidosis presumably arises because of impaired conversion of lactic acid to glucose, an important reaction normally performed in the liver. Patients with renal or liver disease, alcoholism, or conditions that predispose them to tissue anoxia and excess lactic acid production, such as chronic cardiopulmonary dysfunction, are at greatest risk. Metformin also inhibits vitamin B_{12} absorption.

Thiazolidinediones

Thiazolidinediones increase target tissue sensitivity to insulin. **Troglitazone** was the first thiazolidinedione introduced, but it was removed from the market in several countries because of hepatotoxicity. **Rosiglitazone** and **pioglitazone** appear to carry less risk of serious liver dysfunction. The mechanism of action of the thiazolidinediones is not fully understood, but they stimulate the peroxisome proliferator-activated receptor-gamma nuclear receptor (PPAR-γ receptor). This nuclear receptor regulates the transcription of genes encoding proteins involved in carbohydrate and lipid metabolism.

The thiazolidinediones increase glucose uptake in muscle and adipose tissue, inhibit hepatic gluconeogenesis, and have effects on lipid metabolism and the distribution of body fat. Thiazolidinediones reduce both fasting and postprandial hyperglycemia. They are used as monotherapy or in combination with insulin or other oral antidiabetic drugs. Durations of action of thiazolidinediones are presented in Table 24–4.

ADVERSE EFFECTS.   When these drugs are used alone, hypoglycemia is extremely rare. Liver function should be monitored. Thiazolidinediones can cause volume expansion, which presents as edema and mild anemia, especially when combined with exogenous insulin. Heart failure and other cardiovascular complications may occur. Some evidence suggests an increased risk of fractures. Because pioglitazone and troglitazone appear to induce cytochrome P450 enzymes, these drugs can reduce serum concentrations of drugs such as oral contraceptives or cyclosporine that are also metabolized by these enzymes.

Gliptins

The gliptins are orally active inhibitors of dipeptidyl peptidase-4, the enzyme that metabolizes endogenous incretins and similar GLP-1–like molecules. Their effects on glucose metabolism thus resemble those of exenatide, which mimics GLP-1. Elimination is via the kidney, so dosage must be reduced in patients with renal impairment. **Sitagliptin** is the first of this class to be approved. The adverse effects of the drug include headache, nasopharyngitis, and upper respiratory tract infections.

α-Glucosidase Inhibitors

Acarbose and **miglitol** are carbohydrate analogs that act within the intestine to inhibit α-glucosidase, an enzyme necessary for the conversion of complex starches, oligosaccharides, and disaccharides to monosaccharides that can be transported out of the intestinal lumen and into the bloodstream. As a result of impaired absorption, postprandial hyperglycemia is reduced. These drugs have no effect on fasting blood sugar. Both drugs can be used as monotherapy, or in combination with other antidiabetic drugs. This drug class has one of the shorter durations of action of the oral antidiabetic drugs (Table 24–4).

ADVERSE EFFECTS.   The primary adverse effects of α-glucosidase inhibitors include flatulence, diarrhea, and abdominal pain resulting from increased fermentation

of unabsorbed carbohydrate by bacteria in the colon. Patients taking an α-glucosidase inhibitor who experience hypoglycemia should be treated with oral glucose (dextrose) and not sucrose because the absorption of sucrose will be delayed.

TREATMENT OF DIABETES MELLITUS

Type 1 Diabetes Mellitus

Therapy of type 1 DM involves dietary instruction and separate or mixed parenteral administration of shorter and longer acting insulins to maintain stable blood glucose levels during the day and night. The patient must also give careful attention to factors that change insulin requirements. These factors include exercise, infection, other forms of stress, and deviations from the regular diet. Large clinical studies indicate that tight control of blood glucose levels (i.e., "glycemic control") by frequent blood glucose testing and insulin injections reduces the incidence of vascular complications, including renal and retinal damage. The risk of hypoglycemic reactions is increased in tight control regimens, but not enough to obviate the benefits of better control.

Type 2 Diabetes Mellitus

Type 2 DM is usually a progressive disease, and treatment for an individual patient generally escalates over time. Initial treatment begins with weight reduction and dietary control because most type 2 diabetics are overweight. Initial drug therapy is usually monotherapy, often with a second-generation sulfonylurea such as glyburide, glipizide, glimepiride, or, increasingly for patients with type 2 DM and obesity, metformin. Although the initial response to monotherapy is usually good, erosion of glycemic control within 5 to 10 years is common. When monotherapy fails to provide adequate glycemic control, oral antidiabetic drugs are used in combination with each other or with insulin. Because type 2 DM involves both insulin resistance and eventual inadequate insulin production, pharmacotherapy often combines an agent that augments insulin's action with one that augments insulin blood levels. The former includes metformin, a thiazolidinedione, or an α-glucosidase inhibitor, and the latter includes insulin secretagogues, exenatide, or insulin. Sulfonylureas, metformin, thiazolidinediones, and some insulin formulations are long-acting drugs that help control both fasting and postprandial blood glucose levels. In contrast, repaglinide, α-glucosidase inhibitors, exenatide, regular insulin, and the ultra-short insulins are short-acting drugs that primarily target postprandial glucose levels. As is the case for type 1 DM, clinical trials have shown that tight glycemic control in patients with type 2 DM reduces the risk of vascular complications.

HYPERGLYCEMIC DRUGS

Glucagon

Glucagon is a hormone secreted by the A cells of the endocrine pancreas. Glucagon acts through G protein–coupled receptors to stimulate adenylyl cyclase and increase intracellular cyclic adenosine monophosphate (cAMP). Activation of glucagon receptors induces positive chronotropic and inotropic effects in the heart, increases hepatic glycogenolysis and gluconeogenesis, and relaxes smooth muscle, particularly smooth muscle in the gastrointestinal tract.

Clinical Uses

Glucagon can be used to treat severe hypoglycemia in patients with DM or insulin-secreting tumors, but its hyperglycemic action requires intact hepatic glycogen stores. The drug is given intramuscularly or intravenously. Glucagon is also valuable for radiographic studies of the bowel or abdomen when temporary reduction of motility is necessary for optimal visualization. In the management of severe adrenergic β-blocker overdose, glucagon may be the most effective method for stimulating the depressed heart because it increases cardiac cAMP without accessing β receptors.

REHABILITATION FOCUS

Because diabetes is so common (especially type 2), physical therapists often treat patients with this disease.

The therapist may work with an overweight patient to develop an exercise program to promote weight loss, conduct exercise stress treadmill testing as a precursor to the exercise program, or treat the patient because of a complication of long-standing DM. These complications include stroke, cardiovascular disease, nephropathy, retinopathy, repeated infections, and various neuropathies and chronic nonhealing wounds associated with vascular insufficiency or reduced sensation in weight-bearing areas.

Initiation of an exercise regimen along with changes in lifestyle, diet, and pharmacotherapy are four cornerstones of the treatment of both type 1 and 2 DM. Lifestyle changes for patients with type 2 DM include weight reduction and smoking cessation. Dietary goals include eating balanced meals at regular intervals with a reduction in simple carbohydrates following the guidelines set forth by the American Diabetes Association. Some patients with type 2 DM can delay pharmacotherapy with appropriate exercise, diet, and lifestyle changes. Patients with type 1 DM may also improve their glycemic control with a regular exercise program. Regular exercise by patients with both types of DM helps maintain cardiovascular and respiratory function and prevent osteoporosis.

Exercise stress testing should precede the design of an exercise program, especially if cardiovascular pathophysiology is present or a risk. Exercise programs for DM patients should include both aerobic and resistive exercise training because both have been shown to benefit this patient population. In healthy young nondiabetic patients, heart rate is the primary guide to aerobic exercise intensity; maximum target heart rate is often set at 60 to 90% of the age-predicted maximum heart rate. However, in patients medicated with β blockers or those with long-standing DM, the Borg Relative Perceived Exertion (RPE) should be used. In the latter case, autonomic neuropathy can affect heart rate, and RPE may be a better indicator of exercise intensity. In diabetic patients, the target heart rate should be adjusted to 55 to 79% of maximum (9 to 11 RPE). Lower target heart rates of 50 to 60% of maximum (7 to 9 RPE) during exercise should be considered if the initial fitness level is low.

Exercise is not always beneficial to the patient with DM and may be detrimental, depending upon current glycemic control. Exercise is contraindicated when ketosis is present because exercise may exacerbate ketoacidosis. Because exercise increases peripheral uptake of glucose, insulin or oral hypoglycemic drug dosages need to be adjusted to prevent hypoglycemic episodes. Hypoglycemia is always a risk in patients being treated with insulin or secretagogue oral antidiabetic drugs. Physical therapists need to be aware of the fact that repeated bouts of hypoglycemia, resulting from exercise or other causes of poor glycemic control, may result in blunted autonomic nervous system warning symptoms.

▪ CLINICAL RELEVANCE FOR REHABILITATION

Adverse Drug Reactions

Insulin, exenatide, and pramlintide

- Hypoglycemia, mainly with insulin
- Nausea and vomiting
- Weight gain, mainly with insulin and pramlintide

Oral Hypoglycemics

- Hypoglycemia with the insulin secretagogues
- Weight gain with the insulin secretagogues
- Lactic acidosis with biguanides
- Myocardial infarction, edema, heart failure, and anemia with thiazolidinediones
- Flatulence, diarrhea, and abdominal pain with the α-glucosidase inhibitors

Effects Interfering with Rehabilitation

- Post–exercise-induced hypoglycemia may be exacerbated by insulin, pramlintide, and insulin secretagogues.

Possible Therapy Solutions

- Monitor blood glucose levels in all DM patients prior to exercise.
- Check blood pressure and heart rate in patients prior to exercise.
- Discuss with patient the importance of regular meals in conjunction with exercise to control glycemic levels.

Potentiation of Functional Outcomes Secondary to Drug Therapy

- Long-term glycemic control with a conditioning program will assist in weight and glycemic control and improve cardiovascular status.

PROBLEM-ORIENTED PATIENT STUDY

Brief History: The patient is a 50-year-old male with a body mass index of 30 and a 15-year history of type 2 DM and hypertension. The patient is a lawyer with a sedentary lifestyle who previously declined his health-care provider's recommendations to participate in aerobic conditioning programs. The patient controls his diet poorly. He quit smoking 2 years ago.

On examination, the resting heart rate is 68 beats per minute and blood pressure is 130/85 mm Hg. His past history of HbA_{1c} ranges from 7.5 to 8.7%, with the high value being the most recent. His recent finger-stick blood glucose levels have ranged from 95 to 280 mg/dL. Recently, he experienced left shoulder pain that was diagnosed as atherosclerotic exertional angina pectoris. Following this

(continued)

PROBLEM-ORIENTED PATIENT STUDY (*Continued*)

diagnosis, he expressed an interest in developing a regular conditioning program along with dietary changes to improve glycemic control. The patient underwent cardiac stress testing and cardiac catheterization. Electrocardiographic changes were noted during the stress test, and catheterization revealed single vessel disease with 40% occlusion. The cardiologist recommended that the patient continue his medications and begin an exercise program. The patient was sent to an outpatient rehabilitation clinic for program development.

Current Medical Status and Drug Therapy: Previously, the patient was using insulin glargine to provide daily background control in combination with insulin lispro to achieve optimal postprandial glycemic control. The oral hypoglycemic was rosiglitazone. Within the past 3 weeks, the patient converted to a single-compartment insulin pump. Insulin lispro is used in the pump at a lower background rate with boluses at mealtime. Since the medication change, fingerstick daily blood glucose levels have been 58 to 120 mg/dL prior to meals and at bedtime. The pharmacotherapy for hypertension includes labetalol, enalapril, and hydrochlorothiazide. Labetalol also provides prophylaxis for angina pectoris, while enalapril provides prophylaxis for DM nephropathy.

Rehabilitation Setting: Due to documented pathology obtained from the electrocardiogram and cardiac catheterization, poor initial fitness level of the patient, and presence of a β-receptor antagonist (labetalol), the target exertion level for the exercise program was set at 7 RPE. The program included 10 minutes of warm-up with resistive weight training, 20 minutes of treadmill walking at the target RPE, followed by stretching during a 10-minute cool-down period. This program was to be conducted every day. The

patient was complaining about his busy day when he arrived for his first supervised session following work this afternoon. The insulin pump was left on with the background infusion at the preestablished value. The patient completed both the warm-up phase and aerobic training without incident. However, during the cool-down period, he appeared confused and could not follow instructions, and noted that he was hungry and wondered whether he should have had a larger lunch. His skin was cool and clammy; however, his heart rate was 78 bpm and blood pressure was 138/89 mm Hg. No assessment of blood glucose was available, but the patient was provided a regular (nondiet) soda. The emergency paramedics were contacted. By the time they arrived, the patient was coherent, standing, and talking. Measurement of finger-stick blood glucose taken by the paramedics was 68 mg/dL. The patient was transferred to the local hospital for further evaluation.

Problem/Clinical Options: The patient had a previous history of poor glycemic control. Periods of both hyperglycemia and hypoglycemia were documented in the medical history. Three weeks previously, the change to the insulin pump tightened glycemic control, decreasing hyperglycemic episodes, but also causing recorded hypoglycemic episodes. Exercise increased the effects of insulin and the pump was left on at the background infusion rate, setting the stage for a hypoglycemic episode. No documentation of glucose concentration was available, but hypoglycemia likely occurred as a result of the combination of a small meal at lunch, stress from a busy day, exercise, and insulin. In addition, the β-receptor antagonist would have blunted sympathetic manifestations of hypoglycemia. A nondiet soda (which contains a fair amount of glucose) was given to the patient counter potential hypoglycemia.

PREPARATIONS AVAILABLE[1]

Oral Hypoglycemic Preparations

Sulfonylureas

Acetohexamide (Dymelor) (rarely used)
Oral: 250-, 500-mg tablets

Chlorpropamide (generic, Diabinese)
Oral: 100-, 250-mg tablets

Glimepiride (Amaryl)
Oral: 1-, 2-, 4-mg tablets

Glipizide (generic, Glucotrol, Glucotrol XL)
Oral: 5-, 10-mg tablets; 5-, 10-mg extended-release tablets

Glyburide (generic, Diabeta, Micronase, Glynase PresTab)
Oral: 1.25-, 2.5-, 5-mg tablets; 1.5-, 3-, 4.5-, 6-mg Glynase PresTab, micronized tablets

Tolazamide (generic, Tolinase)
Oral: 100-, 250-, 500-mg tablets

Tolbutamide (generic, Orinase)
Oral: 500-mg tablets

Meglitinide and Related Drugs

Repaglinide (Prandin)
Oral: 0.5-, 1-, 2-mg tablets

Nateglinide (Starlix)
Oral: 60-, 120-mg tablets

Biguanide and Biguanide Combinations

Metformin (Glucophage, Glucophage XR)
Oral: 500-, 850-, 1000-mg tablets; extended-release (XR): 500-mg tablets

Metformin Combinations

Glipizide plus metformin (Metaglip)
Oral: 2.5/250-, 2.5/500-, 5/500-mg tablets

Glyburide plus metformin (Glucovance)
Oral: 1.25/250-, 2.5/500-, 5/500-mg tablets

Rosiglitazone plus metformin (Avandamet)
Oral: 1/500-, 2/500-, 4/500-mg tablets

Thiazolidinedione Derivatives

Pioglitazone (Actos)
Oral: 15-, 30-, 45-mg tablets

Rosiglitazone (Avandia)
Oral: 2-, 4-, 8-mg tablets

α-Glucosidase Inhibitors

Acarbose (Precose)
Oral: 50-, 100-mg tablets

Miglitol (Glyset)
Oral: 25-, 50-, 100-mg tablets

Incretin Enhancer

Sitaglipin (Januvia)
Oral: 25-, 50-, 100-mg tablets

Amylinomimetic

Pramlinitide (Symlin)
Parenteral: subcutaneous administration
0.6 mg/mL

Incretin Mimetic

Exenatide (Byetta)
Parenteral: 5, 10 mcg/dose in prefilled pens for subcutaneous administration

Glucagon

Glucagon (generic)
Parenteral: 1-mg lyophilized powder to reconstitute for injection

[1]See Table 24–3 for examples of Insulin preparations.

REFERENCES

Diabetes Prevention Program Research Group: Reduction in the incidence of type 2 diabetes with lifestyle intervention or metformin. *N Engl J Med* 2002;346:393.

Expert Committee on the Diagnosis and Classification of Diabetes Mellitus: Report of the expert committee on the diagnosis and classification of diabetes mellitus. *Diabetes Care* 2003;26:3160.

Goldberg RB, et al: A comparison of lipid and glycemic effects of pioglitazone and rosiglitazone in patients with type 2 diabetes and dyslipidemia. *Diabetes Care* 2005;28:1547.

Heinemann L, et al: Time action profile of the long-acting insulin analog insulin glargine (HOE901) in comparison with those of NPH insulin and placebo. *Diabetes Care* 2000;23:644.

Heptulla RA, et al: The role of amylin and glucagon in the dampening of glycemic excursions in children with type 1 diabetes. *Diabetes* 2005;54:1100.

Kolterman O, et al: Pharmacokinetics, pharmacodynamics, and safety of exenatide in patients with type 2 diabetes mellitus. *Am J Health Syst Pharm* 2005;62:173.

Levien TL: Nateglinide therapy for type 2 diabetes mellitus. *Ann Pharmacother* 2001;35:1426.

McGarry D: Dysregulation of fatty acid metabolism in the etiology of type 2 diabetes. *Diabetes* 2002;51:7.

Mudaliar S, et al: New oral therapies for type 2 diabetes mellitus: The glitazones or insulin sensitizers. *Annu Rev Med* 2001;52:239.

Quattrin T, et al: Efficacy and safety of inhaled insulin (Exubera) compared with subcutaneous insulin therapy in patients with type 1 diabetes. *Diabetes Care* 2004;27:2622.

Rehabilitation

American Diabetes Association: http://www.diabetes.org/home.jsp

Castaneda C, et al: A randomized controlled trial of resistance exercise training to improve glycemic control in older adults with type 2 diabetes. *Diabetes Care* 2002;25:2335.

Chakravarthy MV, et al: An obligation for primary care physicians to prescribe physical activity to sedentary patients to reduce the risk of chronic health conditions. *Mayo Clin Proc* 2002;77:165.

Cryer PE, et al: Hypoglycemia in diabetes. *Diabetes Care* 2003;26:1902.

Dagogo-Jack S: Hypoglycemia in type 1 diabetes mellitus: Pathophysiology and prevention. *Treat Endocrinol* 2004;3:91.

Dey L, Attele AS, Yuan CS: Alternative therapies for type 2 diabetes. *Altern Med Rev* 2002;7:45.

Moreno R, et al: Prognosis of medically stabilized unstable angina pectoris with a negative exercise test. *Am J Cardiol* 1998;82:662, A6.

Rosenstock J: Management of type 2 diabetes mellitus in the elderly: Special considerations. *Drugs Aging* 2001;18:31.

Salpeter S, et al: Risk of fatal and nonfatal lactic acidosis with metformin use in type 2 diabetes mellitus. *Cochrane Database Syst Rev* 2003;CD002967.

Stewart KJ: Exercise training: Can it improve cardiovascular health in patients with type 2 diabetes? *Br J Sports Med* 2004;38:250.

Tan D: Treadmill exercise testing in ischemic heart disease. *Ann Acad Med Singapore* 1987;16:331.

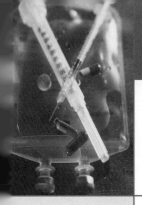

25

DRUGS THAT AFFECT BONE MINERAL HOMEOSTASIS

Calcium and phosphate are the major mineral constituents of bone and are also two of the most important minerals for general cellular function. Accordingly, the body has evolved a complex set of mechanisms by which calcium and phosphate homeostasis is carefully maintained. Approximately 98% of the 1 to 2 kg of calcium and 85% of the 1 kg of phosphorus in the human adult are found in bone, the principal reservoir for these minerals. Mineral homeostasis is dynamic, with constant remodeling of bone and ready exchange of bone minerals with free ions in the extracellular fluid. Bone also serves as the principal structural support for the body and provides space for hematopoiesis in the bone marrow. Abnormalities in bone mineral homeostasis can underlie electrolyte disturbances, resulting in the clinical manifestations of muscle weakness, tetany, and coma. Dysfunction in bone mineral homeostasis can also disturb the structural support of the body in the form of osteoporosis and fractures. Hematopoietic capacity may also be reduced in conditions such as infantile osteopetrosis.

The average American diet provides 600 to 1000 mg of calcium per day, of which a net amount of approximately 100 to 250 mg is absorbed. Absorption principally occurs in the duodenum and upper jejunum, whereas secretion principally occurs in the ileum. The amount of phosphorus in the American diet is about the same as that of calcium. However, the efficiency of phosphate absorption, which mostly occurs in the jejunum, is greater, ranging from 70 to 90%, depending on intake. The movement of calcium and phosphate across the intestinal and renal epithelia is closely regulated. At steady state, renal excretion of calcium and phosphate balances intestinal absorption. Most of the time, over 98% of filtered calcium and 85% of filtered phosphate is reabsorbed by the kidneys.

PHARMACOTHERAPY

The drugs that are used clinically to modulate bone homeostasis can be divided into endogenous molecules and exogenous substances (Figure 25–1).

Endogenous Substances

The two hormones that serve as the principal regulators of calcium and phosphate homeostasis are **parathyroid hormone** (PTH), a protein, and biologically active metabolites of the steroid **vitamin D** (Figure 25–2). Other hormones such as calcitonin, prolactin, growth hormone, insulin, thyroid hormone, glucocorticoids, and gonadal steroids serve secondary roles in calcium and phosphate homeostasis. Several of these hormones, such as calcitonin, glucocorticoids, and

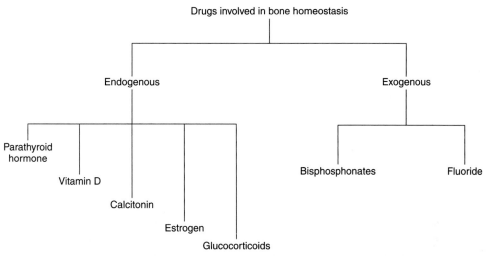

Figure 25–1. Drugs that modulate bone mineral homeostasis may be divided into endogenous molecules and exogenous substances. Parathyroid hormone and vitamin D are of primary importance in this regulation whereas calcitonin, glucocorticoids, and estrogens play modulatory roles. Exogenous agents such as bisphosphonates and fluoride are used to prevent or treat disorders of bone and teeth, respectively.

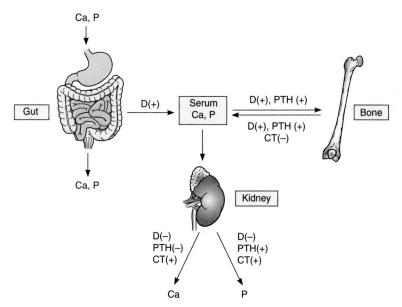

Figure 25–2. Mechanisms that contribute to bone mineral homeostasis. Calcium (*Ca*) and phosphorus (*P*) concentrations in the serum are controlled principally by two hormones: 1,25-dihydroxyvitamin D (calcitriol; *D*) and parathyroid hormone (*PTH*). Serum concentrations are regulated by the action of D and PTH on absorption from the gut and bone and on excretion in the urine. Both hormones remove calcium and phosphorus from bone, increasing serum ion concentrations (+); vitamin D also increases absorption from the gut (+). Vitamin D decreases (–) urinary excretion of both calcium and phosphorus, while PTH reduces (–) calcium but increases (+) phosphorus excretion. Calcitonin (*CT*) is a less critical hormone for calcium homeostasis, but in pharmacologic concentrations, CT can reduce (–) serum calcium and phosphorus by inhibiting bone resorption and stimulating their renal excretion (+). Feedback effects are not shown.

estrogens, have efficacy in the treatment of bone mineral disorders. In addition, calcium, phosphate, and other ions such as sodium alter calcium and phosphate homeostasis.

Vitamin D

Vitamin D, a derivative of 7-dehydrocholesterol, is formed in the skin under the influence of ultraviolet light. Vitamin D is also found in some foods and is a nutritional additive in milk and in calcium supplements. Active metabolites of vitamin D are formed in the liver (25-hydroxyvitamin D, or **calcifediol**) and the kidney (1,25-dihydroxyvitamin D [1,25[OH]$_2$D$_3$], or **calcitriol**, plus other metabolites). Because it is a fat-soluble vitamin, excess vitamin D is stored in adipose tissue. The metabolites of vitamin D differ in the number of hydroxyl groups attached to the steroid ring (Table 25–1). The actions of these metabolites include increased intestinal calcium and phosphorus absorption, decreased renal excretion of minerals, and a net increase in blood levels of both calcium and phosphorus (Figure 25–2, Table 25–2). These actions are mediated by activation of one or possibly a family of nuclear receptors that regulate gene expression. Of the vitamin D metabolites, 1,25[OH]$_2$D is the most potent in stimulating intestinal calcium and phosphate absorption and bone *resorption*. In contrast, bone *formation* can be increased by the administration of a different metabolite, 24,25-dihydroxyvitamin D (**secalcifediol**, 24,25(OH)$_2$D$_3$). Vitamin D supplements and synthetic derivatives are used in the treatment of deficiency states, such as nephrotic syndrome and nutritional rickets. They are also used, in combination with calcium supplementation and other drugs, in the prevention and treatment of osteoporosis in older women and men. Moreover, a number of calcitriol analogs are being synthesized in an effort to examine their clinical usefulness in a variety of nonclassic conditions. For example, **calcipotriene (calcipotriol)** is currently used to treat psoriasis, a hyperproliferative skin disorder. **Doxercalciferol** and **paricalcitol** have recently been approved for treating secondary hyperparathyroidism in patients with renal failure.

Parathyroid Hormone

By regulating calcium and phosphate flux across cellular membranes in bone and kidney, PTH increases serum calcium while decreasing serum phosphate (Figure 25–2, Table 25–2). By an indirect mechanism, PTH increases the activity and number of osteoclasts, cells responsible for bone resorption. PTH activates G protein–coupled receptors on bone–forming osteoblasts, inducing a membrane-bound protein called RANK ligand. RANK ligand increases both the number and activity of osteoclasts. Thus, bone remodeling is actually initiated by osteoclastic bone resorption and followed by osteoblastic bone formation. Although PTH enhances both bone resorption and bone formation, the net effect of excess PTH is increased bone resorption. However, when administered in low, intermittent doses, PTH increases bone formation without stimulating bone resorption. Based on this effect, recombinant

Table 25–1. Vitamin D and its clinically available metabolites and analogs	
Chemical and Generic Names	**Abbreviation**
Vitamin D$_2$; ergocalciferol	D$_2$
Vitamin D$_3$; cholecalciferol	D$_3$
25-Hydroxyvitamin D$_3$; calcifediol	25(OH)D$_3$
1,25-Dihydroxyvitamin D$_3$; calcitriol	1,25(OH)$_2$D$_3$
24,25-Dihydroxyvitamin D$_3$; secalcifediol	24,25(OH)$_2$D$_3$
Dihydrotachysterol	DHT
Calcipotriene (calcipotriol)	None
1 α-Hydroxyvitamin D$_2$; doxercalciferol	1 α(OH)D$_2$
19-nor-1,25-Dihydroxyvitamin D$_2$; paricalcitol	19-nor-1,25(OH)D$_2$

Table 25–2. Actions of parathyroid hormone and vitamin D on gut, bone, and kidney

	Vitamin D	PTH
Intestine	Increased calcium and phosphate absorption by 1,25(OH)$_2$D	Increased calcium and phosphate absorption (by increased 1,25 [OH]$_2$D production)
Kidney	Calcium and phosphate excretion may be decreased by 25(OH)D and 1,25(OH)$_2$D	Decreased calcium excretion, increased phosphate excretion
Bone	Increased calcium and phosphate resorption by 1,25(OH)$_2$D; bone formation may be increased by 24,25(OH)$_2$D	Calcium and phosphate resorption increased by high doses. Low intermittent doses increase bone formation
Net effect on serum levels	Serum calcium and phosphate both increased	Serum calcium increased, serum phosphate decreased

PTH 1-34 (**teriparatide**) has been approved by the United States Food and Drug Administration (FDA) for the treatment of osteoporosis in postmenopausal women. In the kidney, PTH increases calcium and magnesium resorption while reducing the resorption of phosphate, amino acids, bicarbonate, sodium, chloride, and sulfate. Another important action of PTH in the kidney is its stimulation of calcitriol production.

Interaction of PTH and Vitamin D Metabolites

A summary of the principal actions of PTH and vitamin D on intestine, kidney, and bone is presented in Table 25–2. The net effect of PTH is to raise serum calcium and reduce serum phosphate; the net effect of vitamin D is to raise serum levels of both. Regulation of calcium and phosphate homeostasis is achieved through a variety of feedback loops. In the parathyroid gland, specialized G protein–coupled receptors sense extracellular calcium concentration and couple this with intracellular calcium concentration. For example, when extracellular calcium falls, intracellular calcium falls in parallel and parathyroid cells secrete more PTH. Conversely, a rise in intracellular calcium concentration in parathyroid cells inhibits PTH secretion. Phosphate ion indirectly stimulates PTH secretion by forming complexes with calcium in the serum. These complexes decrease the concentration of ionized calcium, which is the form of calcium that binds to the calcium-sensing receptor. In the kidney, high levels of calcium and phosphate reduce calcitriol production and increase secalcifediol production. Since calcitriol is far more potent than secalcifediol at increasing serum calcium and phosphate, the net effect of calcitriol's action is feedback inhibition of vitamin D's main action. Calcitriol inhibits PTH secretion through a direct action on PTH gene transcription. This provides yet another negative feedback loop because PTH is a major stimulus for calcitriol production. The ability of calcitriol to inhibit PTH secretion directly can be exploited by administering analogs that have less effect on serum calcium. Such drugs are proving useful in the management of the secondary hyperparathyroidism that accompanies renal failure, and may be useful in selected cases of primary hyperparathyroidism.

Calcitonin

Calcitonin is a peptide hormone secreted by the parafollicular cells of the thyroid gland. The principal effect of calcitonin is to lower serum calcium and phosphate by actions on bone and kidney (Figure 25–2). Calcitonin inhibits osteoclastic bone resorption. During the initial stages of exogenous calcitonin administration, bone formation is not impaired. However, with continued use, both formation and resorption of bone are reduced. In the kidney, calcitonin reduces resorption of a number of ions including calcium, phosphate, sodium, potassium, and magnesium. Tissues other than bone and kidney are also affected by calcitonin.

In pharmacologic dosages, calcitonin reduces gastric acid output by inhibiting gastrin secretion, and increases secretion of sodium, potassium, chloride, and water into the gut. Although calcitonin does not significantly increase bone mass, it reduces the rate of bone loss, making it a useful drug for the treatment of osteoporosis. Its ability to block bone resorption and lower serum calcium also make it useful for treating Paget's disease and hypercalcemia. Calcitonin is administered by injection or nasal spray.

Estrogens

These compounds were previously discussed (Chapter 22) in relation to their regulation of sexual development, metabolic activity, and reproduction. Estrogens and selective estrogen receptor modulators (SERMs) such as **tamoxifen** or **raloxifene** prevent or delay bone loss in postmenopausal women. However, long-term estrogen treatment increases cardiovascular and cancer risks. Although it is not as effective as estrogen at increasing bone density, raloxifene reduces bone fractures and may reduce the risk of breast cancer.

Glucocorticoids

The glucocorticoids have multiple influences on metabolism that inhibit bone mineral maintenance (Chapter 23). Glucocorticoids alter bone mineral homeostasis by antagonizing vitamin D–stimulated intestinal calcium transport, stimulating renal calcium excretion, and blocking bone formation. As a result, chronic systemic use of glucocorticoids is a common cause of osteoporosis in adults and stunted skeletal development in children. However, glucocorticoids are useful in the intermediate-term treatment of hypercalcemia associated with lymphomas and granulomatous diseases such as sarcoidosis.

Exogenous Agents

A variety of other types of drugs are used to regulate bone mineral homeostasis. The bisphosphonates were developed for that purpose. The antibiotic plicamycin and the thiazide diuretics were developed for other clinical uses, but have found clinical value in treating disorders of bone mineral homeostasis.

Bisphosphonates

The bisphosphonates (**alendronate, etidronate, ibandronate, pamidronate, risedronate, tiludronate, zoledronate**) are short-chain organic polyphosphate compounds that reduce both resorption and formation of bone by acting on the basic hydroxyapatite crystal structure of bone. The bisphosphonates have other complex cellular effects, including inhibiting vitamin D production, inhibiting calcium absorption from the gastrointestinal tract, and directly inhibiting osteoclast function. In postmenopausal women, chronic bisphosphonate therapy slows osteoporosis progression and reduces fractures. The older drugs (etidronate, pamidronate) cause bone mineralization defects and lose their effectiveness over a 12-month period. Alendronate and risedronate cause fewer bone problems and are effective for at least 5 years. These two drugs are commonly used for treating postmenopausal and glucocorticoid-induced osteoporosis and for Paget's disease. Alendronate, used in combination with hormone replacement therapy, further increases bone mass in postmenopausal patients.

Oral bioavailability of bisphosphonates is low (<10%), and food impairs their absorption. Esophageal ulceration may also occur. Patients should take these drugs with large quantities of water, remain upright for 30 minutes, and avoid situations that permit esophageal reflux (i.e., activities that increase intra-abdominal pressure). In the prevention or treatment of osteoporosis, once-weekly administration of a relatively large dose of a bisphosphonate is as efficacious as daily administration of a smaller dose and does not result in more toxicity. Annual intravenous administration of zoledronate has similarly been found to be effective.

Fluoride

Appropriate concentrations of fluoride ion in drinking water (0.5 to 1.0 ppm) or as an additive in toothpaste have a well-documented ability to reduce dental caries. Chronic exposure to fluoride ion, especially in high concentrations, may increase new bone synthesis. What is not clear, however, is whether this new bone has normal strength. Clinical trials of fluoride in patients with osteoporosis have not demonstrated a reduced incidence of fractures. Acute fluoride toxicity, usually caused by ingestion of rat poison, is manifested by gastrointestinal and neurologic symptoms. Chronic toxicity (fluorosis) includes ectopic bone formation (exostoses) and calcified bumps on bones.

Thiazide Diuretics

This drug class was previously discussed in relation to the treatment of hypertension (Chapter 7). Thiazides increase the effectiveness of parathyroid hormone in stimulating renal reabsorption of calcium. In the distal tubule, thiazides block sodium reabsorption at the luminal surface. The resultant fall in intracellular sodium causes a greater calcium-sodium exchange at basolateral membranes, bringing sodium into distal tubule cells and transporting calcium out into the interstitial space. The net effect of thiazide diuretics is enhanced renal calcium reabsorption. Thiazides are useful in reducing hypercalciuria and nephrolithiasis in subjects with idiopathic hypercalciuria. They are not used to treat osteoporosis.

Plicamycin (Mithramycin)

This antibiotic is used to reduce serum calcium and bone resorption in Paget's disease and hypercalcemia. Because of the risk of complications, such as thrombocytopenia, hemorrhage, and hepatic and renal damage, plicamycin is not commonly prescribed. The drug is mainly restricted to short-term treatment of serious hypercalcemia.

■ SELECTED CLINICAL DISORDERS INVOLVING BONE MINERAL-REGULATING HORMONES

Osteoporosis

Osteoporosis is an abnormal loss of bone that predisposes an individual to fractures. Compact bone is affected more than trabecular bone. Osteoporosis is most common in postmenopausal women and elderly men. Osteoporosis can result from chronic administration of glucocorticoids or other drugs, endocrine diseases such as thyrotoxicosis or hyperparathyroidism, malabsorption syndrome, alcohol abuse and cigarette smoking, and idiopathic conditions.

The ability of some agents to reverse the bone loss of osteoporosis is shown in Figure 25–3. The postmenopausal form of osteoporosis may be accompanied by lower calcitriol levels and reduced intestinal calcium

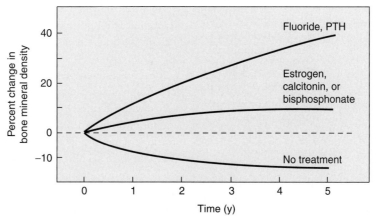

Figure 25–3. Typical changes in bone mineral density with time after the onset of menopause, with and without treatment. In the untreated condition, bone is lost during aging in both men and women. Fluoride and PTH promote new bone formation and can increase bone mineral density throughout the period of treatment. In contrast, estrogen, calcitonin, and bisphosphonates block bone resorption. This leads to a transient increase in bone mineral density because bone formation is not initially decreased. However, with time, both bone formation and bone resorption are decreased and bone mineral density reaches a new plateau.

transport. This form of osteoporosis is secondary to the reduced estrogen production that accompanies menopause; it can be treated with estrogen. However, concerns about increases in breast and endometrial cancer risk and cardiovascular adverse effects have dramatically reduced enthusiasm for this form of therapy. The selective estrogen receptor modulator (SERM) **raloxifene** (Chapter 22) avoids the increased risk of breast and uterine cancer associated with estrogen supplementation while maintaining the benefit to bone. Raloxifene appears to protect against spine fractures, but not hip fractures. In contrast, bisphosphonates and teriparatide protect against both fracture types. Raloxifene does not prevent hot flushes and imposes the same increased risk of venous thrombosis as estrogen.

To counter the reduced intestinal calcium transport associated with osteoporosis, vitamin D therapy is sometimes employed along with dietary calcium supplementation, but there is little evidence that pharmacologic doses of vitamin D are of much additional benefit beyond cyclic estrogens and calcium supplementation. However, in several large studies, vitamin D supplementation (400 to 800 IU/day) and calcitriol and its analog $1\alpha(OH)D_3$ have been shown to increase bone mass and, in several recent studies, to reduce fractures. Use of these agents for osteoporosis is not approved by the FDA.

Calcitonin is approved for the treatment of postmenopausal osteoporosis. It has been shown to increase bone mass and reduce fractures, but only in the spine.

Bisphosphonates are efficacious inhibitors of bone resorption. They increase bone density and reduce the risk of fractures in the hip, spine, and other locations. Alendronate, risedronate, and zoledronate are approved for osteoporosis treatment. These drugs are effective in treating osteoporosis of various causes in men as well as women.

Despite early promise that **fluoride** might be useful in the prevention or treatment of postmenopausal osteoporosis, this form of therapy remains controversial. A new formulation of fluoride (slow release of a lower dose) appears to avoid much of the toxicity of earlier formulations and may reduce fracture rates. This formulation is under consideration for approval by the FDA.

Teriparatide, the recombinant form of PTH 1–34, has recently been approved for treatment of osteoporosis.

Teriparatide is given subcutaneously in a dosage of 20 mcg daily. Like fluoride, teriparatide stimulates new bone formation. However, in contrast to fluoride, teriparatide-stimulated new bone appears structurally normal and is associated with a substantial reduction in the incidence of fractures.

Chronic Renal Failure

The major problems of chronic renal failure that impact bone mineral homeostasis are reduction of calcitriol and secalcifediol production, retention of phosphate (with associated reduction in ionized calcium levels), and secondary hyperparathyroidism. With reduced calcitriol production, less calcium is absorbed from the intestine and less bone is resorbed. The most common clinical presentation is hypocalcemia and hyperphosphatemia. The resulting hypocalcemia usually furthers the hyperparathyroidism. The skeletal system shows a mixture of **osteomalacia,** abnormal bone formation due to inadequate mineralization, and **osteitis fibrosa,** excessive bone resorption with fibrotic replacement of resorption cavities. Some patients may become hypercalcemic. The most common cause of the hypercalcemia is severe **secondary hyperparathyroidism.** Vitamin D supplementation is often prescribed for dialysis patients in chronic renal failure. The choice of supplement depends upon the type and extent of bone disease and hyperparathyroidism. Regardless of the drug employed, careful attention to serum calcium and phosphate levels is required. Calcium supplements and phosphate restriction are combined with vitamin D metabolites. Serum PTH levels are monitored to determine whether therapy is correcting or preventing secondary hyperparathyroidism. Vitamin D metabolites are monitored to assess compliance, absorption, and metabolism.

Other Clinical Disorders

Other clinical disorders involving bone mineralization include **nutritional rickets,** which can be corrected with vitamin D supplementation or exposure to sunlight. A number of disorders involving the gastrointestinal system, such as biliary cirrhosis, may result in abnormal calcium and phosphate homeostasis that ultimately leads to bone disease. This bone involvement may be the result of abnormal calcium or vitamin D intestinal absorption, or systemic toxins from **cholestasis** that inhibit osteoblast function. Clinically, the bone disease secondary to gastrointestinal dysfunction manifests as osteoporosis and osteomalacia, but without osteitis fibrosa. Treatment includes supplementation with vitamin D or its analogs and dietary calcium supplementation.

Patients with **nephrotic syndrome** lose vitamin D metabolites in the urine and subsequently may develop bone disease. Treatment includes vitamin D.

Paget's disease is a localized bone disease characterized by uncontrolled osteoclastic bone resorption with secondary increases in bone formation. The goal of treatment is to reduce bone pain and stabilize or prevent other problems such as progressive deformity, hearing loss, high-output cardiac failure, and immobilization hypercalcemia. Calcitonin and bisphosphonates are first-line agents for treatment of Paget's disease. Patients who fail to respond to these drugs may respond to plicamycin.

REHABILITATION FOCUS

Physical therapists develop exercise programs, which when combined with pharmacotherapy and diet, may delay osteoporosis. Therapists also see patients with osteoporosis for treatment of pain and dysfunction resulting from osteoporosis-induced fractures.

Multiple exercise formats can delay osteoporosis. Weight-bearing exercises (e.g., walking, stair climbing), resistive exercises (e.g., weight lifting, swimming), and aerobic exercises have been shown to delay bone loss and osteoporosis. Of these, resistive training may provide the strongest stimulus for bone remodeling and reduced bone loss. In contrast to pharmacotherapy and diet modification, exercise can reduce the occurrence of comorbidities associated with osteoporosis (such as diabetes mellitus), and maintain and improve cardiovascular and respiratory status. Exercise can also improve strength and balance, which have the added benefit of preventing falls and associated fractures. Finally, exercise may enhance pharmacologically increased bone formation, suggesting that the combination of exercise and drug therapy may optimize building bone mass.

CLINICAL RELEVANCE FOR REHABILITATION

Adverse Drug Reactions

- Bisphosphonates may cause esophageal ulceration.
- Calcitonin administration may cause gastrointestinal distress.
- SERMs such as raloxifene may cause hot flushes and nausea.
- Teriparatide administration may cause chest pain and dyspnea, dizziness, and gastrointestinal distress.

Effects Interfering with Rehabilitation

- Patients taking bisphosphonates within 30 minutes prior to therapy may experience esophageal pain if they are horizontal during the treatment session.
- Therapy sessions may exacerbate gastrointestinal distress due to calcitonin administration.
- Therapy sessions may exacerbate gastrointestinal distress or hot flushes of SERM medications such as raloxifene.
- Therapy sessions may exacerbate adverse effects of teriparatide administration.

Possible Therapy Solutions

- Have patients take bisphosphonates after or at least 1 hour prior to therapy sessions.
- Have patients take calcitonin on a day when therapy is not scheduled.
- Schedule therapy sessions for days when SERM drugs or teriparatide are not administered, or on a day prior to drug administration.

Potentiation of Functional Outcomes Secondary to Drug Therapy

- In postmenopausal women with osteoporosis, exercise without estrogen replacement therapy is effective in increasing or maintaining bone mineral density at certain sites.
- Pharmacotherapy and exercise programs individually, and in combination, help to prevent osteoporosis.

PROBLEM-ORIENTED PATIENT STUDY

Brief History: The patient is a 55-year-old disabled male with a 20-year history of rheumatoid arthritis (RA) and a body mass index of 27. He has bilateral knee joint replacements, the most recent performed 2 years ago. The patient ambulates with two single-point canes to increase mobility and decrease knee pain. He is not currently involved in a regular conditioning program. Three weeks ago, the patient was diagnosed with locally invasive prostate cancer. In conjunction with beginning pharmacotherapy for prostate cancer, the patient received a bone density study, which revealed osteoporosis. Owing to the results of the bone densitometry, the oncologist referred the patient to rehabilitation for development of a conditioning program.

Current Medical Status and Drug Therapy: Previous and current pharmacotherapy for RA included intermittent use of anti-inflammatory glucocorticoids (Chapter 23) and regular medication with nonsteroidal anti-inflammatory drugs and disease-modifying antirheumatic drugs (Chapter 34). The pharmacotherapy for prostate cancer is designed to suppress testosterone production and destroy the in situ cancer cells. Suppression of endogenous testosterone production will be accomplished by continuous dosing with goserelin plus flutamide for the first several weeks to prevent flare-up (Chapter 22). Radiation therapy will be initiated to destroy in situ cancer cells in the prostate. To help prevent further bone loss, over-the-counter vitamin D and calcium carbonate and the prescription drug alendronate will be given with initiation of the cancer pharmacotherapy. These are to be continued as long as goserelin is administered.

Rehabilitation Setting: The patient ambulates independently into the clinic with both canes. He states that recurring acute painful RA flare-ups prevent him from aerobic activities. The near constant knee pain limits him to household and limited community ambulation. His upper body function usually does not limit his activities; however, this is also limited during acute RA flare-ups. After evaluation, the physical therapist recommends a conditioning program that includes upper extremity resistive exercises, as pain and acute episodes of RA allow. Since ambulation or resistive exercises including the lower extremities were limited by pain, the therapist develops an aquatherapy program. Aquatherapy includes ambulation on the clinic's underwater treadmill at a water level that the patient finds comfortable. The program is developed at the clinic, and will be continued at the local recreation center where the patient can walk at a comfortable speed in the shallow end of the pool. The patient will return once every-other-week for treatment modification. The therapist encourages the patient to attempt swimming when he feels more comfortable in the water.

Problem/Clinical Options: In recognition of the patient's current low bone mineral density, which probably stems from his intermittent glucocorticoid use and minimal physical activity, the oncologist made the referral for the development of a conditioning program. In addition, the antiandrogen pharmacotherapy for prostate cancer will suppress bone mineralization, further increasing the potential for osteoporosis. The purpose of the vitamin D, calcium, and alendronate is to minimize any further bone mineralization loss. An appropriate conditioning program in conjunction with anti-osteoporosis drugs will help minimize further bone loss, and may increase bone mineralization. Although aquatic activity is not as effective as resistive exercises in preventing bone demineralization in the lower extremities, the patient's current limitations preclude resistive exercises. Aquatic therapy has the added benefits of maintaining cardiovascular and respiratory functions.

PREPARATIONS AVAILABLE

Vitamin D, Metabolites, and Analogs

Calcifediol (Calderol)
Oral: 20-, 50-mcg capsules

Calcitriol
Oral (Rocaltrol): 0.25-, 0.5-mcg capsules, 1 mcg/mL solution
Parenteral (Calcijex): 1 mcg/mL for injection

Cholecalciferol (D3) (vitamin D3, Delta-D)
Oral: 400, 1000 IU tablets

Dihydrotachysterol (DHT) (DHT, Hytakerol)
Oral: 0.125-mg tablets, capsules; 0.2-, 0.4-mg tablets; 0.2 mg/mL intensol solution

Doxercalciferol (Hectoral)
Oral: 2.5-mcg capsules

Ergocalciferol (D2) (vitamin D2, Calciferol, Drisdol)
Oral: 50,000 IU capsules; 8000 IU/mL drops
Parenteral: 500,000 IU/mL for injection

Paricalcitol (Zemplar)
Parenteral: 5 mcg/mL for injection

Calcium

Calcium acetate (25% calcium) (PhosLo)
Oral: 668-mg (167-mg calcium) tablets; 333.5-mg (84.5-mg calcium), 667-mg (169-mg calcium) capsules

Calcium carbonate (40% calcium) (generic, Tums, Cal-Sup, Os-Cal 500, others)
Oral: Numerous forms available containing 260–600 mg calcium per unit

Calcium chloride (27% calcium) (generic)
Parenteral: 10% solution for IV injection only

Calcium citrate (21% calcium) (generic, Citracal)
Oral: 950-mg (200-mg calcium), 2376-mg (500-mg calcium)

Calcium glubionate (6.5% calcium) (Calcionate, Calciquid)
Oral: 1.8 g (115-mg calcium)/5 mL syrup

Calcium gluceptate (8% calcium) (Calcium Gluceptate)
Parenteral: 1.1 g/5 mL solution for IM or IV injection

Calcium gluconate (9% calcium) (generic)
Oral: 500-mg (45-mg calcium), 650-mg (58.5-mg calcium), 975-mg (87.75-mg calcium), 1-g (90-mg calcium) tablets
Parenteral: 10% solution for IV or IM injection

Calcium lactate (13% calcium) (generic)
Oral: 650-mg (84.5-mg calcium), 770-mg (100-mg calcium) tablets

Tricalcium phosphate (39% calcium) (Posture)
Oral: 1565-mg (600-mg calcium) tablets (as phosphate)

Phosphate and Phosphate Binder

Phosphate
Oral (Fleet Phospho-soda): solution containing 2.5 g phosphate/5 mL (816 mg phosphorus/5 mL; 751 mg sodium/5 mL)
Oral (K-Phos-Neutral): tablets containing 250 mg phosphorus, 298 mg sodium
Oral (Neutra-Phos): For reconstitution in 75 mL water, packet containing 250 mg phosphorus; 164 mg sodium; 278 mg potassium
Oral (Neutra-Phos-K): For reconstitution in 75 mL water, packet containing 250 mg phosphorus; 556 mg potassium; 0 mg sodium
Parenteral (potassium or sodium phosphate): 3 mmol/mL

Sevelamer (Renagel)
Oral: 403-mg capsules

Other Drugs

Alendronate (Fosamax)
Oral: 5-, 10-, 35-, 40-, 70-mg tablets

Calcitonin-Salmon
Nasal spray (Miacalcin): 200 IU/puff
Parenteral (Calcimar, Miacalcin, Salmonine): 200 IU/mL for injection

Etidronate (Didronel)
Oral: 200-, 400-mg tablets
Parenteral: 300-mg/6 mL for IV injection

Pamidronate (generic, Aredia)
Parenteral: 30, 60, 90 mg/vial

Plicamycin (mithramycin) (Mithracin)
Parenteral: 2.5 mg per vial powder to reconstitute for injection

Risedronate (Actonel)
Oral: 5-, 30-, 35-mg tablets

Sodium fluoride (generic)
Oral: 0.55-mg (0.25-mg F), 1.1-mg (0.5 mg F), 2.2-mg (1-mg F) tablets; drops

Teriparatide (Forteo)
Subcutaneous: 250 mcg/mL from prefilled pen (3 mL)

Tiludronate (Skelid)
Oral: 200-mg tablets

Zoledronic acid (Zometa)
Parenteral: 4 mg/vial

REFERENCES

Berenson JR, et al: American Society of Clinical Oncology clinical practice guidelines: The role of bisphosphonates in multiple myeloma. *J Clin Oncol* 2002;20:3719.

Fisher JE, et al: In vivo effects of bisphosphonates on the osteoclast mevalonate pathway. *Endocrinology* 2000; 141:4793.

Incidence and costs to Medicare of fractures among Medicare beneficiaries ≥ 65 years—United States, July 1991–June 1992. *MMWR Morb Mortal Wkly Rep* 1996;45:877.

LaCroix AZ, et al: Low-dose hydrochlorothiazide and preservation of bone mineral density in older adults. *Ann Intern Med* 2000;133:516.

Liberman, UA, et al: Effect of oral alendronate on bone mineral density and the incidence of fractures in postmenopausal osteoporosis. *N Engl J Med* 1995;333: 1437.

Manolagas SC: Birth and death of bone cells: Basic regulatory mechanisms and implications for the pathogenesis and treatment of osteoporosis. *Endocr Rev* 2000;21:115.

McClung MR, et al: Effect of risedronate on the risk of hip fracture in elderly women. *N Engl J Med* 2001;344:333.

Neer RM, et al: Effect of parathyroid hormone (1-34) on fractures and bone mineral density in postmenopausal women with osteoporosis. *N Engl J Med* 2001;344: 1434.

Orwoll E, et al: Alendronate for the treatment of osteoporosis in men. *N Engl J Med* 2000;343:604.

Rodan GA, Martin TJ: Therapeutic approaches to bone diseases. *Science* 2000;289:1508.

Rehabilitation

Bonaiuti D, et al: Exercise for preventing and treating osteoporosis in postmenopausal women. *Cochrane Database Syst Rev* 2002;CD000333.

Chau DL, et al: Osteoporosis and diabetes. *Curr Diab Rep* 2003;3:37.

Chilibeck PD: Exercise and estrogen or estrogen alternatives (phytoestrogens, bisphosphonates) for preservation of bone mineral in postmenopausal women. *Can J Appl Physiol* 2004;29:59.

Clarke MS: The effects of exercise on skeletal muscle in the aged. *J Musculoskelet Neuronal Interact* 2004; 4:175.

Going S, et al: Effects of exercise on bone mineral density in calcium-replete postmenopausal women with and without hormone replacement therapy. *Osteoporos Int* 2003;14:637.

Iwamoto J, et al: Effect of exercise training and detraining on bone mineral density in postmenopausal women with osteoporosis. *J Orthop Sci* 2001;6:128.

Lane JM, Nydick M: Osteoporosis: current modes of prevention and treatment. *J Am Acad Orthop Surg* 1999; 7:19.

Layne JE, Nelson ME: The effects of progressive resistance training on bone density: A review. *Med Sci Sports Exerc* 1999;31:25.

Melton SA, et al: Water exercise prevents femur density loss associated with ovariectomy in the retired breeder rat. *J Strength Cond Res* 2004;18:508.

Moyad MA: Promoting general health during androgen deprivation therapy (ADT): A rapid 10-step review for your patients. *Urol Oncol* 2005;23:56.

Smith MR: Diagnosis and management of treatment-related osteoporosis in men with prostate carcinoma. *Cancer* 2003;97:789.

Swezey RL: Exercise for osteoporosis—is walking enough? The case for site specificity and resistive exercise. *Spine* 1996;21:2809.

Takata S, Yasui N: Disuse osteoporosis. *J Med Invest* 2001; 48:147.

Valentine JF, Sninsky CA: Prevention and treatment of osteoporosis in patients with inflammatory bowel disease. *Am J Gastroenterol* 1999;94:878.

Winett RA, Carpinelli RN: Potential health-related benefits of resistance training. *Prev Med* 2001;33:503.

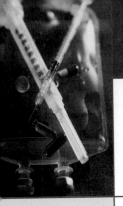

26

ANTIHYPERLIPIDEMIC DRUGS

Atherosclerosis is the abnormal accumulation of lipids and products resulting from an inflammatory response in the walls of arteries, and is the leading cause of death in the Western world. Heart attacks, angina pectoris, peripheral arterial disease, and strokes are common sequelae of atherosclerosis. In some cases, lowering serum lipid concentrations has been shown to prevent the sequelae of atherosclerosis and decrease mortality in patients with a history of cardiovascular disease and hyperlipidemia. The five drug classes discussed in this chapter (Figure 26–1) are used to decrease serum concentrations of lipids in the blood (hyperlipidemia) and to prevent or reverse associated atherosclerosis, or, in the case of hypertriglyceridemia, prevent pancreatitis. Although the drugs are generally safe and effective, adverse effects include drug–drug interactions and rare toxic reactions in skeletal muscle and the liver.

HYPERLIPOPROTEINEMIA

Lipids, mainly cholesterol and triglycerides, are transported in human plasma by macromolecular complexes termed lipoproteins. Lipoproteins are composed of a lipid core surrounded by apolipoproteins that regulate the uptake and off-loading of lipids and interactions with cell membrane receptors. The lipoproteins that are primarily responsible for delivering cholesterol and triglycerides to peripheral tissues originate in the liver and contain a key apoprotein called B-100. These B-100–containing lipoproteins include **very low-density lipoprotein (VLDL)**, **low-density lipoprotein (LDL)**, and **intermediate-density lipoprotein (IDL)** (Figure 26–2). The uptake by cells of B-100–containing lipoproteins can occur by receptor-mediated endocytosis or by scavenger receptors. Receptor-mediated uptake is a carefully regulated process that protects cells from being overloaded with lipids. In contrast, uptake by scavenger receptors is an unregulated process that can overwhelm the ability of a cell to sequester potentially toxic lipids safely. Macrophages in arterial walls use scavenger receptors to take up circulating lipoproteins, especially particles with apolipoproteins that have been modified by free radicals. When these macrophages become overloaded with lipids, they are transformed into distressed foam cells that initiate a local inflammatory response. Engorged foam cells, foam cells that have burst, and the products of the inflammatory responses form the core of an atherosclerotic plaque. Whereas plaques can slowly occlude coronary and cerebral vessels, clinical symptoms are more frequently precipitated by rupture of unstable plaques, leading to occlusive thrombi.

Another lipoprotein, **high-density lipoprotein (HDL)**, exerts several antiatherogenic effects. HDL participates in pathways that retrieve cholesterol from the artery wall and inhibit the

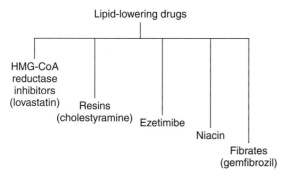

Figure 26–1. The five classes of lipid-lowering drugs. These classes are based on the mechanisms of action of these drugs.

oxidation of atherogenic lipoproteins. Low levels of HDL are an independent risk factor for coronary artery disease, whereas high levels are protective.

Plasma lipids are measured in serum after a 10-hour fast. Desirable and elevated levels are presented in Table 26–1. The risk of atherosclerotic heart disease increases with high concentrations of atherogenic lipoproteins such as LDL ("bad cholesterol") and low concentrations of HDL ("good cholesterol"). Additional risk factors include personal and family history of atherosclerosis, obesity, cigarette smoking, and excessive alcohol intake. Evidence from clinical trials suggests that LDL cholesterol levels of 60 to 70 mg/dL may be optimal for patients with coronary disease. Ideally, triglyceride levels should be below 150 mg/dL.

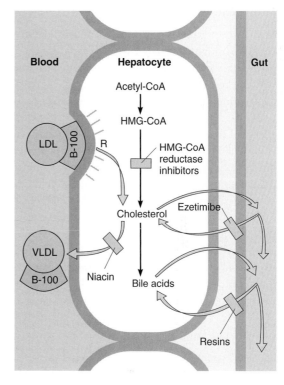

Figure 26–2. Schematic diagram of lipoprotein handling by hepatocytes. The sites of action of several antihyperlipidemic drugs are shown. LDL receptors (R) are increased by treatment with resins and HMG-CoA reductase inhibitors. For identification of abbreviations of the lipoproteins, some drug classes, and additional discussion, see text.

Table 26-1. National cholesterol education program: adult treatment guidelines (2002)

	Optimal	Near Optimal to Above Optimal	Borderline to High[1]	High	Very High
Total Cholesterol	<200		200–239	≥240	
LDL Cholesterol	<100	100–129	130–159	160–189	≥190
HDL Cholesterol				≥60	
Men	≥40				
Women	≥50				
Triglycerides	<150		150–199	200–499	≥500

All values given in mg/dL. Additional information may be found at http://www.nhlbi.nih.gov/guidelines/cholesterol/atp3full.pdf
HDL = high-density lipoprotein; LDL = low-density lipoprotein.
[1]Considered to be high if coronary disease or more than two risk factors are present.

Pathogenesis

Premature or accelerated development of atherosclerosis is strongly associated with elevated levels of total cholesterol and LDL cholesterol. The link between hypertriglyceridemia, an elevated level of triglycerides in the serum while fasting, and atherosclerosis is less well defined. However, it is clear that severe hypertriglyceridemia such as that associated with chylomicronemia, a recessive genetic disorder that prevents the normal uptake or metabolism of chylomicrons, is correlated with a high incidence of acute pancreatitis. Regulation of plasma lipoprotein levels involves a balance among dietary fat intake, hepatic processing, and utilization by peripheral tissues. Primary disturbances in regulation occur in various familial diseases. Secondary disturbances are associated with a Western diet, many endocrine conditions, and diseases of the liver or kidneys. The primary hyperlipoproteinemias are presented in Table 26–2.

TREATMENT STRATEGIES

Dietary measures are the first method of management and may be sufficient to reduce lipoprotein levels to a safe range. Cholesterol, saturated fats, and *trans* fats are the primary dietary factors that contribute to elevated LDL levels, whereas total fat and caloric restriction are important in management of triglycerides. Diets are designed to reduce the total intake of these substances. Homocysteine, which initiates proatherogenic changes in vascular endothelium, can be reduced in many patients by restriction of total protein intake to the amount required for amino acid replacement. Finally, omega-3 fatty acids found in fish oils (but not those found in plants) can induce profound lowering of triglycerides in some patients. In contrast, omega-6 fatty acids found in vegetable oils may increase triglycerides.

Drug therapy can modify hepatic cholesterol synthesis (hydroxymethylglutaryl-coenzyme *A* [HMG-CoA] reductase inhibitors), reduce cholesterol (ezetimibe)

Table 26-2. The primary hyperlipoproteinemias and their drug treatment

Condition	Single Drug	Drug Combination
Primary chylomicronemia (familial lipoprotein lipase or cofactor deficiency)	Dietary management	Niacin plus fibrate
Familial hypertriglyceridemia	Niacin or fibrate	Niacin plus fibrate
Familial combined hyperlipidemia		
VLDL increased	Niacin or fibrate	
LDL increased	Niacin, reductase inhibitor, or ezetimibe	Two or three of the individual drugs
VLDL, LDL increased	Niacin or reductase inhibitor	Niacin or fibrate plus statin or ezetimide
Familial dysbetalipoproteinemia	Fibrate or niacin	Fibrate plus niacin, or niacin plus reductase inhibitor
Familial hypercholesterolemia		
Heterozygous	Reductase inhibitor, resin, niacin, ezetimibe	Two or three of the individual drugs
Homozygous	Niacin, reductase inhibitor, ezetimibe	Niacin plus reductase inhibitor plus ezetimibe

LDL = low-density lipoprotein; VLDL = very low-density lipoprotein.

and bile acid (resins) absorption from the intestine, decrease secretion of lipoproteins (niacin), and increase peripheral clearance of lipoproteins (fibrates) (Figure 26–2). All of these drugs are given orally. In some cases, drug therapy for hyperlipidemia can cause slow physical regression of plaques. The well-documented reduction in acute coronary events following vigorous drug treatment is attributable chiefly to reduction of inflammatory activity in the vessels, which is evident within 2 to 3 months after starting therapy.

HMG-CoA Reductase Inhibitors (Statins)

Mechanism and Effects

Lovastatin and **simvastatin** are prodrugs. The other HMG-CoA reductase inhibitors (**atorvastatin, fluvastatin, pravastatin, rosuvastatin**) are active as given. In the body, the active drugs are structural analogs that competitively inhibit mevalonate synthesis by HMG-CoA reductase, a process essential for cholesterol biosynthesis in the liver (Figure 26–2). Although inhibition of hepatic cholesterol synthesis directly reduces total serum cholesterol, a much greater effect derives from the hepatic response to the reduction in intracellular cholesterol. The liver compensates by

increasing the number of high-affinity LDL receptors, which clear LDL from the blood (Figure 26–2). HMG-CoA reductase inhibitors also have direct antiatherosclerotic effects, and they have been shown to prevent bone loss. They also produce modest decreases in plasma triglycerides and small increases in HDL cholesterol.

Clinical Use

Statins can reduce LDL cholesterol levels dramatically (Table 26–3), especially when used in combination with other drugs (Table 26–2). The statins are commonly used because they are effective and well tolerated. Large clinical trials have shown that they reduce the risk of coronary events and mortality in patients with ischemic heart disease. Fluvastatin has lower maximal efficacy than the other drugs in this group.

Adverse Effects

Mild elevations of aminotransferases released from hepatocytes into the blood are common, but are not often associated with significant hepatic damage. Patients with preexisting liver disease may have more severe reactions. Creatine kinase is an intracellular

Table 26-3.	Lipid-modifying effects of antihyperlipidemic drugs		
Drug	**LDL Cholesterol**	**HDL Cholesterol**	**Triglyceride**
Statins			
Atorvastatin	–25% to –40%	+5% to +10%	↓↓
Fluvastatin	–20% to –30%	+5% to +10%	↓
Lovastatin[1]	–25% to –40%	+5% to +10%	↓
Resins	–15% to –25%	+5%	± or ↑[2]
Ezetimibe	–13% to –19%	+3%	±
Niacin	–15% to –40%	+25% to +35%	↓↓
Fibrates	–10% to –15%	+15% to +20%	↓↓

[1]Pravastatin and simvastatin have effects similar to those of lovastatin.

[2]Resins can increase serum triglyceride concentrations in some patients with familial combined hypercholesterolemia.

± = variable, if any.

Modified, with permission, from Tierney LM, McPhee SJ, Papadikis MA, eds: *Current Medical Diagnosis and Treatment*, 3rd ed. New York: McGraw-Hill, 2004.

enzyme found in various cell types; it is released when such cells are damaged. An increase in creatine kinase (subtype CK-MM) release from skeletal muscle is noted in about 10% of patients; in a few patients, severe muscle pain (myalgia), joint pain (arthralgia), and even rhabdomyolysis may occur. HMG-CoA reductase inhibitors are metabolized by the cytochrome P450 system; drugs or foods (e.g., grapefruit juice) that inhibit cytochrome P450 activity increase the risk of hepatotoxicity and myopathy. Because of evidence that the HMG-CoA reductase inhibitors are teratogenic, these drugs should be avoided in pregnancy. In addition, cholesterol is required for maturation of the nervous system in young children, so the drugs are rarely used in children under the age of 8 years.

Resins

Mechanism and Effects
Bile acid–binding resins (**cholestyramine, colestipol, colesevelam**) are large nonabsorbable polymers that bind bile acids in the intestine (Figure 26–2). By preventing the reabsorption of bile acids secreted by the liver, these agents divert hepatic cholesterol to synthesis of new bile acids, thereby reducing the amount of cholesterol in the tightly regulated hepatic pool. A compensatory increase in the synthesis of hepatic high-affinity LDL receptors increases the removal of LDL lipoproteins from the blood. The resins cause a modest reduction in LDL cholesterol, but have little effect on HDL cholesterol or triglycerides (Table 26–3). In some patients with familial combined hyperlipidemia, resins increase VLDL.

Clinical Use
The resins are used in patients with hypercholesterolemia (Table 26–2). They have also been used to reduce pruritus in patients with cholestasis and bile salt accumulation. They should not be used in hypertriglyceridemia.

Adverse Effects
Adverse effects include bloating, constipation, and an unpleasant gritty taste. Resins impair the absorption of some vitamins (e.g., vitamin K, dietary folates) and drugs (e.g., digitalis, thiazides, warfarin, pravastatin, fluvastatin).

Ezetimibe

Mechanism and Effects
Ezetimibe is a prodrug that is converted in the liver to the active glucuronide form. The drug inhibits an enzyme involved in the gastrointestinal uptake of cholesterol and phytosterols, plant sterols that normally enter gastrointestinal epithelial cells but then are immediately transported back into the intestinal lumen (Figure 26–2). By preventing absorption of dietary cholesterol and cholesterol that is excreted in bile, ezetimibe reduces the cholesterol in the tightly regulated hepatic pool. A compensatory increase in the synthesis of hepatic high-affinity LDL receptors increases the removal of LDL lipoproteins from the blood. As monotherapy, ezetimibe reduces LDL cholesterol by about 18% (Table 26–3). When combined with a reductase inhibitor, ezetimibe is even more effective.

Clinical Use
Ezetimibe is used for treatment of hypercholesterolemia (Table 26–2) and phytosterolemia, a rare genetic disorder that results from impaired export of phytosterols. In spite of its clear effects on cholesterol levels, some recent findings cast doubt on ezetimibe's ability to reduce or reverse plaque formation in humans.

Adverse Effects
Ezetimibe is well tolerated. When combined with reductase inhibitors, it may increase the risk of hepatic toxicity. Serum concentrations of the glucuronide form are increased by fibrates and reduced by cholestyramine.

Niacin (Nicotinic Acid)

Mechanism and Effects
Niacin, but not nicotinamide (another form of vitamin B_3), directly reduces VLDL secretion from the liver and inhibits hepatic synthesis of apolipoproteins or cholesterol (Figure 26–2). Consequently, LDL formation is reduced, and there is a decrease in serum LDL cholesterol (Table 26–3). Increased clearance of VLDL by lipoprotein lipase in the periphery has also been demonstrated and probably accounts for the reduction in serum triglyceride concentrations.

In addition, the levels of HDL often increase. Niacin also decreases circulating fibrinogen and increases tissue plasminogen activator. This combination of effects decreases the risk of formation of thrombi and increases their dissolution.

Clinical Use

Because niacin lowers serum LDL cholesterol and triglyceride concentrations and increases HDL cholesterol concentrations, niacin has wide clinical utility (Table 26–2).

Adverse Effects

Cutaneous flushing is a common adverse effect. Pretreatment with aspirin or other nonsteroidal anti-inflammatory drugs (NSAIDs) reduces the intensity of this flushing, suggesting that it is mediated by prostaglandin release. Tolerance to the flushing reaction usually develops within a few days. Dose-dependent nausea and abdominal discomfort often occur. Pruritus and other skin conditions have been reported. Moderate elevations of liver enzymes and even severe hepatotoxicity may occur. Hyperuricemia occurs in about 20% of patients. Niacin has been shown to induce minor insulin resistance in diabetic and nondiabetic patients. Finally, niacin may potentiate the action of some antihypertensive drugs.

Fibric Acid Derivatives (Fibrates)

Mechanism and Effects

Fibric acid derivatives (e.g., **gemfibrozil, fenofibrate, clofibrate**) are ligands for the peroxisome proliferator-activated receptor-alpha (PPAR-α) protein, a receptor that regulates transcription of genes involved in lipid metabolism. This interaction with PPAR-α results in increased activity of lipoprotein lipase and enhanced clearance of triglyceride-rich lipoproteins (Figure 26–2). Cholesterol biosynthesis in the liver is secondarily reduced. The fibrates reduce serum triglyceride concentrations and produce a modest increase in HDL cholesterol (Table 26–3). There may be a small reduction in LDL cholesterol.

Clinical Use

Gemfibrozil and other fibrates are used to treat hypertriglyceridemia (Table 26–2). Because these drugs have only modest effects on LDL cholesterol, they are often combined with other antilipidemic drugs for treatment of patients with elevated concentrations of both LDL and VLDL.

Adverse Effects

Nausea is the most common adverse effect produced by all members of this drug group. Skin rashes are common with gemfibrozil. A few patients show decreases in white blood count or hematocrit, and these drugs can potentiate the action of anticoagulants. Because there is an increased risk of cholesterol gallstones, fibrates should be used with caution in patients with a history of cholelithiasis. When used in combination with statin drugs, the fibrates significantly increase the risk of myopathy.

COMBINATION THERAPY

All patients with hyperlipidemia are initially treated with dietary modification. To achieve the desired effect on various lipoproteins (LDL, VLDL, and HDL), a drug or drug combination is often added to dietary control to achieve the maximum lipid lowering possible with minimum toxicity. The most common combinations are listed in Table 26–2.

Certain drug combinations present challenges. Because resins interfere with the absorption of certain reductase inhibitors (pravastatin, cerivastatin, atorvastatin, and fluvastatin), these must be taken at least 1 hour before or 4 hours after the resins. The combination of reductase inhibitors with either fibrates or niacin increases the risk of myopathy.

REHABILITATION FOCUS

Hyperlipidemia leading to atherosclerosis and subsequent pathophysiologic sequelae is a major public health problem. Patients treated with cholesterol-lowering drugs may be in rehabilitation for many reasons from improving cardiac function following a myocardial infarct to improving glycemic control associated with diabetes mellitus. Optimal improvement in blood lipid profiles occurs when patients make lifestyle changes (exercise, weight reduction, and dietary reduction in saturated and *trans* fat intake) along with antilipidemic drug therapy. Several drug classes used to treat hyperlipidemia may have adverse effects that clinically manifest as myalgia, arthralgia, and muscle weakness. Careful differential diagnosis should clarify whether these manifestations are the result of musculoskeletal dysfunction or from drug-related adverse effects.

■ CLINICAL RELEVANCE FOR REHABILITATION

Adverse Drug Reactions

- Several of the lipid-lowering drug classes can cause myalgia, arthralgia, and muscle weakness.

Effects Interfering with Rehabilitation

- Arthralgia, myalgia, and muscle weakness may decrease patient function because of pain and may adversely affect functional outcomes of treatment.
  - The clinician should differentiate pain associated with exercise from that associated with the adverse effects of these drugs.

Possible Therapy Solutions

- If the patient presents with any of these manifestations, contact the referring health-care provider.

Potentiation of Functional Outcomes Secondary to Drug Therapy

- Antihyperlipidemic drugs in conjunction with diet and aerobic activity will maximize reduction in blood lipid levels.

PROBLEM-ORIENTED PATIENT STUDY

Brief History: The patient is a 43-year-old Hispanic male with a body mass index of 27. He is employed on an assembly line at an automotive plant. Four weeks ago, he was involved in an industrial accident in which he experienced muscular strains in the upper extremities and low back. He was evaluated in the onsite clinic at the plant. He was initially referred to rehabilitation for pain relief while he was on light duty at work. Subsequently, he enrolled in a work-hardening program to return to full-time regular work status.

Current Medical Status and Drug Therapy: The patient has hypertriglyceridemia and above optimal LDL cholesterol levels. He is currently being treated with gemfibrozil and niacin to lower these values.

Rehabilitation Setting: Three weeks ago, he complained of bilateral muscle and joint pain in both arms and diffuse pain in his back. He also stated that he had muscle weakness in both arms.

During the first week of rehabilitation, he received supportive therapy for pain relief to improve function for light-duty work. Last week, he began the work-hardening program. During that week, he complained that the previous pain and muscle weakness increased. He was counseled that the pain may be related to initiation of the work-hardening program. His complaints of pain and weakness were noted in the chart as delayed-onset muscle soreness. He continued the work-hardening program and was reevaluated. Upon questioning, he denied any changes in his medications since his initial evaluation. He also denied taking over-the-counter medications or supplements. However, he added that he began taking "red-yeast-rice" approximately 5 weeks ago because he heard that it lowers "bad cholesterol." When asked why this was not on the initial evaluation form, he stated: "the form only asked for prescription medicines, and red-yeast-rice was not prescribed."

(continued)

PROBLEM-ORIENTED PATIENT STUDY (*Continued*)

Problem/Clinical Options: The bilateral muscle and joint pain and weakness in the upper extremities and the low back pain would be expected to decrease after 3 weeks if these symptoms were a result of his accident. The patient was referred back to the original health-care provider for further evaluation with the additional information regarding the patient's consumption of red-yeast-rice. Blood analyses revealed an elevation of creatine kinase (subtype CK-MM) and mild elevation of myoglobin. He was diagnosed with myopathy, likely associated with the combination of red-yeast-rice and antihyperlipidemic medications. Red-yeast-rice contains lovastatin (monacolin K) and other naturally occurring statins. When combined with his prescription drugs (niacin and gemfibrozil), this resulted in myopathy and associated clinical manifestations.

PREPARATIONS AVAILABLE

Atorvastatin (Lipitor)
Oral: 10-, 20-, 40-, 80-mg tablets

Cholestyramine (generic, Questran, Questran Light)
Oral: 4-g packets anhydrous granules cholestyramine resin; 210-g (Questran Light), 378-g (Questran) cans

Colesevelam (Welchol)
Oral: 62-mg tablets

Colestipol (Colestid)
Oral: 5-g packets granules; 300-, 500-g bottles; 1-g tablets

Ezetimibe (Zetia)
Oral: 10-mg tablets

Fenofibrate (Tricor)
Oral: 54-, 160-mg tablets

Fluvastatin (Lescol)
Oral: 20-, 40-mg capsules; extended release (Lescol XL): 80-mg capsules

Gemfibrozil (generic, Lopid)
Oral: 600-mg tablets

Lovastatin (generic, Mevacor)
Oral: 10-, 20-, 40-, 80-mg tablets; extended-release tablets (Altocar) 10-, 20-, 40-, 60-mg

Niacin, nicotinic acid, vitamin B$_3$ (generic, others)
Oral: 100-, 250-, 500-, 1000-mg tablets

Pravastatin (Pravachol)
Oral: 10-, 20-, 40-, 80-mg tablets

Rosuvastatin (Crestor)
Oral: 5-, 10-, 20-, 40-mg tablets

Simvastatin (Zocor)
Oral: 5-, 10-, 20-, 40-, 80-mg tablets

REFERENCES

Cannon CP, et al: Intensive vs moderate lipid lowering with statins after acute coronary syndromes. *N Engl J Med* 2004;350:1495.

Libby P, et al: A: Inflammation and atherosclerosis. *Circulation* 2002;105:1135.

Sacks FM, et al: The effect of pravastatin on coronary events after myocardial infarction in patients with average cholesterol levels. Cholesterol and Recurrent Events Investigators. *N Engl J Med* 1996; 335:1001.

Schwartz GG, et al: Effects of atorvastatin on early recurrent ischemic events in acute coronary syndromes: The

MIRACL study: A randomized controlled trial. *JAMA* 2001;285:1711.

Third Report of the National Cholesterol Education Program (NCEP) Expert Panel on Detection, Evaluation, and Treatment of High Blood Cholesterol in Adults (Adult Treatment Panel III) http://www.nhlbi.nih.gov/guidelines/cholesterol/atp3full.pdf

Dietary Treatment

Kromhout D, et al: Prevention of coronary heart disease by diet and lifestyle. *Circulation* 2002;105:893.

Rehabilitation

Baardman T, et al: Changes in plasma lipoproteins after cardiac rehabilitation in patients not on lipid-lowering drugs. *Eur Heart J* 1990;11:722.

Courville KA, et al: Lipid-lowering therapy for elderly patients at risk for coronary events and stroke. *Am Heart Hosp J* 2005;3:256.

Heber D, et al: Cholesterol-lowering effects of a proprietary Chinese red-yeast-rice dietary supplement. *Am J Clin Nutr* 1999;69:231.

Lavie CJ: Treatment of hyperlipidemia in elderly persons with exercise training, nonpharmacologic therapy, and drug combinations. *Am J Geriatr Cardiol* 2004; 13:29.

Lenz TL: Therapeutic lifestyle changes and pharmaceutical care in the treatment of dyslipidemias in adults. *J Am Pharm Assoc (Wash)* 2005;45:492.

Mackinnon LT, Hubinger LM: Effects of exercise on lipoprotein(a). *Sports Med* 1999;28:11.

Smith DJ, Olive KE: Chinese red rice-induced myopathy. *South Med J* 2003;96:1265.

Varady KA, Jones PJ: Combination diet and exercise interventions for the treatment of dyslipidemia: An effective preliminary strategy to lower cholesterol levels? *J Nutr* 2005;135:1829.

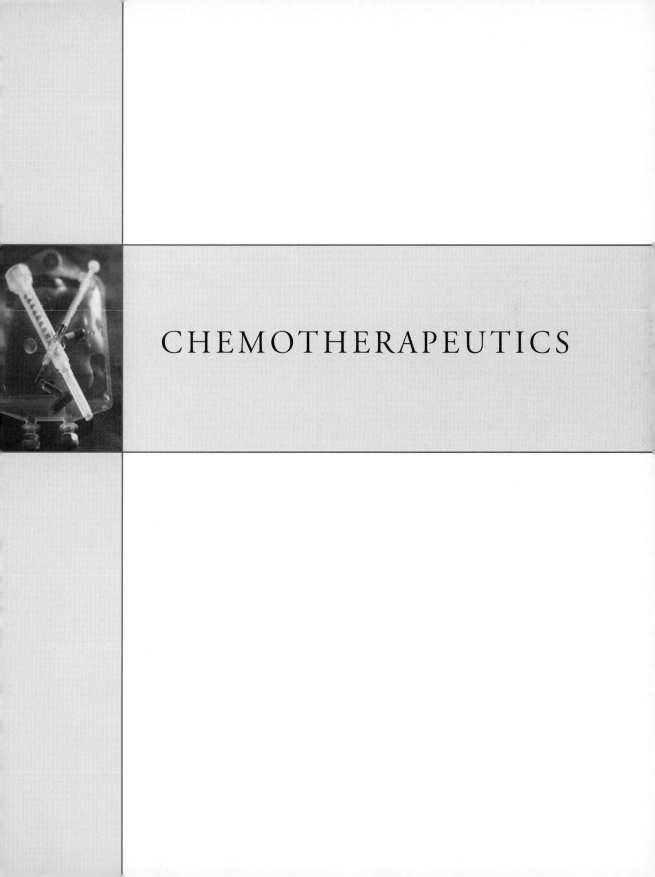

CHEMOTHERAPEUTICS

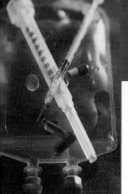

27

ANTIBACTERIAL AGENTS

Infectious diseases are among the most common forms of illness. Thus, many patients undergoing physical rehabilitation may be taking one or more antimicrobial drugs. Most agents (but not all) have little direct impact on the functional rehabilitation outcomes, but they will certainly have an impact on the overall health status of the patient.

The next four chapters address agents used to treat infections caused by various parasites including bacteria, viruses, fungi, protozoa, and helminths (worms). Once these pathogens gain access inside the human body, they can cause illnesses ranging from minor infections to life-threatening illnesses. Antimicrobial drugs are among the most dramatic examples of advances of modern medicine; many infectious diseases once considered incurable and lethal are now amenable to treatment. Antimicrobial drugs are classified and identified according to the primary type of infectious organism they are used to treat (e.g., antibacterial, antiviral, antifungal).

The remarkably powerful and specific activity of antimicrobial drugs is due to *selective toxicity*—that is, drugs are designed to target structures selectively that are either unique to microorganisms or much more important in them than in humans. Therefore, a general understanding of microbial structure and function is necessary to understand the mechanisms of action of antimicrobial agents. Notably, selective toxicity is not perfect, and antimicrobials may exert some adverse effects in humans.

▓ BACTERIAL PATHOGENICITY

Bacterial infections harm humans in several ways. Bacteria can directly damage or destroy human cells by releasing toxins, and they can compete with human cells for vital nutrients. In addition, in immunocompetent individuals, bacteria trigger a host immune response that may damage not only pathogenic bacteria but also human cells and tissues.

It is also important to understand that not all bacteria living in the human body are harmful. In fact, some bacteria normally coexist within humans and actually benefit their human hosts. For example, *Escherichia coli* microorganisms normally inhabit the gastrointestinal tract and are thus considered part of the normal flora. *E coli* assist in digestion of food, synthesize essential nutrients such as vitamin K, and inhibit the growth of other organisms. As an illustration of the latter function, antibiotic therapy often results in the eradication of normal gut flora. After antibiotic treatment is completed, overgrowth of other microorganisms (e.g., yeasts) often occurs.

BACTERIAL STRUCTURE AND NOMENCLATURE

The target site for antibacterial drugs, or antibiotics, is either the cell wall or structures involved in bacterial reproduction.

Bacteria are single-celled *prokaryotes* (cells without a distinct nucleus) that have a characteristic cellular organization. Fungi, protozoa, and multicellular organisms have nuclei containing their genetic material and are called *eukaryotes*. Viruses, on the other hand, are not strictly cellular at all and comprise a very different form of life. Bacterial deoxyribonucleic acid (DNA) forms a long circular molecule called a nucleoid. In addition, genetic information may be present in DNA molecules termed *plasmids*. Plasmids replicate independently of chromosomal DNA and may carry genes that affect resistance to antimicrobials (i.e., plasmid-mediated resistance). Both nucleoid DNA and plasmids are subject to mutations that can be passed on to daughter cells. In addition, bacteria can exchange genetic material by a process called conjugation, thus allowing passage of drug resistance genes without mutation. Both nucleoid and plasmid DNA are transcribed into messenger ribonucleic acid (RNA) by the enzyme RNA polymerase.

Ribosomal function is the same in prokaryotic and eukaryotic cells—that is, ribosomes translate messenger RNA into a new protein chain, the final product of the gene. However, ribosomal structure is characterized as 70S in prokaryotes and as 80S in eukaryotes. (The "S" unit refers to how a molecule sediments under centrifugal force in an ultracentrifuge.) The bacterial 70S ribosome is specifically targeted by certain antibacterials such as the aminoglycosides. Two major subunits comprise the ribosome: 30S and 50S in prokaryotes and 40S and 60S in eukaryotes.

In all bacteria except mycoplasmas, the cell is completely surrounded by a cell wall, a structure not found in eukaryotes. The cell wall lies external to a cytoplasmic membrane, which is similar to the cell membranes of eukaryotic cells. The cell wall's rigidity maintains cell integrity, protecting bacteria from lysis due to high internal osmotic pressure.

Bacteria are classified as *gram positive* or *gram negative* according to their cell wall structure. The primary structural component of the cell wall is a peptidoglycan, a polymer of sugars and charged amino acids, which make the peptidoglycan highly polar. In gram-positive bacteria, the peptidoglycan forms a very thick hydrophilic layer external to the cell membrane. The thick hydrophilic surface of gram-positive bacteria can be digested by lysozyme, an enzyme present in body secretions and intracellular organelles, but provides protection against most other enzymes and bile in the intestine. Penicillin and cephalosporin antibiotics inhibit bacterial cell wall synthesis by disrupting peptidoglycan formation. In gram-negative bacteria, the peptidoglycan layer is thinner and anchored to an overlying outer membrane (Figure 27–1). The outer membrane is relatively hydrophobic. To enable hydrophilic nutrients to enter the cell, gram-negative bacteria have special pores formed by proteins called porins.

The cell wall is a primary determinant of the ultimate shape of the bacterium, which is an important characteristic for bacterial identification. In general, bacterial shapes are categorized as spherical (cocci), rods (bacilli), or helical (spirilla). Although each bacterium is named according to its genus and species (e.g., *Staphylococcus aureus*), bacteria are often categorized by common characteristics such as histologic staining properties and shape. For example, gram-positive cocci include bacteria that stain in a certain manner (determined by the gram-positive cell wall) and are spherical in shape (cocci). This group includes *S aureus* and *Streptococcus pneumoniae*.

The most common way to classify antibiotics is on the basis of their site of action: inhibitors of bacterial cell wall synthesis, inhibitors of bacterial protein synthesis, and inhibitors of bacterial DNA synthesis. Antimycobacterial drugs are discussed separately.

PRINCIPLES OF ANTIBIOTIC THERAPY

Some antibiotics are *bactericidal* (kill bacteria), while others are *bacteriostatic* (inhibit bacterial growth). Bacteriostatic antibiotics are successful in treating infections in patients with intact immune systems because they prevent the bacterial population from increasing, and allow host defense mechanisms to eradicate the remaining population. For bacteriostatic drugs (e.g.,

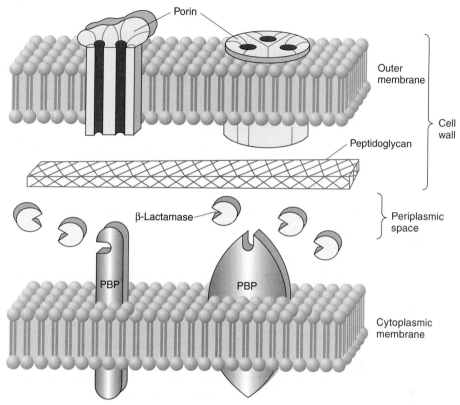

Figure 27–1. A simplified diagram of the cell envelope of a gram-negative bacterium. The outer membrane, a lipid bilayer, is present in gram-negative but not gram-positive bacteria. It is penetrated by porins, proteins that form channels providing hydrophilic access to the cytoplasmic membrane. The peptidoglycan layer is unique to bacteria and is much thicker in gram-positive bacteria than in gram-negative bacteria. Together, the outer membrane and the peptidoglycan layer constitute the cell wall. Penicillin-binding proteins (PBPs) are membrane proteins that cross-link peptidoglycan. β-Lactamases, if present, reside in the periplasmic space or on the outer surface of the cytoplasmic membrane, where they may destroy β-lactam antibiotics that penetrate the outer membrane.

clindamycin, macrolides, sulfonamides, tetracyclines), the concentrations that inhibit growth are much lower than those that kill bacteria. Bactericidal drugs (e.g., **aminoglycosides, β-lactams, fluoroquinolones, streptogramins, vancomycin,** and most antimycobacterial agents) are preferred for treating infections in immunocompromised patients because they are able to eradicate an infection even in the absence of normal host defense mechanisms. For bactericidal drugs, there is little difference between concentrations that inhibit growth and those that kill bacteria.

Dosage regimens with antibiotics have traditionally used multiple daily doses to maintain serum concentrations above the **minimal inhibitory concentration (MIC)** for as long as possible. However, the in vivo effectiveness of some antibiotics (e.g., aminoglycosides) results from a *concentration-dependent* killing action. As the plasma level is increased above the MIC, these agents kill an increasing proportion of bacteria and do so at a more rapid rate. Many other antibiotics (e.g., penicillins and cephalosporins) cause *time-dependent* killing of bacteria, wherein their in vivo efficacy is directly related to time above MIC and becomes independent of concentration once the MIC has been reached.

Some agents exert a *postantibiotic effect* in which inhibition of bacterial growth continues after plasma levels have fallen to low levels. The mechanisms of the postantibiotic effect are unclear, but may reflect delayed time required by bacteria to synthesize new enzymes and cellular components, persistence of antibiotic at target sites, or enhanced susceptibility of bacteria to host defense mechanisms. The postantibiotic effect contributes to the efficacy of once-daily administration of aminoglycosides, and may also contribute to the efficacy of the fluoroquinolones.

ANTIBIOTIC RESISTANCE

The emergence of *microbial resistance* poses an increasing challenge to the use of all antimicrobial drugs. The mechanisms underlying microbial resistance to antibiotics include production of drug-inactivating enzymes, changes in the structure of target receptors, increased antibiotic efflux via drug transporters, and decreases in cell wall permeability to antibiotics. Strategies designed to combat microbial resistance include the use of additional agents that protect against enzymatic inactivation, the use of antibiotic combinations, the introduction of new (and often expensive) chemical derivatives of established antibiotics, and efforts to avoid indiscriminate use or misuse of antibiotics.

The most common cause of resistance is the use of inappropriate antibiotics for viral or other nonsusceptible infections. This presents resident and environmental organisms with selective pressure to develop resistance to the drug being used. A secondary cause of resistance is the use of inadequate dosage or duration of an appropriate drug. Such treatment eliminates only the most susceptible organisms, leaving the more resistant ones to proliferate.

INHIBITORS OF BACTERIAL CELL WALL SYNTHESIS

The major antibiotics in this class are penicillins and cephalosporins. These agents only kill bacterial cells that are actively growing and synthesizing new cell walls. They are called β-lactams, or β-lactam antibiotics, because they share an unusual four-member ring structure called a β-lactam ring. The β-lactam antibiotics include some of the most effective, widely used, and well-tolerated antimicrobial agents. The selective toxicity of β-lactams and other cell wall synthesis inhibitors is due to specific actions on the synthesis of cell walls—structures that are unique to bacteria. More than 50 antibiotics that act as cell wall synthesis inhibitors are currently available, with individual spectra of activity that afford a wide range of clinical applications. Figure 27–2 outlines this broad class of cell wall synthesis inhibitors, and Table 27–1 lists the key drugs in this class.

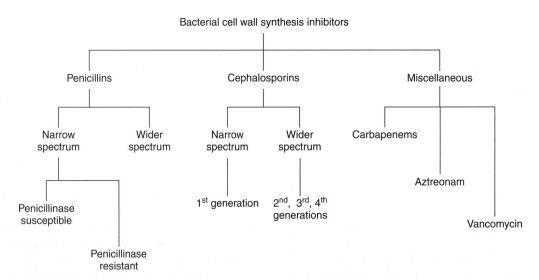

Figure 27–2. Key classes of drugs that inhibit bacterial cell wall synthesis.

Table 27–1.	Key inhibitors of cell wall synthesis	
Subclass	**Prototype**	**Other Significant Agents**
Penicillins		
Limited spectrum	Penicillin G	Penicillin V
β-lactamase–resistant	Methicillin	Nafcillin, oxacillin
Wider spectrum	Ampicillin	Amoxicillin, piperacillin, ticarcillin
Cephalosporins		
First-generation	Cefazolin	Cephradine
Second-generation	Cefamandole	Cefaclor, cefotetan, cefoxitin
Third-generation	Cefoperazone	Cefotaxime, ceftazidime, ceftriaxone
Fourth-generation	Cefepime	
Carbapenems	Imipenem	Ertapenem, meropenem
Monobactam	Aztreonam	
β-lactamase inhibitors	Clavulanic acid	Sulbactam, tazobactam
Other agents	Vancomycin	Bacitracin, cycloserine, fosfomycin

Penicillins

All penicillins are derivatives of 6-aminopenicillanic acid and contain a β-lactam ring structure that is essential for antibacterial activity. Penicillin subclasses have additional chemical modifications that confer differences in antimicrobial activity, susceptibility to acid and enzymatic hydrolysis, and biodisposition. Penicillins vary in their resistance to gastric acid and, therefore, vary in their oral bioavailability. Except for amoxicillin, oral penicillins should generally not be given with food to minimize binding to food proteins and acid inactivation. Thus, patients should be advised to take penicillins 1 to 2 hours before or after meals. Penicillins are not metabolized extensively; they are usually excreted unchanged in the urine via glomerular filtration and tubular secretion. **Ampicillin** and nafcillin are excreted partly in the bile. The plasma half-lives of most penicillins vary from 30 to 60 minutes. Two forms of **penicillin G**, the prototype of a subclass of penicillins with a limited antibacterial spectrum, are administered intramuscularly and have long plasma half-lives because the active drug is released very slowly into the bloodstream. Most penicillins cross the blood-brain barrier only when the meninges are inflamed (e.g., in meningitis).

Mechanisms of Action and Resistance

The β-lactams exert bactericidal effects by inhibiting cell wall synthesis. Inhibition of cell wall synthesis occurs as follows (Figure 27–1): (1) binding of the β-lactam agent to specific receptor proteins called **penicillin-binding proteins (PBPs)** located in the bacterial cytoplasmic membrane, enzymes that cross-link linear peptidoglycan chains that form part of the cell wall; and (2) activation of autolytic enzymes that cause lesions in the bacterial cell wall.

Bacteria have developed several mechanisms to resist destruction by β-lactam drugs. The most common mechanism of resistance is the production of β-**lactamases (penicillinases)** by many bacteria (especially *Staphylococcus* species and many gram-negative organisms). β-Lactamases hydrolyze the β-lactam ring of these antibiotics, resulting in the loss of antibacterial activity. To prevent the inactivation of the β-lactam ring, pencillins are sometimes administered in combination with inhibitors of bacterial β-lactamases (e.g., **clavulanic acid, sulbactam, tazobactam**). Another mechanism of resistance is structural change in target PBPs. This is an important mechanism because altered PBPs are responsible for methicillin resistance (in staphylococci) and penicillin resistance (in pneumococci and enterococci). In some gram-negative bacteria, resistance may be due to impaired penetration of antibiotics to their target PBPs. To cross the outer membrane that distinguishes gram-negative from gram-positive bacteria, β-lactams must enter gram-negative bacteria via porins (Figure 27–1). Altered porin structures may contribute to resistance by impeding β-lactam access to PBPs. Finally, some gram-negative bacteria may produce efflux pumps that effectively expel some β-lactam agents that get past the outer membrane.

Clinical Uses

Penicillins can be divided into very narrow, narrow, and wider spectrum agents, with spectrum referring to the number of organisms against which they provide antibacterial activity. They may also be classified by whether the agents are susceptible to bacterial β-lactamase (penicillinase) (Figure 27–2).

Among the narrow-spectrum *penicillinase–susceptible agents,* **penicillin G** is the prototype. Clinical uses include treatment for infections caused by common streptococci, meningococci, gram-positive bacilli, and spirochetes. Many strains of pneumococci are now resistant to penicillins. Most strains of *Staphylococcus aureus* and a significant number of strains of *Neisseria gonorrhoeae* are resistant via production of β-lactamases. **Penicillin V**, the oral equivalent of penicillin G, is only used in minor oropharyngeal infections.

The very narrow-spectrum penicillinase–resistant subclass includes the prototype **methicillin, nafcillin,** and **oxacillin**. Their primary use is in the treatment of known or suspected staphylococcal infections. However, methicillin-resistant *Staphylococcus aureus* (MRSA) and methicillin-resistant *Staphylococcus epidermidis* (MRSE), two strains important in many hospital-acquired infections, are resistant to other members of this subgroup and are often resistant to multiple antimicrobial drugs.

Wider spectrum penicillinase–susceptible drugs are among the most commonly used penicillins. **Ampicillin** and **amoxicillin** are often used to treat urinary tract infections (UTIs), otitis media, pneumonia, and bacteremias resulting from infections with susceptible bacterial species. **Piperacillin** and **ticarcillin** have activity against several gram-negative bacteria, including *Pseudomonas* (e.g., UTI, pneumonia, bacteremia), *Enterobacter* (e.g., UTI), and in some cases *Klebsiella*

species (e.g., UTI, pneumonia). For infections with penicillinase-producing bacteria, inhibitors of penicillinases (e.g., clavulanic acid) are co-administered to enhance the antibacterial activity of this subclass. Most drugs in this subclass have synergistic actions when used with aminoglycosides, inhibitors of protein synthesis discussed later in this chapter.

Adverse Effects

The penicillins are remarkably nontoxic. However, the potential for allergic reactions is a concern and allergic reactions account for most of the serious adverse effects. All penicillins are cross-sensitizing and cross-reacting, so cross-allergenicity among different penicillins is assumed. About 5 to 10% of individuals with a history of penicillin reaction have an allergic response when given a penicillin again. Allergic reactions include urticaria, severe pruritus, fever, joint swelling, hemolytic anemia, nephritis, and in rare cases anaphylaxis. Methicillin causes nephritis more often than other penicillins, and nafcillin is associated with neutropenia. Ampicillin frequently causes maculopapular skin rash that does not appear to be an allergic reaction.

Large oral doses of penicillins, especially ampicillin, may lead to gastrointestinal upset (e.g., nausea, vomiting, and diarrhea). Gastrointestinal upset may be caused by direct irritation or by overgrowth of gram-positive organisms or yeasts.

Problems Relating to the Use and Misuse of Penicillins

Penicillins are among the most misused antibiotics, having been used irrationally for nonsusceptible infections for over 50 years. As a result, 90% of all staphylococcal strains both in the hospital and in the community are β-lactamase producers, and the prevalence of methicillin-resistant strains of *S aureus* (MRSA) continues to increase. Broad-spectrum penicillins also eradicate normal flora, thereby predisposing the patient to colonization and superinfection with opportunistic, drug-resistant species present within the hospital environment.

Cephalosporins

The cephalosporins also contain the β-lactam ring structure, and are therefore classified as β-lactam antibiotics.

They vary in their antibacterial activity and are designated first-, second-, third-, or fourth-generation drugs according to the order of their introduction into clinical use (Figure 27–2). Several cephalosporins are available for oral use (e.g., cephalexin, cefixime), but most are administered parenterally. Cephalosporins with side chains may undergo hepatic metabolism, but the major elimination mechanism is renal excretion via active tubular secretion. Cefoperazone and ceftriaxone are excreted mainly in the bile. Most first- and second-generation cephalosporins do not enter the cerebrospinal fluid even when the meninges are inflamed.

Mechanisms of Action

Cephalosporins have a broader spectrum of activity than the penicillins because they are less susceptible to many bacterial penicillinases. Cephalosporins' bactericidal activity results from binding to PBPs in bacterial cell membranes and interfering with bacterial cell wall synthesis.

Bacterial resistance to cephalosporins can result from certain β-lactamases, decreases in membrane permeability to cephalosporins, and from altered PBP structures. Methicillin-resistant staphylococci (i.e., MRSA) are also resistant to cephalosporins.

Clinical Uses

Cefazolin (parenteral) and **cephalexin** (oral) are examples of first-generation cephalosporins. Although they are fairly broad-spectrum agents with very minimal toxicities, first-generation cephalosporins are rarely drugs of choice for any infection. Clinical uses include treatment of infections caused by gram-positive cocci, including susceptible staphylococci and common streptococci. Cefazolin may be the drug of choice in infections for which it is the least toxic drug (e.g., *Klebsiella pneumoniae).*

Second-generation agents include **cefotetan, cefoxitin, cefamandole, cefuroxime**, and **cefaclor**. Members of this subclass usually have less activity against gram-positive organisms than first-generation drugs, but have extended gram-negative coverage. Marked differences in activity, pharmacokinetics, and toxicity occur among second-generation agents. Examples of clinical uses include infections caused by *Bacteroides fragilis* (e.g., peritonitis, diverticulitis) *and Haemophilus influenzae* or *Moraxella catarrhalis* (e.g., sinusitis, otitis, lower respiratory infections).

Characteristic features of third-generation drugs (e.g., **ceftazidime, cefoperazone, cefotaxime**) include increased activity against gram-negative organisms resistant to other β-lactam drugs and ability to penetrate the blood-brain barrier (except cefoperazone and cefixime). Individual drugs have activity against *Pseudomonas* (cefoperazone, ceftazidime) and *B fragilis* (**ceftizoxime**). Drugs in this subclass are usually reserved for treatment of serious infections (e.g., bacterial meningitis). The exceptions are **ceftriaxone** (parenteral) and **cefixime** (oral), which are currently drugs of choice to treat gonorrhea. Likewise, in acute otitis media, a single injection of ceftriaxone is usually as effective as a 10-day treatment course with amoxicillin.

The fourth-generation agents have the widest antibacterial spectrum of the cephalosporins. They are more resistant to β-lactamases produced by gram-negative organisms, including *Enterobacter, Haemophilus, Neisseria,* and some penicillin-resistant pneumococci. **Cefepime**, the prototypic fourth-generation agent, combines the gram-positive activity of first-generation agents with the wider gram-negative spectrum of third-generation cephalosporins.

Adverse Effects

Cephalosporins may elicit a variety of hypersensitivity reactions that are identical to those of penicillins, including fever, skin rashes, nephritis, granulocytopenia, hemolytic anemia, and anaphylaxis. However, the chemical nucleus of cephalosporins is sufficiently different from that of penicillins so that some individuals with a history of penicillin allergy may sometimes be treated successfully with a cephalosporin. However, patients with a history of anaphylaxis to penicillins should not receive cephalosporins. Complete cross-hypersensitivity among different cephalosporins should be assumed.

Cephalosporins may cause pain at intramuscular injection sites and phlebitis after intravenous administration. They may increase the nephrotoxicity of aminoglycosides when the two are administered together. Drugs containing a methylthiotetrazole group (e.g., cefamandole, cefoperazone, cefotetan) may cause hypoprothrombinemia and disulfiram-like reactions with ethanol.

Other β-Lactam Drugs

Several other β-lactam drugs are of clinical importance. **Aztreonam** is neither a penicillin nor a cephalosporin. It is a monobactam, named for its chemical structure that contains one β-lactam ring. Aztreonam is resistant to β-lactamases produced by certain gram-negative rods, but has no activity against gram-positive bacteria or anaerobes. It inhibits cell wall synthesis by preferentially binding to a specific penicillin-binding protein (PBP3). It is synergistic with aminoglycosides. Aztreonam is administered intravenously, and is eliminated via renal tubular secretion. Penicillin-allergic patients tolerate aztreonam without reaction. Adverse effects include gastrointestinal upset with possible superinfection, vertigo, headache, and rare hepatotoxicity.

Imipenem, meropenem, and **ertapenem** are **carbapenems** and are chemically different from penicillins. While they retain the β-lactam ring structure, they have low susceptibility to β-lactamases. Carbapenems have wide activity against gram-positive cocci (including some penicillin-resistant pneumococci), gram-negative rods, and anaerobes. The carbapenems are administered parenterally, and are especially useful for infections caused by organisms resistant to other antibiotics.

Because imipenem is inactivated by a renal enzyme, it is administered in combination with cilastatin, an inhibitor of this enzyme. Adverse effects of imipenem-cilastatin include gastrointestinal distress, skin rash, and, at very high plasma levels, central nervous system (CNS) toxicity (confusion, encephalopathy, seizures). There is partial cross-allergenicity with the penicillins. Meropenem is similar to imipenem except that it is not metabolized by renal enzymes and is less likely to cause seizures. Ertapenem has a long half-life, and its intramuscular injection causes pain and irritation.

β-Lactamase Inhibitors

An obvious problem with using β-lactam antibiotics such as penicillins and cephalosporins is that many bacteria produce β-lactamases that inactivate these agents. **Clavulanic acid, sulbactam**, and **tazobactam** are β-lactamase inhibitors that have little or no antibacterial action themselves. They are administered in fixed combinations with certain penicillins to treat infections caused by bacteria that produce β-lactamases. Adverse effects of these drug combinations are caused primarily by the penicillin agent.

Other Inhibitors of Cell Wall Synthesis

Vancomycin is a glycopeptide antibiotic produced by a strain of *Streptococcus*. It binds to a unique set of amino acids used in cross-linking the peptidoglycan cell wall. As a result, chains of the peptidoglycan cannot be cross-linked and the cell wall is disrupted, making the bacterial cell susceptible to lysis. Vancomycin has a narrow spectrum of activity and is used for serious infections caused by drug-resistant gram-positive organisms, including MRSA, penicillin-resistant pneumococci, and *Clostridium difficile.* **Teicoplanin**, another glycopeptide, has similar characteristics.

Some strains of enterococci and staphylococci have become resistant to vancomycin (i.e., vancomycin-resistant enterococci [VRE] and vancomycin-resistant *S aureus* [VRSA]). Resistance to vancomycin is due to a single amino acid change in the bacterial binding site for vancomycin, which significantly decreases its binding affinity. The prevalence of VRE is increasing and poses a serious clinical problem because such organisms usually exhibit multiple-drug resistance. Likewise, strains of MRSA have been reported with intermediate resistance to vancomycin, leading to treatment failures.

Vancomycin is not absorbed from the gastrointestinal tract, but may be given orally to treat bacterial enterocolitis. When given parenterally, vancomycin penetrates most tissues and is eliminated unchanged in the urine. Dosage modification is mandatory in patients with renal impairment. Toxic effects of vancomycin include chills, fever, phlebitis, ototoxicity, and nephrotoxicity. Rapid intravenous infusion may cause diffuse flushing ("red man syndrome").

Daptomycin, a new lipopeptide agent, is chemically different from vancomycin and has a different mechanism of action, but a similar spectrum of activity and indications. It is active against several strains of VRE and VRSA. Daptomycin is described in Chapter 30.

Other inhibitors of cell wall synthesis include **bacitracin** and **cycloserine**. Bacitracin is a peptide antibiotic that interferes with a late stage in cell wall synthesis in gram-positive organisms. Because of its marked nephrotoxicity, this antibiotic is limited to topical use for skin lesions. Bacitracin solutions in saline can also be used for irrigation of joints, wounds, or the pleural cavity. Cycloserine prevents formation of a functional bacterial peptidoglycan. Because of its potential neurotoxicity (tremors, seizures, psychosis), cycloserine is only used to treat strains of *Mycobacterium tuberculosis* (the causative agent of tuberculosis) that are resistant to first-line antituberculous drugs.

■ INHIBITORS OF BACTERIAL PROTEIN SYNTHESIS

The basic process by which mammalian and bacterial cells make proteins is similar. In both mammalian and bacterial cells, the specific genetic information contained within DNA is transcribed into messenger RNA (mRNA). Next, mRNA is translated into a new polypeptide or protein chain. The role of ribosomes in this process is to move along the mRNA chain, recruit transfer RNA (tRNA) molecules that carry different amino acids, and join incoming amino acids to the growing polypeptide chain. One critical difference between protein synthesis in mammalian and bacterial cells is the structure of their ribosomes.

Differences in ribosomal subunits, chemical composition, and functional specificities of component nucleic acids and proteins form the basis of selective toxicity of certain antibiotics against bacterial protein synthesis with much less effect on mammalian cells.

Although drugs in this class vary dramatically in their structure and spectrum of antimicrobial efficacy (Figure 27–3), each agent inhibits bacterial protein synthesis by acting at the level of the bacterial ribosome. **Chloramphenicol, tetracyclines**, and **aminoglycosides** were the first inhibitors of bacterial protein synthesis to be discovered. Because they had a broad spectrum of antibacterial activity and were thought to have low toxicities, they were overused. As a result, many once highly susceptible bacterial species have become resistant, and these drugs are now only used for more selected targets. **Erythromycin**, an older macrolide antibiotic, has a narrower spectrum of action but continues to be active against several important pathogens. Newer drugs (e.g., **streptogramins, linezolid, telithromycin**) have activity against certain gram-positive bacteria that have developed resistance to older antibiotics.

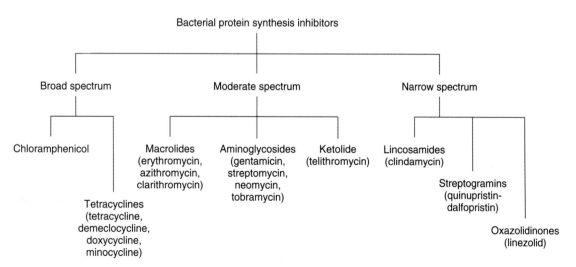

Figure 27–3. Diagram classifying inhibitors of bacterial protein synthesis based on spectrum of antibacterial activity.

Mechanisms of Action

Most antibiotics in this subclass are bacteriostatic. Figure 27–4 illustrates the specific binding sites on the 70S bacterial ribosomal complex for chloramphenicol, tetracyclines, and the macrolides. With the exception of tetracyclines and aminoglycosides, the binding sites for these antibiotics are on the 50S ribosomal subunit. Chloramphenicol, clindamycin, and the macrolides prevent a step called transpeptidation, in which the next new amino acid is added to the nascent peptide chain. Tetracyclines bind to the 30S ribosomal subunit at a site that blocks the binding of amino acid–carrying tRNA (charged tRNA) to the acceptor site of the ribosome-mRNA complex.

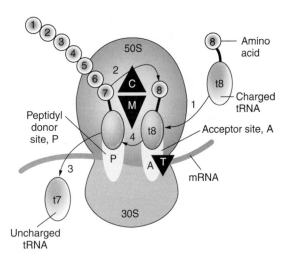

Figure 27–4. Steps in bacterial protein synthesis and targets of chloramphenicol, the macrolides, and tetracyclines. Individual amino acids are shown as numbered circles. The 70S bacterial ribosomal mRNA complex is shown with its 50S and 30S subunits. In step 1, the charged tRNA carrying amino acid 8 binds to the acceptor site A on the 70S ribosome. Transpeptidation occurs when the peptidyl tRNA at the donor site (with amino acids 1 through 7) binds the growing amino acid chain to amino acid 8 (step 2). The uncharged tRNA left at the donor site is released (step 3), and the new 8–amino acid chain with its tRNA shifts to the peptidyl site (transpeptidation, step 4). The antibiotic binding sites are shown schematically as triangles. Chloramphenicol (C) and the macrolides (M) bind to the 50S subunit and block transpeptidation (step 2). Tetracyclines (T) bind to the 30S subunit and prevent binding of the incoming charged tRNA unit (step 1).

The streptogramins are bactericidal for most susceptible organisms. They bind to the 50S ribosomal subunit, and prevent extrusion of the nascent polypeptide chain. In addition, streptogramins inhibit the activity of enzymes that synthesize tRNA, leading to a decrease in free tRNA within the cell. Linezolid also binds to the 50S subunit. It blocks formation of the tRNA-ribosome-mRNA complex. The action of the aminoglycosides is described below.

Chloramphenicol

Chloramphenicol has a simple and distinctive structure, and no other antimicrobials have been discovered in this chemical class. It is effective orally as well as parenterally and is distributed throughout all tissues. It readily crosses the placental and blood-brain barriers. The drug undergoes enterohepatic cycling, and is mostly inactivated by the liver. Chloramphenicol has a wide spectrum of antimicrobial activity and is usually bacteriostatic. It is not active against *Chlamydia*. Although chloramphenicol does not bind to ribosomal RNA of mammalian cells, it can inhibit the functions of mammalian mitochondrial ribosomes, which are more similar to bacterial ribosomes. Clinically significant resistance to chloramphenicol occurs through the formation of plasmid-encoded enzymes that inactivate the drug.

CLINICAL USES. Because of its toxicity and bacterial resistance, chloramphenicol has very few uses as a systemic drug. It is a back-up drug for severe infections caused by *Salmonella* species and for the treatment of penicillin-resistant pneumococcal or meningococcal meningitis, or in patients who have major hypersensitivity reactions to penicillin. Chloramphenicol is commonly used as a topical agent for eye infections because of its broad spectrum and ability to penetrate ocular tissue.

ADVERSE EFFECTS. Patients taking chloramphenicol occasionally develop nausea, vomiting, and diarrhea. Oral or vaginal candidiasis may occur as a result of alteration of normal microbial flora. Chloramphenicol commonly causes dose-related reversible suppression of red blood cell production. Idiosyncratic aplastic anemia, which involves suppression of production of all blood cells, can also occur, but is rare and unrelated to dose. Unfortunately, it occurs more frequently with prolonged use and is usually irreversible.

If newborn infants are given high dosages, chloramphenicol may accumulate because infants lack effective mechanisms for metabolism of the drug. The resulting **gray baby syndrome** includes vomiting, flaccidity, hypothermia, gray color, cyanosis, and cardiovascular collapse.

Because chloramphenicol inhibits hepatic enzymes that metabolize several drugs, it has significant interactions when taken with other drugs. Half-lives are prolonged, and serum concentrations of phenytoin, tolbutamide, chlorpropamide, and warfarin are increased. Like other bacteriostatic inhibitors of microbial protein synthesis, chloramphenicol can antagonize bactericidal drugs such as penicillins or aminoglycosides.

Tetracyclines

Tetracyclines (**tetracycline, doxycycline, minocycline, demeclocycline**) are broad-spectrum bacteriostatic antibiotics that inhibit protein synthesis in gram-positive and gram-negative bacteria, *Rickettsia* (the cause of Rocky Mountain spotted fever and some other difficult to treat infections), *Chlamydia, Mycoplasma, Borrelia* (the cause of Lyme disease), and some protozoa. Drugs in this class have only minor differences in their activities against specific organisms. Susceptible organisms accumulate tetracyclines intracellularly via energy-dependent transport systems in their cell membranes. Tetracyclines have little effect on mammalian protein synthesis because an active efflux mechanism prevents their intracellular accumulation.

Oral absorption is variable, especially for the older drugs, and may be impaired by foods and multivalent cations (calcium, iron, aluminum). Tetracyclines have a wide tissue distribution and cross the placental barrier. All of the tetracyclines undergo enterohepatic cycling. Doxycycline is excreted mainly in feces; the other tetracyclines are eliminated primarily in the urine. The half-lives of doxycycline and minocycline are longer than those of other tetracyclines.

Plasmid-mediated resistance to tetracyclines is widespread. Resistance mechanisms include decreased activity of the uptake systems and, most importantly, the development of mechanisms such as efflux pumps for active extrusion of tetracyclines. Plasmids that include genes involved in producing efflux pumps for tetracyclines commonly include resistance genes for multiple antibiotics.

CLINICAL USES. A tetracycline is the drug of choice in infections caused by *Mycoplasma pneumoniae* (in adults), *Chlamydia, Rickettsia,* and *Vibrio* (e.g., cholera). Specific tetracyclines are used in the treatment of gastrointestinal ulcers caused by *Helicobacter pylori* (tetracycline), in Lyme disease (doxycycline), and in the meningococcal carrier state (minocycline). Doxycycline is also used for the prevention of malaria and in the treatment of amebiasis . Demeclocycline inhibits the renal actions of antidiuretic hormone (ADH) and is used in the management of patients with ADH-secreting tumors.

Tetracyclines are alternative drugs in the treatment of syphilis. They are also used in the treatment of respiratory infections caused by susceptible organisms, for prophylaxis against infection in chronic bronchitis, in the treatment of leptospirosis , and in the treatment of acne.

ADVERSE EFFECTS. Hypersensitivity reactions (i.e., fever, rashes) to tetracyclines are uncommon. Most of the adverse reactions are due to direct toxicity of the tetracycline agent or due to alterations in microbial flora.

Effects on the gastrointestinal system range from mild nausea and diarrhea to severe, possibly life-threatening colitis. Disturbances in the normal flora are due to suppression of tetracycline-susceptible organisms and overgrowth of resistant organisms, especially pseudomonas, staphylococci, and candida. This can result in intestinal disturbances, anal pruritus, vaginal or oral candidiasis, or enterocolitis.

Tetracyclines bind to calcium deposited in newly formed bone or teeth in young children. Thus, fetal exposure to tetracyclines may lead to tooth enamel dysplasia and discoloration and irregularities in bone growth. Although usually contraindicated in pregnancy, there may be situations in which the benefit of administering tetracyclines outweighs the risk. If taken for long periods of time in children under 8 years of age, tetracyclines may cause similar changes in teeth and bone.

High doses of tetracyclines, especially in pregnant patients and those with preexisting hepatic disease, may impair liver function and lead to hepatic necrosis. Likewise, in patients with kidney disease, tetracyclines may exacerbate renal dysfunction.

Systemic tetracyclines (especially demeclocycline) may enhance skin sensitivity to ultraviolet light, particularly in fair-skinned individuals.

Dose-dependent reversible dizziness and vertigo have been reported with doxycycline and minocycline.

Macrolides

The macrolide antibiotics are large cyclic lactone ring structures with attached sugars. The macrolides include the prototypic drugs **erythromycin, azithromycin**, and **clarithromycin**. The macrolides have good oral bioavailability, but azithromycin absorption is impeded by food. Macrolides distribute to most body tissues, but azithromycin is unique in that the levels achieved in tissues and in phagocytes are considerably higher than those in the plasma. The elimination of erythromycin (via biliary excretion) and clarithromycin (via hepatic metabolism and urinary excretion of intact drug) is fairly rapid (half-life 2 to 5 hours). Azithromycin is eliminated slowly (half-life 2 to 4 days), mainly in urine as unchanged drug.

CLINICAL USES. Erythromycin has activity against many species of *Campylobacter, Chlamydia, Mycoplasma, Legionella*, gram-positive cocci (including β-lactamase–producing staphylococci), and some gram-negative organisms. The antibacterial action may be bacteriostatic or bactericidal; the latter effect occurring more commonly at higher concentrations for susceptible organisms. Erythromycin does not have activity against penicillin-resistant *Streptococcus pneumoniae* or methicillin-resistant *S aureus* (MRSA).

The spectra of activity of azithromycin and clarithromycin are similar to erythromycin, but include greater activity against *Chlamydia, Mycobacterium avium* complex, and *Toxoplasma* species. Because of its long half-life, a 4-day course of treatment with azithromycin has been effective in community-acquired pneumonia. Clarithromycin is approved for prophylaxis against and treatment of *M avium* complex and as a component of drug regimens for ulcers caused by *Helicobacter pylori*.

Resistance to macrolide antibiotics in gram-positive organisms involves efflux pump mechanisms and the production of an enzyme (methylase) that alters the drugs' ribosomal binding site. Cross-resistance among individual macrolides is complete; that is, if an organism is resistant to one macrolide agent, it will be resistant to all other macrolides. In the case of methylase-producing bacterial strains, there is partial cross-resistance with other drugs that bind to the same ribosomal site as macrolides, including clindamycin and streptogramins. Resistance in Enterobacteriaceae is due to formation of drug-metabolizing esterases.

ADVERSE EFFECTS. Gastrointestinal irritation (anorexia, nausea, vomiting) is often associated with oral administration. Stimulation of gut motility is the most common reason for discontinuing erythromycin and choosing another antibiotic. This action is sometimes exploited therapeutically in patients with inadequate gastrointestinal motility. A hypersensitivity-based acute cholestatic hepatitis (fever, jaundice, impaired liver function) may occur with erythromycin estolate. This condition usually resolves. Hepatitis is rare in children, but there is an increased risk with erythromycin estolate in pregnant patients. Because erythromycin inhibits several forms of hepatic cytochrome P450, it increases the plasma levels of anticoagulants, carbamazepine, cisapride, digoxin, and theophylline. Similar drug interactions have also occurred with clarithromycin. Drug interactions are uncommon with azithromycin because this agent does not inhibit hepatic cytochrome P450.

Telithromycin

Telithromycin is a ketolide structurally related to macrolides. It has the same mechanism of action as erythromycin and a similar moderate spectrum of antimicrobial activity. However, some macrolide-resistant microbial strains are susceptible to telithromycin because it binds more tightly to ribosomes and is a poor substrate for bacterial efflux pumps that mediate resistance. Clinical uses include community-acquired bacterial pneumonia and other upper respiratory tract infections. Telithromycin is given orally once daily and is eliminated in the bile and the urine.

Clindamycin

Clindamycin inhibits bacterial protein synthesis via a mechanism similar to that of the macrolides, although it is not chemically related. Mechanisms of resistance include alteration of the drug's ribosomal binding site and enzymatic inactivation of the drug. Cross-resistance between clindamycin and the macrolides is common. Good tissue penetration occurs after oral absorption. Clindamycin is eliminated partly by metabolism and partly by biliary and renal excretion.

CLINICAL USES. The main use of clindamycin is in the treatment of severe infections caused by certain anaerobes such as *Bacteroides* (most common bacteria in the colon) that often participate in mixed infections. Clindamycin (sometimes in combination with an aminoglycoside or cephalosporin) is used to treat penetrating wounds of the abdomen and the gut, infections originating in the female genital tract (e.g., septic abortion and pelvic abscesses), or aspiration pneumonia. Clindamycin has been used as a back-up drug against gram-positive cocci, and is currently recommended for prophylaxis of endocarditis in patients with cardiac valve disease who are allergic to penicillin. Clindamycin plus primaquine is an effective alternative to trimethoprim-sulfamethoxazole for moderate to moderately severe *Pneumocystis jiroveci* pneumonia in AIDS patients. It is also used in combination with pyrimethamine for AIDS-related toxoplasmosis of the brain.

ADVERSE EFFECTS. Adverse effects of clindamycin include gastrointestinal irritation, skin rashes, neutropenia, and hepatic dysfunction. Severe diarrhea and enterocolitis have followed clindamycin administration. Antibiotic-associated colitis due to superinfection with *C difficile* is a potentially fatal complication and must be recognized promptly and treated.

Streptogramins

Quinupristin-dalfopristin is a combination of two streptogramins. The combination has rapid bactericidal activity that lasts longer than the half-lives of the individual compounds. Antibacterial activity includes penicillin-resistant pneumococci, methicillin-resistant and vancomycin-resistant staphylococci (MRSA and VRSA, respectively), and resistant *Enterococcus faecium*. Administered intravenously, the combination product may cause pain at the infusion site and an arthralgia-myalgia syndrome. Streptogramins are potent inhibitors of CYP3A4 and increase plasma levels of many drugs, including cisapride, cyclosporine, diazepam, nonnucleoside reverse transcriptase inhibitors, and warfarin.

Linezolid

Linezolid is the first of a new class of antibiotics called oxazolidinones. Linezolid is mainly bacteriostatic, and is active against gram-positive cocci, including strains resistant to β-lactams and vancomycin (e.g., vancomycin-resistant *E faecium*). Linezolid binds to a unique site on one of the ribosomal subunits, and there is currently no cross-resistance with other protein synthesis inhibitors. Although rare to date, resistance can occur with a decreased affinity of linezolid for its binding site. Linezolid is available in both oral and parenteral formulations. The primary adverse effect is hematologic; thrombocytopenia and neutropenia occur, most commonly in immunosuppressed patients.

Aminoglycosides

Aminoglycosides exert bactericidal activity and are useful mainly against aerobic gram-negative microorganisms. One of the primary advantages of aminoglycosides is that they can often be used in a once-daily dosing protocol, which can save time and lends itself to outpatient therapy with these agents. In addition, once-daily dosing can be more effective and less toxic than traditional dosing regimens. Aminoglycosides have greater efficacy when administered as a single large dose because their bactericidal effectiveness is concentration dependent. That is, as the plasma level is increased above the MIC, aminoglycosides kill an increasing proportion of bacteria and do so more rapidly. Aminoglycosides can also exert a postantibiotic effect, so that that their killing action continues when plasma levels have declined below measurable levels. The single large daily dose of an aminoglycoside generally results in fewer adverse effects because toxicity depends both on a critical plasma concentration and on the time that such a level is exceeded. With single large doses, the time above such a threshold is shorter than with administration of multiple smaller doses.

The aminoglycosides include **gentamicin, amikacin, neomycin, tobramycin**, and others. They are structurally related amino sugars attached by glycosidic linkages. All of the aminoglycosides are polar compounds, so they are not absorbed after oral administration. Therefore, they must be given intramuscularly or intravenously for systemic effect. They have limited tissue penetration and do not readily cross the blood-brain barrier. The major mode of excretion is via the kidney, and plasma levels of these drugs are greatly affected by changes in renal function. With normal renal function, the elimination half-life of aminoglycosides is 2 to 3 hours. Patients receiving aminoglycosides for more than 1 day must have plasma levels of the drug monitored for safe and effective dosage selection and adjustment. Even with once-daily dosing, plasma levels may be monitored, especially in patients with decreased kidney function.

MECHANISM OF ACTION. To kill susceptible bacteria, aminoglycosides must penetrate the bacterial cell envelope . This process is partly dependent on oxygen-dependent active transport; therefore, these agents have minimal activity against strict anaerobes. To assist entry of aminoglycosides into bacterial cells, aminoglycosides may be co-administered with a cell wall synthesis inhibitor such as a β-lactam agent. Once inside the bacterial cell, aminoglycosides bind to the 30S ribosomal subunit and interfere with protein synthesis in at least three ways: (1) they block formation of the initiation complex; (2) they cause misreading of mRNA; and (3) they inhibit translocation (Figure 27–5).

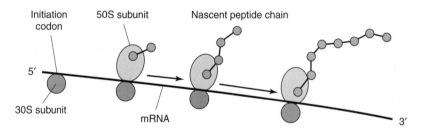

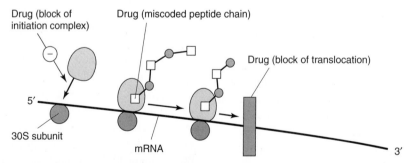

Figure 27–5. Putative mechanisms of action of the aminoglycosides. Normal protein synthesis is shown in the top panel. At least three different aminoglycoside effects have been described (*bottom panel*): block of formation of the initiation complex; miscoding of amino acids in the emerging peptide chain due to misreading of the mRNA; and block of translocation on mRNA. Block of movement of the ribosome may occur after the formation of a single initiation complex, resulting in an mRNA chain with only a single ribosome on it, a so-called monosome.

CLINICAL USES. Aminoglycosides are mostly used against gram-negative enteric (i.e., intestinal) bacteria. The main differences among the individual aminoglycosides lie in their activities against specific organisms, particularly gram-negative rods. Gentamicin, tobramycin, and amikacin are important drugs for the treatment of serious infections caused by aerobic gram-negative bacteria, including *E coli* and *Enterobacter, Klebsiella* (especially important in respiratory infections and urinary tract infections)*, Proteus, Providencia, Pseudomonas,* and *Serratia* (important in septicemia and pulmonary infections) species. These aminoglycosides also have activity against other species (e.g., *H influenzae, Moraxella catarrhalis, Shigella*), although they are not drugs of choice for infections caused by these organisms. When used alone, aminoglycosides are not reliably effective for treating infections caused by gram-positive cocci. Antibacterial synergy may occur when aminoglycosides are used in combination with cell wall synthesis inhibitors. For example, aminoglycosides may be combined with penicillins to treat pseudomonal, listerial (important in some cases of meningitis), and enterococcal infections.

Streptomycin is an aminoglycoside that is often used in the treatment of tuberculosis, plague, and tularemia (rabbit fever). Because of the risk of irreversible ototoxicity, streptomycin should not be used when other drugs will serve. Owing to its toxic potential, **neomycin** is only used topically or locally (e.g., in the gastrointestinal tract to eliminate bowel flora). **Netilmicin** is usually reserved for treatment of serious infections caused by organisms resistant to the other aminoglycosides.

ADVERSE EFFECTS. All aminoglycosides are ototoxic and nephrotoxic. Auditory or vestibular damage (or both) may occur and may be irreversible. Auditory impairment, which may manifest as tinnitus and high-frequency hearing loss initially, is more likely with amikacin and kanamycin. Vestibular dysfunction, which may manifest as vertigo, ataxia, and loss of balance, is more likely with gentamicin and tobramycin. These toxic risks are proportionate to plasma levels of the drug. Precautions taken to reduce these risks include once-daily dosing (versus traditional dosing regimens), monitoring plasma levels of aminoglycosides with appropriate dose modification, and avoiding the additive ototoxicity of loop diuretics during dosing. Because ototoxicity has been reported after fetal exposure, aminoglycosides are contraindicated in pregnancy unless their potential benefits are judged to outweigh risk.

Renal toxicity usually takes the form of acute tubular necrosis, which is often reversible. It is more common in elderly patients and in those concurrently receiving amphotericin B, cephalosporins, or vancomycin. Gentamicin and tobramycin are the most nephrotoxic aminoglycosides.

Allergic skin reactions may occur in patients, and contact dermatitis may occur in personnel handling these drugs. Neomycin is the most likely culprit.

Although rare, respiratory paralysis may occur at high doses. It is usually reversible by prompt treatment with calcium and neostigmine, but ventilatory support may be required.

INHIBITORS OF BACTERIAL DNA SYNTHESIS

The **sulfonamides, trimethoprim,** and **fluoroquinolones** make up the group of drugs that exert antibacterial effects by interfering with bacterial DNA synthesis (Figure 27–6). Individual key drugs in this class of drugs are listed in Table 27–2.

Sulfonamides and Trimethoprim

Mechanism of Action and Pharmacokinetics
Sulfonamides and trimethoprim are called **antifolate drugs** because they interfere with folic acid synthesis. Folic acid and folate are the names of forms of vitamin B_9. Folic acid is the synthetic form found in fortified foods and supplements, and folate is the anionic form found naturally in foods. Folic acid is necessary for DNA replication; thus, it is necessary for production and maintenance of new cells. While mammals can use exogenous (i.e., dietary) folate, many bacteria cannot and rely on enzymes to synthesize folate from its precursor, para-aminobenzoic acid (PABA). Antifolate drugs inhibit folic acid synthesis at different stages (Figure 27–7). The selective toxicity of antifolate drugs results from the fact that mammalian cells utilize dietary folic acid, so inhibition of folic acid synthesis will primarily affect bacteria.

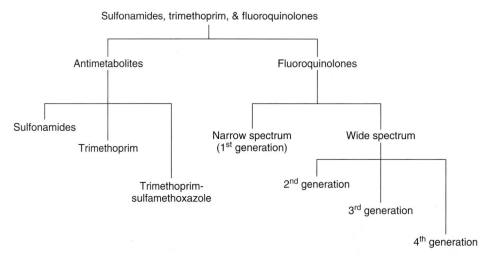

Figure 27–6. Classification of inhibitors of bacterial DNA synthesis: sulfonamides, trimethoprim, and fluoroquinolones.

Used as single agents, sulfonamides are bacteriostatic inhibitors of folic acid synthesis (Figure 27–7). They competitively inhibit dihydropteroate synthase and can also act as substrates for this enzyme, resulting in the synthesis of nonfunctional forms of folic acid. Trimethoprim selectively inhibits bacterial dihydrofolate reductase, which prevents formation of the active form of folic acid. Bacterial dihydrofolate reductase is 4 to 5 orders of magnitude more sensitive to trimethoprim inhibition than the mammalian form of dihydrofolate reductase. Because microbial resistance is common if sulfonamides are used as single antimicrobial agents, a sulfonamide is frequently used in combination with trimethoprim, with the combination being known as TMP-SMZ or TMP-SMX. This combination causes a *sequential blockade* of folic acid synthesis in which both drugs inhibit sequential steps in bacterial metabolism. This results in a synergistic, often bactericidal, action against a wide spectrum of microorganisms. Resistance to the combination occurs but has been relatively slow in development.

Table 27–2.	Key inhibitors of bacterial DNA synthesis	
Subclass	**Prototype**	**Other Significant Agents**
Sulfonamides		
Oral agents	Sulfisoxazole	
Local agents	Sulfacetamide	
Combination	Trimethoprim-sulfamethoxazole (TMP-SMX)	
Fluoroquinolones		
First generation	Norfloxacin	
Second generation	Ciprofloxacin	Ofloxacin
Third generation	Levofloxacin	
Fourth generation	Moxifloxacin	

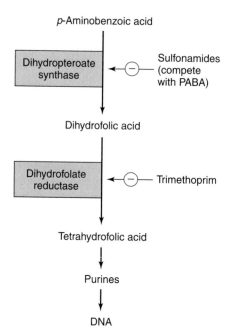

p-Aminobenzoic acid

Dihydropteroate synthase ←―(−)― Sulfonamides (compete with PABA)

Dihydrofolic acid

Dihydrofolate reductase ←―(−)― Trimethoprim

Tetrahydrofolic acid

Purines

DNA

Figure 27–7. Inhibitory effects of sulfonamides and trimethoprim on folic acid synthesis. Inhibition of 2 successive steps in the formation of tetrahydrofolic acid constitutes sequential blockade and results in antibacterial synergy.

The sulfonamides are weakly acidic compounds that have a chemical nucleus resembling PABA, the substrate with which they compete. Members of this group differ mainly in their pharmacokinetic properties and clinical uses. Shared pharmacokinetic features include modest tissue penetration, hepatic metabolism, and excretion of both intact drug and acetylated metabolites in the urine. They can be divided into three major groups: (1) oral absorbable; (2) oral nonabsorbable; and (3) topical. The oral absorbable sulfonamides can be classified as short-acting (e.g., sulfisoxazole), intermediate-acting (e.g., sulfamethoxazole), or long-acting (e.g., sulfadoxine) on the basis of their half-lives. Sulfonamides bind to plasma proteins at sites shared by bilirubin and by other drugs.

Trimethoprim is structurally similar to folic acid. It is a weak base and is trapped in acidic environments, reaching high concentrations in prostatic and vaginal fluids. A large fraction of trimethoprim is excreted unchanged in the urine.

Clinical Uses

Among the oral absorbable sulfonamides, **sulfisoxazole** and **sulfamethoxazole** are used almost exclusively for treating urinary tract infections. Oral sulfadiazine plus pyrimethamine (a dihydrofolate reductase inhibitor) work synergistically as a first-line treatment for toxoplasmosis. As topical agents, several sulfonamides are used to treat bacterial ophthalmic and wound infections. **Sodium sulfacetamide** ophthalmic solution or ointment is effective for treating bacterial conjunctivitis. In the prevention of infection of burn wounds, mafenide acetate can be used to treat topical infections. However, **silver sulfadiazine** is the preferred agent because mafenide acetate can cause metabolic acidosis.

The combination of trimethoprim-sulfamethoxazole is the drug regimen of choice for infections such as *Pneumocystis jiroveci* pneumonia, toxoplasmosis, and nocardiosis (Chapter 29). TMP-SMX is also a possible back-up drug for cholera, typhoid fever, and shigellosis, and has been used in the treatment of infections caused by MRSA and *Listeria monocytogenes*.

Adverse Effects

Adverse effects of the sulfonamides include hypersensitivity reactions, hepatotoxicity, nephrotoxicity, and gastrointestinal discomfort such as nausea, vomiting, and diarrhea. Allergic reactions, including skin rashes and fever, are common. Cross-allergenicity among the individual sulfonamides should be assumed and may rarely occur with chemically related drugs (e.g., oral hypoglycemics, thiazides). Common drug interactions include competition with warfarin and methotrexate for plasma protein binding, which transiently increases the plasma levels of these drugs. Sulfonamides can displace bilirubin from plasma proteins, with the risk of severe newborn jaundice and kernicterus if used in the third trimester of pregnancy. Persons with glucose-6-phosphate dehydrogenase (G6PD) deficiency may suffer hemolysis if sulfonamides are given.

Trimethoprim may cause the predictable adverse effects of an antifolate drug, including megaloblastic anemia, leukopenia, and granulocytopenia. These effects are usually ameliorated by supplementary folinic acid. The combination of TMP-SMX may also cause any of the adverse effects associated with sulfonamides. AIDS patients given TMP-SMX have a high incidence of adverse effects, including fever, rashes, leukopenia, and diarrhea.

Fluoroquinolones

Mechanism of Action and Pharmacokinetics

Fluoroquinolones selectively inhibit two enzymes critical for bacterial DNA synthesis: **topoisomerase II (DNA gyrase)** and **topoisomerase IV**. Inhibition of DNA gyrase prevents relaxation of positively supercoiled DNA; uncoiling is required for normal transcription, whereas inhibition of topoisomerase IV interferes with the separation of replicated chromosomal DNA during cell division.

Fluoroquinolones are usually bactericidal against susceptible organisms. Like aminoglycosides, the fluoroquinolines also exhibit postantibiotic effects.

Resistance has emerged to the older fluoroquinolones, but has been offset to some extent by the introduction of newer generations with expanded activity against common pathogenic organisms.

All of the fluoroquinolones have good oral bioavailability (although some antacids may interfere) and penetrate most body tissues. Elimination of most fluoroquinolones is through the kidneys; dosage reductions are usually needed in renal dysfunction. Moxifloxacin is eliminated partly by hepatic metabolism and also by biliary excretion. Half-lives of fluoroquinolones are usually 3 to 8 hours, but the agents eliminated by nonrenal routes have half-lives from 10 to 20 hours.

Fluoroquinolines are classified by "generation" based on their antimicrobial spectrum of activity (Table 27–2). **Norfloxacin**, a first-generation agent, is the least active fluoroquinolone against both gramnegative and gram-positive organisms. **Ciprofloxacin** and **ofloxacin** (second-generation fluoroquinolones) have excellent activity against gram-negative bacteria and moderate to good activity against gram-positive cocci. Third-generation fluoroquinolones (e.g., **levofloxacin**) are slightly less active against gram-negative bacteria, but have greater activity against gram-positive cocci, including *S pneumoniae* and some strains of

enterococci and MRSA. The most recently introduced fourth-generation drugs (e.g., **moxifloxacin**) are the broadest spectrum fluoroquinolones to date, with enhanced activity against anaerobes.

Clinical Uses

Fluoroquinolones are effective in the treatment of urogenital and gastrointestinal tract infections even when caused by multidrug-resistant bacteria. Fluoroquinolones (except norfloxacin, which does not achieve adequate systemic concentrations) have been used widely for respiratory tract, skin, bone, joint, and soft tissue infections. However, their effectiveness may be variable because of the emergence of resistance. Ciprofloxacin and ofloxacin are alternatives to thirdgeneration cephalosporins in gonorrhea, and are administered in single oral doses. Ofloxacin will eradicate accompanying organisms such as *Chlamydia*. Levofloxacin has good activity against organisms associated with community-acquired pneumonia. Fluoroquinolones have also been used in the meningococcal carrier state, in the treatment of tuberculosis, and in prophylactic management of neutropenic patients.

Adverse Effects

Overall, fluoroquinolones are very well tolerated. Gastrointestinal distress is the most common side effect. In addition, they may cause skin rashes, headache, dizziness, insomnia, abnormal liver function tests, and phototoxicity. Although rare, tendonitis has been reported, which may be serious because of the risk of tendon rupture. They are not recommended for use in children or in pregnancy because they have caused cartilage problems in developing animals. Fluoroquinolones may increase plasma levels of theophylline and other methylxanthines, enhancing their toxicity.

ANTIMYCOBACTERIAL DRUGS

Mycobacteria are slow-growing aerobic gram-positive bacteria that are widespread in the environment and in animals. The peptidoglycan layer has a different chemical basis than gram-positive or gram-negative bacteria. The outer envelope contains a variety of complex lipids called mycolic acids, which create a waxy layer that provides resistance to drying and other environmental factors. Thus, mycobacteria can survive for prolonged periods in the environment and are effectively transmitted by airborne droplets. After entering host cells, mycobacteria survive as intracellular parasites in macrophages.

Major human pathogens include *Mycobacterium tuberculosis* and *M leprae*, the causative agents of tuberculosis and leprosy, respectively. Mycobacteria other than tuberculosis are associated with several other conditions, usually in immunocompromised individuals. In AIDS patients in the United States, *M avium* complex is an increasingly important pathogen.

Mycobacterial infections are generally slowly developing chronic conditions. Because mycobacterial cell wall components promote immunologic reactions, a significant portion of the pathology is attributable to the host immune response rather than to direct bacterial toxicity. For all mycobacterial infections, social and environmental factors as well as genetic predisposition play a role.

Chemotherapy for tuberculosis, leprosy, and other atypical mycobacteria is complicated by numerous factors, including (1) limited information about the mechanisms of antimycobacterial drug actions; (2) the rapid development of resistance; (3) the intracellular location of mycobacteria; (4) the chronic nature of mycobacterial disease, which requires protracted drug treatment and is associated with drug toxicities; and (5) patient compliance. Chemotherapy of mycobacterial infections almost always involves prolonged use of drug combinations to delay the emergence of resistance and to enhance antimycobacterial efficacy.

Drugs Used in Tuberculosis

The major drugs used in tuberculosis are **isoniazid (INH), rifampin, ethambutol, pyrazinamide,** and **streptomycin** (Table 27–3). Actions of these agents on *M tuberculosis* are bactericidal or bacteriostatic, depending on drug concentration and strain susceptibility. Treatment of pulmonary tuberculosis usually begins with a three- or four-drug combination regimen depending on the known or anticipated rate of resistance to INH. Directly observed therapy (DOT) regimens, in which a health-care provider witnesses ingestion of the antituberculosis agents, are recommended in noncompliant patients and in drug-resistant tuberculosis.

Isoniazid

Isoniazid is structurally similar to pyridoxine (vitamin B_6). The drug is well absorbed orally and penetrates cells to act on intracellular mycobacteria. It is metabolized by the liver and the rate of metabolism varies among ethnic groups. Fast metabolizers may require higher dosage than slow metabolizers for equivalent therapeutic effects.

MECHANISM OF ACTION. Antitubercular action involves inhibition of an acyl carrier protein reductase involved in synthesis of mycolic acid required for the outer envelope of the peptidoglycan layer. Because resistance can emerge rapidly if the drug is used alone, INH is always used together with other antituberculosis drugs in active infections.

CLINICAL USE. INH is the single most important drug used in tuberculosis and is a component of most drug combination regimens for this disease (Table 27–3).

Table 27-3.	Antimicrobials used in the treatment of tuberculosis and recommended duration of therapy	
Regimen (in approximate order of preference)		**Duration (months)**
Isoniazid, rifampin, pyrazinamide		6
Isoniazid, rifampin		9
Rifampin, ethambutol, pyrazinamide		6
Rifampin, ethambutol		12
Isoniazid, ethambutol		18
All other		≥24

INH is given as the sole drug in the treatment of latent infection (formerly known as prophylaxis) including purified protein derivative (PPD) skin test converters, and for individuals who have close contact with patients with active disease.

ADVERSE EFFECTS. Neurotoxic effects are common and include peripheral neuritis, restlessness, muscle twitching, and insomnia. Pyridoxine can be given to reduce this toxicity without impairing the antibacterial action. INH is hepatotoxic and may cause abnormal liver function tests, jaundice, and hepatitis. Fortunately, hepatotoxicity is rare in children. INH may inhibit the hepatic metabolism of drugs (e.g., phenytoin). Hemolysis and a lupus-like syndrome have been reported.

Rifampin

Rifampin is bactericidal against susceptible *M tuberculosis* organisms. When given orally, it is well absorbed and distributed to most body tissues, including the CNS. The drug undergoes enterohepatic cycling and is partially metabolized in the liver. Both free drug and metabolites are eliminated mainly in the feces.

MECHANISM OF ACTION. Rifampin inhibits DNA-dependent RNA polymerase (encoded by the *rpo* gene) in *M tuberculosis* and many other microorganisms. If rifampin is used alone, changes in drug sensitivity of the polymerase emerges rapidly, leading to resistance.

CLINICAL USE. In tuberculosis, rifampin is always used in combination with other drugs (Table 27–3) because resistance develops rapidly when it is used alone in active infections. Rifampin can be used as the sole drug in treatment of latent tuberculosis in INH-intolerant patients or in individuals who have close contact with patients carrying INH-resistant strains. Other uses of rifampin include the meningococcal and staphylococcal carrier states. In leprosy, rifampin given monthly delays the emergence of resistance to dapsone.

ADVERSE EFFECTS. Rifampin imparts a harmless orange color to urine, sweat, tears, and contact lenses (soft lenses may be permanently stained). Occasional adverse effects include rashes, thrombocytopenia, nephritis, and liver dysfunction.

Rifampin commonly causes light-chain proteinuria and may impair antibody responses. If given less often than twice weekly, rifampin may cause a flu-like syndrome (chills, fever, myalgias) and anemia.

Rifampin strongly induces liver drug-metabolizing enzymes and enhances the elimination rate of many drugs, including anticonvulsants, contraceptive steroids, cyclosporine, ketoconazole, methadone, terbinafine, and warfarin. **Rifabutin** is less likely to cause drug interactions than rifampin and is equally effective as an antimycobacterial agent. Rifabutin is usually preferred over rifampin in treating tuberculosis in AIDS patients.

Ethambutol

This antituberculous drug is well absorbed orally and distributed to most tissues, including the CNS when the meninges are inflamed. A large fraction is eliminated unchanged in the urine. Dose reduction is necessary in renal failure.

MECHANISM OF ACTION. Ethambutol interferes with mycobacterial cell wall synthesis by inhibiting arabinosyl transferases involved in the synthesis of arabinogalactan, a component of the organisms' cell walls. Resistance occurs rapidly via mutations in the *emb* gene if the drug is used alone.

CLINICAL USE. The main use of ethambutol is in tuberculosis, including tubercular meningitis. To avoid resistance, ethambutol is always given in combination with other antituberculous drugs (Table 27–3).

ADVERSE EFFECTS. The most common adverse effects are dose-dependent visual disturbances, including decreased visual acuity, red-green color blindness, optic neuritis, and possible retinal damage (from prolonged use at high doses). Most of these effects regress if the drug is stopped promptly. Other neurotoxic effects include headache, confusion, and peripheral neuritis. Ethambutol is relatively contraindicated in children too young to permit assessment of visual acuity and red-green color discrimination.

Pyrazinamide

Pyrazinamide is well absorbed orally and penetrates most body tissues, including inflamed meninges. The drug is partly metabolized to pyrazinoic acid, and both parent molecule and metabolite are excreted in the urine. Plasma half-life of pyrazinamide is increased in hepatic or renal failure.

MECHANISM OF ACTION. The mechanism of action of pyrazinamide is unknown; however, its bacteriostatic action appears to require metabolic conversion via pyrazinamidases (encoded by the *pncA* gene) present in *M tuberculosis*. Resistant mycobacteria lack these enzymes, and resistance develops rapidly if the drug is used alone. There is minimal cross-resistance with other antimycobacterial drugs.

CLINICAL USE. Pyrazinamide, when combined with other antituberculous drugs (INH and rifampin), is an important front-line drug used in "short-course" (i.e., 6 months) treatment regimens as a "sterilizing" agent active against residual intracellular organisms that may cause relapse.

ADVERSE EFFECTS. Approximately 40% of patients develop nongouty polyarthralgia (i.e., pain at multiple joints). Hyperuricemia occurs commonly but is usually asymptomatic. Other adverse effects include myalgia, gastrointestinal irritation, maculopapular rash, hepatic dysfunction, porphyria, and photosensitivity reactions.

Streptomycin

This aminoglycoside is now used more frequently than before because of the growing prevalence of strains of *M tuberculosis* resistant to other drugs. Streptomycin is used principally in drug combinations for the treatment of life-threatening tuberculous disease, including meningitis, miliary dissemination (mycobacterial invasion of multiple organs via the bloodstream), and severe organ tuberculosis. The pharmacodynamic and pharmacokinetic properties of streptomycin are similar to those of other aminoglycosides.

Alternative Drugs

Several drugs with antimycobacterial activity are used in cases that are resistant to first-line agents; they are considered second-line drugs because they are no more effective, and their toxicities are often more serious than those of the major drugs. Second-line agents include **amikacin, ciprofloxacin, ofloxacin,**
ethionamide, para-aminosalicylic acid (PAS), capreomycin, and **cycloserine.** As with first-line agents, these drugs are always used in combinations.

Drugs Used in Leprosy

Mycobacterium leprae is the causative agent of leprosy (Hansen's disease). *M leprae* grows intracellularly, typically within skin and endothelial cells and Schwann cells of peripheral nerves. Onset of leprosy is gradual and the spectrum of disease is broad, depending on the host's immune response. Leprosy requires close and prolonged contact for transmission. Transmission is directly related to overcrowding and poor hygiene, and occurs by direct contact and aerosol inhalation. Although rare in the United States, the worldwide prevalence of cases is estimated at over 1 million, with highest concentration being in Southeast Asia, Africa, and Central and South America.

Several drugs closely related to the sulfonamides have been used effectively in long-term treatment of leprosy. **Dapsone** (diaminodiphenylsulfone) remains the most active drug against *M leprae*. Like the sulfonamides, its mechanism of action involves inhibition of folic acid synthesis. Resistance can develop, especially if low doses are given. Dapsone can be given orally, penetrates tissues well, undergoes enterohepatic cycling, and is eliminated in the urine, partly as acetylated metabolites. It is usually well tolerated. Common adverse effects include gastrointestinal irritation, fever, skin rashes, and methemoglobinemia. Hemolysis may occur, especially in patients with G6PD deficiency.

Dapsone is rarely used alone in leprosy. Drug regimens usually include combinations of dapsone with rifampin (or rifabutin, see discussion above) with or without **clofazimine.** Clofazimine causes gastrointestinal irritation and pinkish brown skin discoloration.

Acedapsone is a repository form of dapsone that provides inhibitory plasma concentrations for several months. In addition to its use in leprosy, dapsone is an alternative drug for the treatment of *P jiroveci* pneumonia in AIDS patients.

Drugs for Atypical Mycobacterial Infections

Infections resulting from atypical mycobacteria (e.g., *M marinum, M avium-intracellulare, M ulcerans*), although sometimes asymptomatic, may be treated with the described antimycobacterial drugs (e.g., ethambutol, rifampin) or other antibiotics (e.g., erythromycin, amikacin).

M avium complex (MAC) is a cause of disseminated infections in AIDS patients. Currently, clarithromycin or azithromycin is recommended for primary prophylaxis in patients with CD4 counts less than 50/μL. Treatment of MAC infections requires a combination of drugs; one favored regimen consists of azithromycin or clarithromycin with ethambutol and rifabutin.

REHABILITATION FOCUS

A large number of antibacterial agents are currently in clinical use. Many factors are considered in the choice of a particular drug. These include the species of bacterium (if known), the bacterium's drug susceptibility (if known), the location of the infection (which often points to the most likely organism), the severity of infection, and the adverse effects of the drug under consideration in a patient with impaired elimination mechanisms (e.g., renal or liver dysfunction).

One serious problem of antibacterial therapy is the potential for increasing the prevalence of resistant strains. The number of resistant bacterial strains continues to increase and mechanisms for the development of bacterial resistance are complex. As health-care professionals, physical therapists should educate patients about the role each individual plays in limiting the development of drug-resistant bacteria. Specifically, patients can be reminded that (1) antibacterial drugs should be used cautiously and not overused, and (2) once a drug regimen has been initiated, it should be completed in its entirety.

Physical therapists routinely treat patients receiving antibacterial agents for conditions either directly or indirectly related to their need for rehabilitative intervention. For example, therapists often treat patients with infections directly related to rehabilitation, such as burns, open wounds, and surgery. Other infections not directly related to rehabilitation include pneumonia and urinary tract infections. These infections are common in both hospitalized patients and patients receiving outpatient or home health care.

Because such a large proportion of patients receiving rehabilitation services will be taking antibacterial agents, physical therapists should have a general understanding of the various types of antibacterial agents, their type of action (e.g., bactericidal or bacteriostatic), and their adverse effects.

Finally, physical therapists must understand their role in preventing the spread of infections. Handwashing between patients, adequately cleaning or sterilizing rehabilitation equipment (e.g., walkers, whirlpools) between patients, and maintaining appropriate sterile technique when working with open infections can limit therapists' transferring infection among patients.

CLINICAL RELEVANCE FOR REHABILITATION

Adverse Drug Reactions

The most common adverse effects associated with many of the antibacterial agents include hypersensitivity and allergic reactions and gastrointestinal disturbances.

- Hypersensitivity or allergic reactions: skin rashes, itching, wheezing, ultraviolet sensitivity, fever, anaphylaxis
- Gastrointestinal problems: nausea, vomiting, diarrhea, superinfection with resistant organisms, colitis
- Many antibiotics (especially chloramphenicol, erythromycin, clarithromycin, fluoroquinolones, and rifampin) have significant drug interactions, increasing or decreasing plasma levels of other drugs.
- IV infusions of cephalosporins and vancomycin may cause phlebitis.
- Some antibiotics inhibit production of red blood cells (e.g., chloramphenicol), white blood cells (e.g., clindamycin, linezolid, trimethoprim) or platelets (e.g., linezolid).

- Doxycycline and minocycline may cause dizziness and vertigo.
- Vancomycin and aminoglycosides are ototoxic.
- Fluoroquinolones may cause tendonitis.
- Antimycobacterial drugs commonly cause neurotoxic effects (e.g., isoniazid, ethambutol), visual changes (e.g., ethambutol, pyrazinamide), and nongouty polyarthralgia (e.g., pyrazinamide).

Effects Interfering with Rehabilitation
- Hypersensitivity reactions and gastrointestinal problems may hinder rehabilitation intervention.
- If plasma levels of other drugs increase, patients may experience increased adverse effects. If plasma levels of other drugs decrease, their efficacy may be decreased.
- Phlebitis causing pain, tenderness, and edema in the affected extremity may limit mobility.
- Anemia limits exercise tolerance. Leukocytopenia increases patients' susceptibility to infection. Thrombocytopenia increases patients' susceptibility to bleeding and bruising.
- Dizziness and vertigo may limit mobility and balance, increasing the risk of falling.
- High-frequency hearing loss, more common with amikacin and kanamycin, may limit patients' ability to follow directions of therapist. Vertigo, ataxia, and loss of balance, more common with gentamicin and tobramycin, may limit mobility and increase risk of falling.
- Tendonitis may limit range of motion and strengthening of involved joints.
- Neurotoxic and visual disturbances may hinder participation in rehabilitation programs.

Possible Therapy Solutions
- Alter therapy times around gastrointestinal problems if symptoms occur routinely with continued therapy.
- The physical therapist should know all of the drugs the patient is taking, be aware of the agents with high potential to cause significant drug interactions, and recognize adverse effects, or decreases in drug efficacy.

- Phlebitis after parenteral antibiotic administration should be reported to the primary health-care provider. Weight bearing on the affected extremity should be as tolerated, following any restrictions set by the primary health-care provider.
- Aerobic exercise goals should be lowered in patients with anemia. Oxygen saturation should be monitored by pulse oximetry during exercise to ensure adequate oxygenation.
- Physical therapists should take extra infection control precautions when working with patients with leukocytopenia: sanitizing all equipment prior to patient use, treating patient in his/her own room in preference to areas with larger pathogenic exposures (e.g., therapy gym), and avoiding patient contact if the therapist is ill.
- In patients with thrombocytopenia, sharp wound debridement, deep tissue massage, and resistive exercise that puts significant pressure on bony or small surface areas (e.g., resistive tubing around ankle, resisted seated knee extension) should be avoided.
- For dizziness, increase the assistance provided or the stability of the assistive device and caution patients to move slowly, especially when transitioning between positions.
- If the patient reports (or the therapist observes) decreased hearing acuity or vestibular function, these symptoms should be reported to the primary health-care provider immediately.
- Tendonitis as a result of fluoroquinolones should be reported to the primary health-care provider. Strengthening exercises around involved joints should be avoided to avoid risk of tendon rupture.
- Neurotoxic and visual disturbances consequent to antimycobacterial drugs should be reported to the primary health-care provider. In the absence of serious toxicity, the patient should be strongly encouraged to continue with the drug regimen because compliance is required for eradication of the infectious agent. If symptoms are limiting activity, rehabilitation goals may need to be postponed until the drug regimen has been completed.

PROBLEM-ORIENTED PATIENT STUDY

Brief History: The patient is a 53-year-old white female with a 40-year history of insulin-dependent type 1 diabetes mellitus. Two weeks ago, she suffered a myocardial infarction (MI) for which she was hospitalized for several days. In addition to her insulin, she has been taking the anticoagulant warfarin since her MI. Prior to her MI, the patient had been referred to an outpatient wound clinic for evaluation and treatment of neuropathic ulcers on both feet.

Current Medical Status and Drugs: The patient attends the wound clinic for her first treatment, 2.5 weeks after her MI. When the patient takes off her shoes and socks, the physical therapist notes that the ulcer on her right foot has increased in size since the evaluation and that the right lower extremity is edematous. The therapist contacts the primary health-care provider with the patient's change in status. The wound is cultured and is positive for *S aureus*. The patient is given oral erythromycin to treat the wound infection and resulting phlebitis.

Rehabilitation Setting: After another week, the patient returns to the wound clinic. The physical therapist notes that the wound circumference on the right foot is back to the baseline measurements

taken prior to her MI. However, the wound bed appears to have an increased amount of necrotic tissue. The physician working at the wound clinic writes an order for whirlpool cleansing and wet-to-dry dressings for debridement. After discussion between the physician and the physical therapist of the proposed treatment plan, changes are made to the treatment plan to include enzymatic debridement instead of wet-to-dry dressings and modification of orthotics to inhibit wound progression.

Problem/Clinical Options: The patient was prescribed an anticoagulant after her MI to lessen the likelihood of thrombus formation. Subsequently, she was given erythromycin to treat the bacterial infection in her right lower extremity. Erythromycin inhibits several hepatic cytochrome P450 isoforms, and therefore has significant drug interactions. Specifically, erythromycin increases the plasma level of anticoagulants, leading to an increased risk of bleeding. The proposed treatment plan of wet-to-dry dressings for wound debridement would result in significant tissue tearing, with resultant bleeding that may be increased with the patient's current medications. In contrast, enzymatic debridement of necrotic tissue would make bleeding almost negligible.

PREPARATIONS AVAILABLE

β-Lactam Antibiotics and Other Cell Wall Synthesis Inhibitors

Penicillins

Amoxicillin (generic, Amoxil, others)
Oral: 125-, 200-, 250-, 400-mg chewable tablets; 500-, 875-mg tablets; 250-, 500-mg capsules; powder to reconstitute for 50, 125, 200, 250, 400 mg/mL solution

Amoxicillin/potassium clavulanate (generic, Augmentin)[1]
Oral: 250-, 500-, 875-mg tablets; 125-, 200-, 250-, 400-mg chewable tablets; 1000-mg

extended-release tablet powder to reconstitute for 125, 200, 250 mg/5 mL suspension

Ampicillin (generic)
Oral: 250-, 500-mg capsules; powder to reconstitute for 125-, 250-mg suspensions
Parenteral: powder to reconstitute for injection (125, 250, 500 mg, 1, 2 g per vial)

Ampicillin/sulbactam sodium (generic, Unasyn)[2]
Parenteral: 1, 2 g ampicillin powder to reconstitute for IV or IM injection

Carbenicillin (Geocillin)
Oral: 382-mg tablets

Dicloxacillin (generic)
Oral: 250-, 500-mg capsules

Mezlocillin (Mezlin)
Parenteral: powder to reconstitute for injection (in 1-, 2-, 3-, 4-g vials)

Nafcillin (generic)
Oral: 250-mg capsules
Parenteral: 1, 2 g per IV piggyback units

Oxacillin (generic)
Oral: 250-, 500-mg capsules; powder to reconstitute for 250 mg/5 mL solution
Parenteral: powder to reconstitute for injection (0.5, 1, 2, 10 g per vial)

Penicillin G (generic, Pentids, Pfizerpen)
Oral: 0.2-, 0.25-, 0.4-, 0.5-, 0.8-million unit tablets; powder to reconstitute 400,000 units/5 mL suspension
Parenteral: powder to reconstitute for injection (1-, 2-, 3-, 5-, 10-, 20-million units)

Penicillin G benzathine (Permapen, Bicillin)
Parenteral: 0.6-, 1.2-, 2.4-million units per dose

Penicillin G procaine (generic)
Parenteral: 0.6-, 1.2-million units/mL for IM injection only

Penicillin V (generic, V-Cillin, Pen-Vee K, others)
Oral: 250-, 500-mg tablets; powder to reconstitute for 125 , 250 mg/5 mL solution

Piperacillin (Pipracil)
Parenteral: powder to reconstitute for injection (2, 3, 4 g per vial)

Piperacillin and tazobactam sodium (Zosyn)[3]
Parenteral: 2-, 3-, 4-g powder to reconstitute for IV injection

Ticarcillin (Ticar)
Parenteral: powder to reconstitute for injection (1, 3, 6 g per vial)

Ticarcillin/clavulanate potassium (Timentin)[4]
Parenteral: 3 g powder to reconstitute for injection

Cephalosporins and Other β-Lactam Drugs

Narrow Spectrum (First-Generation) Cephalosporins

Cefadroxil (generic, Duricef)
Oral: 500-mg capsules; 1-g tablets; 125, 250, 500 mg/5 mL suspension

Cefazolin (generic, Ancef, Kefzol)
Parenteral: powder to reconstitute for injection (0.25, 0.5, 1 g per vial or IV piggyback unit)

Cephalexin (generic, Keflex, others)
Oral: 250-, 500-mg capsules and tablets; 1-g tablets; 125, 250 mg/5 mL suspension

Cephalothin (generic, Keflin)[5]
Parenteral: powder to reconstitute for injection and solution for injection (1 g per vial or infusion pack)

Cephapirin (Cefadyl)
Parenteral: powder to reconstitute for injection (1 g per vial or IV piggyback unit)

Cephradine (generic, Velosef)
Oral: 250-, 500-mg capsules; 125, 250 mg/5 mL suspension
Parenteral: powder to reconstitute for injection (0.25, 0.5, 1, 2 g per vial)

Intermediate Spectrum (Second-Generation) Cephalosporins

Cefaclor (generic, Ceclor)
Oral: 250-, 500-mg capsules; 375-, 500-mg extended-release tablets; powder to reconstitute for 125, 187, 250, 375 mg/5 mL suspension

Cefamandole (Mandol)
Parenteral: 1, 2 g (in vials) for IM, IV injection

Cefmetazole (Zefazone)
Parenteral: 1-, 2-g powder for IV injection

Cefonicid (Monocid)
Parenteral: powder to reconstitute for injection (1, 10 g per vial)

Cefotetan (Cefotan)
Parenteral: powder to reconstitute for injection (1, 2, 10 g per vial)

Cefoxitin (Mefoxin)
Parenteral: powder to reconstitute for injection (1, 2, 10 g per vial)

Cefprozil (Cefzil)
Oral: 250-, 500-mg tablets; powder to reconstitute 125, 250 mg/5mL suspension

Cefuroxime (generic, Ceftin, Kefurox, Zinacef)
Oral: 125-, 250-, 500-mg tablets; 125, 250 mg/5 mL suspension
Parenteral: powder to reconstitute for injection (0.75, 1.5, 7.5 g per vial or infusion pack)

Loracarbef (Lorabid)
Oral: 200-, 400-mg capsules; powder for 100, 200 mg/5 mL suspension

Broad-Spectrum (Third- and Fourth-Generation) Cephalosporins

Cefdinir (Omnicef)
Oral: 300-mg capsules; 125 mg/5 mL suspension

Cefditoren (Spectracef)
Oral: 200-mg tablets

Cefepime (Maxipime)
Parenteral: powder for injection 0.5, 1, 2 g

Cefixime (Suprax)
Oral: 200-, 400-mg tablets; powder for oral suspension, 100 mg/5 mL

Cefoperazone (Cefobid)
Parenteral: powder to reconstitute for injection (1, 2 g per vial, 10 g bulk)

Cefotaxime (Claforan)
Parenteral: powder to reconstitute for injection (0.5, 1, 2 g per vial)

Cefpodoxime proxetil (Vantin)
Oral: 100-, 200-mg tablets; 50-, 100-mg granules for suspension in 5 mL

Ceftazidime (generic, Fortaz, Tazidime)
Parenteral: powder to reconstitute for injection (0.5, 1, 2 g per vial)

Ceftibuten (Cedax)
Oral: 400-mg capsules; 90, 180 mg/5 mL powder for oral suspension

Ceftizoxime (Cefizox)
Parenteral: powder to reconstitute for injection and solution for injection (0.5, 1, 2 g per vial)

Ceftriaxone (Rocephin)
Parenteral: powder to reconstitute for injection (0.25, 0.5, 1, 2, 10 g per vial)

Carbapenems and Monobactam

Aztreonam (Azactam)
Parenteral: powder to reconstitute for injection (0.5, 1, 2 g)

Ertapenem (Invanz)
Parenteral: 1 g powder to reconstitute for intravenous (0.9% NaCl diluent) or intramuscular (1% lidocaine diluent) injection

Imipenem/cilastatin (Primaxin)
Parenteral: powder to reconstitute for injection (250, 500, 750 mg imipenem per vial)

Meropenem (Merrem IV)
Parenteral: powder for injection (0.5, 1 g per vial)

[1]Clavulanate content varies with the formulation; see package insert.
[2]Sulbactam content is half the ampicillin content.
[3]Tazobactam content is 12.5% of the piperacillin content.
[4]Clavulanate content 0.1 g.
[5]Not available in the United States.

Other Drugs Discussed in This Chapter

Cycloserine (Seromycin Pulvules)
Oral: 250-mg capsules

Fosfomycin (Monurol)
Oral: 3-g packet

Vancomycin (generic, Vancocin, Vancoled)
Oral: 125-, 250-mg Pulvules; powder to reconstitute for 250 mg/5 mL, 500 mg/6 mL solution
Parenteral: 0.5-, 1-, 5-, 10-g powder to reconstitute for IV injection

Inhibitors of Bacterial Protein Synthesis

Chloramphenicol

Chloramphenicol (generic, Chloromycetin)
Oral: 250-mg capsules; 150 mg/5 mL suspension
Parenteral: 100-mg powder to reconstitute for injection

Tetracyclines

Demeclocycline (Declomycin)
Oral: 150-, 300-mg tablets; 150-mg capsules

Doxycycline (generic, Vibramycin, others)
Oral: 50-, 100-mg tablets and capsules; powder to reconstitute for 25 mg/5 mL suspension; 50 mg/5 mL syrup
Parenteral: 100-, 200-mg powder to reconstitute for injection

Methacycline (Rondomycin)
Oral: 150-, 300-mg capsules

Minocycline (Minocin)
Oral: 50-, 100-mg tablets and capsules; 50 mg/5 mL suspension

Tetracycline (generic, Achromycin V, others)
Oral: 100-, 250-, 500-mg capsules; 250-, 500-mg tablets; 125 mg/5 mL suspension
Parenteral: 100-, 250-mg powder to reconstitute for IM injection; 250-, 500-mg powder to reconstitute for IV injection

Macrolides

Azithromycin (Zithromax)
Oral: 250-mg capsules; powder for 100, 200 mg/5 mL oral suspension

Clarithromycin (Biaxin)
Oral: 250-, 500-mg tablets, 500-mg extended-release tablets; granules for 125, 250 mg/5 mL oral suspension

Erythromycin (generic, Ilotycin, Ilosone, E-Mycin, Erythrocin, others)
Oral (base): 250-, 333-, 500-mg enteric-coated tablets
Oral (base) delayed-release: 333-mg tablets, 250-mg capsules
Oral (estolate): 500-mg tablets; 250-mg capsules; 125, 250 mg/5 mL suspension
Oral (ethylsuccinate): 200-, 400-mg film-coated tablets; 200, 400 mg/5 mL suspension
Oral (stearate): 250-, 500-mg film-coated tablets
Parenteral: lactobionate, 0.5-, 1-g powder to reconstitute for IV injection

Ketolides

Telithromycin (Proteck)
Oral: 800-mg tablets

Lincomycins

Clindamycin (generic, Cleocin)
Oral: 75-, 150-, 300-mg capsules; 75 mg/5 mL granules to reconstitute for solution
Parenteral: 150 mg/mL in 2-, 4-, 6-, 60-mL vials for injection

Streptogramins

Quinupristin and dalfopristin (Synercid)
Parenteral: 30:70 formulation in 500 mg vial for reconstitution for IV injection

Oxazolidinones

Linezolid (Zyvox)
Oral: 400-, 600-mg tablets; 100-mg powder for solution
Parenteral: 2 mg/mL for IV infusion

Aminoglycosides and Spectinomycin

Amikacin (generic, Amikin)
Parenteral: 50, 250 mg (in vials) for IM, IV injection

Gentamicin (generic, Garamycin)
Parenteral: 10, 40 mg/mL vials for IM, IV injection

Kanamycin (Kantrex)
Oral: 500-mg capsules
Parenteral: 500, 1000 mg for IM, IV injection; 75 mg for pediatric injection

Neomycin (generic, Mycifradin)
Oral: 500-mg tablets; 125 mg/5 mL solution

Netilmicin (Netromycin)
Parenteral: 100 mg/mL for IM, IV injection

Paromomycin (Humatin)
Oral: 250-mg capsules

Spectinomycin (Trobicin)
Parenteral: 2 g powder to reconstitute for IM injection

Streptomycin (generic)
Parenteral: 400 mg/mL for IM injection

Tobramycin (generic, Nebcin)
Parenteral: 10, 40 mg/mL for IM, IV injection; powder to reconstitute for injection

Inhibitors of Bacterial DNA Synthesis

Sulfonamides, Trimethoprim, and Fluoroquinolones

General-Purpose Sulfonamides

Sulfadiazine (generic)
Oral: 500-mg tablets

Sulfamethizole (Thiosulfil Forte)
Oral: 500-mg tablets

Sulfamethoxazole (generic, Gantanol, others)
Oral: 500-mg tablets; 500 mg/5 mL suspension

Sulfanilamide (AVC)
Vaginal cream: 15%

Sulfisoxazole (generic, Gantrisin)
Oral: 500-mg tablets; 500 mg/5 mL syrup
Ophthalmic: 4% solution

Sulfonamides for Special Applications

Mafenide (Sulfamylon)
Topical: 85 mg/g cream; 5% solution

Silver sulfadiazine (generic, Silvadene)
Topical: 10-mg/g cream

Sulfacetamide sodium (generic)
Ophthalmic: 1, 10, 15, 30% solutions; 10% ointment

Trimethoprim

Trimethoprim (generic, Proloprim, Trimpex)
Oral: 100-, 200-mg tablets

Trimethoprim-sulfamethoxazole co-trimoxazole, TMP-SMZ (generic, Bactrim, Septra, others)
Oral: 80 mg trimethoprim + 400 mg sulfamethoxazole per single-strength tablet; 160 mg trimethoprim + 800 mg sulfamethoxazole per double-strength tablet; 40 mg trimethoprim + 200 mg sulfamethoxazole per 5 mL suspension
Parenteral: 80 mg trimethoprim + 400 mg sulfamethoxazole per 5 mL for infusion (in 5 mL ampules and 5-, 10-, 20-, 30-, 50-mL vials)

Quinolones and Fluoroquinolones

Cinoxacin (generic, Cinobac)
Oral: 250-, 500-mg capsules

Ciprofloxacin (Cipro, Cipro I.V.)
Oral: 250-, 500-, 750-mg tablets; 50, 100 mg/mL suspension
Parenteral: 2, 10 mg/mL for IV infusion
Ophthalmic (Ciloxan): 3 mg/mL solution; 3.3 mg/g ointment

Enoxacin (Penetrex)
Oral: 200-, 400-mg tablets

Levofloxacin (Levaquin)
Oral: 250, 500, 750 mg for injection
Parenteral: 250, 500 mg for IV injection
Ophthalmic (Quixin): 5 mg/mL solution

Lomefloxacin (Maxaquin)
Oral: 400-mg tablets

Moxifloxacin (Avelox, Avelox I.V.)
Oral: 400-mg tablets
Parenteral: 400 mg in IV bag

Nalidixic acid (NegGram)
Oral: 250-, 500-, 1000-mg caplets; 250 mg/5 mL
suspension

Norfloxacin (Noroxin)
Oral: 400-mg tablets

Ofloxacin (Floxin)
Oral: 200-, 300-, 400-mg tablets
Parenteral: 200 mg in 50 mL 5% D/W for IV
administration; 20, 40 mg/mL for IV injection
Ophthalmic (Ocuflox): 3 mg/mL solution

Antimycobacterial Drugs

Drugs Used in Tuberculosis

Aminosalicylate sodium (Paser)
Oral: 4 g delayed-release granules

Capreomycin (Capastat Sulfate)
Parenteral: 1-g powder to reconstitute for injection

Cycloserine (Seromycin Pulvules)
Oral: 250-mg capsules

Ethambutol (Myambutol)
Oral: 100-, 400-mg tablets

Ethionamide (Trecator-SC)
Oral: 250-mg tablets

Isoniazid (generic)
Oral: 50-, 100-, 300-mg tablets; syrup, 50 mg/5 mL
Parenteral: 100 mg/mL for injection

Pyrazinamide (generic)
Oral: 500-mg tablets

Rifabutin (Mycobutin)
Oral: 150-mg capsules

Rifampin (generic, Rifadin, Rimactane)
Oral: 150-, 300-mg capsules
Parenteral: 600-mg powder for IV injection

Rifapentine (Priftin)
Oral: 150-mg tablets

Streptomycin (generic)
Parenteral: 1 g lyophilized for IM injection

Drugs Used in Leprosy

Clofazimine (Lamprene)
Oral: 50-mg capsules

Dapsone (generic)
Oral: 25-, 100-mg tablets

REFERENCES

Bain KT, Wittbrodt ET: Linezolid for the treatment of resistant gram-positive cocci. *Ann Pharmacother* 2001; 35:566.

Blondeau JM: Expanded activity and utility of the new fluoroquinolones: A review. *Clin Ther* 1999; 21:3.

Centers for Disease Control and Prevention: Vancomycin resistant *Staphylococcus aureus*—Pennsylvania, 2002. *JAMA* 2002;288: 2116.

Centers for Disease Control and Prevention. Prevention and treatment of tuberculosis in patients infected with human immunodeficiency virus: Principles of therapy and revised recommendations. *MMWR Morb Mortal Wkly Rep* 1998;47(RR-20):1.

Davidson R, et al: Resistance to levofloxacin and failure of treatment of pneumococcal pneumonia. *N Engl J Med* 2002;346:747.

Diagnosis and treatment of disease caused by nontuberculous mycobacteria. *Am J Respir Crit Care Med* 1997;156(2 Part 2):S1.

Fulton B, Perry CM: Cefopodoxime proxetil: A review of its use in the management of bacterial infections in pediatric patients. *Paediatr Drugs* 2001; 3:137.

Gee T, et al: Pharmacokinetics and tissue penetration of linezolid following multiple oral doses. *Antimicrob Agents Chemother* 2001;45:1843.

Havlir DV, Barnes PF: Tuberculosis in patients with human immunodeficiency virus infection. *N Engl J Med* 1999; 340:367.

Jasmer RM, et al: Latent tuberculosis infection. *N Engl J Med* 2002;347:1860.

Nicolau DP, et al: Once-daily aminoglycoside dosing: Impact on requests and costs for therapeutic drug monitoring. *Ther Drug Monit* 1996;18:263.

Radanst JM, et al: Interaction of fluoroquinolones with other drugs: Mechanisms, variability, clinical significance, and management. *Clin Infect Dis* 1992; 14:272.

Suh B, Lorber B: Quinolones. *Med Clin North Am* 1995; 79:869.

Targeted tuberculin testing and treatment of latent tuberculosis infection. *Am J Respir Crit Care Med* 2000;161 (4 Part 2):S221.

Wilson WR, et al: Antibiotic treatment of adults with infective endocarditis due to streptococci, enterococci, staphylococci, and HACEK microorganisms. *JAMA* 1995;274:1706.

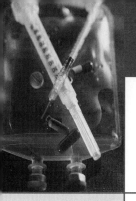

28

ANTIVIRAL AGENTS

■ VIRUSES

Viruses are obligate intracellular parasites. That is, unlike bacteria, viruses depend on living host cells to replicate and function. Since viruses rely on the synthetic machinery of host cells, viruses can be extremely small. In many cases, the entire viral particle, or virion, consists only of nucleic acids (deoxyribonucleic acid [DNA] or ribonucleic acid [RNA]) surrounded by a protein shell, or capsid. Some viruses have an additional glycoprotein coat called an *envelope.*

Viral infections range from common minor illnesses, such as the common cold and cold sores, to life-threatening diseases, such as AIDS, Ebola, and severe acute respiratory syndrome (SARS). In addition, some viruses can cause certain types of cancer. For example, human papillomavirus is the primary causative agent of cervical cancer.

Viral transmission can occur in many ways. The most common ways that virions enter the body are via inhaled droplets (e.g., rhinovirus, the causative agent of the common cold), contaminated food or water (e.g., hepatitis A), direct contact from infected hosts (e.g., HIV), or direct inoculation by bites of infected *vectors* (e.g., dengue fever, transmitted by mosquitoes).

■ ANTIVIRAL AGENTS

Viruses are complicated chemotherapy targets for several reasons. Since viruses rely on host cells' machinery to function, the selective pharmacologic destruction of a virus without destroying human cells is difficult. Early treatment is critical, but frequently not possible because viral replication often peaks before clinical symptoms develop. Many antiviral agents also rely on a normal immune system to destroy the virus. Thus, immune suppression often lengthens viral illnesses. Finally, mutations that cause changes in viral structure and enzymes often lead to the emergence of drug-resistant viral strains. Some viruses (influenza A and B, hepatitis B virus [HBV]) can be effectively controlled by *vaccines* (see section Vaccines and Immune Globulins: Active and Passive Immunizations below).

Antiviral drugs can potentially exert their actions at several stages of viral replication, including (1) viral attachment and entry into the host cell; (2) uncoating of viral nucleic acid; (3) synthesis of early viral regulatory proteins; (4) synthesis of RNA or DNA nucleic acids; (5) late protein synthesis and processing; (6) viral packaging and assembly, and (7) virion release (Figure 28–1).

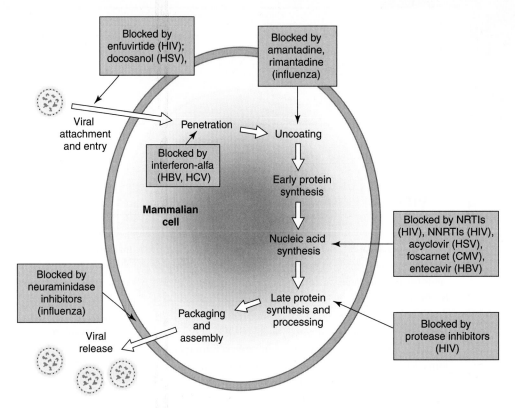

Figure 28–1. The major sites of drug action on viral replication. Diseases in parentheses, see text.

One of the most important trends in viral chemotherapy, especially in the management of HIV infection, has been the introduction of combination drug therapy, in which more than one stage of viral replication is inhibited. The benefits of combination antiviral therapy include greater clinical effectiveness and the prevention or delay of drug resistance.

The antiviral agents covered in this chapter include drugs against herpes, HIV, influenza, HBV, and hepatitis C (HCV) (Figure 28–2).

ANTIHERPES DRUGS

Second to flu (influenza) and common cold viruses, herpes viruses are among the leading causes of human viral disease. The term *herpes* is derived from the Greek word *herpein*, which means to creep. This refers to the creeping or spreading quality of skin lesions caused by many herpes viruses. Although eight types of human herpes viruses have been identified, the most common herpes viruses are herpes simplex virus type 1 (HSV-1), herpes simplex virus type 2 (HSV-2), varicella-zoster virus (VZV), Epstein-Barr virus (EBV), and cytomegalovirus (CMV).

Once infected by any herpes virus, the infection remains for the life of the individual. Herpes infections are well-known for remaining silent—or latent—for months or even years. Then, in response to some trigger (e.g., sun exposure, concurrent viral illness, immunosuppression), the virus is reactivated and the patient once again becomes symptomatic.

Most adult Americans harbor HSV-1, the HSV strain primarily responsible for orofacial (e.g., cold sores) and ocular infections. It is estimated that one in five Americans over the age of 12 years carries HSV-2, which generally causes genital infections. Notably, HSV-1 and HSV-2 can cause outbreaks at either body site by direct contact with infectious secretions or

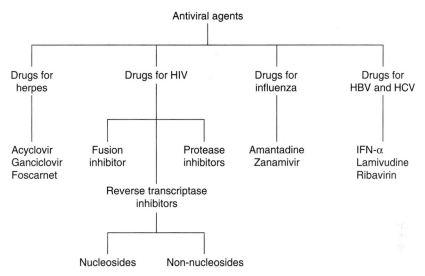

Figure 28–2. Drugs classes used in the treatment of viral infections and diseases.

mucous membranes. During the primary infection, HSV spreads from infected epithelial and mucosal cells to nearby sensory nerve endings and is transported along the axon to the cell body. The virus enters the nucleus of a neuron, where it persists indefinitely in a latent state. Recurrent HSV infection occurs as a result of reactivation of the virus in the sensory ganglion. The virus migrates down the nerve axon and produces vesicular lesions, as well as intermittent asymptomatic viral shedding. Lesions usually heal within 2 weeks. Relapsing episodes are often physically and psychologically distressing. Pregnant women who are shedding the virus may transmit it during delivery, with severe and potentially fatal consequences to the neonate.

In its primary infection, VZV causes **chickenpox** (herpes varicella) in children and is rapidly spread via airborne droplets and contact with lesions. Herpes zoster, also known as **shingles,** is a reactivation of a previous infection with VZV. Roughly 2 to 3 days before vesicular skin lesions appear, the patient often experiences pain along affected dermatomes. The area generally remains painful until lesions heal in 2 to 3 weeks. Herpes zoster cannot be contracted from someone who has herpes zoster because the infection always comes from latent VZV infection in the patient's own spinal cord ganglia. However, the primary infection—

chickenpox can be transmitted from a person with herpes zoster to someone who has not already had chickenpox (or the chickenpox vaccine). Vaccines are currently available for both chickenpox and shingles (see section Vaccines and Immune Globulins: Active and Passive Immunizations).

Cytomegalovirus (CMV) may be acquired congenitally, perinatally, or postnatally. It is the most common congenital (present at birth) infection in the United States, and its incidence increases with age. Indeed, CMV is estimated to infect the majority of adults by 40 years of age. While multiple organs can be affected, CMV is usually asymptomatic in healthy adults. However, in immunocompromised individuals, especially those with AIDS, CMV infections cause various illnesses. In individuals with AIDS, the most common manifestation is an eye infection called *CMV retinitis.*

Most drugs active against herpes viruses inhibit viral DNA polymerases, enzymes that assist in viral replication. Often, antiviral drugs are bioactivated by virus-specific or host enzymes to active drug forms. It is important to note that anti-herpes agents act against the replicating virus by incorporating into the viral DNA, and therefore are ineffective against latent (non-replicating) virus. Three oral antiherpes drugs are licensed for the treatment of HSV and VZV infections: **acyclovir, valacyclovir,** and **famciclovir.** They share similar mechanisms of action and indications for clinical use, and all are fairly well tolerated.

Acyclovir

Mechanism of Action and Pharmacokinetics

Acyclovir (acycloguanosine) is derived from the nucleoside guanosine. Acyclovir is activated first by virus-specific and then by host enzymes to form acyclovir triphosphate, which competes with deoxyguanosine triphosphate for the viral DNA polymerase. The drug then becomes incorporated into the viral DNA, but because acycloguanosine lacks the necessary position for nucleotide attachment, the DNA chain terminates. Resistance of HSV has been reported, mainly among immunocompromised patients. Resistance is often associated with mutations in the viral enzyme thymidine kinase, which is involved in the initial bioactivation of acyclovir. Strains resistant to acyclovir are cross-resistant to similar drugs such as ganciclovir, valacyclovir, and famciclovir. Resistant infections are often managed by foscarnet, cidofovir, or trifluridine, which use a different mechanism of antiviral action, but these drugs are significantly more toxic than acyclovir.

Acyclovir is available in oral, topical, and intravenous forms. Because of its short half-life, oral acyclovir must be taken several times per day. Patients with renal impairment require reduced dosages because the kidneys are primarily responsible for eliminating acyclovir.

Clinical Uses and Toxicity

Oral acyclovir has multiple uses. It is most commonly used for the treatment of mucocutaneous and genital herpes lesions (Table 28–1) and prophylaxis in immunocompromised patients. Oral therapy is the most effective route of administration for treating primary HSV infection and recurrent genital herpes. In initial episodes of genital herpes, oral acyclovir shortens the duration of symptoms, the time for lesions to heal, and the duration of viral shedding. In recurrent genital herpes, the time course is also shortened. Daily oral suppressive therapy decreases the frequency of symptomatic genital herpes outbreaks and asymptomatic viral shedding. This latter point is especially important in decreasing the risk of transmission to sexual partners. Intravenous acyclovir is the treatment of choice for serious HSV infections such as herpes simplex encephalitis and neonatal HSV infections, serious VSV infections, and VSV infections in immunocompromised patients.

Oral administration of acyclovir is generally well tolerated, with headache and gastrointestinal distress occasionally reported. Toxic effects with intravenous administration include delirium, tremor, seizures, hypotension, and nephrotoxicity.

Table 28–1.	**Clinical uses of antiviral drugs**	
Virus	**Drug(s) of Choice**	**Alternative or Adjunctive Drugs**
CMV	Ganciclover	Cidofovir, foscarnet, fomivirsen
HSV, VZV	Acyclovir or similar[1]	Cidofovir, foscarnet, vidarabine
HBV	IFN-α or lamivudine	Adefovir
HCV	IFN-α	Ribavirin
Influenza A	Amantadine or oseltamivir	Rimantidine
Influenza B	Oseltamivir	Zanamivir

CMV = cytomegalovirus; HSV = herpes simplex virus; VZV = varicella-zoster virus; HBV = hepatitis B virus; HCV = hepatitis C virus; IFN-α = interferon-α.

[1]Anti-HSV drugs similar to acyclovir include famciclovir, penciclovir, and valacyclovir.

Acyclovir Congeners

Several antiherpes drugs, such as **valacyclovir, famciclovir**, and **penciclovir,** are congeners—drugs that share similar chemical structures and characteristics— of acyclovir. Consequently, acyclovir congeners share many of acyclovir's clinical uses. After oral administration, valacyclovir is converted to acyclovir by the liver. Greater plasma levels can be achieved with valacyclovir than with acyclovir; thus, the duration of action is longer. Although valacyclovir is as effective as acyclovir in the cutaneous healing rate for herpes zoster (shingles), valacyclovir has been shown to be associated with a shorter duration of zoster-associated pain. Oral famciclovir is converted to penciclovir by the liver. It is well tolerated, and it is similar to acyclovir in its pharmacokinetic properties and clinical uses. Penciclovir is the active metabolite of famciclovir. Topical penciclovir is an effective treatment for recurrent genital herpes infection of the labia.

Ganciclovir

Mechanism of Action and Pharmacokinetics

Ganciclovir inhibits viral DNA polymerases of cytomegalovirus (CMV) and HSV. The first step in bioactivation of ganciclovir is a phosphorylation step catalyzed by virus-specific enzymes in both HSV-infected and CMV-infected cells. Ganciclovir is usually given intravenously and penetrates well into tissues, including the central nervous system (CNS) and the eye. It is also available as an intraocular implant. Valganciclovir, a prodrug of ganciclovir, has greater oral bioavailability than ganciclovir. Thus, valganciclovir has largely replaced oral ganciclovir because patients are required to take fewer pills per day.

Clinical Uses and Toxicity

Ganciclovir's activity against CMV is about 100 times greater than that of acyclovir. It is often used in immunocompromised patients for the treatment and prophylaxis of CMV infections, especially CMV retinitis, a vision-threatening infection of the eye. The most common systemic toxic effect of ganciclovir (and valganciclovir) is myelosuppression, a decrease in the ability of bone marrow to produce blood cells. Rare side effects include neurotoxicity (confusion, seizures) and nephrotoxicity.

Cidofovir

Mechanism of Action and Pharmacokinetics

Cidofovir is bioactivated exclusively by host cell enzymes. It inhibits the DNA polymerases of HSV, CMV, adenovirus, and human papillomavirus. Cidofovir is active against many acyclovir and ganciclovir-resistant strains because its bioactivation does not require viral kinases. To date, clinical resistance to cidofovir is rare. Cidofovir is generally administered topically or intravenously. It has a long intracellular half-life of 17 to 65 hours, permitting long intervals between doses.

Clinical Uses and Toxicity

Intravenous cidofovir is used to treat CMV retinitis and mucocutaneous HSV infections, including strains resistant to acyclovir. It is also effective in treating genital warts. Cidofovir is dose-dependently nephrotoxic. Patients receiving cidofovir will also receive a drug that blocks active tubular secretion (probenecid) to decrease its nephrotoxicity. Concurrent administration of other potentially nephrotoxic drugs (e.g., nonsteroidal anti-inflammatory drugs [NSAIDs]) should be avoided.

Foscarnet

Mechanism of Action and Pharmacokinetics

Foscarnet inhibits viral DNA polymerase, RNA polymerase, and HIV reverse transcriptase. It is only administered intravenously, and it penetrates well into tissues, including the CNS.

Clinical Uses and Toxicity

Foscarnet is an alternative drug for the prophylaxis and treatment of CMV infections, and it has activity against ganciclovir- and cidofovir-resistant strains. It is also effective against acyclovir-resistant HSV and VZV herpes strains, and may suppress resistant infections in AIDS patients. Toxic effects can be severe. These include nephrotoxicity, electrolyte imbalances (especially hypocalcemia), genitourinary ulcerations, and CNS effects (headache, hallucinations, seizures).

Idoxuridine, Trifluridine, and Vidarabine

Idoxuridine, trifluridine, and vidarabine are frequently used topically in the treatment of herpes keratitis, an eye infection that can be recurrent and may lead to blindness. Idoxuridine and trifluridine are too toxic for systemic use. Despite marked toxic potential, vidarabine has been used intravenously for severe HSV infections, especially those resistant to acyclovir. Toxic systemic effects include gastrointestinal irritation, hepatic dysfunction, and CNS toxicity (paresthesias, tremor, convulsions).

ANTI-HIV DRUGS

Human immunodeficiency virus (HIV) strikes the immune system, specifically targeting CD4 T lymphocytes. Depletion of CD4 cells ultimately leads to profound immunosuppression. Acquired immune deficiency syndrome (AIDS) is symptomatic disease, characterized by the development of a wide spectrum of opportunistic infections and malignancies either acquired or reactivated as a result of the immunosuppression caused by HIV. Worldwide, HIV/AIDS is a global health problem, affecting over 40 million people, with over 70% of infected individuals living in sub-Saharan Africa. In the United States, it is estimated that 1 million people are currently living with HIV/AIDS. While primary routes of infection in developed countries include male homosexual intercourse and intravenous drug use, primary routes of infection in developing countries include heterosexual contact and vertical transmission from mother to child.

To understand the drugs used in the treatment of HIV, the life cycle of HIV must be briefly examined (Figure 28–3). HIV is a retrovirus, meaning that it is an enveloped virus with a single-stranded RNA, not DNA, genome. Before HIV can enter CD4 cells, viral glycoproteins in the envelope bind to CD4 and chemokine receptors. Next, the virus fuses with the host cell membrane and uncoats as it enters the host cell. After uncoating, viral replication depends on the viral **reverse transcriptase** enzyme, which transcribes the viral genome from RNA into DNA. This newly formed double-stranded DNA is integrated into the human host's genome by an integrase enzyme. Integrated viral DNA is then transcribed by a host polymerase enzyme into messenger RNA, which is translated into proteins that assemble into immature noninfectious virions that bud from the host cell membrane. Proteolytic cleavage allows maturation into fully infectious virions.

As we mark the completion of the first 25 years of the HIV/AIDS epidemic, there is no cure for HIV infection or AIDS. However, pharmacologic therapy can dramatically improve the length and quality of life for infected individuals, and can delay the onset of AIDS. Without pharmacologic treatment, most patients die within a few years after the onset of symptoms. Currently, the standard of care in treating HIV infection involves initiating highly active antiretroviral therapy (HAART) that requires three to four antiretroviral drugs. If possible, HAART is initiated before symptoms appear. The goal of combination regimens is to inhibit or stop viral replication at a number of different steps (Figure 28–3). Compared with the administration of a single antiretroviral agent, combination therapy increases the efficacy of drug therapy, decreases the risk of developing drug resistance, and reduces viral load. Six classes of antiretroviral agents are currently available: nucleoside reverse transcriptase inhibitors (NRTIs), nonnucleoside reverse transcriptase inhibitors (NNRTIs), protease inhibitors (PIs), a fusion inhibitor, an integrase inhibitor, and an entry receptor blocker (Table 28–2).

Drug combinations are tailored to each patient depending on many variables, including potency and susceptibility, patient tolerance, convenience, and adherence to drug regimen. With the exception of the fusion inhibitor, the anti-HIV agents are all available as oral formulations. Drug management of HIV/AIDS is subject to change as newer agents become available. New pharmacotherapies are being sought that offer the advantages of once-daily dosing, smaller pill size, lower incidence of adverse effects, new viral targets, and activity against virus that is resistant to other agents.

Nucleoside Reverse Transcriptase Inhibitors

The NRTIs were the first group of drugs used to treat HIV infection. NRTIs selectively inhibit the HIV viral

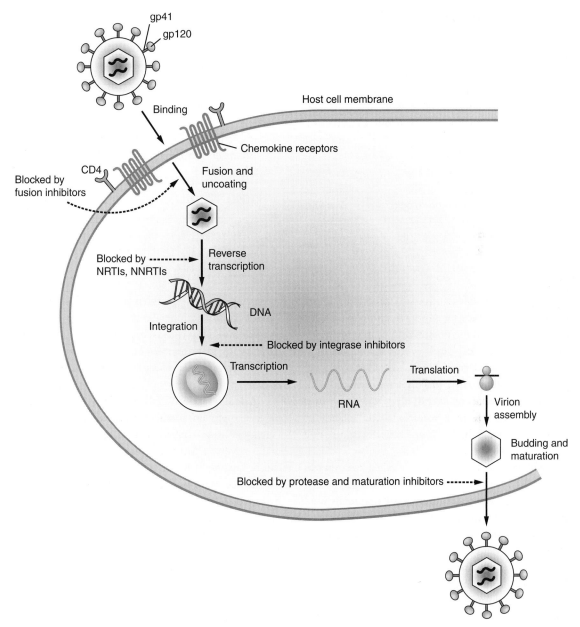

Figure 28–3. Life cycle of HIV and the major target sites of antiretroviral agents.

reverse transcriptase (Figure 28–3). The reverse transcriptase incorporates the phosphorylated NRTI (instead of a natural nucleotide) into the growing DNA chain, thus preventing complete conversion of viral RNA into DNA. If used as single agents to treat HIV, resistance emerges rapidly. However, resistance is rare in combination regimens. The NRTIs include **zidovudine, didanosine, zalcitabine, lamivudine, stavudine,** and **abacavir**. Details about each of these drugs follow.

Table 28–2.	Antiretroviral drugs	
Subclass	**Prototype**	**Other Significant Agents**
Nucleoside reverse transcriptase inhibitors	Zidovudine	Abacavir, didanosine, lamivudine, stavudine, zalcitabine, tenofovir[1]
Nonnucleoside reverse transcriptase inhibitors	Delavirdine	Efavirenz, nevirapine
Protease inhibitors	Indinavir	Amprenavir, lopinavir, nelfinavir, ritonavir, saquinavir
Fusion inhibitor	Enfuvirtide	
Integrase inhibitor	Raltegravir	
Entry receptor blocker	Maraviroc	

[1]Tenofovir is a nucleotide reverse transcriptase inhibitor.

Severe toxic effects are associated with most NRTIs, with the exception of lamivudine (3TC). All of the NRTIs have the potential to cause a rare, but serious, lactic acidosis and severe hepatic steatosis, likely due to mitochondrial damage in liver cells. Risk factors include obesity, prolonged treatment with NRTIs, and preexisting liver dysfunction. Symptoms include severe nausea, vomiting, and persistent abdominal pain. NRTI administration will often be suspended in these cases.

Zidovudine (ZDV), formerly called azidothymidine, or AZT, was the first antiretroviral drug approved for HIV treatment. Zidovudine is still frequently used in combination drug regimens. It is also used in prophylaxis against HIV infection through accidental needle sticks and via vertical transmission from mother to fetus. Zidovudine is active orally and is distributed to most tissues, including the CNS. The primary adverse effect is myelosuppression, which may be severe enough to require transfusions. Gastrointestinal distress, headaches, myalgia, agitation, and insomnia may also occur, but tend to decrease or resolve during therapy.

Didanosine (ddI) should be taken on an empty stomach to maximize bioavailability. The major clinical toxicity of didanosine (and to a lesser extent zalcitabine and stavudine) is dose-dependent pancreatitis. This occurs more frequently in alcoholic patients and those with hypertriglyceridemia. Other adverse effects include painful peripheral distal neuropathy, diarrhea, and CNS toxicity (headache, irritability, insomnia). Patients on didanosine also must have frequent retinal examinations because of reports of retinal changes and optic neuritis.

Zalcitabine (ddC) has relatively high oral bioavailability, but plasma levels decrease significantly when the drug is taken with food or antacids. The major adverse effect is peripheral neuropathy, which can be treatment limiting in 10 to 20% of patients. The neuropathy appears to be slowly reversible if treatment is discontinued promptly. Other major toxicities include oral and esophageal ulcerations and pancreatitis. Headache, arthralgias, myalgias, nausea, and rash may occur, but tend to resolve during therapy.

Unlike didanosine and zalcitabine, the bioavailability of **lamivudine** (3TC) is high and not food-dependent. It is commonly used as a component in HAART, as well as in the treatment of hepatitis B infections (see discussion below). Lamivudine is one of the best-tolerated NRTIs. Potential adverse effects are generally mild and include headache, fatigue, and gastrointestinal discomfort.

Stavudine (d4T) also has good oral bioavailability that is not food dependent. The major adverse effect of stavudine is dose-related peripheral sensory neuropathy. The incidence of these symptoms increases with coadministration of other neuropathy-inducing NRTIs such as didanosine and zalcitabine. Symptoms usually resolve completely if stavudine is discontinued. Other potential adverse effects include pancreatitis and arthralgias. As discussed above, all NRTIs have the potential to cause lactic acidosis with hepatic steatosis. However, these toxicities tend to occur more frequently in patients receiving stavudine than in those receiving other NRTIs.

Abacavir has good oral bioavailability that is unaffected by food. In a small percentage of patients taking abacavir, potentially fatal hypersensitivity reactions can occur. Symptoms usually occur in the first 6 weeks of therapy and include fever, malaise, vomiting, diarrhea, and anorexia.

Tenofovir (a nucleotide) inhibits the HIV reverse transcriptase and becomes incorporated into the DNA, causing chain termination. Its bioavailability increases after ingestion of a high-fat meal, so patients are advised to ingest tenofovir with a meal. Gastrointestinal irritation is the most common adverse effect, but this rarely requires discontinuation of therapy.

Nonnucleoside Reverse Transcriptase Inhibitors

The NNRTIs interrupt transcription of viral RNA into DNA by a different mechanism than the NRTIs. The NNRTIs bind directly to the viral reverse transcriptase (Figure 28–3), change the shape of the enzyme, and inhibit DNA synthesis. Thus, unlike the NRTIs, which become incorporated into the viral DNA, NNRTI agents inactivate the reverse transcriptase to prevent DNA formation. Like the NRTIs, resistance can occur rapidly if these drugs are used as monotherapy. As a class, adverse effects associated with NNRTI administration include varying levels of gastrointestinal distress and skin rashes. NNRTI agents are metabolized by the cytochrome P450 (CYP450) system, which increases the likelihood of drug-drug adverse interactions. Drugs in the NNRTI class include **nevirapine, delavirdine,** and **efavirenz.**

Oral bioavailability of nevirapine is good, and is not affected by food intake. Nevirapine is typically used as a component in HAART. It is also used prophylactically as a single dose to HIV-infected mothers at the onset of labor and to the neonate. Nevirapine can cause severe hypersensitivity reactions such as Stevens-Johnson syndrome and a life-threatening toxic epidermal necrolysis.

Delavirdine's oral bioavailability is good, but it is reduced by antacids. Delavirdine causes rash in about 20% of patients, although the rash is not life-threatening. Other adverse effects include headache, nausea, fatigue, and diarrhea. Because it has been shown to cause birth defects in animals, women should take precautions against pregnancy while taking delavirdine.

Efavirenz is generally used in combination with two NRTIs. The bioavailability of efavirenz increases after a high-fat meal. Adverse effects include CNS dysfunction (dizziness, drowsiness, headache, confusion, agitation, delusions, nightmares), skin rash, and increases in plasma cholesterol. Dosing at bedtime may be helpful for decreasing perception of some of the CNS effects. Pregnancy should also be avoided in women taking efavirenz because of fetal abnormalities observed in animals.

Protease Inhibitors

Assembly of infectious HIV virions depends on HIV-1 protease (Figure 28–3). Protease inhibitors (PIs) result in production of immature, noninfectious virions. As a class, the PIs in HAART drug combinations lead to the development of carbohydrate and lipid metabolic dysregulation. This syndrome includes hyperglycemia, insulin resistance, and hyperlipidemia. A lipodystrophy, or selective redistribution of fat, also occurs. Thus, patients may acquire a cushingoid appearance: buffalo hump, gynecomastia, abdominal obesity, and peripheral wasting. Incidence of the syndrome is about 30 to 50% of those patients on a HAART regimen containing PIs, with a median onset time of about 1 year after onset of treatment. Owing to these side effects, AIDS patients receiving PIs within a HAART regimen often receive counseling about heart disease as a new complication. Like the NNRTI agents, PIs are metabolized by the CYP450 system, increasing the likelihood of drug-drug adverse interactions. Six PIs are available for HIV treatment, and these are used in combinations with NRTIs and NNRTIs.

Indinavir must be taken on an empty stomach for maximal absorption. To avoid renal damage (nephrolithiasis), patients should consume at least 48 oz of water daily. Other adverse effects include nausea, diarrhea, and thrombocytopenia.

Bioavailability of **ritonavir** increases when given with food. The most common adverse effects are gastrointestinal disturbances, paresthesias (peripheral and circumoral), altered (bitter) taste, and hypertriglyceridemia. During the first weeks of therapy, nausea, vomiting, and abdominal pain usually occur and patients should be warned to expect these symptoms.

Saquinavir should be taken with food to improve its bioavailability and to decrease gastrointestinal distress. Other adverse effects include rhinitis, headache, and neutropenia.

Nelfinavir has higher absorption when taken with food. Its primary adverse effect is dose-limiting diarrhea, although this symptom often responds to antidiarrheal medications.

Amprenavir is rapidly absorbed from the gastrointestinal tract, and it can be taken with or without food; however, high-fat meals may decrease absorption and should be avoided. Common side effects are gastrointestinal distress, perioral paresthesias, depression, and rash. In a small percentage of cases, amprenavir has caused life-threatening rashes, including Stevens-Johnson syndrome, severe enough for the drug to be discontinued.

Lopinavir is often administered with ritonavir because of enhanced efficacy and improved tolerability. Absorption is enhanced with food. Adverse effects include nausea, vomiting, diarrhea, pancreatitis, and asthenia (decrease in strength).

Fusion Inhibitor

Enfuvirtide represents a new class of antiretroviral agents. The drug binds to a portion of the viral envelope and prevents conformational changes required for fusion of the viral and human cellular membranes (Figure 28–3). Unlike other anti-HIV drugs, enfuvirtide is not available in oral formulations. It is administered subcutaneously in combination with other antiretrovirals in treatment-experienced patients with persistent HIV-1 replication despite current therapy. Injection site reactions and hypersensitivity may occur.

Integrase Inhibitor

Raltegravir is an inhibitor of viral integrase, the enzyme required for integration of the viral DNA with that of the host. Block of this step (Figure 28–3) prevents replication of the viral genome. The drug is active by the oral route and is not affected by food. The drug is well tolerated but headache and gastrointestinal disturbances have been reported.

HIV Entry Receptor Blocker

Maraviroc combines with a chemokine receptor on lymphocytes and prevents the binding of HIV to cell-surface receptors, a step required for entry into host cells (Figure 28–3). It is orally active and always used with other anti-HIV drugs. Toxicity includes hypersensitivity reactions and hepatotoxicity.

ANTI-INFLUENZA DRUGS

There are three types of influenza viruses: A, B, and C. Influenza A and B produce similar clinical infections, manifested by fever, chills, malaise, myalgia, headache, nasal congestion, nonproductive cough, and sore throat. Influenza C is usually a minor illness. Influenza A and B infections are typically self-limiting, and most patients recover within 7 days. Anti-influenza agents can decrease the duration and severity of fever and systemic symptoms. They can also be used for prophylaxis of clinical infection. Complications of influenza, including pneumonia, occur more frequently in older adults, residents of long-term health-care facilities, and individuals with chronic illnesses such as diabetes mellitus and pulmonary or cardiovascular diseases. Available vaccines for the most current influenza A and B viral strains are recommended before the beginning of influenza season (typically fall or winter) for susceptible individuals as well as health-care workers.

Amantadine and Rimantadine

Amantadine and rimantadine inhibit an early replication step of the influenza A virus (not influenza B). These agents prevent viral uncoating within infected host cells (Figure 28–1). Both drugs are about 70 to

90% effective in preventing clinical illness. If treatment begins about 1 to 2 days after the onset of clinical flu symptoms, both drugs reduce the duration of fever and systemic complaints by 1 to 2 days. Rapid development of resistance occurs in up to 50% of treated individuals, and transmission of resistant virus to household members has been documented. Although the mechanism of action is not clearly defined, amantadine is also used to alleviate motor abnormalities in Parkinson's disease (Chapter 17). The most common adverse effects include gastrointestinal irritation, dizziness, ataxia, and slurred speech.

Oseltamivir and Zanamivir

These drugs inhibit neuraminidases produced by influenza A and B. By cleaving attachments between viral proteins and surface proteins of infected cells, viral neuraminidases promote virion release and prevent clumping of newly released virions. Thus, neuraminidase inhibitors hinder viral spread. Both drugs are approved for the treatment of acute uncomplicated influenza infection. Unlike amantadine and rimantidine, oseltamivir and zanamivir are active against both influenza A and influenza B. When a 5-day drug course is initiated within 36 to 48 hours after the onset of symptoms, use of either drug shortens the severity and duration of illness, and may also decrease the incidence of respiratory complications in children and adults. Oseltamivir is used orally, and zanamivir is used intranasally or by oral inhalation using the Diskhaler device provided. Taken prophylactically, oseltamivir significantly decreases the incidence of influenza. Gastrointestinal symptoms may occur with oseltamivir, which may be decreased by administration with food. Zanamivir may induce bronchospasm in asthmatic patients.

■ ANTIHEPATITIS DRUGS

Each of the recognized hepatitis viruses (A to E) belongs to a distinct virus family, but all of them have a long incubation period between initial infection and onset of symptoms. Hepatitis can easily be spread before symptoms appear, and many cases are likely unreported because initial symptoms may be mild.

Both HBV and HCV are bloodborne viral infections. Sharing of intravenous drug use equipment and sexual contact with an infected person are the most frequent sources of HBV transmission, whereas intravenous drug use is the primary means of HCV transmission. Treatment of these infections is critical because there are millions of chronic carriers of HBV and HCV. Untreated carriers are not only infectious to others, but they can also develop long-term complications such as chronic hepatitis, cirrhosis of the liver, and hepatocellular carcinoma.

All currently available agents for use in the treatment of HBV and HCV are suppressive rather than curative. In general, antihepatitis drugs are more effective at hindering disease progression in HBV infection than in HCV infection. Compliance with drug treatment is also problematic. Adverse effects may be intolerable, and dosing regimens are often rigorous, requiring injections once daily or three times weekly for several months in the case of interferons. Drugs used for treatment of viral hepatitis fall into two broad categories: **immune modulators** (interferons) and **replication inhibitors** (lamivudine, adefovir, ribavirin) (Table 28–1). Given the morbidity and mortality associated with these infections, improved chemotherapies are critically needed. Although a vaccine is available for HBV, none is yet available for HCV.

Interferon-α and Pegylated Interferon-α

Mechanism of Action and Pharmacokinetics
Interferons are endogenous cytokines that are part of the body's innate immune defenses. These proteins act through host cell surface receptors to increase the formation of antiviral proteins. Interferons are classified according to the cell type from which they were derived. Each of the three distinct major classes of human interferons (α, β, γ) has unique physicochemical properties, biologic effects, and producer cells. The antiviral action of interferon-α (IFN-α) is primarily due to activation of a host cell ribonuclease that degrades viral RNA. In addition, IFN-α promotes formation of natural killer cells that destroy virally infected liver cells.

There are several preparations of IFN-α available for treatment of both HBV and HCV. The interferons are available as subcutaneous or intramuscular injections, which are given either daily or three times per week. The attachment of polyethylene glycol to IFN-α (termed pegylated IFN-α) extends its duration of action, allowing for less frequent dosing.

Clinical Uses and Toxicity

IFN-α is used in the treatment of chronic HBV as a monotherapy or in combination with lamivudine. IFN-α used with ribavirin for acute HCV infection reduces progression to chronic HCV. For chronic HCV, pegylated IFN-α with ribavirin is superior to nonpegylated IFN-α as monotherapy. IFN-α is also used in the treatment of Kaposi sarcoma, papillomatosis, and topically for genital warts. Interferons also prevent dissemination of herpes zoster in cancer patients. Typical adverse effects of IFN-α include a flu-like syndrome within 6 hours after dosing in about 30% of patients, which tends to resolve with continued administration. Gastrointestinal symptoms, profound fatigue, neutropenia, myalgia, rash, and hypotension can also occur. Severe neuropsychiatric symptoms (severe depression, mental confusion) have been reported.

Adefovir

Mechanism of Action, Pharmacokinetics, and Clinical Use

Although initially developed for treatment of HIV, adefovir is currently approved for treatment of HBV. Similar to tenofovir (see section on anti-HIV drugs), adefovir is a nucleotide analog. It competitively inhibits HBV DNA polymerase, causing chain termination after incorporation into viral DNA. It suppresses HBV replication and improves liver histology and fibrosis at 1 year. However, after cessation of therapy, HBV DNA reappears. Oral bioavailability is good, and it is unaffected by meals.

Toxicity

The primary toxicity is dose-dependent nephrotoxicity, which is more likely in patients with renal dysfunction and those receiving the drug for more than 1 year. As with the NRTIs, adefovir may cause lactic acidosis and hepatomegaly.

Lamivudine

Lamivudine is a NRTI agent used in treatment of HIV (see discussion above). At lower doses than those used for HIV, lamivudine is used for treatment of chronic HBV infection. Although lamivudine's use as a monotherapy rapidly suppresses HBV replication and is relatively nontoxic, resistance emerges rapidly. If patients still have detectable levels of HBV DNA, they are often switched to IFN-α or adefovir.

Ribavirin

Mechanism of Action and Pharmacokinetics

Ribavirin inhibits the replication of many DNA and RNA viruses, including influenza A and B, parainfluenza, HCV, and HIV. The precise mechanism of action is not known, but it inhibits the formation of viral DNA, prevents capping of viral mRNA, and blocks RNA-dependent RNA polymerases of some viruses. Ribavirin is available orally, intravenously, and as an aerosol. Oral bioavailability increases with high-fat meals and decreases with antacid consumption.

Clinical Uses and Toxicity

Ribavirin is used with IFN-α to treat patients with chronic HCV infection with liver disease. Monotherapy with ribavirin alone is not effective. In viral hemorrhagic fevers, early intravenous ribavirin decreases mortality. Ribavirin is also used in the treatment of respiratory syncitial virus (RSV) in children. Systemic use may cause a dose-dependent hemolytic anemia. Aerosolic formulations may cause conjunctival and bronchial irritation. Ribavirin is absolutely contraindicated in pregnancy because it is a human teratogen.

■ VACCINES AND IMMUNE GLOBULINS: ACTIVE AND PASSIVE IMMUNIZATIONS

Vaccines consist of whole virions or virus fragments that are completely inactivated (dead) or partially inactivated (live attenuated). Active immunization consists of inoculation with a vaccine that triggers the host immune system to produce antibodies and cell-mediated immunity against this antigen. Thus, active immunization provides immunity to subsequent exposure to that particular virus. The ideal vaccine prevents the viral disease, prevents the virus carrier state, and produces long-lasting immunity with a minimum number of immunizations, absence of toxicity, and convenience for mass immunizations (e.g., inexpensive and easy to administer). Live attenuated products stimulate natural resistance and impart longer lasting immunity than dead antigens. However, the risk of contracting the viral disease is greater than with completely inactivated antigens. Examples of live attenuated vaccines include those for measles, mumps, and rubella (MMR), poliovirus (the oral vaccine), and varicella. Vaccines containing dead viral antigens include those for rabies, both hepatitis A and B viruses, and poliovirus (the parenteral vaccine). Currently, vaccines are available for many viral infections. Whereas some vaccinations are required by law (e.g., measles, poliomyelitis), others are only administered to high-risk populations (e.g., influenza). Selected examples of commonly used material for active immunization in the United States are given in Table 28–3.

Unlike active immunization, which requires time to develop because the individual's immune system must produce its own antibodies, **passive immunization** allows an individual to gain immediate immunity because it consists of the transfer of preformed **immunoglobulins** to an individual. Since the recipient does not produce his/her own antibodies, passive immunization is temporary. Passive immunization products generally contain high titers of antibodies either directed against a specific antigen, or may simply contain antibodies found in most of the population. Passive immunization is used for (1) individuals who are unable to form antibodies (e.g., congenital agammaglobulinemia); (2) prevention of disease when time does not permit active immunization (e.g., post-exposure); (3) treatment of certain diseases normally prevented by immunization (e.g., tetanus); and (4) treatment of conditions for which active immunization is unavailable or impractical (e.g., snakebite). Antibodies can be derived from animal or human sources. Immunizations derived from human antibodies have the advantages of avoiding the risk of

hypersensitivity reactions and having a longer half-life than those from animal sources. Selected materials for passive immunization are presented in Table 28–4.

■ REHABILITATION FOCUS

Although many antiviral agents limit the extent of systemic damage, especially when initiated early in the course of viral infection, very few completely cure viral infections. Patients taking antiviral agents face particular challenges in adhering to complicated drug regimens. HAART regimens generally require HIV/AIDS patients to take more than a dozen pills per day–some on an empty stomach, some with meals, and others with large quantities of water. Antihepatitis interferon compounds require injections one to three times per week, often for extended periods of time. In addition, the adverse effects of systemic antiviral agents may cause patients to abandon a complete course of treatment.

Physical therapists can assist patients' compliance with drug regimens. Therapists can arrange drugs in a single readily accessible location, teach patients to use a timer to signal dosing times, develop a color-coded system with pill boxes to remind patients which drugs need to be taken separately from or with food, and remind and educate patients about the importance of adherence to the antiviral regimen.

In arranging therapy sessions, therapists must be sensitive to the profound impact that antiviral drugs have on patients' ability to participate. Nausea, vomiting, diarrhea, or malaise may delay treatment sessions. In an inpatient setting, frequent brief sessions may be more effective and tolerable than a single longer session. Pain due to peripheral neuropathies or myalgia may alter a treatment plan toward pain alleviation, in which therapists can assist by adjunctive use of heat modalities and transcutaneous electrical nerve stimulation (TENS). Flexibly managing therapy sessions around patients' best time optimizes their ability to reach rehabilitation goals.

Because HIV directly targets the immune system, AIDS patients are among the most immunocompromised individuals. In addition to HAART, AIDS patients are often taking prophylactic medications to

Table 28–3. Materials commonly used for active immunization in the United States[1]

Vaccine	Type of Agent	Route of Administration	Indications
Diphtheria-tetanus-acellular pertussis (DTaP)	Toxoids and inactivated bacterial components	Intramuscular	1. For all children 2. Booster every 10 years in adolescents and adults
Haemophilus influenzae type b conjugate (Hib)	Bacterial polysaccharide conjugated to protein	Intramuscular	1. For all children 2. Asplenia and other at-risk conditions
Hepatitis A	Inactivated virus	Intramuscular	1. Travelers to hepatitis A endemic areas 2. Homosexual and bisexual men 3. Illicit drug users 4. Chronic liver disease or clotting factor disorders 5. Persons with occupational risk for infection 6. Persons living in, or relocating to, endemic areas 7. Household and sexual contacts of individuals with acute hepatitis A
Hepatitis B	Inactive viral antigen, recombinant	Intramuscular (subcutaneous injection is acceptable in individuals with bleeding disorders)	1. For all infants 2. Preadolescents, adolescents, and young adults 3. Persons with occupational, lifestyle, or environmental risk 4. Hemophiliacs 5. Hemodialysis patients 6. Postexposure prophylaxis
Influenza, inactivated	Inactivated virus or viral components	Intramuscular	1. Adults ≥50 years of age 2. Persons with high risk conditions (e.g., asthma) 3. Health care workers and others in contact with high-risk groups 4. Residents of nursing homes and other residential chronic care facilities 5. All children aged 6–23 months
Influenza, live attenuated	Live virus	Intranasal	Healthy persons aged 5–49 years who desire protection against influenza

(continued)

Table 28–3. **Materials commonly used for active immunization in the United States[1] (*Continued*)**

Vaccine	Type of Agent	Route of Administration	Indications
Measles	Live virus	Subcutaneous	1. Adults and adolescents born after 1956 without a history of measles or live virus vaccination on or after their first birthday 2. Postexposure prophylaxis in unimmunized persons
Measles-mumps-rubella (MMR)	Live virus	Subcutaneous	For all children
Meningococcal conjugate vaccine	Bacterial polysaccharides conjugated to diphtheria toxoid	Intramuscular	1. All adolescents 2. Preferred over polysaccharide vaccine in persons aged 11–55 years
Meningococcal polysaccharide vaccine	Bacterial polysaccharides of serotypes A/C/Y/W-135	Subcutaneous	1. Military recruits 2. Travelers to areas with epidemic meningococcal disease 3. Individuals with asplenia, complement deficiency, or properdin deficiency 4. Control of outbreaks in closed or semi-closed populations 5. College freshmen who live in dormitories 6. Microbiologists who are routinely exposed to isolates of *Neisseria meningitidis*
Mumps	Live virus	Subcutaneous	Adults born after 1956 without history of mumps or live virus vaccination on or after their first birthday
Pneumococcal conjugate vaccine	Bacterial polysaccharides conjugated to protein	Intramuscular or subcutaneous	
Pneumococcal polysaccharide vaccine	Bacterial polysaccharides of 23 serotypes	Intramuscular or subcutaneous	1. Adults ≥65 years of age 2. Persons at increased risk for pneumococcal disease or its complications
Poliovirus vaccine, inactivated (IPV)	Inactivated viruses of all three serotypes	Subcutaneous	1. For all children 2. Previously unvaccinated adults at increased risk for occupational or travel exposure to polioviruses

(*continued*)

Table 28–3. Materials commonly used for active immunization in the United States[1] (*Continued*)

Vaccine	Type of Agent	Route of Administration	Indications
Rabies	Inactivated virus	Intramuscular (IM) or intradermal (ID)	1. **Preexposure** prophylaxis in persons at risk for contact with rabies virus 2. **Postexposure** prophylaxis (administer with rabies immune globulin)
Rubella	Live virus	Subcutaneous	Adults born after 1956 without history of rubella or live virus vaccination on or after their first birthday
Tetanus-diphtheria (Td or DT)[2]	Toxoids	Intramuscular	1. All adults who have not been immunized as children 2. Postexposure prophylaxis if >5 years has passed since last dose
Typhoid, Ty21a oral	Live bacteria	Oral	Risk of exposure to typhoid fever
Varicella	Live virus	Subcutaneous	1. For all children 2. Persons past their 13th birthday without history of varicella infection 3. Postexposure prophylaxis in susceptible persons
Yellow Fever	Live virus	Subcutaneous	1. Laboratory personnel who may be exposed to yellow fever virus 2. Travelers to areas where yellow fever occurs

[1]Dosage for the specific product, including variations for age, are best obtained from the manufacturer's package insert.
[2]Td = Tetanus and diphtheria toxoids for use in persons ≥7 years of age (contains less diphtheria toxoid than DPT and DT). DT = Tetanus and diphtheria toxoids for use in persons <7 years of age (contains the same amount of diphtheria toxoid as DPT).

prevent opportunistic infections from other viruses, bacteria, fungi, and miscellaneous pathogens. Therapists should be alert to new signs and symptoms of acute infections, and report these to the primary health-care provider immediately to facilitate aggressive treatment in early infectious stages. Physical therapists must vigilantly practice standard precautions when working with HIV/AIDS patients. This also includes staying home or avoiding patient care when illness strikes the therapist to prevent pathogen transmission.

■ CLINICAL RELEVANCE FOR REHABILITATION

Adverse Drug Reactions

Antiherpes drugs
- Ganciclovir may cause myelosuppression.
- Cidofovir and foscarnet can cause nephrotoxicity.
- Foscarnet (and less commonly, ganciclovir) can cause CNS toxicity including headache, hallucinations, and seizures.

Table 28–4.   Selected passive immunizations[1]

Indication	Product	Dosage	Comments
Bone marrow transplantation	Immune globulin (intravenous)[2]	500 mg/kg IV on days 7 and 2 prior to transplantation and then once weekly through day 90 after transplantation.	Prophylaxis to decrease the risk of infection, interstitial pneumonia, and acute graft-versus-host disease in adults undergoing bone marrow transplantation.
Chronic lymphocytic leukemia (CLL)	Immune globulin (intravenous)[2]	400 mg/kg IV every 3–4 weeks. Dosage should be adjusted upward if bacterial infections occur.	CLL patients with hypogammaglobulinemia and a history of at least one serious bacterial infection.
Cytomegalovirus (CMV)	Cytomegalovirus immune globulin (intravenous)	Consult the manufacturer's dosing recommendations.	Prophylaxis of CMV infection in bone marrow, kidney, liver, lung, pancreas, heart transplant recipients.
HIV-infected children	Immune globulin (intravenous)[2]	400 mg/kg IV every 28 days.	HIV-infected children with recurrent serious bacterial infections or hypogammaglobulinemia.
Idiopathic thrombocytopenic purpura (ITP)	Immune globulin (intravenous)[2]	Consult the manufacturer's dosing recommendations for the specific product being used.	Response in children with ITP is greater than in adults. Corticosteroids are the treatment of choice in adults, except for severe pregnancy-associated ITP.
Primary immunodeficiency disorders	Immune globulin (intravenous)[2]	Consult the manufacturer's dosing recommendations for the specific product being used.	Primary immunodeficiency disorders include specific antibody deficiencies (e.g., X-linked agammaglobulinemia) and combined deficiencies (e.g., severe combined immunodeficiencies).

[1]Passive immunotherapy or immunoprophylaxis should always be administered as soon as possible after exposure. Prior to the administration of animal sera, patients should be questioned and tested for hypersensitivity.
[2]See the following references for an analysis of additional uses of intravenously administered immune globulin: Ratko TA, et al: Recommendations for off-label use of intravenously administered immunoglobulin preparations. *JAMA* 1995;273:1865; and Dalakas MC: Intravenous immune globulin therapy for neurologic diseases. *Ann Intern Med* 1997;126:721.

Anti-HIV drugs

- Many anti-HIV drugs cause gastrointestinal distress (nausea, vomiting, diarrhea, abdominal pain), malaise, fatigue, and CNS dysfunction (headache, agitation, dizziness, confusion).

- The NNRTIs and PIs are metabolized by the cytochrome P450 system, increasing likelihood of drug-drug interactions.
- Food decreases bioavailability of some NRTIs (didanosine, zalcitabine) and the PI indinavir.

- An empty stomach decreases bioavailability of some NNRTIs (efavirenz), and PIs (ritonavir, saquinavir, nelfinavir, lopinavir).
- Antacids decrease bioavailability of zalcitabine, delavirdine, and amprenavir.

NRTIs
- All NRTIs (especially stavudine) have the potential to cause serious lactic acidosis and severe hepatic steatosis.
  - Zidovudine can cause severe myelosuppression.
  - Didanosine, zalcitabine, and stavudine can cause dose-dependent pancreatitis.
  - Didanosine, zalcitabine, and stavudine can cause peripheral neuropathy.
  - Didanosine can produce retinal changes.

NNRTIs
- Most NNRTIs tend to produce a rash, which can be life-threatening with nevirapine.

PIs
- The PIs often cause carbohydrate and lipid metabolic dysregulation.
  - Indinavir can cause kidney damage.
  - Ritonavir and amprenavir can cause paresthesias.
  - Amprenavir can cause life-threatening rashes.
  - Lopinavir can cause asthenia (weakness).

Anti-influenza drugs
- Amantadine and oseltamivir can cause gastrointestinal upset.
- Amantadine can cause dizziness and ataxia.
- Zanamivir may induce bronchospasm in asthmatic patients.

Anti-hepatitis drugs
- IFN-α can cause flu-like symptoms within six hours after parenteral dosing.
- IFN-α can cause hypotension and severe neuropsychiatric symptoms.
- Aerosolic ribavirin can cause conjunctival and bronchial irritation.

Effects Interfering with Rehabilitation
- Myelosuppression (ganciclovir, zidovudine) can result in decreased resistance to nosocomial infections (due to leukopenia), increased fatigue and shortness of breath (due to anemia), and easy bruising or excessive bleeding from minor wounds (due to thrombocytopenia).
- Concurrent use of NSAIDs for musculoskeletal pain and inflammation should be avoided when patients are taking nephrotoxic drugs (e.g., cidofovir, foscarnet).
- Gastrointestinal and CNS effects can affect participation and functional performance of patients in rehabilitation programs.
- HIV/AIDS patients on HAART who take over-the-counter drugs or supplements risk decreased or increased blood drug levels, resulting in either undermedication or increased adverse effects associated with overmedication.
- Severe nausea, vomiting, abdominal pain, rapid respirations or shortness of breath in HIV/AIDS patients receiving NRTIs may indicate onset of lactic acidosis.
- HIV/AIDS patients receiving NRTIs who complain of constant pain in the upper abdomen with possible radiation to the back may be experiencing acute pancreatitis.
- Painful peripheral neuropathies (didanosine, zalcitabine, stavudine), paresthesias (ritonavir, amprenavir), dizziness and ataxia (amantadine), and asthenia (lopinavir) can affect mobility and gait, and limit participation in rehabilitation.
- Retinal changes (didanosine) can affect vision, balance, and mobility.
- Protease inhibitor-induced metabolic dysregulation increases patients' risk profile for cardiovascular disease.
- Patients taking zanamivir or ribavirin may have respiratory dysfunction.
- Participation in therapies may be limited within the first hours after IFN-α administration.

Possible Therapy Solutions
- If the patient has myelosuppression, physical therapists should practice excellent standard precautions to prevent infection transmission. Exercise intensity and duration should be reduced to account for decreased oxygen-carrying capacity of the blood. In addition, extreme caution should be taken to avoid inadvertent or sustained pressure on any area of the patient, due to decreased clotting ability.

- If patients taking nephrotoxic drugs experience musculoskeletal pain after exercise or therapies, drug alternatives such as heat or ice should be used instead of NSAIDs.
- Therapy should be timed to occur during periods when adverse effects are lowest. Therapists should discuss with the referring health-care provider or pharmacist whether certain drugs can be taken at night to decrease perception of some CNS effects and minimize their impact on patients' functional performance and ability to participate in therapy.
- Physical therapists can assist with reinforcing optimal drug dosing schedules for patients on HAART. For example, therapists can make pictures or tables in convenient locations, such as above the bedside or in the kitchen, to remind patients which pills should be taken on an empty stomach and which should be taken with meals. Didanosine, zalcitabine, and indinavir should be taken on an empty stomach. Efavirenz, tenofovir, ritonavir, saquinavir, nelfinavir, and lopinavir should be taken with meals. Antacids should not be taken with zalcitabine, delavirdine, and amprenavir.
- Because of the large potential for drug-drug interactions with HIV/AIDS patients on HAART, physical therapists should take a complete drug history and educate the patient regarding the potential for any drug, including herbal supplements and cold medicines, to interfere with drug metabolism. Therapists should strongly encourage the patient to discuss all current drug use with the referring health-care provider.
- Symptoms consistent with lactic acidosis or pancreatitis should be immediately reported to referring health-care provider, and therapy discontinued until symptoms resolve.
- Patient reports of vision changes, peripheral neuropathy, and paresthesias should be reported to referring health-care provider to determine if dose reduction alleviates symptoms.
- Any rash or progression or spread of a current rash should be immediately reported to the primary health-care provider because of the ability for many antiviral drugs to produce life-threatening rashes.
- Patients taking PIs should be monitored for signs of cardiovascular disease. If tolerated, exercise prescriptions should be modified to increase participation in aerobic exercise.
- Physical therapists should carefully monitor respiratory function during therapy with patients taking zanamivir or ribavirin, especially if patients have chronic obstructive pulmonary disease. Worsening of symptoms should be reported to the primary health-care provider. Short-acting bronchodilators should be immediately available in the case of bronchospasm.

PROBLEM-ORIENTED PATIENT STUDY

Brief History: The patient is a 44-year-old male who has been HIV positive for 10 years. On his most recent physician visit, it was noted that he was hyperglycemic and hyperlipidemic. In addition, although his weight has not changed in the past year, he notes that his legs appear thinner and his waist is definitely larger.

Current Medical Status and Drugs: The patient's HAART regimen includes two NRTIs, one NNRTI,

and a protease inhibitor. Since the patient's HIV infection has responded very well to this drug regimen, his physician is currently reluctant to switch to a protease inhibitor–sparing regimen. Instead, she has referred him to rehabilitation to assess the efficacy of a nonpharmacological approach to the hyperglycemia, hyperlipidemia, and lipodystrophy syndrome.

Rehabilitation Setting: The physical therapist prescribes an exercise program for the patient that includes

(continued)

PROBLEM-ORIENTED PATIENT STUDY (*Continued*)

aerobic and progressive resistance training. His exercise program includes 40 minutes of moderate aerobic activity and 20 minutes of resistance training three to four times per week. Larger muscle groups, especially the lower extremities, are targeted for strengthening. The therapist monitors his vital signs, and progresses exercises appropriately to his tolerance. The patient has been stringently following his exercise program for 4 months. He is quite pleased with the results, as he notes that his belt fits better now and he is noting more strength and mass in his legs. At his physician's reassessment, his metabolic profile has also improved significantly: decreased lipidemia, decreased fasting blood glucose, and decreased resting blood pressure.

Problem/Clinical Options: Without question, HAART has increased the lifespan and improved

the quality of life of individuals with HIV infection. As HIV/AIDS patients live longer, other morbidities have emerged, including cardiovascular disease. Protease inhibitors traditionally included in HAART regimens are often associated with development of dyslipidemia, insulin resistance, and lipodystrophy. Similar to the management of these conditions in HIV-uninfected individuals, exercise can be used to help prevent potential cardiovascular and metabolic complications in HIV-infected people. Recommendations include smoking cessation, reduction in dietary fat, and increasing exercise. Specifically, resistance and aerobic exercises have been shown to help HIV-infected individuals gain lean body mass, decrease truncal adiposity, and decrease total cholesterol and triglyceride concentrations.

PREPARATIONS AVAILABLE

Abacavir (Ziagen)
Oral: 300-mg tablets; 20 mg/mL solution
Oral (Trizir): 300-mg tablets in combination with 150 mg lamivudine and 300 mg zidovudine

Acyclovir (generic, Zovirax)
Oral: 200-mg capsules; 400-, 800-mg tablets; 200 mg/5 mL suspension
Parenteral: 50 mg/mL; powder to reconstitute for injection (500, 1000 mg/vial)
Topical: 5% ointment

Adefovir (Hepsera)
Oral: 10-mg tablets

Amantadine (generic, Symmetrel)
Oral: 100-mg capsules, tablets; 50 mg/5 mL syrup

Amprenavir (Agenerase)
Oral: 50-, 150-mg capsules; 15 mg/mL solution

Cidofovir (Vistide)
Parenteral: 375 mg/vial (75 mg/mL) for IV injection

Delavirdine (Rescriptor)
Oral: 100-, 200-mg tablets

Didanosine (dideoxyinosine, ddI)
Oral (Videx): 25-, 50-, 100-, 150-, 200-mg tablets; 100-, 167-, 250-mg powder for oral solution; 2-, 4-g powder for pediatric solution
Oral (Videx-EC): 125-, 200-, 250-, 400-mg delayed-release capsules

Efavirenz (Sustiva)
Oral: 50-, 100-, 200-mg capsules; 600-mg tablets

Enfuvirtide (Fuzeon)
Parenteral: 90 mg/mL for injection

Famciclovir (Famvir)
Oral: 125-, 250-, 500-mg tablets

Fomivirsen (Vitravene)
Intravitreal: 6.6 mg/mL for injection

Foscarnet (Foscavir)
Parenteral: 24 mg/mL for IV injection

Ganciclovir (Cytovene)
Oral: 250-, 500-mg capsules
Parenteral: 500 mg/vial for IV injection
Intraocular implant (Vitrasert): 4.5 mg ganciclovir/implant

Idoxuridine (Herplex)
Ophthalmic: 0.1% solution

Imiquimod (Aldera)
Topical: 5% cream

Indinavir (Crixivan)
Oral: 100-, 200-, 333-, 400-mg capsules

Interferon alfa-2a (Roferon-A)
Parenteral: 3-, 6-, 9-, 36-million IU vials

Interferon alfa-2b (Intron-A)
Parenteral: 3-, 5-, 10-, 18-, 25-, and 50-million IU vials

Interferon alfa-2b (Rebetron)
Parenteral: 3-million IU vials (supplied with oral ribavirin, 200-mg capsules)

Interferon alfa-n3 (Alferon N)
Parenteral: 5-million IU/vial

Interferon alfacon-1 (Infergen)
Parenteral: 9- and 15-mcg vials

Lamivudine (Epivir)
Oral (Epivir): 150-, 300-mg tablets; 10 mg/mL oral solution
Oral (Epivir-HBV): 100-mg tablets; 5 mg/mL solution
Oral (Combivir): 150-mg tablets in combination with 300 mg zidovudine
Oral (Trizir): 300-mg tablets in combination with 150 mg lamivudine and 300 mg zidovudine

Lopinavir/ritonavir (Kaletra)
Oral: 133.3 mg/33.3 mg capsules; 400 mg/100 mg per 5 mL solution

Maraviroc (Selzentry)
Oral: 150, 300 mg tablets

Nelfinavir (Viracept)
Oral: 250-mg tablets; 50 mg/g powder

Nevirapine (Viramune)
Oral: 200-mg tablets; 50 mg/5 mL suspension

Oseltamivir (Tamiflu)
Oral: 75-mg capsules; powder to reconstitute as suspension (12 mg/mL)

Peginterferon alfa-2a (pegylated interferon-alfa 2a, Pegasys)
Parenteral: 180 mcg/mL

Peginterferon alfa-2b (pegylated interferon-alfa 2b, PEG-Intron)
Parenteral: powder to reconstitute as 100, 160, 240, 300 mcg/mL injection

Penciclovir (Denavir)
Topical: 1% cream

Raltegravir (Isentress)
Oral: 400-mg tablets

Ribavirin
Aerosol (Virazole): powder to reconstitute for aerosol; 6 g/100 mL vial
Oral (Rebetol): 200-mg capsules
Oral (Rebetron): 200 mg in combination with 3-million units interferon alfa-2b (Intron-A)

Rimantadine (Flumadine)
Oral: 100-mg tablets; 50 mg/5 mL syrup

Ritonavir (Norvir)
Oral: 100-mg capsules; 80 mg/mL oral solution

Saquinavir
Oral (Invirase): 200-mg hard gel capsules
Oral (Fortovase): 200-mg soft gel capsules

Stavudine (Zerit)
Oral: 15-, 20-, 30-, 40-mg capsules; powder for 1 mg/mL oral solution

Tenofovir (Viread)
Oral: 300-mg tablets

Trifluridine (Viroptic)
Topical: 1% ophthalmic solution

Valacyclovir (Valtrex)
Oral: 500-, 1000-mg tablets

Valgancyclovir (Valcyte)
Oral: 450-mg capsules

Zalcitabine (dideoxycytidine, ddC) (Hivid)
Oral: 0.375-, 0.75-mg tablets

Zanamivir (Relenza)
Inhalational: 5 mg/rotadisk

Zidovudine (azidothymidine, AZT) (Retrovir)
Oral: 100-mg capsules, 300-mg tablets, 50 mg/5 mL syrup
Oral (Combivir): 300-mg tablets in combination with 150 mg lamivudine
Oral (Trizir): 300-mg tablets in combination with 150 mg lamivudine and 300 mg zidovudine
Parenteral: 10 mg/mL

REFERENCES

Baker DE: Pegylated interferons. *Rev Gastroenterol Disord* 2001;1:87.

Cocohoba JM, McNicholl IR: Valganciclovir: An advance in cytomegalovirus therapeutics. *Ann Pharmacother* 2001;36:2075.

Drugs for non-HIV viral infections. *Med Lett Drugs Ther* 2002;44:9.

Geary RS, et al: Fomivirsen: Clinical pharmacology and potential drug interactions. *Clin Pharmacokinet* 2002; 41:255.

Johnson MA, et al: Clinical pharmacokinetics of lamivudine. *Clin Pharmacokinet* 1999;36:41.

Kimberlin DW, et al: Safety and efficacy of high-dose intravenous acyclovir in the management of neonatal herpes simplex virus infections. *Pediatrics* 2001;108:230.

Lauer GM, Walker BD: Hepatitis C infection. *N Engl J Med* 2001;345:41.

Malik AH, Lee WM: Chronic hepatitis B virus infection: Treatment strategies for the next millenium. *Ann Intern Med* 2000;132:723.

Martin DF, et al: A controlled trial of valganciclovir as induction therapy for cytomegalovirus retinitis. *N Engl J Med* 2002;346:1119.

Piscitelli SC, Gallicano KD: Interactions among drugs for HIV and opportunistic infections. *N Engl J Med* 2001;344:984

Qazi NA, et al: Lopinavir/ritonavir (ABT-378/r). *Expert Opin Pharmacother* 2002;3:315.

Recommendations for use of antiretroviral drugs in pregnant HIV-1–infected women for maternal health and interventions to reduce perinatal HIV-1 transmission in the United States. *Med Lett Drugs Ther* 2002; 51(RR-18):1.

Sexually Transmitted Diseases Treatment Guidelines—2002. *Med Lett Drugs Ther* 2002;51(RR-6):1.

Whitley RJ: Herpes simplex virus infection. *Semin Pediatr Infect Dis* 2002;13:6.

Yeni PG, et al: Antiretroviral treatment for adult HIV infection in 2002. Updated recommendations of the International AIDS Society—USA Panel. *JAMA* 2002; 288:222.

Relevant Websites

www.aidsinfo.nih.gov
www.cdc.gov
www.hivinsite.com

Rehabilitation

Fisher SD, et al: Impact of HIV and highly active antiretroviral therapy on leukocyte adhesion molecules, arterial inflammation, dyslipidemia, and atherosclerosis. *Atherosclerosis* 2006;185:1.

Goodman CC, Boissonnault WG, Fuller KS: *Pathology: Implications for the Physical Therapist,* 2nd ed. Philadelphia: Saunders, 2003.

Jones SP, et al: Short-term exercise training improves body composition and hyperlipidaemia in HIV-positive individuals with lipodystrophy. *AIDS* 2001;15:2049.

Roubenoff R, et al: Feasibility of increasing lean body mass in HIV-infected adults using progressive resistance training. *Med Sci Sports Exerc* 1998;30:S183.

Roubenoff R, et al: A pilot study of exercise training to reduce trunk fat in adults with HIV-associated fat redistribution. *AIDS* 1999;13:1373–5.

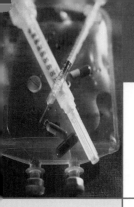

29

ANTIFUNGAL AND
ANTIPARASITIC AGENTS

In the most general scientific sense, a "*parasite*" includes all of the known infectious agents such as viruses, bacteria, fungi, protozoa (single-celled eukaryotes of the animal kingdom), and helminths (worms) that live in or on host tissue, generally at the expense of the host. Certain species of parasites cause human infections. Some infections, especially fungal, are common in both industrialized and underdeveloped nations and cause varying degrees of illness and debility. Diseases caused by protozoan and helminthic parasites are among the leading causes of disease and death in tropical and subtropical regions. Many of these infections are intensified by inadequate water sanitation and hygiene, and their management is hampered by difficulty in controlling the vector (e.g., mosquito, in the case of malaria). This chapter describes the most commonly used drugs to treat fungal, protozoan, and helminthic infections.

ANTIFUNGAL AGENTS

Most human mycoses—diseases caused by fungal infections—are minor or superficial. However, the incidence and severity of human fungal infections have increased dramatically over the last few decades. This shift reflects the enormous number of immunocompromised patients (secondary to HIV and immunosuppressive drugs) who are at increased risk for invasive fungal infections, as well as the widespread use of broad-spectrum antimicrobials, which eliminate competitive nonpathogenic bacteria. In addition, fungi (especially *Candida* species) may be introduced into tissues that are normally resistant to invasion by, for example, central intravascular devices or hemodialysis.

Fungal infections are difficult to treat for several reasons. First, selective toxicity against fungal cells (and not the human host's cells) is more difficult to achieve than for bacteria. Second, many antifungal agents suffer from problems with solubility, stability, and absorption. Third, fungi readily develop resistance.

For years, the mainstay of pharmacotherapy against systemic fungal infections has been the polyene class of drugs, especially amphotericin B. These drugs are toxic and azole agents (a different chemical class) have been developed as alternative antifungal drugs. However, owing to widespread use, azole-resistant organisms are becoming more widespread. Recently, the newest class of antifungals–the echinocandins–has demonstrated improved safety, efficacy, and tolerability.

Antifungals are generally classified on the basis of their target site of action. The major classes of antifungal agents—**azoles**, polyenes, **echinocandins**, and **terbinafine**–kill fungi by disrupting the synthesis or function of fungal cellular membranes. In contrast, the fungicidal

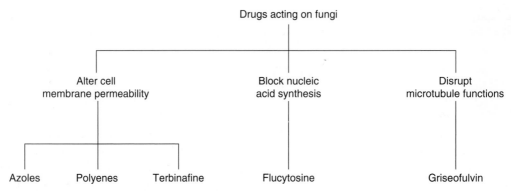

Figure 29–1. Fungal infections are difficult to treat, particularly in the immunocompromised patient. Most fungi are resistant to conventional antimicrobial agents, and only a few drugs are available for the treatment of systemic fungal diseases. Amphotericin B (a polyene) and the azoles are the primary drugs used in systemic infections. They are selectively toxic to fungi because they interact with or inhibit the synthesis of ergosterol, a sterol unique to fungal cell membranes. Echinocandins (not shown) interfere with cell wall function.

actions of the less important agents, **flucytosine** and **griseofulvin**, are due to interference with intracellular functions (Figure 29–1 and 29–2). Clinically, antifungal drugs fall into several categories: drugs (oral or parenteral) for systemic infections, oral drugs for mucocutaneous infections (mucous membranes and skin), and topical drugs for mucocutaneous infections (Table 29–1).

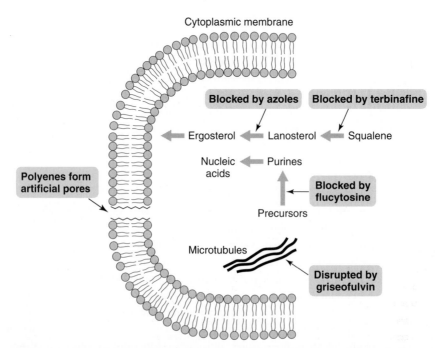

Figure 29–2. Sites of action of some antifungal drugs. The cell cytoplasmic membrane shown is that of a typical fungus. Because ergosterol is not a component of mammalian membranes, significant selective toxicity is achieved with the azole drugs. Echinocandins (not shown) cause disruption of the cell wall.

Table 29–1.	Some important antifungal drugs		
Class	**Drug**	**Indications**	**Toxicities**
Allylamines (topical)	Terbinafine, naftifine, butenafine hydrochloride	*Tinea cruris, tinea corporis*	
Allylamines (oral)	Terbinafine	Onychomycosis	Rash, gastrointestinal irritation, taste disturbances, rare cases of hepatic failure
Azoles	Fluconazole	Treatment and prophylaxis for cryptococcal meningitis	Gastrointestinal disturbances, rash, varying degree of hepatic damage, drug interactions, visual disturbances (voriconazole)
	Itraconazole	*Blastomyces* and *Sporothrix* infections, subcutaneous chromoblastomycosis	
	Voriconazole	Invasive aspergillosis, candidemia	
	Posaconazole	Prophylaxis of invasive aspergillosis, treatment of oropharyngeal candidiasis	
Azoles (topical)	Clotrimazole, miconazole, ketoconazole	*Tinea pedis, tinea cruris, tinea corporis,* vaginal yeast infections, oral candidal infections	
Echinocandin	Caspofungin, micafungin, anidulafungin	*Candida* infections, life-threatening fungal infections that are resistant to amphotericin and azoles	
Flucytosine		*Cryptococcus neoformans* and some *Candida* species	Bone marrow impairment (anemia, leukopenia, thrombocytopenia)
Griseofulvin		Dermatophytoses	Skin rash, hives, gastrointestinal irritation, photosensitivity, drug interactions
Polyenes (primarily parenteral)	Amphotericin B	Almost all life-threatening systemic fungal functions	1. Infusion-related: fever, chills, muscle spasms, hypotension 2. Slower: renal damage
Polyenes (topical)	Nystatin	Localized candidal infections in oropharynx, vagina, and areas where opposing skin rub together	

Drugs for Systemic Fungal Infections

Amphotericin B

CHEMISTRY AND PHARMACOKINETICS. Amphotericin B is a polyene agent and one of the most important drugs for the treatment of systemic mycoses. It is available in oral, topical, and parenteral forms. Because it is poorly absorbed, oral amphotericin B is only effective against fungi in the lumen of the gastrointestinal tract. Topical forms are used for oral or cutaneous candidiasis. Amphotericin B is generally administered intravenously as a nonlipid colloidal suspension, as a lipid complex, or in a liposomal formulation. Development of the latter form has reduced its nephrotoxicity by decreasing nonspecific binding to human cell membranes, permitting the use of larger doses. Amphotericin B is widely distributed to all tissues except the central nervous system (CNS). Therefore, treatment of CNS fungal infections may necessitate intrathecal administration. Amphotericin B is primarily eliminated by hepatic metabolism. Hepatic impairment, renal impairment, and dialysis have little effect on drug concentrations.

MECHANISM OF ACTION AND CLINICAL USES. Amphotericin B kills fungi by binding to ergosterol (a major sterol constituent unique to fungal cell membranes) and forming pores, which results in leakage of cellular contents and cell death (Figure 29–2). Some binding to human cellular membranes occurs, probably accounting for amphotericin B's serious toxicity.

Amphotericin B has the widest antifungal spectrum of any agent. It is considered the drug (or codrug) of choice for treating almost all life-threatening systemic infections caused by *Aspergillus, Blastomyces, Candida albicans, Cryptococcus, Histoplasma,* and *Mucor*. It is often used as the initial agent within a treatment regimen for serious fungal infections, and is then replaced by an azole for chronic treatment or relapse prevention. Amphotericin B is typically administered by slow intravenous infusion continued to a defined total dose rather than a defined time span. Doses vary depending on the particular infection, but it is not uncommon for patients to receive daily IV treatment for 6 to 12 weeks.

TOXICITY. Toxic side effects of amphotericin B are divided into two categories: immediate reactions related to drug infusion and reactions that occur more slowly. Infusion-related adverse effects of amphotericin B are extremely common. These include fever, chills, vomiting, muscle spasms, headache, and significant hypotension occurring during infusion of the drug. Slowing the infusion rate or decreasing the daily dose may reduce these effects. In addition, premedication with antipyretics, antiemetics, antihistamines, meperidine (an opioid analgesic), or glucocorticoids may be provided to partially overcome infusion-related effects.

The most significant slower toxicity associated with amphotericin B is renal damage. Nearly all patients experience some renal impairment, with reversible and irreversible components. The irreversible form of nephrotoxicity usually results from prolonged administration. Strategies to decrease nephrotoxicity include concomitant saline infusion, dose reduction (made possible by adding another antifungal agent), and the use of liposomal formulations of amphotericin B. Anemia may also result because of decreased renal production of erythropoietin. Intrathecal administration may cause seizures and neurologic damage.

Azoles

CHEMISTRY AND PHARMACOKINETICS. The azoles are a class of antifungals named after the five-membered carbon-nitrogen ring in their structure. The azoles used for systemic fungal infections include **ketoconazole, fluconazole, itraconazole, posaconazole,** and **voriconazole**. Fluconazole, posaconazole, and voriconazole are more reliably absorbed orally than the other azoles. The azoles are distributed to most body tissues, but drug levels achieved in the CNS are very low (with the exception of fluconazole and possibly posaconazole). The liver metabolizes ketoconazole, itraconazole, posaconazole, and voriconazole, and the kidneys eliminate fluconazole.

MECHANISM OF ACTION. The azoles disrupt membrane function of fungal cells by interfering with the synthesis of ergosterol (Figure 29–2), a process utilizing cytochrome P450 enzymes similar to human P450 isoforms. Resistance to azoles is becoming more widespread owing to increased use of this class of drugs for long-term prophylaxis of systemic mycoses in immunocompromised and neutropenic patients.

TOXICITY. As a group, the azoles are relatively nontoxic. The most common adverse effects include minor gastrointestinal disturbances and rash. Varying degrees of hepatotoxicity may occur, especially in patients with impaired liver function. All azoles inhibit human hepatic cytochrome P450s to some extent because of their similarity to the fungal target enzymes. Thus, patients taking azoles (especially ketoconazole) in combination with other drugs may have higher plasma concentrations of drugs that are primarily metabolized by the cytochrome P450 system. In addition, inhibition of human cytochrome P450 (especially by ketoconazole) interferes with synthesis of adrenal and other steroids, which may lead to gynecomastia, menstrual irregularities, or infertility. Because it causes more adverse effects than the other azoles, ketoconazole is rarely used for systemic fungal infections, and is now mostly used for chronic mucocutaneous and dermatologic fungal infections.

Specific Azoles

FLUCONAZOLE. Because of its high oral bioavailability, relatively good gastrointestinal tolerance, and fewer effects on hepatic enzymes, fluconazole has the highest therapeutic index of all the azoles. Fluconazole is the treatment of choice for initial treatment and secondary prophylaxis for cryptococcal meningitis, and is also used in treating active infection due to *Cryptococcus neoformans*. It is effective against esophageal and oropharyngeal candidiasis, vaginal candidiasis, candidemia, and most infections caused by *Coccidioides*.

ITRACONAZOLE. Itraconazole is effective against many systemic fungal infections caused by *Blastomyces* and *Sporothrix* and for subcutaneous chromoblastomycosis (chronic, localized skin and subcutaneous tissue infection that follows traumatic implantation of one of several different fungal species). It can be used as the primary or alternative drug for treating infections caused by *Aspergillus*, *Coccidioides*, *Cryptococcus*, and *Histoplasma*. It is also used extensively in the treatment of dermatophytoses and onychomycosis.

POSACONAZOLE. This newest azole has been recommended for prophylaxis of invasive aspergillosis in high-risk immunocompromised patients and for treatment of oropharyngeal candidiasis, including cases refractory to itraconazole and fluconazole. The full clinical usefulness and toxic potential of posaconazole are not yet established.

VORICONAZOLE. Voriconazole is well absorbed orally and has an even wider spectrum of antifungal activity than itraconazole. It is replacing amphotericin B for the treatment of invasive aspergillosis because of greater efficacy with less toxicity. Voriconazole has also been used as an alternative drug in candidemia and in AIDS patients for the treatment of candidal esophagitis and stomatitis. In addition to the adverse effects common to the azoles, voriconazole has been reported to cause transient visual disturbances in more than 30% of patients.

Flucytosine

CHEMISTRY AND PHARMACOKINETICS. Flucytosine (5-fluorocytosine, 5-FC) is related to the anticancer drug fluorouracil. Unlike amphotericin B, it is effective orally and is distributed to most body tissues, including the CNS. To avoid toxic accumulation, serum concentrations are monitored regularly and dose reductions are made for patients with renal impairment.

MECHANISM OF ACTION AND CLINICAL USES. Flucytosine is preferentially taken up by fungal cells, where it is enzymatically converted to a compound that inhibits deoxyribonucleic acid (DNA) and ribonucleic acid (RNA) synthesis, thus preventing formation of fungal proteins (Figure 29–2). When used as a single-drug therapy, resistance to flucytosine emerges rapidly. Co-treatment with amphotericin B decreases the likelihood of resistance and produces synergistic fungicidal effects.

The antifungal spectrum of flucytosine is fairly narrow; it is active against yeasts such as *Cryptococcus neoformans* and some *Candida* species. To provide optimal fungicidal effects and reduce resistance, flucytosine is given in combination with amphotericin B or fluconazole. These drug combinations may be used to treat susceptible candidal septicemia, endocarditis and urinary tract infections, cryptococcal meningitis (one of the most common opportunistic CNS infections in AIDS patients), and pulmonary infections.

TOXICITY. The most common adverse effects result from the metabolism of flucytosine to the anticancer drug fluorouracil. Reversible impairment of bone marrow function results in anemia, leukopenia, and thrombocytopenia. Less commonly, flucytosine causes liver dysfunction. Patients' blood concentrations and renal function are monitored during drug therapy to avoid toxic accumulation.

Echinocandins

CHEMISTRY AND PHARMACOKINETICS. Echinocandins represent the newest class of antifungal agents, with a novel mechanism of action. Currently, three agents are available in this category: **caspofungin**, **micafungin**, and **anidulafungin**. Because these drugs are not well absorbed orally, they are only administered intravenously. Caspofungin distributes widely to most tissues except the cerebrospinal fluid (CSF). However, despite low CSF concentrations, positive results have been reported with caspofungin in the treatment of cerebral aspergillosis. Doses are decreased in patients with severe hepatic impairment.

MECHANISM OF ACTION AND CLINICAL USES. The echinocandins inhibit an enzyme present in fungal, but not mammalian cells. The result is impaired synthesis of β(1–3) glucan, an essential component of fungal cell walls. The echinocandins are used for the treatment of patients with candidemia and other forms of *Candida* infections (esophageal candidiasis, peritonitis, and intra-abdominal abscess). Early studies suggest that the potential for development of resistance to the echinocandins is low, suggesting that this class of antifungal agents may be used as therapy in life-threatening fungal infections (e.g., invasive aspergillosis) with strains that are no longer susceptible to conventional antifungals such as amphotericin B and the azoles.

TOXICITY. To date, excellent tolerability and safety have been reported with the echinocandins. Compared with the other systemic antifungal agents, very few drug interactions have been reported with caspofungin.

Systemic Drugs Used in Mucocutaneous Fungal Infections

Mucocutaneous fungal infections include the superficial infections of skin, mucous membranes (including the oropharynx and vagina), and the nails. These disorders are confined to the cutaneous surface, with little likelihood for systemic proliferation. Commonly, these include infections with *Candida* organisms, usually *C albicans*. The severity of diseases may range from relatively minor cosmetic inconveniences such as onychomycosis (chronic fungal infection that affects toenails more commonly than fingernails) to oral thrush, which is a painful candidal infection that is often the first manifestation of local or systemic immunosuppression. Although mucocutaneous fungal infections are superficial, topical drug application alone is often ineffective because of insufficient penetration into affected tissues. This is especially true with onychomycosis, in which topical antifungal agents are unlikely to penetrate through all nail layers.

Griseofulvin

Griseofulvin is used to treat dermatophytoses—fungal infections of the skin, hair, and nails. Griseofulvin's oral absorption is variable, but can be optimized when patients take ultramicrosize formulations with a high-fat meal. Griseofulvin interferes with microtubule formation in dermatophytes (Figure 29–2). It is deposited in keratin precursor cells, which are gradually exfoliated and replaced with noninfected tissue. Griseofulvin remains bound to new keratin, protecting the skin from new infection. To allow for replacement of infected keratin by newly resistant keratin, griseofulvin must be administered for long periods of time: 2 to 6 weeks for skin and hair infections and for at least 6 months for toenail infections. However, the use of griseofulvin is plagued by high relapse rates, especially for onychomycosis. The most common adverse reactions include skin rashes and urticaria (hives). Other side effects include gastrointestinal irritation, mental confusion, headache, and photosensitivity. Drug interactions occur with warfarin, phenobarbital, and alcohol. In addition, griseofulvin may increase the rate at which hepatic enzymes metabolize estrogens, possibly decreasing effectiveness of contraceptives and producing menstrual irregularities.

Terbinafine

Terbinafine

Terbinafine has generally replaced griseofulvin in the treatment of onychomycosis. Terbinafine inhibits a fungal enzyme and results in accumulation of a substance toxic to the fungus. Terbinafine offers a shorter treatment regimen, higher cure rate, lower relapse rate, and fewer adverse effects than griseofulvin. Daily oral treatment for 12 weeks may result in a clinical cure rate as high as 60 to 75%. Adverse reactions include gastrointestinal upset, headache, rash, and taste disturbances. Rare cases of hepatic failure have been reported with the use of terbinafine in individuals with and without preexisting liver disease. Consequently, liver enzyme levels and a complete blood count are obtained before terbinafine is initiated and repeated every 4 to 6 weeks during treatment.

Topical Antifungal Drugs

A number of dermatologic fungal infections such as ringworm, jock itch, and athlete's foot as well as some localized (oral, vaginal) candidal infections may be successfully treated with topical antifungal agents. Topical agents can be divided into three major categories: polyenes, azoles, and allylamines.

Nystatin is a polyene agent similar to amphotericin B. It acts by disrupting fungal cell membrane permeability, resulting in cell death. Because its toxicity precludes systemic use, nystatin is only used topically; the drug is not significantly absorbed from skin or mucous membranes. Nystatin (as powder, cream, ointment, or vaginal tablet) is commonly used to treat localized candidal infections in the oropharynx, in the vagina, and in areas where opposing skin surfaces may rub together, such as around the perineum or under the breasts. Localized infections can be cured rapidly, often within 24 to 72 hours after treatment initiation.

The most common topical azole agents are **clotrimazole** and **miconazole**. Both are available with a prescription as well as over-the-counter (OTC) as creams, powders, sprays, or vaginal suppositories. Clotrimazole and miconazole creams are used for the effective treatment of *tinea pedis* (athlete's foot), *tinea cruris* (jock itch), and *tinea corporis* (ringworm). Vaginal clotrimazole suppositories are used in the treatment of vaginal yeast infections. Oral clotrimazole lozenges (called

troches) are used to treat oral candidiasis infections that commonly occur in immunocompromised individuals. Systemic absorption is minimal and adverse effects are rare.

Topical allylamine creams are available by prescription for the treatment of dermatologic fungal infections such as *tinea cruris* and *tinea corporis*. These include terbinafine, **naftifine**, and **butenafine hydrochloride**.

■ ANTIPARASITIC AGENTS

A large number of protozoa and helminths are capable of infecting humans. Drugs designed to kill these parasites must take into account their complex life cycles and the differences between their metabolic pathways and those of the host. Thus, drugs acting against protozoa are usually inactive against helminths and vice versa. Because protozoa and helminths are eukaryotes, they are metabolically more similar to humans than are bacteria. Although some antibacterial agents have antiprotozoal activity (e.g., metronidazole and doxycycline), most are ineffective against eukaryotic parasites.

Rational approaches to antiparasitic chemotherapy use the principle of selective toxicity, which exploits the biochemical and physiologic differences between parasite and human host cells. Many antiparasitic agents act on targets (usually enzymes) that are either unique to the parasite, or that possess sufficient differences between host and parasite to allow safe drug activity. Despite differences between host and parasite, many of the more effective antiparasitic drugs have significant toxicity and their use has to balance benefit against risk.

Climatic changes and international travel have facilitated the spread of many parasitic diseases, while starvation and poor sanitation that accompany poverty and war have promoted the reemergence of others. Drug resistance has also dramatically influenced the ability to treat and control many parasitic diseases.

Antiprotozoal Drugs

Protozoa are unicellular eukaryotic organisms. The parasitic protozoa that cause disease in humans either require the invasion of a suitable host to complete all or part of their life cycle, or they present as free-living protozoa that

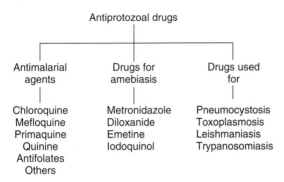

Figure 29–3. Diseases caused by protozoans constitute a worldwide health problem. Antiprotozoal drugs are used to combat malaria, amebiasis, toxoplasmosis, pneumocystosis, trypanosomiasis, and leishmaniasis.

may become pathogenic in immunocompromised individuals. Conditions caused by protozoa include malaria, amebiasis, toxoplasmosis, pneumocystosis, trypanosomiasis, and leishmaniasis (Figure 29–3).

Drugs for Malaria

In terms of annual mortality, malaria remains the most important tropical parasitic disease. The World Health Organization estimates that malaria kills over 2.5 million people yearly, with the majority of deaths occurring in children under the age of 5 years in sub-Saharan Africa. Although four *Plasmodium* species infect humans (*P falciparum, P malariae, P ovale, P vivax*), *P falciparum* is responsible for the most serious life-threatening complications and death. Transmission most commonly occurs when an infected mosquito injects the infectious form of the parasite, the *sporozoite*, into the individual's blood. Sporozoites circulate to the liver and infect liver cells. Here, they reproduce to form merozoites, which eventually leave the liver, reenter the bloodstream, and invade red blood cells (RBCs). Parasites mature within RBCs, are released, and continue infecting more RBCs. At this stage of infection, clinical disease is manifested by recurrent flu-like attacks, fever, severe anemia, and, in some cases, cerebral malaria and death.

In *P falciparum* and *P malariae* infections, only one cycle of liver cell invasion and multiplication occurs. Liver infection ceases spontaneously in less than 4 weeks. In this case, drugs that eliminate parasites

within RBCs (e.g., *chloroquine, quinine*) can cure most of these infections if the parasite is not drug resistant. On the other hand, *P ovale* and *P vivax* can remain dormant in the liver for months or years. Subsequent malaria relapses can occur after successful pharmacotherapy directed against the erythrocytic parasites. To cure these infections, an antimalarial agent that eliminates liver parasites must be used in conjunction with agents that eliminate erythrocytic parasites. No single available antimalarial agent can reliably bring about a radical cure; that is, eliminate both hepatic and erythrocytic stages.

The major drugs used in malarial prophylaxis and treatment are shown in Table 29–2. For many agents, antimalarial activity is due to either intracellular accumulation of a compound toxic to the parasite (e.g., **chloroquine**), interference with parasitic DNA replication (e.g., **quinine**), or inhibition of critical enzymes involved in folic acid synthesis (e.g., **pyrimethamine, proguanil, sulfadoxine**). For other drugs, the antimalarial mechanism of action is not clear (e.g., **halofantrine** and **doxycycline**). Since parasites are increasingly resistant to multiple drugs, no chemoprophylactic regimen is fully protective, and treatment for malaria depends on knowledge of changing resistance patterns.

The first line of defense against malaria is limiting contact with mosquitoes by using mosquito repellent, keeping arms and legs covered, staying indoors during mosquitoes' feeding hours (dusk and throughout the night), and sleeping under mosquito netting. Physical therapists involved in the Peace Corps, Health Volunteers Overseas, or other international organizations are likely to practice in malaria endemic areas. Prior to leaving home, individuals should consult the Centers for Disease Control and Prevention (CDC) (http:// www.cdc.gov/travel/destinat.htm; or telephone 877-FYI-TRIP) for current recommendations regarding specific antimalarial chemoprophylaxis, resistance patterns, and treatment if malaria is contracted.

CHLOROQUINE, MEFLOQUINE, AND ANTIFOLATE AGENTS (PYRIMETHAMINE/SULFADOXINE). Chloroquine, long considered the drug of choice for prophylaxis and treatment of malaria, is no longer considered the first-line antimalarial agent in many countries owing to worldwide prevalence of

Table 29–2.	Drugs used in malaria		
Drug	**Use in Acute Attacks?**	**Use for Eradication of Liver Stages?**	**Use for Prophylaxis?**
Chloroquine	Yes	No	Yes, except in regions where *P falciparum* is resistant
Quinine, mefloquine	Yes, in resistant *P falciparum*	No	Yes, mefloquine[1] is used in regions with chloroquine-resistant *P falciparum*
Primaquine	No	Yes	Yes, if exposed to *P vivax* or *P ovale*
Antifols	Yes, but only in resistant *P falciparum*	No	Not usually advised as single agents
Artemisinins	Yes	No	No

[1]Doxycycline or atovaquone-proguanil (Malarone) are also recommended for chemoprophylaxis in regions where chloroquine-resistant *P falciparum* are endemic.

chloroquine-resistant parasites. In regions where *P falciparum* is not resistant, chloroquine is used for chemoprophylaxis and for acute attacks of falciparum and nonfalciparum malaria. Chloroquine is generally well tolerated, even with prolonged use. The most common adverse effects are gastrointestinal upset, skin rash or itching, and headaches. Consumption of calcium- and magnesium-containing antacids should be avoided because they significantly decrease oral chloroquine absorption. Dosing after meals may reduce some adverse effects. Long-term administration of high doses may cause severe skin lesions, peripheral neuropathies, myocardial depression, retinal damage, auditory impairment, and toxic psychosis.

Common alternatives for treating chloroquine-resistant strains include **mefloquine**, combined **pyrimethamine/sulfadoxine** (antifolate agents), and **atovaquone/proguanil (Malarone)**, but resistance is emerging to mefloquine in some regions (parts of Southeast Asia), and significant resistance to the antifolate agents is now common for *P falciparum* and less common for *P vivax*. Malarone is becoming the preferred prophylactic agent for travelers to Africa and has shown efficacy for treatment of active malaria. Common adverse effects of mefloquine and the antifolate compounds

include gastrointestinal distress and rash. Mefloquine causes headache and dizziness. Severe neuropsychiatric disturbances such as depression, confusion, acute psychosis, or seizures have also been reported with mefloquine. Toxicities for the antifolate compounds include hemolysis and kidney damage. The toxicity of malarone includes gastrointestinal disturbances, headache, and rash.

QUININE. Quinine is the original antimalarial drug that is derived from the bark of the native South American cinchona tree. Quinine remains the drug of choice for life-threatening malaria. Quinine acts rapidly against all four species of human malaria parasites in erythrocytes. Its main use is in treating chloroquine-resistant falciparum malaria. However, quinine is often used in combination with a second drug (**doxycycline** or **clindamycin**) to limit toxicity by shortening its duration of use (generally to 3 days). Quinine is generally not used in chemoprophylaxis because of toxicity and potential increases in parasitic resistance to these agents. Therapeutic doses of quinine commonly cause *cinchonism*. Milder symptoms of cinchonism such as gastrointestinal distress, headache, vertigo, blurred vision, and tinnitus do not warrant discontinuation of the drug. Higher doses of quinine result in cardiac conduction disturbances. In some individuals with hypersensitivity, severe blood disorders can occur. Therapy is discontinued in hypersensitive patients and those with severe cinchonism.

PRIMAQUINE. Primaquine is the only drug available to eradicate liver stage parasites of *P vivax* and *P ovale* and should be used in conjunction with an antimalarial effective against parasites within RBCs. It is generally well tolerated, but sometimes causes nausea, headache, and epigastric pain. Because it can produce severe hemolysis in patients with glucose-6-phosphate dehydrogenase (G6PD) deficiency, persons for whom this agent is being considered must be evaluated for G6PD enzyme levels and the drug should not be used in those who are G6PD deficient.

ARTEMISININ. The most important newer antimalarial compounds are derivatives of artemisinin (an extract of the Chinese herbal remedy quinghaosu). These agents combine rapid antimalarial activity with an absence of clinically important resistance: they are the only drugs reliably effective against quinine-resistant strains. Because of their short half-lives, artemisinin and its analogs artesunate and artemether are generally used with another antimalarial agent and are not useful in chemoprophylaxis. Although they appear to be better tolerated than most antimalarials, the artemisinins are currently available in the United States and Canada only on special request, but are widely available in Africa and Asia.

Drugs for Amebiasis

Amebiasis is infection with *Entamoeba histolytica*. Although amebiasis occurs worldwide, it is most prevalent in tropical and subtropical areas, especially in crowded and unsanitary living conditions. The organism lives and reproduces on the mucosal surface of the large intestine. Encysted forms periodically pass out in the feces, and can survive in the external environment and act as infective forms. Infection with *E histolytica* occurs as a result of inadequate sanitation, or when food or drink is contaminated by infected food handlers. Ingested cysts adhere to intestinal epithelial cells and invade the mucosal lining. *E histolytica* can cause asymptomatic intestinal infection, mild to moderate colitis, mild diarrhea, severe intestinal infection (amebic dysentery), liver abscess, and other extraintestinal infections.

Drugs for amebiasis (Table 29–3) include tissue amebicides (**chloroquine, emetines, metronidazole**),

Table 29–3.	Drugs used in the treatment of protozoal infections other than malaria
Drugs of Choice	**Primary Indications**
Diloxanide furoate	Asymptomatic intestinal amebiasis
Melarsoprol	Drug of choice in African sleeping sickness (late, CNS stage of trypanosomiasis); also used in mucocutaneous forms of the disease
Metronidazole plus diloxanide or iodoquinol	Mild to severe intestinal amebiasis
Metronidazole plus diloxanide, followed by paromomycin	Hepatic abscess form of amebiasis
Nifurtimox	Trypanosomiasis caused by *Trypanosoma cruzi*
Pentamidine	Hemolymphatic stage of trypanosomiasis; also used in *Pneumocystis jiroveci* pneumonia
Pyrimethamine plus sulfadiazine	Drug combination of choice in toxoplasmosis
Sodium stibogluconate	Drug of choice for leishmaniasis (all species)
Suramin	Drug of choice for hemolymphatic stage of trypanosomiasis (*T brucei gambiense, T rhodesiense*)
Trimethoprim-sulfamethoxazole	Drug combination of choice in *P jiroveci* infections

which act on organisms in the bowel wall and the liver; and luminal amebicides (**diloxanide furoate, iodoquinol, paromomycin**), which act only in the lumen of the bowel. Drug choice depends on the type of amebic infection.

DILOXANIDE FUROATE. For asymptomatic disease (carriers with no symptoms in nonendemic areas), diloxanide furoate is the first choice. This drug is well tolerated, with usually mild gastrointestinal symptoms.

METRONIDAZOLE. For mild to severe intestinal infection, liver abscess, and other extraintestinal amebic disease, metronidazole is generally used in conjunction with a luminal amebicide. Adverse effects of metronidazole include gastrointestinal irritation, headache, and, less frequently, leukopenia, dizziness, and ataxia. (See Chapter 30 for further discussion of metronidazole.)

EMETINE AND DEHYDROEMETINE. Emetine and dehydroemetine may still be used as back-up drugs for treatment of severe intestinal or hepatic amebiasis in hospitalized patients. However, because they may cause severe toxicity (including gastrointestinal distress, muscle weakness, and cardiovascular dysfunction), they have been mostly replaced by metronidazole.

Drugs for Pneumocystosis and Toxoplasmosis
Pneumocystis jiroveci (formerly called *P carinii*) is the cause of human pneumocystosis. Although now recognized as a fungus, *P jiroveci* is responsive to antiprotozoal drugs, not antifungals. Commonly found in normal humans, the fungus causes symptomatic disease only in immune-deficient individuals. Thus, there is a high incidence of *P jiroveci* pneumonia in patients receiving immunosuppressive therapy and in patients with AIDS.

TRIMETHOPRIM PLUS SULFAMETHOXAZOLE. Trimethoprim plus sulfamethoxazole (TMP-SMZ) is the first-line therapy for *P jiroveci* pneumonia. TMP-SMZ is also used as a chemoprophylactic drug combination for prevention of *P jiroveci* infection in immunocompromised individuals. While chemoprophylactic doses are generally much better tolerated than treatment for active infection, high-dose therapy entails significant toxicity in up to 50% of AIDS patients. Important toxicities include gastrointestinal distress, rash, fever, neutropenia, and thrombocytopenia. These adverse effects may be severe enough to warrant discontinuance of TMP-SMZ. Because of the high prevalence of serious adverse effects with TMP-SMZ, several drugs have been used as alternative agents against *P jiroveci* infection. Notably, none is as effective as TMP-SMZ.

PENTAMIDINE. Pentamidine is a well-established alternative drug for *P jiroveci* infection. For prophylaxis, pentamidine is administered as an inhaled aerosol. Although well tolerated in this form, it is not as effective as daily TMP-SMZ. For treatment of active *P jiroveci* infection, pentamidine must be administered parenterally. Serious adverse effects result from parenteral administration, including respiratory stimulation followed by respiratory depression, severe hypotension, hypoglycemia, anemia, neutropenia, hepatitis, and pancreatitis.

ATOVAQUONE. Atovaquone is an oral drug initially developed as an antimalarial, but it has also been approved for the treatment of mild to moderate *P jiroveci* pneumonia. Although less effective than TMP-SMZ or pentamidine, it is better tolerated. Adverse effects include fever, rash, cough, nausea, vomiting, diarrhea, and abnormal liver function tests.

Drugs for Toxoplasmosis
Toxoplasmosis is infection with *Toxoplasma gondii*. Infection occurs by ingesting oocysts released in the feces of infected cats (primary hosts) or by eating raw meat containing tissue cysts. Infection with this protozoan is widespread, but is not serious unless it is acquired (or reactivated) in immunosuppressed patients or acquired during pregnancy, when the organism invades all fetal tissues, especially the CNS. Damage to the eye is the most common consequence, although the brain may also be affected.

The antifolate agents **pyrimethamine** with **sulfadiazine** (or with **clindamycin** in patients allergic to sulfonamides) are used for treatment of congenital toxoplasmosis and acute infection in immunocompromised individuals. In AIDS-related *Toxoplasma* encephalitis, high-dose treatment must be given for many weeks and is associated with gastric irritation, neurologic symptoms (headaches, insomnia, tremors, seizures) and serious blood abnormalities. **Spiramycin** is an antibiotic that is used to treat toxoplasmosis acquired during pregnancy. Treatment lowers the risk of development of congenital toxoplasmosis.

Drugs For Trypanosomiasis

The protozoan genus *Trypanosoma* contains three species that cause human disease. Infections with *T gambiense* and *T rhodesiense* cause African trypanosomiasis (African sleeping sickness), and *T cruzi* infection causes American trypanosomiasis (Chagas disease). Trypanosomiasis is transmitted by the bite of infected insect vectors, which are the tsetse fly for African trypanosomiasis and reduviid bugs for American trypanosomiasis. Currently available drugs for all forms of trypanosomiasis are seriously deficient in both efficacy and safety. Availability of these drugs is also a concern: the CDC classifies several of these drugs as investigational agents, supplying them only upon request. Some of these drugs include **bithionol, dehydroemetine, diethylcarbamazine, melarsoprol, nifurtimox, sodium stibogluconate**, and **suramin**.

SURAMIN AND PENTAMIDINE. After a bite by an infected tsetse fly, widespread lymph node enlargement occurs and the organism establishes in the blood and rapidly multiplies. Suramin is the first-line therapy for this acute hemolymphatic stage of African trypanosomiasis. Because suramin does not enter the CNS, it is not effective against advanced disease when the CNS becomes involved. Suramin is administered intravenously and causes adverse effects including skin rashes, gastrointestinal distress, and neurologic complications. Pentamidine may be used as an alternative to suramin or in combination with suramin for the early hemolymphatic stage. Adverse effects (described above for its use against pneumocystosis) are noted in half of patients receiving therapeutic doses.

MELARSOPROL AND EFLORNITHINE. Once African trypanosomiasis has infected the CNS, drugs that cross the blood-brain barrier must be administered. Even though melarsoprol is extremely toxic (it is an arsenic derivative), it is still considered the drug of choice because of the severity of African trypanosomiasis at this stage. Immediate toxicity includes fever, vomiting, abdominal pain, and arthralgias. The drug may also cause a reactive encephalopathy that can be fatal. To avoid the toxicity of melarsoprol as well as increasing treatment failures that may be due to drug resistance, eflornithine has been introduced as a second option for treating advanced disease. It is available orally and intravenously, and is effective against some forms of African trypanosomiasis. Toxicity is markedly less than that from melarsoprol, but adverse effects still include gastrointestinal distress, blood abnormalities, and seizures.

NIFURTIMOX AND BENZNIDAZOLE. Chagas disease, caused by *T cruzi* infection, is one of the main causes of death due to heart failure in Latin American countries. *T cruzi* primarily invades cardiac muscle cells and macrophages. Initial infection usually results in a transient febrile illness. After invasion of host cells, the disease pursues a very slow course. The two major symptoms of Chagas disease, myocarditis and intestinal tract dilation, can take years to develop. Two drugs are available to treat Chagas disease: nifurtimox and benznidazole. Both drugs are commonly used to treat the acute infection, but are often unsuccessful at complete eradication of the protozoan, thus allowing progression to the cardiac and gastrointestinal syndromes. The toxicities of both drugs, including gastrointestinal irritation and severe CNS effects, are a major drawback in their use, frequently forcing discontinuation of the treatment. Benznidazole is not commercially available in the United States and Canada.

Drugs for Leishmaniasis

Leishmania parasites are transmitted by the bite of infected sandflies. Infection results in cutaneous (skin), mucocutaneous (skin, nose, mouth), or visceral (liver and spleen) leishmaniasis. More than 12 million people are known to be infected with leishmaniasis, with the cutaneous and mucocutaneous forms being much more prevalent than the life-threatening visceral disease. The cutaneous disease is particularly prevalent in Afghanistan, Algeria, Brazil, Iraq, Iran, Peru, Saudi Arabia, and Syria. More than 90% of the world's cases of visceral leishmaniasis are in India, Bangladesh,

Nepal, Sudan, and Brazil. The disease is often known by many local names (e.g., Oriental sore, espundia, Baghdad boil, Delhi sore, and kala-azar). Those at increased risk of leishmaniasis (particularly cutaneous leishmaniasis) include Peace Corps volunteers, people who do research outdoors at night, and soldiers. The cutaneous and mucocutaneous leishmania infections range from localized self-healing ulcers to disseminated lesions that give rise to chronic disfiguring conditions. Lesions may eventually heal with significant scarring, but will leave the individual relatively immune to reinfection. In contrast, visceral infection develops slowly and is characterized by hepatomegaly and splenomegaly. Left untreated, visceral leishmaniasis almost always results in death.

SODIUM STIBOGLUCONATE. This drug, based on the heavy metal antimony, has been the mainstay of treatment for leishmaniasis. The drug must be administered parenterally (intravenous or intramuscular), and intramuscular injections can be very painful. Although few adverse effects occur initially, the toxicity of sodium stibogluconate increases over the course of therapy. The most commonly encountered adverse effects include gastrointestinal symptoms, fever, headache, myalgias, arthralgias, and rash. It is potentially cardiotoxic (QT prolongation), but these effects are generally reversible. Cure rates for the cutaneous and mucocutaneous forms are generally good with several weeks of therapy. However, treatment for the visceral disease (kala-azar) is ineffective at times, has shown increasing resistance, and is associated with treatment-related deaths in a small percentage of cases. Alternative drugs such as **pentamidine** and **miltefosine** (for visceral leishmaniasis), **fluconazole** or **metronidazole** (for cutaneous lesions), and **amphotericin B** (for mucocutaneous leishmaniasis) have been used when therapy is ineffective.

MILTEFOSINE. This drug, originally developed as an antineoplastic drug, is the first effective oral drug used in the treatment of cutaneous and visceral leishmaniasis. The cure rate of miltefosine, especially for the visceral disease, is very promising, and the drug is generally well tolerated. Adverse effects include nausea and vomiting. Because the drug has demonstrated teratogenicity, miltefosine should not be given to pregnant women. Miltefosine is currently not approved for use in the United States.

Anthelmintic Drugs

The helminths include all groups of parasitic worms. Three main groups parasitize human organs, most often the gastrointestinal tract: tapeworms (*Cestoda*), flukes (*Trematoda* or *Digenea*), and **roundworms** (*Nematoda*). Tapeworms and flukes are relatively flat and have specialized structures to secure attachment to the host's intestine or blood vessels. Roundworms have long cylindrical bodies and generally lack specialized attachment structures. Transmission may be direct by swallowing infective stages or by larvae actively penetrating the skin or indirect by injection from infected insect vectors. Some of the drugs used in helminthic infections are outlined in Figure 29–4, and listed in Table 29–4.

Drugs That Act Against Nematodes (Roundworms)
It is estimated that more than 1 billion people worldwide are infected by intestinal nematodes, with much higher prevalence in moist subtropical and tropical climates. Medically important intestinal nematodes responsive to anthelmintic drugs include

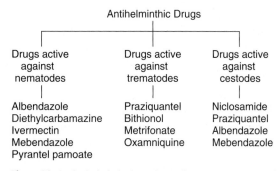

Figure 29–4. Anthelmintic drugs have diverse mechanisms of action and properties. Many act against specific parasites, and few are devoid of toxicity to host cells. Reactions to dead and dying parasites may cause serious toxicity in patients. Anthelmintic drugs are divided into three groups on the basis of the type of worm primarily affected–nematodes, trematodes, and cestodes. The drugs of choice and alternative agents for some important helminthic infections are listed in Table 29–4.

Table 29–4.	Major helminthic infections and the drugs used to treat them	
Infecting Organism	**Drugs of Choice**	**Alternative Drugs**
Nematodes		
Ascaris lumbricoides (roundworm)	Albendazole, mebendazole	Pyrantel pamoate, piperazine
Necator americanus, Ancylostoma duodenale	Albendazole, mebendazole	Pyrantel pamoate
Trichuris trichiura (whipworm)	Albendazole	Mebendazole, pyrantel pamoate
Strongyloides stercoralis (threadworm)	Ivermectin	Thiabendazole, albendazole
Enterobius vermicularis (pinworm)	Albendazole or mebendazole	Pyrantel pamoate
Cutaneous larva migrans	Ivermectin	Albendazole, diethylcarbamazine
Wuchereria bancrofti, Brugia malayi	Ivermectin + albendazole	Diethylcarbamazine
Onchocerca volvulus	Ivermectin	Suramin
Trematodes (flukes)		
Schistosoma haematobium	Praziquantel	Metrifonate
Schistosoma mansoni	Praziquantel	Oxamniquine
Schistosoma japonicum	Praziquantel	None
Paragonimus westermani	Praziquantel	Bithionol
Fasciola hepatica	Bithionol	Praziquantel, emetine, dehydroemetine
Cestodes (tapeworms)		
Taenia saginata	Niclosamide or praziquantel	Mebendazole
Taenia solium	Niclosamide or praziquantel	
Diphyllobothrium latum	Niclosamide or praziquantel	
Cysticercosis	Albendazole	Praziquantel
Echinococcus granulosus (hydatid disease)	Albendazole	Mebendazole

Enterobius vermicularis (pinworm), *Trichuris trichiura* (whipworm), *Ascaris lumbricoides* (roundworm), *Ancylostoma* and *Necator* species (hookworms), and *Strongyloides stercoralis* (threadworm). Pinworms are the most common intestinal nematode in developed countries and are also the least pathogenic. Eggs that are laid on the perianal skin cause itching, and transmission generally occurs from contaminated fingers. While hookworm (*Ancylostoma* and *Necator* species) infections are rare in the United States, threadworm (*Strongyloides stercoralis*) infections are endemic in rural areas of the southeastern states and the Appalachian region. Not as common as intestinal nematodes, tissue nematodes still infect over a half billion people worldwide. Tissue nematodes responsive to anthelmintic therapy include *Ancylostoma*, *Dracunculus*, *Onchocerca*, and *Toxocara* species and *Wuchereria bancrofti*.

ALBENDAZOLE. This is an oral drug with a wide anthelmintic spectrum. It is the drug of choice for roundworm (ascariasis), hookworm, pinworm, and whipworm infections. It is an alternative drug for threadworm and filariasis (endemic in some tropical areas and responsible for elephantiasis when the lymphatics are infected) infections. Dosing of albendazole varies depending on the parasitic infection being treated. During short courses of therapy, albendazole has relatively few adverse effects.

MEBENDAZOLE. This is another primary drug for ascariasis, pinworm, and whipworm infections, with cure rates of 90 to 100%. It has a low incidence of adverse effects, primarily limited to gastrointestinal irritation. Its use is contraindicated in pregnancy, as it may be embryotoxic.

IVERMECTIN. This is the drug of choice for onchocerciasis, a chronic disease endemic in West and sub-Saharan Africa, as well Saudi Arabia and Yemen. Chronic infection often results in serious ophthalmologic complications, including blindness. Ivermectin immobilizes sensitive parasites by inhibiting neurotransmitter function in parasites. It does not cross the blood-brain barrier, and does not interfere with human neurotransmission. Ivermectin is generally given as a single-dose oral therapy. Adverse effects include fever, headache, dizziness, rash, pruritus, tachycardia, hypotension, and pain in joints, muscles, and lymph glands. These symptoms are often of short duration and manageable with antihistamines and nonsteroidal anti-inflammatory drugs (NSAIDs).

Drugs That Act Against Trematodes (Flukes)
The medically important trematodes include several parasites that have an enormous impact on human populations, such as *Clonorchis sinensis* (human liver fluke, endemic in Southeast Asia), *Schistosoma* species (blood flukes, estimated to affect more than 200 million persons worldwide), and *Paragonimus westermani* (lung fluke, endemic in Asia and India).

PRAZIQUANTEL. This drug has a wide anthelmintic spectrum. It kills susceptible worms by increasing cell membrane permeability, resulting in paralysis of their musculature, and eventual phagocytosis by human immune cells and death. Praziquantel is the safest and most effective drug for treating schistosomiasis (all species) and most other trematode and cestode infections. It is effective against adult worms

and immature stages. Common mild and transient adverse effects include headache, dizziness, and malaise. These generally do not require treatment, but may be more frequent or serious in patients with heavy worm burdens.

Drugs That Act Against Cestodes (Tapeworms)
Cestode eggs are passed into soil from a primary host (humans in most cestode infestations), and ingested by and hatched in an intermediate host (e.g., cow, pig) in which they enter tissue and encyst. Primary hosts then ingest cysts in the flesh of the intermediate host. In some cestodes (*Echinococcus* and *Spirometra* species), humans are the intermediate hosts and larvae live within tissues and migrate through different organ systems. The four medically important cestodes are *Taenia saginata* (beef tapeworm), *T solium* (pork tapeworm, which can cause larval forms in the brain and eyes), *Diphyllobothrium latum* (fish tapeworm), and *Echinococcus granulosus* (dog tapeworm, which is endemic in South America, Iceland, Australia, New Zealand, and southern parts of Africa and can cause cysts in the liver, lungs, and brain). The primary drugs for treatment of cestode infections are **praziquantel** (see above) and **niclosamide**. Niclosamide is used to treat infections caused by beef, pork, and fish tapeworms. It is not effective in cysticercosis, an infection caused by the pork tapeworm *T solium* (**albendazole** or praziquantel is used) or disease caused by *E granulosus* (albendazole is used). Toxic effects are mild, but include gastrointestinal distress, headache, rash, and fever.

▇ REHABILITATION FOCUS

This chapter includes an extremely broad spectrum of antiparasitic agents–from antifungal drugs to antimalarial and anthelmintic drugs. Most physical therapists will treat patients taking antifungal agents, whether it is the athlete using a topical antifungal for athlete's foot or the AIDS patient receiving an intravenous agent to treat a systemic mycosis. Less commonly, physical therapists will encounter infections such as malaria and leishmaniasis that are endemic in tropical regions throughout the world. However, therapists traveling to these regions or caring for returning military personnel will often be involved in the management of infected individuals. For example, many individuals in malarial endemic regions will be receiving chemoprophylaxis or treatment for active malaria while participating in rehabilitation programs. An understanding of the medications' potential adverse effects allows the therapist to optimize the delivery (e.g., intensity and timing) of therapy sessions. In some cases, individuals suffering from advanced stages of these diseases are not appropriate rehabilitation candidates. However, the physical therapist still serves as a valuable member of the health-care team in providing education regarding limiting the spread of infection.

CLINICAL RELEVANCE FOR REHABILITATION

Adverse Drug Reactions

Systemic drugs used for fungal infections
- Amphotericin B almost always produces infusion-related adverse effects including fever, chills, vomiting, muscle spasms, headache, and significant hypotension.
- Amphotericin B may cause anemia.
- Flucytosine may cause reversible anemia and thrombocytopenia.
- All azole agents inhibit hepatic drug-metabolizing enzymes (cytochrome P450s) to some extent.
- Voriconazole may cause transient visual disturbances.

Antiparasitic drugs
- At therapeutic doses, many antiparasitic agents produce skin rashes, varying degrees of gastrointestinal distress, and neurologic complications ranging from headaches and tremors to confusion, acute psychosis, and seizures.

Anthelmintic drugs
- Many anthelmintics cause dizziness, tachycardia, hypotension, joint and muscle pain, and malaise.

Effects Interfering with Rehabilitation

Systemic drugs used for fungal infections
- Infusion-related effects of amphotericin B can limit patients' ability to participate in rehabilitation.

- Anemia and thrombocytopenia may result in decreased capacity to exercise and to control bleeding after injury, respectively.
- Inhibition of cytochrome P450s can cause higher plasma concentrations of other drugs, resulting in a potential increase or prolongation of therapeutic or adverse effects.
- Transient visual disturbances can interfere with functional performance of patients participating in rehabilitation.

Antiparasitic drugs
- The severity of many parasitic infections, as well as adverse effects of the drugs used to treat them, can interfere with functional performance of patients.

Anthelmintic drugs
- Many anthelmintics cause dizziness, tachycardia, hypotension, joint and muscle pain, and malaise.

Possible Therapy Solutions

Systemic drugs used for fungal infections
- If a patient is receiving intravenous amphotericin B, rehabilitation services should be scheduled away from this time.
- If decreased exercise tolerance or excessive bruising is noted with patients receiving amphotericin B or flucytosine, contact the referring health-care provider.
- If a patient taking any azole agent demonstrates new symptoms or if a patient is considering (or currently) taking an OTC drug or herbal supplement, contact the referring health-care provider for concerns regarding drug interactions.
- Visual disturbances should be reported to the referring health-care provider.

Antiparasitic drugs
- Therapy may need to be postponed until parasitic infection has been brought under control.

Anthelmintic drugs
- During short courses of therapy, adverse effects of many anthelmintic drugs are usually short in duration. Rehabilitation can be postponed until adverse effects cease or improve.

PROBLEM-ORIENTED PATIENT STUDY

Brief History: The patient is a 22-year-old male who returned from a military rotation in Iraq 2 months ago. He was admitted to a military rehabilitation hospital 4 days ago for an amputee rehabilitation program. He sustained a below the knee amputation (BKA) of the right lower extremity 1 week ago, secondary to a traumatic injury that occurred during a military operation. Prior to his injury, he was functionally independent and an avid basketball player.

Current Medical Status and Drugs: At admission, the patient was noted to have several crusted raised lesions that were up to 1 inch in diameter on his face, neck, and left forearm. The patient reported that the lesions were much larger and painful several weeks ago. An infectious disease physician sampled skin scrapings of the lesion and diagnosed the condition as cutaneous leishmaniasis, commonly known as "Baghdad boil." The patient was started on a 20-day intravenous course of sodium stibogluconate, which he receives once per day, immediately prior to afternoon physical therapy sessions. Rehabilitation precautions include non-weight-bearing on the right stump. The patient's current drugs include pain medication as needed.

Rehabilitation Setting: The patient is very motivated to return to his prior level of function and has been participating in rehabilitation therapy twice per day since the first day of admission. During the first week of rehabilitation, the patient met each therapy goal regarding edema control, stump maintenance, stretching, strengthening, and pregait activities. He was making remarkable gains in therapy, until 5 days after he started IV sodium stibogluconate. His energy level began declining, and he has been unable to complete an hourly physical therapy session. Today, while exercising in the parallel bars, he had to sit down

twice secondary to dizziness. He complains of severe hip and knee pain, as well as gluteal, quadriceps, and back muscle soreness. Although some of the patient's complaints may be due to his vigorous participation in rehabilitation, the therapist notes that some symptoms may be adverse effects of the drug therapy for cutaneous leishmaniasis. The therapist encourages the patient that these symptoms are likely to dissipate once the full course of drug therapy has ended. The patient states that the drug treatment "has been far worse than these little sores." He states his intention to tell the doctor that he is no longer going to take the prescribed medication, so that he can "get on with rehab."

Problem/Clinical Options: The physician should be notified of the patient's symptoms, as well as their limiting impact on physical rehabilitation goals. Over half of patients receiving IV sodium stibogluconate experience fatigue, arthralgias, and myalgias. While symptoms necessitate interruption of treatment in only a small percentage of cases, these side effects are generally reversible. First, the patient should be educated about the cost to benefit ratio of continuing drug therapy. Untreated cutaneous leishmaniasis lesions can leave large, unsightly scars. In some cases, localized skin infections can spread to the mouth or nose (mucosal leishmaniasis) and cause potentially disfiguring scars. Second, attempts should be made to schedule therapy sessions as far apart from IV drug sessions as possible to determine whether adverse effects are attenuated during therapy sessions. Finally, the therapist can encourage and reassure the patient that the drug therapy is limited to a maximum of 20 days, and that the distressing symptoms will likely not persist or interfere with long-term rehabilitation goals.

PREPARATIONS AVAILABLE

Antifungal Agents

Amphotericin B
Parenteral:
Conventional formulation (Amphotericin B, Fungizone): 50-mg powder for injection
Lipid formulations:
(Abelcet): 100 mg/20 mL suspension for injection
(AmBisome): 50-mg powder for injection
(Amphotec): 50-, 100-mg powder for injection
Topical: 3% cream, lotion, ointment

Butaconazole (Femstat, Mycelex-3)
Topical: 2% vaginal cream

Butenafine (Mentax)
Topical: 1% cream

Caspofungin (Cancidas)
Parenteral: 50-, 70-mg powder for injection

Clotrimazole (Lotrimin, others)
Topical: 1% cream, solution, lotion; 100-, 200-mg vaginal suppositories

Econazole (Spectazole)
Topical: 1% cream

Fluconazole (Diflucan)
Oral: 50-, 100-, 150-, 200-mg tablets; powder for 10, 40 mg/mL suspension
Parenteral: 2 mg/mL in 100- and 200-mL vials

Flucytosine (Ancobon)
Oral: 250-, 500-mg capsules

Griseofulvin (Grifulvin, Grisactin, Fulvicin P/G)
Oral microsize: 125-, 250-mg capsules; 250-mg tablets, 125 mg/5 mL suspension
Oral ultramicrosize[1]: 125-, 165-, 250-, 330-mg tablets

Itraconazole (Sporanox)
Oral: 100-mg capsules; 10 mg/mL solution
Parenteral: 10 mg/mL for IV infusion

Ketoconazole (generic, Nizoral)
Oral: 200-mg tablets
Topical: 2% cream, shampoo

Miconazole (Micatin, others)
Topical: 2% cream, powder, spray; 100-, 200-mg vaginal suppositories

Naftifine (Naftin)
Topical: 1% cream, gel

Natamycin (Natacyn)
Topical: 5% ophthalmic suspension

Nystatin (generic, Mycostatin)
Oral: 500,000-unit tablets
Topical: 100,000 units/g cream, ointment, powder; 100,000 units vaginal tablets

Oxiconazole (Oxistat)
Topical: 1% cream, lotion

Sulconazole (Exelderm)
Topical: 1% cream, lotion

Terbinafine (Lamisil)
Oral: 250-mg tablets
Topical: 1% cream, gel

Terconazole (Terazol 3, Terazol 7)
Topical: 0.4%, 0.8% vaginal cream; 80-mg vaginal suppositories

Tioconazole (Vagistat-1)
Topical: 6.5% vaginal ointment

Tolnaftate (generic, Aftate, Tinactin)
Topical: 1% cream, gel, solution, aerosol powder

Voriconazole (Vfend)
Oral: 50-, 200-mg tablets
Parenteral: 200-mg vials, reconstituted to a 5 mg/mL solution

Antiparasitic Agents

Albendazole (Albenza)
Oral: 200-mg tablets

Atovaquone (Mepron)
Oral: 750 mg/5 mL suspension

Atovaquone-proguanil (Malarone)
Oral: 250 mg atovaquone + 100 mg proguanil tablets; pediatric 62.5 mg atovaquone + 25 mg proguanil tablets

Chloroquine (generic, Aralen)
Oral: 250-, 500-mg tablets (equivalent to 150, 300 mg base, respectively)
Parenteral: 50 mg/mL (equivalent to 40 mg/mL base) for injection

Clindamycin (generic, Cleocin)
Oral: 75-, 150-, 300-mg capsules; 75 mg/5 mL suspension
Parenteral: 150 mg/mL for injection

Dehydroemetine[2]

Doxycycline (generic, Vibramycin)
Oral: 20-, 50-, 100-mg capsules; 50-, 100-mg tablets; 25 mg/5 mL suspension; 50 mg/5 mL syrup
Parenteral: 100, 200 mg for injection

Eflornithine (Ornidyl)
Parenteral: 200 mg/mL for injection

Halofantrine (Halfan)
Oral: 250-mg tablets

Iodoquinol (Yodoxin)
Oral: 210-, 650-mg tablets

Mefloquine (generic, Lariam)
Oral: 250-mg tablets

Melarsoprol (Mel B)[2]

Metronidazole (generic, Flagyl)
Oral: 250-, 500-mg tablets; 375-mg capsules; extended-release 750-mg tablets
Parenteral: 5 mg/mL

Nifurtimox[2]

Nitazoxanide (Alinia)
Oral: powder for 100 mg/5 mL oral solution

Paromomycin (Humatin)
Oral: 250-mg capsules

Pentamidine (Pentam 300-, Pentacarinat, pentamidine isethionate)
Parenteral: 300-mg powder for injection

Primaquine (generic)
Oral: 26.3 mg (equivalent to 15 mg base) tablet

Pyrimethamine (Daraprim)
Oral: 25-mg tablets

Quinidine gluconate (generic)
Parenteral: 80 mg/mL (equivalent to 50 mg/mL base) for injection

Quinine (generic)
Oral: 260-mg tablets; 200-, 260-, 325-mg capsules

Sodium stibogluconate[2]

Sulfadoxine and pyrimethamine (Fansidar)
Oral: 500 mg sulfadoxine plus 25 mg pyrimethamine tablets

Suramin[2]

Anthelmintic Agents

Albendazole (Albenza, Zentel)[3]
Oral: 200-mg tablets; 100 mg/5 mL suspension

Bithionol (Bitin)[4]
Oral: 200-mg tablets

Diethylcarbamazine (Hetrazan)[4]
Oral: 50-mg tablets

Ivermectin (Mectizan, Stromectol)[5]
Oral: 3-, 6-mg tablets

Levamisole (Decaris, Ethnor, Ketrax, Solaskil)
Oral: 50-, 150-mg tablets and syrup

Mebendazole (generic, Vermox)
Oral: 100-mg chewable tablets; outside the United States, 100 mg/5 mL suspension

Metrifonate (trichlorfon, Bilarcil)[6]
Oral: 100-mg tablets

Niclosamide (Niclocide)[6]
Oral: 500-mg chewable tablets

Oxamniquine (Vansil, Mansil)
Oral: 250-mg capsules; outside the United States, 50mg/mL syrup

Oxantel pamoate (Quantrel)[6]; oxantel/pyrantel pamoate (Telopar)[6]

Oral: tablets containing 100 mg (base) of each drug; suspensions containing 20 or 50 mg (base) per mL

Piperazine (generic, Vermizine)

Oral: piperazine citrate tablets equivalent to 250 mg of the hexahydrate; piperazine citrate syrup equivalent to 500 mg of the hexahydrate per 5 mL

Praziquantel (Biltricide; others outside the United States)

Oral: 600-mg tablets (other strengths outside the United States)

Pyrantel pamoate (Antiminth, Combantrin, Pin-rid, Pin-X)

Oral: 50 mg (base)/mL suspension; 62.5 mg (base) capsules (available without prescription in the United States)

Suramin (Bayer 205, others)[4]

Parenteral: ampules containing 0.5- or 1-g powder to be reconstituted as a 10% solution and used immediately

Thiabendazole (Mintezol)

Oral: 500-mg chewable tablets; suspension, 500 mg/mL

[1]Ultramicrosize formulations of griseofulvin are approximately 1.5 times more potent, milligram for milligram, than the microsize preparations.

[2]Available in the United States only from the Drug Service, CDC, Atlanta (404-639-3670).

[3]Albendazole is approved in the United States for the treatment of cysticercosis and hydatid disease.

[4]Not marketed in the United States but is available from the Parasitic Disease Drug Service, Centers for Disease Control and Prevention, Atlanta: 404-639-3670.

[5]Approved for use in the United States for the treatment of onchocerciasis and strongyloidiasis. See Chapter 1 for comment on the unlabeled use of drugs.

[6]Not available in the United States.

REFERENCES

Antifungal Agents

Diekema DJ, et al: Activities of caspofungin, itraconazole, posaconazole, ravuconazole, voriconazole, and amphotericin B against 448 recent clinical isolates of filamentous fungi. *J Clin Microbiol* 2003;41:3623.

Groll A, et al: Clinical pharmacology of systemic antifungal agents: A comprehensive review of agents in clinical use, current investigational compounds, and putative targets for antifungal drug development. *Adv Pharmacol* 1998;44:343.

Herbrecht R, et al: Voriconazole versus amphotericin B for primary therapy of invasive aspergillosis. *N Engl J Med* 2002;347:408.

McPhee SJ, Papadakis MA, Tierney LM Jr: *2007 Current Medical Diagnosis & Treatment*, 46th ed. New York: McGraw-Hill, 2007.

Rezabek GH, Friedman AD: Superficial fungal infections of the skin: Diagnosis and current treatment recommendations. *Drugs* 1992;43:674.

Saag MS, Dismukes WE: Azole antifungal agents: Emphasis on new triazoles. *Antimicrob Agents Chemother* 1988;32:1.

Sarosi GA, Davies SF: Therapy for fungal infections. *Mayo Clin Proc* 1994;69:1111.

Vazquez JA: The safety of anidulafungin. *Expert Opin Drug Saf* 2006;5(6):751.

Wagner C, et al: The echinocandins: comparison of their pharmacokinetics, pharmacodynamics and clinical applications. *Pharmacology* 2006;78(4):161.

Wong-Beringer A, et al: Lipid formulations of amphotericin B. Clinical efficacy and toxicities. *Clin Infect Dis* 1998;27:603.

Antiparasitic Agents

General

Drugs for parasitic infections. *Med Lett Drugs Ther* 2002;44:33. (Issue available at www.medicalletter.com/freedocs/parasitic.pdf.)

Rosenblatt JE: Antiparasitic agents. *Mayo Clin Proc* 1999; 74:1161.

Malaria

Adjuk M, et al: Amodiaquine-artesunate versus amodiaquine for uncomplicated *Plasmodium falciparum* malaria in African children: A randomised, multicentre trial. *Lancet* 2002;359:1365.

Bindschedler M, et al: Comparison of the cardiac effects of the antimalarials coartemether and halofantrine in healthy participants. *Am J Trop Med Hyg* 2002;66:293.

Dorsey G, et al: Sulfadoxine/pyrimethamine alone or with amodiaquine or artesunate for treatment of uncomplicated malaria: A longitudinal randomised trial. *Lancet* 2002;360:2031.

Foley M, Tilley L: Quinoline antimalarials: mechanisms of action and resistance and prospects for new agents. *Pharmacol Ther* 1998;79:55.

Guerin PJ, et al: Malaria: Current status of control, diagnosis, treatment, and a proposed agenda for research and development. *Lancet Infect Dis* 2002;2:564.

Hill DR, et al: Primaquine: Report from CDC expert meeting on malaria chemoprophylaxis I. *Am J Trop Med Hyg* 2006;75(3):402.

Ling J, et al: Randomized, placebo-controlled trial of atovaquone/proguanil for the prevention of *Plasmodium falciparum* or *Plasmodium vivax* malaria among migrants to Papua, Indonesia. *Clin Infect Dis* 2002;35:825.

Mutabingwa T, et al: Chlorproguanil-dapsone for treatment of drug-resistant falciparum malaria in Tanzania. *Lancet* 2001;358:1218.

Nosten F, Brasseur P: Combination therapy for malaria. *Drugs* 2002;62:1315.

Olliaro P: Mode of action and mechanisms of resistance for antimalarial drugs. *Pharmacol Ther* 2001;89:207.

Price R, et al: Adverse effects in patients with acute falciparum malaria treated with artemisinin derivatives. *Am J Trop Med Hyg* 1999;60:547.

Ridley RG: Medical need, scientific opportunity and the drive for antimalarial drugs. *Nature* 2002;415:686.

Rosenthal PJ (ed): *Antimalarial Chemotherapy: Mechanisms of Action, Resistance, and New Directions in Drug Discovery.* Totowa, NJ: Humana Press, 2001.

Staedke SG, et al: Amodiaquine, sulfadoxine/pyrimethamine, and combination therapy for treatment of uncomplicated falciparum malaria in Kampala, Uganda: a randomised trial. *Lancet* 2001;358:368.

Sulo J, et al: Chlorproguanil-dapsone versus sulfadoxine-pyrimethamine for sequential episodes of uncomplicated falciparum malaria in Kenya and Malawi: A randomised clinical trial. *Lancet* 2002;360:1136.

van Agtmael MA, et al: Artemisinin drugs in the treatment of malaria: From medicinal herb to registered medication. *Trends Pharmacol Sci* 1999;20:199.

van Vugt M, et al: Artemether-lumefantrine for the treatment of multidrug-resistant falciparum malaria. *Trans R Soc Trop Med Hyg* 2000;94:545.

Winstanley P: Modern chemotherapeutic options for malaria. *Lancet Infect Dis* 2001;1:242.

Amebiasis

Blessmann J, Tannich E: Treatment of asymptomatic intestinal *Entamoeba histolytica* infection. *N Engl J Med* 2002;347:1384.

Freeman CD, et al: Metronidazole: A therapeutic review and update. Drugs 1997;54:679.

Petri WA, Singh U: Diagnosis and management of amebiasis. *Clin Infect Dis* 1999;29:1117.

Other Protozoal Infections

Aronson NE, et al: Safety and efficacy of intravenous sodium stibogluconate in the treatment of leishmaniasis: Recent U.S. military experience. *Clin Infect Dis* 1998;27:1457.

Burchmore RJ, et al: Chemotherapy of human African trypanosomiasis. *Curr Pharm Des* 2002;8:256.

Burri C, et al: Efficacy of new, concise schedule for melarsoprol in treatment of sleeping sickness caused by *Trypanosoma brucei gambiense:* A randomised trial. *Lancet* 2000;355:1419.

Castro JA, et al: Toxic side effects of drugs used to treat Chagas' disease (American trypanosomiasis). *Hum Exp Toxicol* 2006;25(8);471.

Croft SL, Yardley V: Chemotherapy of leishmaniasis. *Curr Pharm Des* 2002;8:319.

Guerin PJ, et al: Visceral leishmaniasis: Current status of control, diagnosis, and treatment, and a proposed research and development agenda. *Lancet Infect Dis* 2002;2:494.

Hepburn NC: Management of cutaneous leishmaniasis. *Curr Opin Infect Dis* 2001;14:151.

Katz DE, Taylor DN: Parasitic infections of the gastrointestinal tract. *Gastroenterol Clin North Am* 2001;30:797.

Legros D, et al: Treatment of human African trypanosomiasis—present situation and needs for research and development. *Lancet Infect Dis* 2002;2:437.

Nitazoxanide (Alinia)—a new antiprotozoal agent. *Med Lett Drugs Ther* 2003;45:29.

Okhuysen PC: Traveler's diarrhea due to intestinal protozoa. *Clin Infect Dis* 2001;33:110.

Sobel JD, et al: Tinidazole therapy for metronidazole-resistant vaginal trichomoniasis. *Clin Infect Dis* 2001; 33:1341.

Sundar S, et al: Oral miltefosine for Indian visceral leishmaniasis. *N Engl J Med* 2002;347:1739.

Urbina JA: Specific treatment of Chagas disease: Current status and new developments. *Curr Opin Infect Dis* 2001;14:717.

Anthelmintic Drugs

Anadol D, et al: Treatment of hydatid disease. *Paediatr Drugs* 2001;3:123.

Ayles HM, et al: A combined medical and surgical approach to hydatid disease: 12 years' experience at the Hospital for Tropical Diseases, London. *Ann R Coll Surg Engl* 2002;84:100.

Bockarie MJ, et al: Mass treatment to eliminate filariasis in Papua New Guinea. *N Engl J Med* 2002;347:1841.

Burnham G: Onchocerciasis. *Lancet* 1998;351:1341.

Carpio A: Neurocysticercosis: An update. *Lancet Infect Dis* 2002;2:751.

Caumes E: Treatment of cutaneous larva migrans. *Clin Infect Dis* 2000;30:811.

Cioli D: Chemotherapy of schistosomiasis: An update. *Parasitol Today* 1998;14:418.

Drugs for parasitic infections. *Med Lett Drugs Ther* 2002;44:33. Issue available at http://www.medicalletter.com/freedocs/parasitic.pdf

Dunyo SK, et al: A randomized double-blind placebo-controlled field trial of ivermectin and albendazole alone and in combination for the treatment of lymphatic filariasis in Ghana. *Trans R Soc Trop Med Hyg* 2000; 94:205.

Forrester JE, et al: Randomized trial of albendazole and pyrantel in symptomless trichuriasis in children. *Lancet* 1998;352:1103.

Garcia HH, Del Brutto OH: *Taenia solium* cysticercosis. *Infect Dis Clin North Am* 2000;14:97.

Gardon J, et al: Effects of standard and high doses of ivermectin on adult worms of *Onchocerca volvulus*: a randomised controlled trial. *Lancet* 2002;360:203.

Horton J: Albendazole: A review of anthelmintic efficacy and safety in humans. *Parasitology* 2000;121:S113.

Jackson TF, et al: A comparison of mebendazole and albendazole in treating children with *Trichuris trichiura* infection in Durban, South Africa. *S Afr Med J* 1998;88:880.

Stephenson I, Wiselka M: Drug treatment of tropical parasitic infections: recent achievements and developments. *Drugs* 2000;60:985.

Rehabilitation

Aronson NE, et al: Safety and efficacy of intravenous sodium stibogluconate in the treatment of leishmaniasis: Recent U.S. military experience. *Clin Infect Dis* 1998;27:1457.

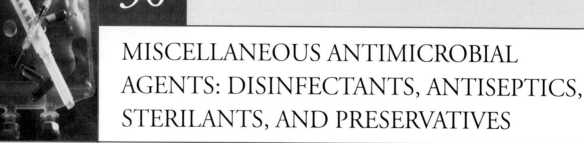

30

MISCELLANEOUS ANTIMICROBIAL AGENTS: DISINFECTANTS, ANTISEPTICS, STERILANTS, AND PRESERVATIVES

The agents discussed in this chapter include miscellaneous antimicrobials, including those specific for urinary infections, and disinfectants and antiseptics (Figure 30–1). Because physical therapists often treat patients with infections and use equipment that can potentially transfer pathogens, the use of antiseptics and disinfectants discussed in the latter half of the chapter is particularly relevant to rehabilitation practice.

MISCELLANEOUS ANTIMICROBIAL AGENTS

Metronidazole

Chemistry and Pharmacokinetics
Metronidazole is a nitroimidazole drug used primarily in treating infections caused by anaerobic bacteria and protozoa. Metronidazole can be administered orally, intravenously, or by rectal suppository. The drug penetrates readily into almost all tissues, including the cerebrospinal fluid, achieving levels similar to plasma.

Mechanism of Action and Clinical Uses
Metronidazole kills amoebae, bacteria, and sensitive protozoans. The drug is readily taken up by anaerobic organisms and cells, where it acts by disrupting DNA and inhibiting nucleic acid synthesis. Metronidazole is the treatment of choice for anaerobic or mixed intra-abdominal infections, pseudomembranous colitis, and brain abscess involving susceptible organisms. Metronidazole may be used in treating anaerobic infections such as might be present in empyema, lung abscess, bone and joint infections, and diabetic foot ulcers. In the treatment of diabetic lower extremity infections in older males, once-daily use of metronidazole combined with another antibiotic has been shown to be as effective as the traditional antibiotic regimen given every 6 hours with significantly less associated cost. Metronidazole is also used to treat infections caused by *Clostridium difficile*, a gram-positive bacillus that can precipitate pseudomembranous colitis, which is clinically manifested as severe diarrhea (*C difficile*–associated diarrhea, CDAD). *C difficile* is one of the most rapidly increasing communicable infections, possibly exceeding methicillin-resistant *Staphylococcus aureus* (MRSA) and other drug-resistant microorganisms.

Metronidazole has many other uses. As an oral tablet or topical vaginal gel, it effectively treats bacterial vaginosis. As part of a multidrug regimen, metronidazole is commonly used in the eradication of *Helicobacter pylori* in peptic ulcer disease. As an antiprotozoal drug, metronidazole is the drug of choice for treating giardiasis (traveler's diarrhea) and the common sexually

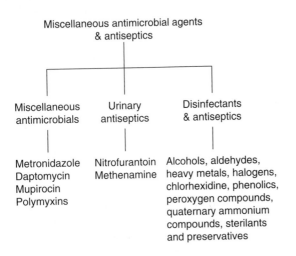

Figure 30–1. These agents are divided into miscellaneous antimicrobials, those specific for urinary infections and disinfectants and antiseptics. Subsequent divisions are based on chemical class or clinical use.

transmitted disease trichomoniasis. Metronidazole is also used as a topical antibiotic for the chronic dermatologic condition rosacea.

Toxicity

The most common adverse effects include nausea or vomiting, gastrointestinal discomfort, diarrhea, headache, dizziness, dry mouth, and altered taste sensation (especially the perception of a sharp metallic taste). Because metronidazole has a disulfiram-like effect, drinking alcoholic beverages while taking metronidazole can cause stomach pain, nausea, vomiting, headache, and flushing of the face. Patients should be instructed to avoid alcohol (including alcohol-containing cough syrups) while taking this drug and for at least 3 days after discontinuing treatment.

Daptomycin

Chemistry, Mechanism of Action, and Pharmacokinetics

Daptomycin is a member of one of the newer classes of antibiotics called cyclic lipopeptides. Daptomycin's structure promotes rapid bactericidal effects via a unique mechanism. By insertion of its lipophilic tail into the bacterial cell membrane, daptomycin causes loss of intracellular potassium, depolarizes the bacterial membrane potential, and results in rapid bacterial cell death. Daptomycin is administered by slow intravenous infusion for the treatment of complicated skin and soft tissue infections due to aerobic gram-positive organisms. Since daptomycin is primarily excreted by the kidneys, dose reductions are required in patients with renal impairment.

Clinical Uses

Daptomycin is effective against most clinically relevant gram-positive bacteria, including infections due to MRSA, vancomycin-resistant *S aureus* (VRSA), and vancomycin-resistant enterococcus (VRE). Daptomycin has also proven effective for *S aureus* bacteremia and endocarditis.

Toxicity

Mild adverse effects include nausea and vomiting, constipation, diarrhea, headache, dizziness, and injection site reactions. During daptomycin treatment, a small but significant percentage of patients develop myopathies (generalized muscle pain, cramps, or weakness) associated with elevations in creatine kinase. Thus, patients given daptomycin should be monitored for skeletal muscle dysfunction and creatine kinase elevation and coadministration with 3-hydroxy-3-methylglutaryl coenzyme A (HMG-CoA) reductase inhibitors ("statins") should be avoided. In addition, transitory paresthesias and peripheral neuropathies have been reported.

Mupirocin

Mechanism of Action and Clinical Uses

Mupirocin (pseudomonic acid A) is an antibiotic originally isolated from the gram-negative bacterium *Pseudomonas fluorescens*. By binding to bacterial isoleucyl transfer-RNA synthetase, mupirocin prevents isoleucine incorporation into bacterial proteins, thus inhibiting bacterial protein synthesis.

Mupirocin is formulated as a topical ointment and indicated for the treatment of secondarily infected traumatic skin lesions and minor skin infections such as impetigo caused by gram-positive bacteria (e.g., *S aureus*, beta-hemolytic streptococci and *Streptococcus pyogenes*). With direct application of mupirocin to the skin or mucous membranes, high local concentrations are achieved. Use of an occlusive dressing following application increases penetration 5- to 10-fold, but the absorbed amount has been estimated to be <0.24% of the applied amount. Systemic absorption of mupirocin through intact skin is minimal; however, any drug reaching the systemic circulation is rapidly metabolized to an inactive metabolite that is eliminated by renal excretion. Most drug elimination is via desquamation of skin cells rather than metabolism.

Nasal carriage of *S aureus* (both methicillin-susceptible and methicillin-resistant strains) is a well-defined risk factor for subsequent nosocomial infection in hospitalized patients. Thus, intranasal application of mupirocin has been used for the elimination of *S aureus* in patients and health-care workers. However, prolonged and widespread mupirocin use is associated with the development of mupirocin resistance. Judicious use of topical mupirocin, including limiting treatment to carriers and considering other treatment regimens, should be emphasized.

Adverse Effects

The most common adverse side effects are local erythema, rash, stinging, and itching. In addition, prolonged usage may result in overgrowth of nonsusceptible organisms, including fungi.

Polymyxins

Mechanism of Action and Clinical Uses

The polymyxins are a group of cationic detergent antibiotics that kill gram-negative bacteria by disrupting the bacterial cell membrane. Owing to significant toxicity associated with systemic administration, the polymyxins are primarily used topically, but have also been used for irrigation of wounds and the urinary bladder. Ointments or drops containing **polymyxin B** in combination with **neomycin** and **hydrocortisone** are often used for eye or ear infections. Over-the-counter topical formulations including polymyxin B with neomycin and/or bacitracin are commonly used for infected superficial skin lesions.

Toxicity

If systemic absorption occurs, serious adverse effects include neurotoxicity (dizziness, ataxia, paresthesias) and nephrotoxicity (acute renal tubular necrosis).

URINARY TRACT ANTISEPTICS

The urinary tract is one of most common sites of bacterial infection, especially among women. Urinary tract antiseptics such as nitrofurantoin and methenamine are oral drugs that lack systemic antibacterial effects because of their rapid metabolism. Because these drugs are excreted into the urine in high enough concentrations to inhibit urinary pathogens, they are useful drugs for the treatment of acute lower urinary tract infections (UTIs) as well as prevention of recurrent UTIs. Urine pH is monitored before starting and throughout therapy because the agents' effectiveness is increased at low pH (<5.5), and low pH is an independent inhibitor of bacterial growth in urine. Thus, these drugs are often administered with urine-acidifying agents such as a protein-rich diet with cranberry juice. In addition, patients are instructed to avoid eating most fruits (especially citrus fruits and juices) and dairy products, which tend to alkalinize the urine. Nitrofurantoin and methenamine are bactericidal for many gram-positive and gram-negative bacteria, although they have no activity against urea-splitting gram-negative bacteria (*Proteus* or *Pseudomonas* species), because these organisms increase urinary pH and thereby decrease the drugs' effectiveness. Both nitrofurantoin and methenamine have the advantage that resistance rarely or slowly develops in susceptible bacterial populations.

Nitrofurantoin

When used to treat uncomplicated acute UTI, the normal adult daily dose of nitrofurantoin is 50 to 100 mg taken four times daily for at least 1 week. For prevention of chronic UTIs, a single 100-mg daily dose may be taken.

Nitrofurantoin should be taken with food to improve drug absorption and to decrease adverse gastrointestinal effects such as vomiting, nausea, and anorexia. In addition to gastrointestinal irritation, skin rashes and photosensitivity are common side effects. Patients should also be informed that nitrofurantoin colors the urine dark yellowish orange or brown, which is a normal and harmless side effect.

Nitrofurantoin may cause hemolytic anemia in patients with glucose-6-phosphate dehydrogenase

(G6PD) deficiencies. This deficiency is the most common human enzymopathy; it is found in roughly 10% of African Americans and 60% of Kurdish Jews. Hemolytic anemia may also occur in neonates with immature enzyme systems within the red blood cells. For this reason, nitrofurantoin is contraindicated in women in the last month of pregnancy (38 to 42 weeks' gestation), in nursing mothers, and in neonates less than 1 month of age.

Peripheral neuropathies have been reported, and may be more likely in patients with renal impairment, diabetes mellitus, and vitamin B deficiency. Progressive pulmonary interstitial pneumonitis and fibrosis have been reported when nitrofurantoin has been given over longer periods of time (≥6 months). Because nitrofurantoin is primarily excreted by the kidneys, urinary concentrations in patients with renal impairment may be subtherapeutic. In patients with severe renal insufficiency, nitrofurantoin is contraindicated because high blood levels may cause toxicity. Finally, in patients with diabetes mellitus, nitrofurantoin may cause inaccurate results with some urine glucose tests.

Methenamine

Methenamine mandelate and methenamine hippurate are methenamine salts. When combined with urine acidification, methenamine acts as a weak base that hydrolyzes in acidic urine to form ammonia and formaldehyde. Urinary formaldehyde may be bactericidal or bacteriostatic depending on urinary pH, volume, and flow. Methenamines may be used in the treatment of UTIs in patients with intermittent catheterization, but they are not effective in patients with indwelling urinary catheters. Both methenamine salts are commonly used for the prevention of UTIs, although evidence regarding their effectiveness in UTI prophylaxis is mixed and may be dependent on patient population. The methenamines should not be taken concurrently with sulfonamide antibacterials because insoluble precipitates may form and increase the likelihood of crystalluria.

DISINFECTANTS, ANTISEPTICS, STERILANTS, AND PRESERVATIVES

Although the terms are often used interchangeably, disinfectants and antiseptics have specific definitions (Table 30–1). Disinfectants are chemical agents that inhibit or kill various microorganisms on nonliving objects in the environment (Table 30–2). They should not be used on living tissue. Antiseptics inhibit microorganism growth and reproduction on inanimate objects, but they are also safe enough to be used on the surfaces of living tissue, such as skin. Notably, disinfectants and antiseptics do not have selective toxicity; each agent displays a different microbicidal profile that must be considered for appropriate and effective use. Sterilization refers to the use of physical or chemical means to destroy all microbial life, including highly resistant bacterial endospores.

Disinfection involves the destruction of infective organisms by physical or chemical means (Table 30–2),

Table 30–1.	Commonly used terms related to chemical and physical killing of microorganisms
Antisepsis	Application of an agent to living tissue for the purpose of preventing infection
Decontamination	Destruction or marked reduction in number or activity of microorganisms
Disinfection	Chemical or physical treatment that destroys most vegetative microbes or viruses, but not spores, in or on inanimate surfaces
Sanitization	Reduction of microbial load on an inanimate surface to a level considered acceptable for public health purposes
Sterilization	A process intended to kill or remove all types of microorganisms, including spores, and usually including viruses with an acceptable low probability of survival
Pasteurization	A process that kills nonsporulating microorganisms by hot water or steam at 65–100°C

Table 30–2.   Activities of disinfectants

	Bacteria				Viruses		Other		
	Gram-positive	Gram-negative	Acid-fast	Spores	Lipophilic	Hydrophilic	Fungi	Amebic cysts	Prions
Alcohols (isopropanol, ethanol)	HS	HS	S	R	S	V	—	—	R
Aldehydes (glutaraldehyde, formaldehyde)	HS	HS	MS	S (slow)	S	MS	S	—	R
Chlorhexidine gluconate	HS	MS	R	R	V	R	—	—	R
Sodium hypochlorite, chlorine dioxide	HS	HS	MS	S (pH 7.6)	S	S (at high conc)	MS	S	MS (at high conc)
Hexachlorophene	S (slow)	R	R	R	R	R	R	R	R
Povidone, iodine	HS	HS	S	S (at high conc)	S	R	S	S	R
Phenols, quaternary ammonium compounds	HS	HS	MS	R	S	R	—	—	R
Strong oxidizing agents, cresols	HS	MS to R	R	R	S	R	R	R	R

HS = highly susceptible; S = susceptible; MS = moderately susceptible; R = resistant; V = variable; — = no data.

reducing the number of potentially infective organisms either by killing, removing, or diluting them. Disinfection is often accomplished by ionizing radiation or dry or moist heat.

The ideal disinfectant would be able to kill all pathogenic microorganisms without harming healthy human tissue. Since the ideal disinfectant does not exist, a combination of agents is often used (e.g., addition of a disinfectant to a detergent), and the choice of which to use depends on the particular situation.

Washing, which dilutes and partially removes potentially infectious organisms, and the use of barriers (e.g., gloves, condom, respirator), which prevent pathogens from gaining entry into the host, are foremost in infection prevention and control.

Hand washing is the single most important way to prevent transmission of pathogens from person to person or from regions of higher microbial load (e.g., mouth, nose, gut) to potential sites of infection. Although hand washing with soap and water effectively removes and dilutes most infectious agents, skin disinfectants are added to detergents for preoperative surgical cleansing of the surgeon's hands and the patient's surgical incision site. To minimize irritation, dryness, and skin sensitization, regular hand washing should be done without disinfectants. In addition, for regular hand washing, it may be preferable to create conditions that are inhospitable to bacterial reproduction rather than to kill bacteria with disinfectants. Because of their rapid reproduction rate, it is possible that survival of bacteria following an antiseptic challenge may result in increased propagation of strains of antiseptic-resistant bacteria. For this reason, the wisdom of the current trend of adding antibacterial agents to regular hand soap and impregnated cloths and fabrics may be questioned.

Appropriate Choice of a Disinfectant, Antiseptic, or Sterilant

The choice of antiseptic, disinfectant, or sterilant (or combination) depends on several factors including, but not limited to, risk of infection associated with the use of each agent, intrinsic resistance of the microorganism,

number of microorganisms present (microbial load), mixed populations of organisms, amount of organic material present (e.g., blood, feces, tissue), stability and concentration of agent, time and temperature of exposure, pH, and hydration and binding of the agent to surfaces.

As noted, disinfectants, antiseptics, and sterilants do not have selective toxicity. Every agent has more or less marked cytotoxic properties. For cleansing wounds, antiseptics are often avoided because they interfere with wound healing. Thus, both the patient and health-care professionals must consider the short-term and long-term toxicity of each agent. The Environmental Protection Agency (EPA) regulates disinfectants and sterilants and the Food and Drug Administration (FDA) regulates antiseptics. Major classes of antiseptics, disinfectants, and sterilants are described below.

Alcohols

The most frequently used alcohols for treatment table disinfection and skin antisepsis are **ethanol** and **isopropyl alcohol (isopropanol)**. Alcohols rapidly kill vegetative bacteria, *Mycobacterium tuberculosis,* and many fungi. Alcohol's biocidal effects are due to its ability to dehydrate cells, disrupt membranes, and coagulate proteins. Exposure to 70 to 80% ethanol or isopropanol (by volume in water) for at least 5 minutes is the best practice for optimal surface and skin disinfection. These high-concentration alcohol mixtures also quickly and effectively inactivate HIV and hepatitis B and C viruses on surfaces. Alcohols are not considered sterilants because they do not inactivate spores, penetrate protein-containing organic material, or inactivate hydrophilic viruses. In addition, rapid evaporation prevents alcohols from having a lasting residual action. Alcohols are useful in situations in which access to running water and soap is limited (e.g., home care setting). To limit their skin-drying effect, emollients are often added to hand-use antiseptic formulations. Because of alcohols' flammability, they should be used and stored in cool and well-ventilated areas. Their complete evaporation must be allowed before use of any flame, cautery, or lasers.

Aldehydes

Formaldehyde and **glutaraldehyde** (sometimes called cold sterilants) are used for high-level disinfection or sterilization of medical instruments that cannot tolerate exposure to the high temperatures required for steam sterilization (autoclaving). Thus, they are used for sterilizing plastic and rubber and equipment that cannot be autoclaved. By cross-linking proteins and nucleic acids, aldehydes inactivate a broad spectrum of microorganisms and viruses. Aldehyde disinfection or sterilization may fail if dilutions are below effective concentrations, if organic material is present, or if the liquid formulation is unable to penetrate into crevices in medical instruments. For this last reason, circulating baths can be used to increase penetration of aldehyde solutions, while decreasing exposure of the operator to irritating fumes.

Formaldehyde is available as a 40% weight/volume solution in water (100% formalin). At a concentration of 8%, formaldehyde exhibits a broad spectrum of activity against bacteria, bacterial toxins, spores, viruses, and fungi. Destruction of spores may take up to 18 hours, but the speed of action may be increased by solution in 70% alcohol. Alcohol probably strips protective lipids, allowing formaldehyde better access to the pathogen. Formalin is used for high-level disinfection of hemodialyzers, preparation of vaccines, and embalming of tissues.

A 2% glutaraldehyde solution is activated by alkali for use as a broad-spectrum disinfectant. Specific applications for its use include disinfecting respiratory therapy equipment, physical therapy whirlpool tubs, and dialysis treatment equipment. Glutaraldehyde is found in commonly used products such as Cidex, Hospex, and Sonacide. While glutaraldehyde has greater sporicidal activity than formaldehyde, it may not be as effective at killing *M tuberculosis*. Once activated by alkali, glutaraldehyde begins to polymerize. Thus, its activated shelf life is about 2 weeks. Test strips are available to measure activity.

Formaldehyde and glutaraldehyde are highly irritating to the skin, eye, and respiratory tract even at low levels for short periods. Formaldehyde gas has a distinctive, pungent, and irritating odor that is detectable even at extremely low concentrations (<1 ppm). The Occupational Safety and Health Administration (OSHA) has declared that formaldehyde is a potential carcinogen and has established an exposure standard that limits the 8-hour time-weighted exposure of employees to 0.75 ppm (permissible exposure limit [PEL]). However, for sensitized individuals, odor may not be an adequate indicator of the presence of formaldehyde and may not provide a reliable warning of hazardous concentrations. Because it is slightly heavier than air, vapors can result in asphyxiation in poorly ventilated, enclosed, or low-lying areas. Glutaraldehyde solutions are pale yellow liquids with a rotten-apple odor. Although OSHA does not currently have a required PEL for glutaraldehyde, the National Institute for Occupational Safety and Health (NIOSH) has established a recommended exposure limit of 0.2 ppm. There are several ways to minimize or limit occupational exposure to the aldehydes, including ensuring the agents are used in fume hoods with exhaust ventilation, using only enough to perform required disinfecting procedure, avoiding skin contact by use of personal protective equipment (PPE) such as gloves, goggles, face shields, and respirators. Gloves should be made of nitrile or butyl rubber because latex gloves do not provide adequate protection.

Heavy Metals

For many years, heavy metal salts were used as antiseptics and disinfectants because of their ability to denature proteins. Most heavy metal ion preparations are now considered to be too toxic for routine use. However, **mercury** and **silver** still have a limited number of applications.

Mercury is an environmental hazard, and many strains of bacteria have developed resistance to mercurials. While the use of mercury-containing preservatives has declined in recent years because of an increasing awareness of the theoretic potential for neurotoxicity, **thimerosal** is still used as a preservative (0.001 to 0.004%) in numerous biologic and drug products, including immune sera, antitoxins, and certain vaccines. Notably, thimerosal was removed from or reduced to trace amounts in all vaccines routinely recommended for children ≤6 years of age except for influenza vaccines. **Mercurochrome**, generically known as merbromin, was a popular topical antiseptic for years. In 1998, the FDA declared merbromin "not generally recognized as safe and effective" because of concerns about its mercury content. Although distribution has effectively been discontinued in the United States, it is still available in most other countries.

Inorganic silver salts are strongly bactericidal. Bacterial (and probably fungal) silver sensitivity relates to silver's ability to irreversibly denature key enzyme systems. Silver exhibits low toxicity in humans, with minimal expected risk from clinical exposure by dermal applications or through urologic and hematogenous routes. **Silver sulfadiazine** (1%) is a widely used safe and effective topical cream used to help prevent gram-positive and gram-negative bacterial colonization of burned skin and tissues. Physical therapists should be aware that a blue-black pseudoeschar forms over the wound surface that must be removed before more cream is applied or wound healing will be hindered.

Over the past 5 years, silver has undergone a renaissance as a topical antibacterial agent in wound healing. It is incorporated into virtually all classes of wound dressings. The popularity of silver-based antimicrobial dressings may be due to new formulations allowing slow and sustained release of silver, newer research indicating that colonized wounds display delayed wound healing, and aggressive manufacturer marketing. The majority of in vivo studies indicate that silver dressings decrease wound bioburden and may be effective against antibiotic-resistant organisms (e.g., *Staphylococcus*, *Pseudomonas*, *Enterococcus*); however, bacterial resistance may occur. Although some evidence suggests that silver retards wound epithelialization, the majority of in vivo evidence suggests that silver is not cytotoxic to viable cells.

Halogens (Iodine, Iodophors, Chlorine)

Iodine and Iodophors

Iodine antiseptics have a wide spectrum of antimicrobial and antiviral activity. Thus far, microorganisms appear unable to develop resistant strains to iodine. Iodine in a 1:20,000 solution is bactericidal within one minute and sporicidal within 15 minutes. It is usually used in an alcohol solution called tincture of iodine as a preoperative antiseptic for intact skin. Although iodine preparations are effective bactericidals, many studies have demonstrated some degree of cytotoxicity, impaired wound healing, and reduced wound strength. In addition, iodine use is decreasing because of serious hypersensitivity reactions and its propensity to stain clothing and dressings.

Iodophors are mixtures of iodine with solubilizing agents such as surfactants or povidone. Iodophor topical solutions release free iodine, but are more gentle to the skin, less likely to provoke hypersensitivity reactions, and less likely to stain fabric than tincture of iodine. Although they maintain germicidal action, the effectiveness of any iodophor depends on the percentage of released free iodine. They may be used as antiseptics or disinfectants, with the latter containing more free iodine. The most common iodophor is **povidone-iodine (polyvinylpyrolidone [PVP])**; marketed as Betadine. Povidone itself has no germicidal action; it controls the release of the inorganic iodine. Povidone-iodine is widely used for cleaning dirty wounds, scrubbing surgeons' hands, and patients' intact preoperative surgical site. Povidone iodine has not been proven to be effective for decontaminating medical equipment.

Chlorine

When chlorine dissolves in water, hypochlorous acid is produced. Chlorine is a fairly universal and inexpensive disinfectant. It is found most commonly as a 5.25% sodium hypochlorite solution in the form of common household bleach. Depending on the concentration, **sodium hypochlorite** is effective against most common pathogens, including HIV, tuberculosis, hepatitis B and C, fungi, antibiotic-resistant strains of staphylococci, and enterococci. The Centers for Disease Control and Prevention (CDC) recommends a 1:10 dilution of 5.25% household bleach (5000 ppm of available chlorine) for disinfecting blood spills. At this concentration, most pathogens and spores are killed or inactivated. The exception is that a concentration range of 1,000 to 10,000 ppm is required to kill mycobacteria. In a recent review of 33 studies, sodium hypochlorite was effective for sterilization at a concentration of 5000 ppm for 5 minutes and for disinfection at 1000 ppm for 10 minutes. Dilutions of sodium hypochlorite in water (pH 7.5 to 8.0) will retain antimicrobial activity for months if kept in tightly closed opaque containers. However, frequent opening and closing markedly reduces its efficacy.

Because chlorine is inactivated by blood, serum, feces, and protein-containing materials, organic material must be removed from the surface to be disinfected prior to use of sodium hypochlorite. Thus, bleach is an excellent disinfectant, but a poor cleaner. After cleaning, a 1:10 solution is effective simply by being wiped on and left to dry. Extreme caution must be taken not to combine sodium hypochlorite with either ammonia or with any acid because irritating chlorine gas evolves. If sodium hypochlorite solution contacts a product containing formaldehyde, a carcinogenic compound results. The best practice is not to add anything to sodium hypochlorite except water. Sodium hypochlorite solutions are caustic to the skin and eyes, so users should wear rubber gloves and—if ventilation is not ideal—goggles. Sodium hypochlorite solutions are corrosive to aluminum, silver, and stainless steel.

Chlorhexidine

Chlorhexidine gluconate is a water-soluble antiseptic whose bacteriostatic and bactericidal properties arise from its ability to disrupt bacterial membranes. It is more effective against gram-positive cocci and mycobacteria and less effective against gram-negative rods. It also has moderate activity against fungi and viruses. Chlorhexidine inhibits spore germination (unlike alcohol-based antiseptics), and is effective in the presence of blood and organic materials (unlike sodium hypochlorite).

One of the primary uses of chlorhexidine is as an oral mouthwash used in the prevention and treatment of gingivitis. This application may be appropriate in patients who cannot independently or adequately brush their teeth because it provides up to 24 hours of antimicrobial activity. Nondental uses for chlorhexidine include preoperative skin preparation and antiseptic hand wash (Hibiclens: 4% chlorhexidine gluconate) against MRSA. Chlorhexidine is inactivated by anionic and nonionic compounds found in many mouthwashes, toothpastes, soaps, and moisturizers. Chlorhexidine mouth rinses should be used approximately

2 hours after use of other dental products. Likewise, hand moisturizers or soaps should not be used after hand washing with chlorhexidine immediately prior to patient care. Because chlorhexidine binds strongly to the skin and mucosa, it has significant residual activity; it inhibits the proliferation or survival of microorganisms after application. Often, low concentrations (0.5% to 1.0%) of chlorhexidine are added to alcohol-based hand-washing preparations to increase the residual activity of alcohol alone. Chlorhexidine is safe for cleansing the skin of adults and infants, and has a low potential for eliciting skin sensitivity. Although uncommon, skin irritation is concentration dependent, so products containing 4% chlorhexidine are the most likely to cause skin reactions with frequent use. Eye contact should be avoided because it can cause corneal damage.

Phenolics

Phenol was the first disinfectant to be used in clinical medical practice. Although effective, it is highly corrosive, toxic upon absorption, and carcinogenic. Many less toxic derivatives of phenol have been developed. Among the most popular are hexachlorophene and chlorhexidine (discussed above).

Phenolic disinfectants are commonly used for hard surface decontamination in hospitals (e.g., floors, counters, beds). Phenolics are bactericidal (including mycobacteria), fungicidal, and capable of inactivating many viruses such as HIV and herpes simplex types 1 and 2. Phenolics do not destroy spores.

Because of its bacteriostatic properties (especially against *S aureus*), **hexachlorophene** was widely used as an antiseptic hand wash in hospitals. It has residual activity for several hours after use and gradually reduces bacterial counts on hands after repetitive use. However, with repeated use, hexachlorophene is absorbed through the skin. In 1972, the FDA warned that hexachlorophene should not be used routinely to bathe infants because of its potential neurotoxic effects. Hexachlorophene should not be used to bathe patients with burns or extensive areas of sensitive skin. Soaps containing 3% hexachlorophene are available by prescription only, and routine use of hexachlorophene is generally not recommended for hand antisepsis.

Peroxygen Compounds

When used at appropriate concentrations, the peroxygen compounds, **hydrogen peroxide** and **peracetic acid**, are useful as disinfectants and sterilants. Their advantages include effectiveness against a wide variety of organisms (bacteria, yeast, fungi, viruses, and spores) and the fact that their decomposition products (oxygen and water) are nontoxic. The primary disadvantage is a rather short-lived antimicrobial effect.

Hydrogen peroxide's killing ability is due to the hydroxyl radical, which is one of the strongest oxidants known. It is an effective disinfectant when used for inanimate objects with low water content. Anaerobes are most sensitive because they do not produce catalase, which breaks down peroxide. In the home, hydrogen peroxide can be found in diluted form (3% to 10%), whereas industrial uses involve concentrated solutions (30% or greater). Hydrogen peroxide is not stable; it must be protected from light and kept in a cool place because light and heat exposure cause degradation. Hydrogen peroxide is used to disinfect surfaces such as respirators, plastic eating utensils, and soft contact lenses. To be an effective sporicidal, concentrations of 10 to 25% are required. Dilute hydrogen peroxide is used as a mouthwash to help control plaque, although it has not been proven to be effective in critically ill patients. Finally, hydrogen peroxide was previously used in first aid kits to disinfect and debride wounds. When applied to a wound, hydrogen peroxide combines with catalase produced in tissues, decomposing into oxygen and water and producing effervescence. It was rationalized that this process helped loosen necrotic or inorganic material that might inhibit wound healing. However, hydrogen peroxide damages healthy cells (keratinocytes and fibroblasts) required for wound healing. Thus, hydrogen peroxide is no longer recommended for wound care.

Peracetic acid is a mixture of hydrogen peroxide and acetic acid in a watery solution. Since it is explosive in pure form, it is used in dilute solution and transported in vented containers to prevent increased pressure as oxygen is released. As with hydrogen peroxide, the hydroxyl radical released from peracetic acid is the lethal species. Peracetic acid is a stronger bactericidal and sporicidal agent than hydrogen peroxide. At room temperature, 250 to 500 ppm peractic acid is effective against most bacteria when applied to contaminated surfaces for 5 minutes. Destruction of spores is increased with both a rise in temperature and an increase in concentration (500 to 300,000 ppm). Effectiveness is slightly decreased by the presence of organic matter, but can be maintained by an increase in concentration. Peracetic acid may be formulated as a liquid spray or mop-on solution. Automatic sterilization systems using low concentrations of peracetic acid (0.1% to 0.5%) have been designed to sterilize medical and dental instruments.

Quaternary Ammonium Compounds

Quaternary ammonium compounds ("quats") are cationic surface-active detergents widely used in hospitals for disinfection of noncritical hard surfaces such as bench tops and floors. They are most likely to be encountered by health-care workers in central supply, housekeeping, and patient and surgical services areas. **Benzalkonium chloride** is the most widely used quat antiseptic. Other quats used as antiseptics are **cetrimide, cetylpyridium chloride**, and **benzethonium chloride**.

Quaternary ammonium compounds are mostly bacteriostatic, sporistatic, and fungistatic, although they are microbicidal against certain pathogens at higher concentrations. Antimicrobial activity probably involves cell membrane disruption. They are ineffective against mycobacteria and gram-negative bacteria. In addition, their antimicrobial activity is antagonized by the presence of organic material, soaps, many nonionic detergents, and calcium, magnesium, ferric, and aluminum ions. Several strains of *S aureus* have recently been described with genetic resistance to quaternary ammonium compounds. Because contamination of stock solutions with gram-negative rods can be a problem, the CDC has recommended that benzalkonium chloride and other similar quaternary ammonium compounds not be used as antiseptics.

Sterilants

When all microbial life, including highly resistant bacterial endospores, must be destroyed, sterilization is required. Sterility is an absolute term meaning there are no relative degrees of sterility. Sterilization can be performed by physical or chemical means. During chemical sterilization, sterilants are applied to materials for appropriate times and temperatures.

The recommended sterilization for biohazardous material is autoclaving—the use of pressurized steam at a temperature of 120°C for a minimum of 30 minutes. Autoclaving medical and surgical instruments can only be done when these materials do not contain plastic or rubber. In the latter case, gas sterilization may be performed. Although few gases are able to kill microbes, ethylene oxide gas is a highly effective disinfectant, and kills spores rapidly. Widespread use of ethylene oxide is limited by its extreme flammability, its cost, and its classification as a mutagen and carcinogen. OSHA's permissible exposure level for ethylene oxide is 1 ppm as a time-weighted measure. Alternative sterilants are increasingly being employed, such as vapor phase hydrogen peroxide, peracetic acid, ozone, gas plasma, chlorine dioxide, formaldehyde, and propylene oxide.

Preservatives

Preservatives are required to prevent microbial growth and contamination in many pharmaceutical, cosmetic, and therapy-related products in multiple-use containers such as ultrasound gel or friction massage cream. The ideal preservative must be effective against a broad spectrum of microorganisms, soluble, stable, and non-irritating to tissues to which they are applied.

Commonly used preservatives include **benzoic acid** and salts, **parabens, sorbic acid** and salts, **propylene glycol,** phenolic compounds, quaternary ammonium salts, alcohols, and mercurials such as thimerosal. To inhibit *S aureus* and *Escherichia coli*, the concentration of propylene glycol must exceed 10%. At this concentration, propylene glycol is a skin sensitizer. Although rare, cases of contact dermatitis from preservatives in ultrasonic gels have been reported. Healthcare professionals should investigate the type and concentration of preservative in any product prior to patient application.

▉ REHABILITATION FOCUS

Physical therapists, like all health-care workers, should follow standard precautions with all patients regardless of their infection status. These practices include routine hand washing before and after contact with each patient and hand drying with clean one-use towels, wearing appropriate PPE (e.g., gloves, gown, eyewear) when treating patients with whom there is potential contact with blood, mucous membranes, or other body fluids. If a specific diagnosis of a transmissible infection has been made, therapists should follow facility guidelines regarding additional precautions that need to be taken based on how the infection is transmitted.

Since physical therapists treat multiple patients with therapy-related equipment, ensuring that this equipment is not an infection reservoir or transport vehicle is of the utmost importance. Therapists must evaluate all equipment and ask how each item can be safely disinfected between each patient.

Although following product recommendations for disinfection of equipment is a straightforward policy, the type of disinfectant chosen is often facility dependent, and disinfection procedures are chosen based upon the frequency of encountering specific pathogens. In outpatient clinics, individual treatment tables and mats can be protected with clean single-use sheets. Between patients, these surfaces should then be wiped down with a broad-spectrum spray disinfectant active against many fungi, viruses, and strains of *Streptococcus* and *Staphylococcus* (e.g., Matt-Kleen, Whizzer). In hospital settings, multiple patient use therapy equipment such as walkers, crutches, and canes must also be disinfected, with careful attention being paid to hand-gripping surfaces and, if possible, a broader-spectrum disinfectant should be used.

The epidemiology of *C difficile* infection provides an important example. It has been shown that patients receiving rehabilitation services in a hospital setting have a 2.6-fold higher chance of developing *C difficile*–associated diarrhea (CDAD), a potentially fatal infection, compared to patients not receiving such services. However, appropriate infection control measures can decrease the incidence of CDAD by 50%. Preventing the spread of *C difficile* spores among patients in institutional settings requires isolation of the *C difficile*–infected patient, use of barrier precautions, appropriate hand hygiene, and use of appropriate sporicidal agents on environmental surfaces. Physical therapists should reduce the increased incidence of CDAD associated with rehabilitation by hand washing with soap and water since alcohol-based hand cleaners do not eradicate *C difficile*. In addition, therapy-related equipment and other hard environmental surfaces that have come in contact with *C difficile*–infected patients should be disinfected with bleach for approximately 10 to 15 minutes to inactivate spores.

In situations in which patients have been identified as having a readily transmissible pathogen, therapists must follow isolation precautions. Ideally, therapy equipment should be dedicated to that particular patient. If equipment must be used with other patients (e.g., whirlpool, ultrasound), consult facility infection control policies regarding what type of disinfectant must be used to eradicate the particular pathogen. If appropriate disinfection cannot take place inside the patient's room, discuss with infection control specialists at the facility regarding the safest way to transport equipment to the location where it can be cleaned to decrease the potential of transmitting infection en route.

Health-care professionals should understand the advantages and disadvantages of each antiseptic or disinfectant in order to choose the most appropriate agent for a given application. It is critical that health-care professionals always ask patients about potential sensitivities to agents, and that therapists recognize signs and symptoms of allergy or sensitivities to agents. Inhibiting or destroying pathogens must be performed while providing adequate protection for the patient and the health-care professional. When wound care is a component of a patient's treatment, the therapist must apply knowledge regarding the potential (e.g., in vitro) or demonstrated effect of antiseptics on the wound-healing process.

Before selecting an antiseptic or disinfectant or working in an environment where these agents are used, the therapist should answer several questions: (1) What are the active ingredients in the agents used in the rehabilitation environment (e.g., quaternary ammonium compounds, phenolics, chlorine bleach, iodine products)? (2) Against which microorganisms

is the agent effective? (3) Is it safe for daily use? (4) Should PPE be worn and what type? (5) Are permissible exposure levels set by OSHA or NIOSH? (6) What conditions must be met for the agent to be the most effective antimicrobial? (7) Will it damage surfaces cleaned with it? (8) Is it safe to mix with another agent to maximize antibacterial effectiveness? (9) Is it a "one-step" disinfectant-cleaner or a disinfectant? (e.g., chlorhexidine vs sodium hypochlorite)? (10) What is the cost of the product?

Finally, product instructions for dilution ratio must always be followed carefully for safety and effectiveness. Inappropriate choice, concentration, or application of any disinfectant or antiseptic agent may result in unsuccessful antimicrobial efficacy, compromised safety, or both.

■ CLINICAL RELEVANCE FOR REHABILITATION

Adverse Drug Reactions

Some of the antimicrobial drugs described in this chapter have potential adverse effects that may negatively impact a patient's rehabilitation progress. Each of the disinfectants and antiseptics discussed also has unique disadvantages. Adverse or potentially toxic reactions or sensitivities to these agents may affect the patient, and also the physical therapist using or coming into contact with them.

Miscellaneous antimicrobial agents
- Dizziness is a common adverse effect of metronidazole and daptomycin.
- Myopathies may occur with daptomycin.
- Peripheral neuropathies may occur with daptomycin and nitrofurantoin.
- Nitrofurantoin may produce inaccurate results in some urine glucose tests.

Disinfectants, antiseptics, sterilants, and preservatives
- Alcohols and chlorhexidine can produce excessive drying of the skin, especially when used frequently. Alcohols are very flammable.
- Silver allergy is a contraindication for using any silver-impregnated or silver-based wound-care product.

- Iodine and iodophors have varying degrees of cytotoxicity depending on the concentration of free iodine. Some patients have allergic reactions to iodine; they often report this as "seafood allergy."
- Sodium hypochlorite (bleach) is inactivated by organic material. In addition, bleach emits unpleasant odors and reacts with other chemicals to create toxic gases.
- Hydrogen peroxide damages healthy keratinocytes and fibroblasts.
- Some preservatives have the potential to act as skin sensitizers.

Effects Interfering with Rehabilitation

Miscellaneous antimicrobial agents

- Dizziness may limit patients' ability to change positions and their ability to participate in aerobic exercise.
- Myopathies may present as muscle pain or decreased muscle strength. Symptoms depend on the severity of the myopathy as well as which muscle groups are involved. Difficulty rising from chairs, climbing or descending stairs, getting out of the bathtub, shaving, and brushing hair suggests proximal muscle weakness. Difficulties with handwriting and grasp indicate distal muscle weakness.
- Peripheral neuropathies may be purely sensory or mixed sensorimotor, manifested by numbness, tingling, pinprick sensation (paresthesias) in fingers and toes, and possibly muscle weakness.
- Some glucose urine tests (e.g., Clinitest) cannot be used as a marker for glucose urine concentration for patients taking nitrofurantoin.

Disinfectants, antiseptics, sterilants, and preservatives

- Excessive skin dryness due to habitual use of alcohols or chlorhexidine can lead to skin irritation or breakdown.
- The flammability of alcohol-based hand antiseptics limits their use to cool, well-ventilated areas free of sparks or flames. This may prevent their use during certain home-based rehabilitation treatments.
- Use of silver-impregnated wound-care products should be avoided in individuals with an allergy or sensitivity to silver.

- Iodine and iodophors impair wound healing and reduce wound strength and may cause serious hypersensitivity reactions.
- To disinfect a surface effectively, body fluids must be removed prior to the use of sodium hypochlorite, creating twice the work for the health-care professional responsible for cleaning and disinfecting biologic spills. Prior to choosing bleach for disinfection, the therapist must also determine whether the chemical used to clean the area is safe to use with sodium hypochlorite.
- Hydrogen peroxide inhibits wound healing.
- Quaternary ammonium compounds and chlorhexidine are rendered ineffective in the presence of soaps and many nonionic detergents.
- Many products commonly used in the rehabilitation setting such as ultrasound gel and friction massage cream contain preservatives that have the potential to cause allergic skin reactions such as contact dermatitis.

Possible Therapy Solutions

Miscellaneous antimicrobial agents

- To prevent loss of balance, patients should be advised not to change positions abruptly, and therapists should provide more assistance in transfers and gait as needed.
- Patient complaints of paresthesias or weakness should be thoroughly evaluated and symptoms and signs reported to the attending physician. Therapists should be alert to the greater likelihood of peripheral neuropathies in patients with renal impairment or diabetes mellitus. Any patient taking daptomycin who complains of muscle pain or presents with muscle weakness should be reported to the physician for possible assessment of elevated creatine phosphokinase levels.
- Diabetic patients taking nitrofurantoin should be advised to use blood glucose monitoring to measure blood glucose levels. If urine monitoring is necessary, urine tests that are not affected by nitrofurantoin (e.g., Clinistix or Tes-Tape) should be used.

Disinfectants, antiseptics, sterilants, and preservatives

- Avoid hand moisturizers after washing hands with chlorhexidine because moisturizing agents antagonize chlorhexidine's antimicrobial properties. For therapists who consistently use alcohol-based hand antiseptics, choose products with added emollients rather than separate hand creams to ameliorate the skin-drying effect. Hand creams can often act as vectors for pathogens.

- When using alcohol-based antiseptics or disinfectants, therapists should ensure that the agent has completely evaporated before the use of any equipment that could potentially create a spark.

- In patients with chronic wounds, therapists should inquire about any known allergies or sensitivities to silver prior to the use of silver-impregnated wound-care products or silver sulfadiazine cream. In addition, therapists should recognize and report any adverse reaction to the attending physician and ensure that the patient's medical record reflects the silver allergy or sensitivity since many wound care and medical products contain silver.

- Iodine, iodophors, and hydrogen peroxide should not be used to disinfect or debride wounds.

- Alcohol-based disinfectants are reasonably inexpensive and safe and can be used if the corrosive effects of bleach are to be avoided. These agents should be used to disinfect treatment tables and rehabilitation equipment between every patient. In the presence of organic material, chlorhexidine is still an effective disinfectant. If sporicidal effects are required, an additional disinfectant must be chosen since chlorhexidine is only sporistatic.

- Physical therapists must know the ingredients in products applied to patients' skin. They must inquire whether patients have known sensitivities or allergies to specific preservatives, be able to recognize skin reactions, and discontinue use appropriately.

PROBLEM-ORIENTED PATIENT STUDY

Brief History: The patient is a 64-year-old female with type I diabetes mellitus since age 10. She was admitted to the hospital 10 days ago for wound care of a neuropathic right foot ulcer infected with MRSA. Prior to admission, she was independent with all activities of daily living (ADLs), transfers, and ambulation without an assistive device.

Current Medical Status and Drugs: At admission, the patient was treated with vancomycin to treat the MRSA infection. After 3 days, the ulcer appeared to be worsening, and it was also determined that the *S aureus* infection was resistant to vancomycin. On day 4 after admission, vancomycin was discontinued and the patient was started on daily intravenous daptomycin. Rehabilitation precautions include no weight bearing (NWB) on the right lower extremity. Patient's current drugs include insulin and daptomycin.

Rehabilitation Setting: The patient has been participating in rehabilitation therapy twice a day since the second day of her admission. On evaluation, the therapist noted decreased strength in bilateral upper and lower extremities (4/5). The patient required moderate assistance for transfer from bed to chair. She was able to ambulate 20 feet with a front-wheeled walker with moderate assistance for balance and maintenance of NWB status on the right lower extremity. For the first 7 days of therapy, the patient made consistent gains in strength and ambulation. She was able to transfer independently and ambulate over 200 feet with a front-wheeled walker with standby assistance. Yesterday, when the therapist arrived at the patient's room, the patient complained of muscle aches and pains and declined therapy. Today, the patient requires minimal assistance to transfer from a chair to standing in the walker because of leg weakness. She declines further therapy today because of persistent muscle pain and cramping.

Problem/Clinical Options: Onset of muscle pain and weakness 7 days into rehabilitation therapy without an abrupt progression in exercise program signals another possible source for the patient's

PROBLEM-ORIENTED PATIENT STUDY (*Continued*)

complaints. The patient's complaints of muscle pain began 5 days after she began intravenous daptomycin for treatment of the infected foot ulcer. Although not common, the adverse effect profile for daptomycin includes reports of myopathy, characterized by generalized muscle pain, cramps, or weakness. Because the patient has had diabetes for more than 50 years,

it is likely that she also has some renal impairment, which may increase the likelihood for adverse effects since daptomycin is primarily excreted by the kidneys. The therapist should report these muscular symptoms to the physician immediately. If the myopathy was induced by daptomycin, it should resolve after daptomycin is discontinued.

PREPARATIONS AVAILABLE

Miscellaneous Antimicrobial Drugs

Methenamine hippurate (Hiprex, Urex)
Oral: 1.0-g tablets

Methenamine mandelate (generic)
Oral: 0.5-, 1-g tablets; 0.5 g/5 mL suspension

Metronidazole (generic, Flagyl)
Oral: 250-, 500-mg tablets; 375-mg capsules; 750-mg extended-release tablets
Parenteral: 5 mg/mL; 500 mg for injection

Mupirocin (Bactroban)
Topical: 2% ointment, cream

Nitrofurantoin (Macrodantin, generic)
Oral: 25-, 50-, 100-mg capsules, 25 mg/5 mL suspension

Polymyxin B (Polymyxin B Sulfate)
Parenteral: 500,000 units per vial for injection
Ophthalmic: 500,000 units per vial

Disinfectants, Antiseptics, and Sterilants

Benzalkonium (generic, Zephiran)
Topical: 17% concentrate; 50% solution; 1:750 solution

Benzoyl peroxide (generic)
Topical: 2.5%, 5%, 10% liquid; 5%, 5.5%, 10% lotion; 5%, 10% cream; 2.5%, 4%, 5%, 6%, 10%, 20% gel

Chlorhexidine gluconate (Hibiclens, Hibistat, others)
Topical: 2%, 4% cleanser, sponge; 0.5% rinse in 70% alcohol
Oral rinse (Peridex, Periogard): 0.12%

Glutaraldehyde (Cidex)
Instruments: 2%, 3.2% solution

Hexachlorophene (pHisoHex)
Topical: 3% liquid; 0.23% foam

Iodine aqueous (generic, Lugol's Solution)
Topical: 2–5% in water with 2.4% sodium iodide or 10% potassium iodide

Iodine tincture (generic)
Topical: 2% iodine or 2.4% sodium iodide in 47% alcohol, in 15, 30, 120 mL and in larger quantities

Nitrofurazone (generic, Furacin)
Topical: 0.2% solution, ointment, and cream

Ortho-phthalaldehyde (Cidex OPA)
Instruments: 0.55% solution

Oxychlorosene sodium (Clorpactin)
Topical: 2 g powder for solution for irrigation, instillation, or rinse

Povidone-iodine (generic, Betadine)
Topical: available in many forms, including aerosol, ointment, antiseptic gauze pads, skin cleanser (liquid or foam), solution, and swabsticks

Silver nitrate (generic)
Topical: 10%, 25%, 50% solution

Thimerosal (generic, Mersol)
Topical: 1:1000 tincture and solution

REFERENCES

Miscellaneous Antimicrobial Agents and Urinary Antiseptics

Aslam S, Musher DM: An update on diagnosis, treatment, and prevention of *Clostridium difficile*-associated disease. *Gastroenterol Clin North Am* 2006;35(2):315.

Clay PG, et al: Clinical efficacy, tolerability, and cost savings associated with the use of open-label metronidazole plus ceftriaxone once daily compared with ticarcillin/clavulanate every 6 hours as empiric treatment for diabetic lower-extremity infections in older males. *Am J Geriatr Pharmacother* 2004;2(3):181.

Edwards DI: Nitroimidazole drugs—action and resistance mechanisms. (Two parts.) J Antimicrob Chemother 1993;31:9, 201.

Fowler VG, et al: Daptomycin versus standard therapy for bacteremia and endocarditis caused by *Staphylococcus aureus*. *N Engl J Med* 2006;355(7):653.

Larson E: Guidelines for use of topical antimicrobial agents. *Am J Infect Dis Control* 1988;16:233.

Lee B, et al: Methenamine hippurate for preventing urinary tract infections. *Cochrane Database Syst Rev* 2002; 1:CD003265.

McDonald LC, et al: Clostridium difficile infection in patients discharged from US short-stay hospitals 1996–2003. *Emerg Infect Dis* 2006;12:409.

Schiotz HA, Guttu K: Value of urinary prophylaxis with methenamine in gynecologic surgery. *Acta Obstet Gynecol Scand* 2002;81(8):743.

Scully BE: Metronidazole. *Med Clin North Am* 1988; 72:623.

Disinfectants, Antiseptics, and Sterilants

Ascenzi JM (ed): *Handbook of Disinfectants and Antiseptics*. New York: Marcel Dekker, 1996.

Best M, et al: Efficacies of selected disinfectants against *Mycobacterium tuberculosis*. *J Clin Microbiol* 1990; 28:2234.

Bischoff WE, et al: Handwashing compliance by health-care workers: The impact of introducing an accessible, alcohol-based hand antiseptic. *Arch Intern Med* 2000;160:1017.

Block SS (ed): *Disinfection, Sterilization and Preservation*, 5th ed. Philadelphia: Lippincott Williams & Wilkins, 2001.

Brett DW: A discussion of silver as an antimicrobial agent: Alleviating the confusion. *Ostomy Wound Manage* 2006;52(1):34.

Doebbing BN, et al: Comparative efficacy of alternative handwashing agents in reducing infections in intensive care units. *N Engl J Med* 1992;327:88.

Fraise AP: Susceptibility of antibiotic-resistant cocci to biocides. *J Appl Microbiol* 2002;92 Suppl:158S.

Gardner JF, Peel MM: *Introduction to Sterilization, Disinfection and Infection Control*, 3rd ed. Churchill Livingston, 1997.

Guideline for Hand Hygiene in Health-Care Settings: *Morbidity and Mortality Recomm Rep* 2002; 51(RR-16):1.

Johnson PD, et al: Efficacy of an alcohol/chlorhexidine hand hygiene program in a hospital with high rates of nosocomial methicillin-resistant *Staphylococcus aureus* (MRSA) infection. *Med J Aust* 2005; 183(10):509.

Kaye ET, Kaye KM: Topical antibacterial agents. *Infect Dis Clin North Am* 1995;9:547.

Kramer SA: Effect of povidone-iodine on wound healing: A review. *J Vasc Nurs* 1999;17(1):17.

Lansdown AB: Silver in health care: Antimicrobial effects and safety in use. *Curr Probl Dermatol* 2006;33:17–34.

Lewis DL, Arens M: Resistance of microorganisms to disinfection in dental and medical devices. *Nat Med* 1995;1:956.

Maki DG, et al: Prospective randomized trial of povidone-iodine, alcohol and chlorhexidine for prevention of infection associated with central venous and arterial catheters. *Lancet* 1991;338:339.

Moorer WR: Antiviral activity of alcohol for surface disinfection. *Int J Dent Hyg* 2003;1(3):138.

Russell AD: Bacterial spores and chemical sporicidal agents. *Clin Microbiol Rev* 1990;3:99.

Rutala WA, et al: Disinfection practices for endoscopes and other semicritical items. *Infect Control Hosp Epidemiol* 1991;12:282.

Rutula WA: Guidelines for selection and use of disinfectants. *Am J Infect Control* 1990;18:99.

Sopwith, et al: Preventing infection from reusable medical equipment: A systematic review. *BMC Infect Dis* 2002;2:4.

Widmer AF, Frei R: Decontamination, disinfection, and sterilization. In *Manual of Clinical Microbiology,* 7th ed. Murray PR, et al, ed. American Society for Microbiology, 1999.

Rehabilitation

Bartlett JG, Perl TM: The new *Clostridium difficile*—what does it mean? *N Engl J Med* 2005;353:2503.

Buchner AM, Sonnenberg A: Medical diagnoses and procedures associated with clostridium difficile colitis. *Am J Gastroenterol* 2001;96:766.

Eguino P, et al: Allergic contact dermatitis due to propylene glycol and parabens in an ultrasonic gel. *Contact Dermatitis* 2003;48(5):290.

Erdmann SM, et al: Allergic contact dermatitis due to methyldibromoglutaronitrile in EuxylK 400 in an ultrasonic gel. *Contact Dermatitis* 2001;44(1):39.

Loo VG, et al: A predominantly clonal multi-institutional outbreak of *Clostridium difficile*–associated diarrhea with high morbidity and mortality. *N Engl J Med* 2005;353:2442.

Perez J, et al: Activity of selected oxidizing microbicides against the spores of *Clostridium difficile:* Relevance to environmental control. *Am J Infect Control* 2005; 33(6):320.

Schwartz DA, Geyer SJ: Clostridial infections. In *Pathology of Infectious Diseases.* Conner DH, et al, eds. Stamford, CT: Appleton & Lange; 1997;1:517–529.

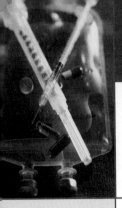

31

CANCER CHEMOTHERAPY

ancer is a disease of cells characterized by a shift in the control mechanisms that govern cell proliferation and differentiation. Cells that have undergone neoplastic transformation often express normal fetal cell surface antigens or display other signs of apparent immaturity. Cancer cells may also exhibit qualitative or quantitative chromosomal abnormalities, including translocations and amplified gene sequences. Cancer cells proliferate excessively and form local tumors that can compress or invade adjacent normal structures. Within local tumors, a small subpopulation of cells can be described as tumor stem cells. These cells retain the ability to undergo repeated cycles of proliferation and can migrate to distant sites in the body to colonize various organs in the process called metastasis. Thus, tumor stem cells can express **clonogenic** (colony-forming) capabilities. Chromosomal abnormalities in tumor stem cells reflect their genetic instability, which leads to progressive selection of subclones that can survive more readily in the host's multicellular environment. Abnormalities in various metabolic pathways and cellular components (e.g., expression of cell-surface drug transporters) accompany neoplastic progression. The invasive and metastatic processes, as well as metabolic abnormalities resulting from the cancer, cause illness and eventual death unless the neoplasm can be eradicated with treatment.

A classification of anticancer drugs is presented in Figure 31–1. Initial division is based on whether the drugs affect DNA (action on DNA and action on mitotic spindle) or modulate hormonal activity (hormonal agents). Drugs affecting DNA may inhibit synthesis or directly damage DNA. As a group, anticancer drugs are more toxic than any other drugs because they act not only on neoplastic cells but also on normal cells that are in dividing or resting states. Therefore, the benefits of anticancer drugs must be carefully weighed against their risks.

CAUSES OF CANCER

The incidence, geographic distribution, and behavior of specific types of cancer are related to multiple factors, including gender, age, genetic make-up, and exposure to environmental carcinogens. Of these, environmental exposure is the only modifiable risk factor. Chemical carcinogens, particularly those in tobacco smoke, as well as azo dyes, aflatoxins, asbestos, and benzene have been clearly implicated in cancer induction in humans and animals. In the laboratory, potential environmental carcinogens can be identified by microbial mutagenesis and animal testing.

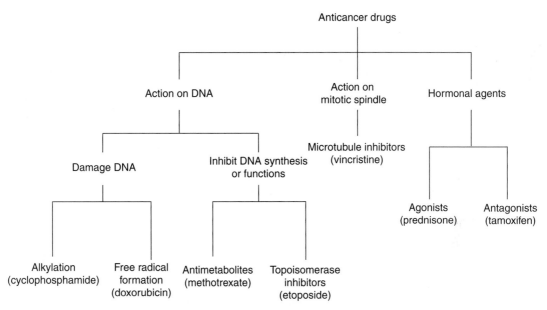

Figure 31–1. Initial classification of anticancer drugs is based on location(s) of action. The first two classes affect DNA or mitosis, whereas the third class modulates hormonal influences on cancer cells. Subsequent divisions of anticancer drugs affecting DNA are based on whether the drug affects DNA directly, or alters DNA synthesis and replication. Drugs that modulate hormonal influence on cancer cells are subsequently divided into agonists or antagonists.

Certain deoxyribonucleic acid (DNA) viruses and type C ribonucleic acid (RNA) viruses have been implicated as cancer-causing (oncogenic) agents in animals and humans. Oncogenic RNA viruses contain a reverse transcriptase that transcribes the RNA of the tumor virus into the DNA code of the infected host cell. In this way, the information governing transformation becomes a stable part of the host cell genome. Expression of virus-induced neoplasia also depends on additional host and environmental factors that modulate the transformation process. Certain cellular genes, known as oncogenes, are homologous to the transforming genes of retroviruses and induce neoplastic transformation. Oncogenes code for specific growth factors and their receptors, and may be amplified (increased number of gene copies) or modified by a single nucleotide polymorphism in malignant cells. Another class of genes, **tumor suppressor genes,** plays an important role in suppressing neoplastic transformation. If a tumor suppressor gene is mutated, deleted, or damaged, neoplastic change is likely to occur. Such changes may be inherited, occur spontaneously, or may be acquired through exposure to exogenous chemicals or radiation.

CANCER THERAPEUTIC MODALITIES

Cancer is the second most common cause of death in the United States, causing over 500,000 fatalities annually. Currently, one-third of cancer patients are cured with local modalities (surgery or radiation therapy), which are quite effective when the tumor has not metastasized by the time of treatment. In the remaining cases, when early micrometastasis is a characteristic feature of the neoplasm, a systemic approach such as chemotherapy is required (often in conjunction with surgery or radiation) for effective cancer management. At present, about 50% of patients with cancer can be cured, with chemotherapy contributing to the cure in 10 to 15% of patients.

CANCER CELL CYCLE KINETICS

Cancer cell cycle kinetics and population kinetics explain, in part, the limited effectiveness of most available anticancer drugs. Figure 31–2 presents a schematic summary of cell cycle kinetics and stages at which particular anticancer drug classes act. This information is relevant to the mode of action, indications, and scheduling of cell cycle–specific drugs (CCS, drugs that are most effective in a particular phase of the cycle) and cell cycle–nonspecific (CCNS, insensitive to the phase of the cell cycle) drugs. Examples of drugs falling into these two major classes are summarized in Table 31–1.

In general, CCS drugs are most effective in hematologic malignancies and in solid tumors in which a relatively large proportion of the cells are proliferating or are in the growth fraction. The growth fraction represents the number of cells within the malignant tumor that are at some stage of division (i.e., other than G_0) compared to the total number of malignant cells (i.e., those in division plus those in G_0) (Figure 31–2). For the growth fraction, the first value is placed in the numerator and the latter value in the denominator. The fraction is then represented as a percentage. The CCNS drugs (many of which bind to and damage cellular DNA) are useful for treating solid tumors with both low and high growth fractions. In all instances, effective agents sterilize (i.e., inactivate) tumor stem cells, which are often only a small fraction of the cells within a tumor. Non–stem cells (i.e., those that have irreversibly differentiated) are considered sterile and are not a significant component of the cancer problem.

RESISTANCE TO ANTICANCER DRUGS

Drug resistance is a major problem in cancer chemotherapy. Mechanisms of resistance include, but are not limited to, the following six examples.

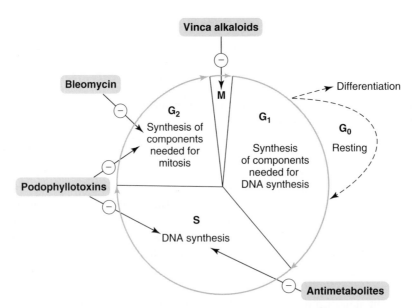

Figure 31–2. Phases of the cell cycle that are susceptible to the actions of cell cycle–specific (CCS) drugs. All dividing cells, normal and neoplastic, traverse these cell cycle phases before and during cell division. CCS drug actions may not be restricted to a specific phase, but tumor cells are usually most responsive to specific drugs (or drug groups) in the phases indicated. Cell cycle–nonspecific (CCNS) drugs act on tumor cells while they are actively cycling and while they are in the resting phase (G_0). G_1, gap or growth; G_2, gap 2; M, mitosis; S, synthesis.

Table 31–1.	Cell cycle specificity of major classes of anticancer drugs	
Cell Cycle–Specific (CCS) Agents	**Cell Cycle–Nonspecific (CCNS) Agents**
Antimetabolites	**Alkylating agents**
Capecitabine	Busulfan
Cladribine	Carmustine
Cytarabine	Cyclophosphamide
Fludarabine	Lomustine
Fluorouracil	Mechlorethamine
Gemcitabine	Melphalan
Mercaptopurine	Thiotepa
Methotrexate	**Anthracyclines**
Thioguanine	Daunorubicin
Antitumor antibiotic	Doxorubicin
Bleomycin	Epirubicin
Podophyllotoxins	Idarubicin
Etoposide	Mitoxantrone
Teniposide	**Antitumor antibiotics**
Taxanes	Dactinomycin
Docetaxel	Mitomycin
Paclitaxel	**Camptothecins**
Vinca alkaloids	Irinotecan
Vinblastine	Topotecan
Vincristine	**Platinum analogs**
Vinorelbine	Carboplatin
	Cisplatin
	Oxaliplatin

1. Cancer cells may increase their rate of DNA repair. This mechanism is particularly important in the case of resistance to alkylating agents.
2. Some tumor cells increase their production of thiol-trapping agents (e.g., glutathione), which inactivate certain anticancer drugs. This mechanism of resistance is seen with several of the alkylating agents and antibiotics.
3. Cancer cells may alter target enzymes. For example, increased synthesis of dihydrofolate reductase and changes in this enzyme are mechanisms of resistance of tumor cells to methotrexate.
4. Cancer cells may decrease conversion of a prodrug into the active form of the drug. Resistance to the purine antimetabolites (mercaptopurine, thioguanine) and the pyrimidine antimetabolites (cytarabine, fluorouracil) can result from decreased activity of tumor cell enzymes required to convert these prodrugs to their cytotoxic metabolites.
5. Cancer cells may increase the inactivation of certain cancer drugs. Increased activity of enzymes capable of inactivating anticancer drugs is a mechanism of tumor cell resistance to most of the purine and pyrimidine antimetabolites.
6. Cancer cells may decrease intracellular drug concentration by increased efflux pump activity. This form of multidrug resistance involves increased expression of a normal gene. For example, MDR1 is a gene that codes for a cell surface P-glycoprotein. As discussed in Chapter 3, this transport protein is normally present in various cells throughout the body. In intestinal cells, the protein is involved in transport of drugs back into the lumen. In some multidrug-resistant malignancies, the activity of this transporter is increased, and the accelerated efflux of many anticancer drugs provides resistance for these cells.

ANTICANCER DRUGS

Alkylating Agents

The alkylating agents include nitrogen mustards (**cyclophosphamide, mechlorethamine**), **nitrosoureas** (**carmustine, lomustine**), and **alkylsulfonates** (**busulfan**). Other drugs that act in part as alkylating agents include **cisplatin, dacarbazine,** and **procarbazine**. The alkylating agents are CCNS drugs. Some are active as given, whereas others are prodrugs that are converted to active metabolites in the body. The reactive molecules covalently bind with one of the four nucleotides in DNA. This binding (alkylation) usually follows intramolecular cyclization in the drug, which creates an intermediate that forms a covalent bond with DNA. When two nucleotides in the double helix DNA are alkylated by the same drug molecule, the two DNA strands are cross-linked. The resulting cross-linked DNA cannot be separated and replicated in mitosis, halting cell division. Alkylating agents may also exert cytotoxic effects by

forming covalent bonds with other cellular constituents such as proteins. Alkylation of DNA also results
in abnormal base pairing and DNA strand breakage.
Several alkylating agents and their acute and delayed
toxicities are listed in Table 31–2. DNA alkylation
probably represents the major interaction that leads

to cell death. Some of the more commonly used alkylating drugs are discussed below.

Cyclophosphamide
Cyclophosphamide is a prodrug that is converted to
one or more highly reactive metabolites by hepatic

Table 31–2.	Alkylating agents and toxicities	
Alkylating Agent	**Acute Toxicity**	**Delayed Toxicity**
Mechlorethamine	Nausea and vomiting, myelosuppression[1]	Moderate depression of peripheral blood count; excessive doses produce severe bone marrow
Chlorambucil	Nausea and vomiting, myelosuppression	depression with leukopenia, thrombocytopenia, and bleeding; alopecia and hemorrhagic cystitis
Cyclophosphamide	Nausea and vomiting, myelosuppression	occasionally occur with cyclophosphamide; cystitis can be prevented with adequate
Melphalan	Nausea and vomiting, myelosuppression	hydration plus mesna[2]; busulfan is associated skin pigmentation, pulmonary fibrosis, and
Thiotepa (triethylenethio- phosphoramide)	Nausea and vomiting, myelosuppression	adrenal insufficiency
Busulfan	Nausea and vomiting, myelosuppression	
Carmustine (BCNU)[3]	Nausea and vomiting	Leukopenia, thrombocytopenia, and rarely hepatitis
Lomustine (CCNU)[3]	Nausea and vomiting	
Altretamine	Nausea and vomiting	Leukopenia, thrombocytopenia, and peripheral neuropathy
Procarbazine	Nausea and vomiting, flu-like syndrome, drug interactions	Bone marrow depression, central nervous system depression, leukemogenic
Dacarbazine	Nausea and vomiting	Bone marrow depression
Cisplatin	Nausea and vomiting, myelosuppression	Nephrotoxicity, peripheral sensory neuropathy, ototoxicity, nerve dysfunction
Carboplatin	Myelosuppression, nausea and vomiting	Rarely: peripheral neuropathy, renal toxicity, and hepatic dysfunction
Oxaliplatin	Nausea and vomiting, laryngopharyngeal dysesthesias	Peripheral sensory neuropathy, diarrhea, myelosuppression, and renal toxicity

[1]Myelosuppression is the depression of bone marrow activity, with reduction of mature blood cells such as erythrocytes, leukocytes, and platelets in the circulating blood.
[2]Mesna prevents urotoxic effects of cyclophosphamide.
[3]If a tumor is resistant to one alkylating agent, it will usually be relatively resistant to other agents of this class except for nitrosoureas such as those presented.

cytochrome P450 enzymes. Clinical uses of cyclophosphamide include non-Hodgkin's lymphoma, breast and ovarian cancers, and neuroblastoma. One advantage of the drug is that it can be taken orally. Toxicities observed with cyclophosphamide include cardiac dysfunction, pulmonary toxicity, and a syndrome of inappropriate antidiuretic hormone release.

Cisplatin, Carboplatin, and Oxaliplatin

These drugs are rarely used alone in cancer chemotherapy, but are included as part of a larger drug treatment regimen. Their mechanism of action is not completely understood, but they are thought to act like alkylating agents. These drugs are used intravenously. They distribute to most tissues and are cleared in unchanged form by the kidney. Cisplatin is commonly used as a component of regimens for cancers of the testicle, bladder, lung, and ovary. Carboplatin has similar uses. Oxaliplatin has activity against colorectal cancer. Their toxicities are listed in Table 31–2. In the case of cisplatin, drug-induced renal damage may be reduced by the use of mannitol (an osmotic diuretic) and forced hydration. Carboplatin and oxaliplatin are less nephrotoxic than cisplatin, but they are more neurotoxic and have greater myelosuppressant actions.

Procarbazine

Procarbazine is orally active and penetrates into most tissues, including the cerebrospinal fluid. The drug is eliminated via hepatic metabolism. Procarbazine forms hydrogen peroxide, which generates free radicals that cause DNA strand scission (breaks). The drug is used as a component of regimens for Hodgkin's disease and non-Hodgkin's lymphomas (common cancers of lymphatic tissue) and for some brain tumors. Procarbazine has multiple toxicities, including peripheral neuropathy and skin reactions. Procarbazine also inhibits many enzymes, including monoamine oxidase and those involved in hepatic drug metabolism. Disulfiram-like reactions have occurred with ethanol.

Other Alkylating Agents

Busulfan is sometimes used in chronic myelogenous leukemia. **Carmustine** and **lomustine** are highly lipid-soluble drugs used as adjuncts in the management of brain tumors. **Dacarbazine** is used in regimens for

Hodgkin's disease. Additional toxicities include skin rash, phototoxicity, and a flu-like syndrome.

Antimetabolites

Antimetabolites used in cancer are structurally similar to endogenous compounds that are important in rapidly dividing cells. They include antagonists of folic acid (**methotrexate**), purines (**mercaptopurine, thioguanine**), and pyrimidines (**fluorouracil, cytarabine**). Antimetabolites are CCS drugs that act primarily in the S phase of the cell cycle (Figure 31–2). Their sites of action on DNA synthetic pathways are shown in Figure 31–3. In addition to cytotoxic effects on neoplastic cells, the antimetabolites also have immunosuppressant effects (Chapter 32). Commonly used antimetabolites and delayed toxicities of these drugs are presented in Table 31–3.

Methotrexate

Both oral and intravenous administration of methotrexate afford good tissue distribution except to the CNS. Methotrexate is not metabolized, and its clearance is dependent on renal function. Adequate hydration is needed to prevent crystallization in renal tubules.

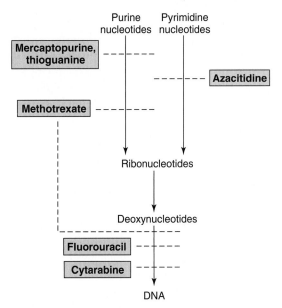

Figure 31–3. Sites of action (*dashed lines*) of antimetabolites on DNA synthetic pathways.

Table 31–3.	Antimetabolites and toxicities

Chemotherapeutic Agent	Delayed Toxicity[1]
Capecitabine	Diarrhea, hand-and-foot syndrome[2], myelosuppression, nausea, and vomiting
Cladribine	Myelosuppression, nausea, vomiting, and immunosuppression
Cytarabine	Nausea, vomiting, bone marrow depression, stomatitis, and cerebellar ataxia
Fludarabine	Myelosuppression, immunosuppression, fever, myalgias, and arthralgias
Fluorouracil (5-FU)	Nausea, mucositis, diarrhea, myelosuppression, hand and foot syndrome, and neurotoxicity
Gemcitabine	Nausea, vomiting, diarrhea, myelosuppression
Mercaptopurine (6-MP)	Myelosuppression, immunosuppression, and hepatotoxicity
Methotrexate (MTX)	Mucositis, diarrhea, bone marrow depression with leukopenia and thrombocytopenia
Thioguanine (6-TG)	Myelosuppression, immunosuppression, and hepatoxicity

[1]These drugs do not cause acute toxicity.
[2]Hand-and-foot syndrome is a form of erythromelalgia manifested as tingling, numbness, pain, erythema, swelling, and increased pigmentation.

Methotrexate acts as an inhibitor of dihydrofolate reductase. This action decreases synthesis of thymidylate, purine nucleotides, and several amino acids, thus interfering with nucleic acid and protein metabolism. The formation of polyglutamate derivatives of methotrexate appears to be important for cytotoxic actions. Tumor cell resistance mechanisms include decreased drug accumulation, changes in the activity of dihydrofolate reductase or its drug sensitivity, and decreased formation of polyglutamates. Clinically, methotrexate is effective in choriocarcinoma, acute leukemias, non-Hodgkin's and cutaneous T-cell lymphomas, and breast cancer. Methotrexate is also used as an immune suppressant in rheumatoid arthritis, psoriasis, and transplant rejection. In combination with mifepristone, it is an effective abortifacient. The most common toxicities are listed in Table 31–3. Long-term use of methotrexate has caused hepatotoxicity and pulmonary infiltrates and fibrosis. Salicylates, nonsteroidal anti-inflammatory drugs, sulfonamides, and sulfonylureas enhance the toxicity of methotrexate.

Mercaptopurine and Thioguanine

Both mercaptopurine (6-MP) and thioguanine (6-TG) have low oral bioavailability because of first-pass metabolism. Mercaptopurine and thioguanine act as purine antimetabolites. Both drugs are activated by hypoxanthine-guanine phosphoribosyltransferases (HGPRTases) to toxic nucleotides that inhibit several enzymes involved in purine metabolism. Resistant tumor cells may have decreased HGPRTase activity, or they may have increased production of alkaline phosphatases that inactivate the toxic nucleotides. Clinical uses of these purine antimetabolites are mainly in the acute leukemias and chronic myelocytic leukemia. Bone marrow suppression is the dose-limiting toxicity. Hepatic dysfunction includes cholestasis, jaundice, and necrosis. The metabolism of 6-MP by xanthine oxidase is inhibited by allopurinol, a drug used in the treatment of gout (Chapter 34).

Fluorouracil

When given intravenously, fluorouracil (5-FU) is widely distributed, including into the cerebrospinal fluid. Elimination is mainly by metabolism. Fluorouracil is converted in cells to 5-fluoro-2'-deoxyuridine-5'-monophosphate, which inhibits thymidylate synthase and leads to "thymineless death" of cells. Resistance mechanisms include decreased activation of

5-FU, increased thymidylate synthase activity, and reduced drug sensitivity of this enzyme. Fluorouracil is used clinically in bladder, breast, colon, head and neck, liver, and ovarian cancers. The drug is also used topically for keratoses and superficial basal cell carcinoma. In addition to the toxicities listed in Table 31–3, alopecia may occur.

Cytarabine

Cytabarine (cytosine arabinoside, ARA-C) is used parenterally and (with slow intravenous infusion) may reach appreciable levels in the cerebrospinal fluid. Cytarabine is eliminated via hepatic metabolism. Cytarabine acts as a pyrimidine antimetabolite; it is activated by kinases to ara-cytidine triphosphate (AraCTP), an inhibitor of DNA polymerases. Of all the antimetabolites, cytarabine is the most specific for the S phase of the tumor cell cycle. Resistance to cytarabine can occur as a result of decreased uptake or decreased conversion to AraCTP. Clinically, cytarabine is a major drug for the treatment of acute myelogenous leukemia. Neurotoxicity is associated with high doses and includes cerebellar dysfunction and peripheral neuritis.

Plant Alkaloids

These important CCS drugs include vinca alkaloids (**vinblastine, vincristine**), podophyllotoxins (**etoposide, teniposide**), camptothecins (**topotecan, irinotecan**), and taxanes (**paclitaxel, docetaxel**). These drugs act in S, G_2, and M phases of the cell cycle (Figure 31–2). The acute and delayed toxicities associated with these anticancer drugs are presented in Table 31–4.

Vinblastine, Vincristine, and Vinorelbine

Vinblastine and vincristine are natural alkaloids, whereas vinorelbine is semisynthetic. These drugs are given parenterally. They penetrate most tissues, but not the cerebrospinal fluid, and are cleared mainly via biliary excretion. These agents block mitotic spindle formation by preventing the assembly of tubulin dimers into microtubules. They act primarily in the M phase of the cell cycle. Resistance can occur from increased drug efflux from tumor cells via overexpression of membrane drug transporters. Clinically, vincristine is used in acute leukemias, lymphomas, Wilms' tumor, and choriocarcinoma. Vinblastine is

Table 31–4.   Plant alkaloid anticancer drugs and toxicities

Drug	Acute Toxicity	Delayed Toxicity
Docetaxel	Hypersensitivity, rash	Neurotoxicity, fluid retention, neutropenia
Etoposide (VP-16), teniposide	Nausea and vomiting, hypotension	Alopecia, bone marrow depression
Irinotecan	Diarrhea, nausea, and vomiting	Diarrhea, bone marrow depression, nausea and vomiting, liver function abnormalities
Paclitaxel	Nausea and vomiting, hypotension, arrhythmias, hypersensitivity	Bone marrow depression, peripheral sensory neuropathy
Topotecan	Nausea and vomiting	Bone marrow depression, arthralgias
Vinblastine	Nausea and vomiting	Alopecia, loss of reflexes, bone marrow depression, gastrointestinal distress
Vincristine	None	Loss of reflexes, muscle weakness, peripheral neuritis, paralytic ileus, mild bone marrow depression, alopecia
Vinorelbine	Nausea and vomiting	Bone marrow depression, fatigue, constipation, hyporeflexia, paresthesias

used for lymphomas, neuroblastoma, testicular carcinoma, and Kaposi's sarcoma. Vinorelbine is used mainly in lung and breast cancers.

Etoposide and Teniposide

Etoposide and teniposide are extracted from the root of the May apple plant. They are usually used parenterally, but etoposide is also well absorbed after oral administration and distributes to most tissues. Elimination is mainly via the kidneys, and dose reductions should be made in patients with renal impairment. Their mechanisms of action are similar: they increase DNA degradation (possibly via interaction with topoisomerase II) and inhibit mitochondrial electron transport. The drugs are most active in the late S and early G_2 phases of the cell cycle. Clinically, these drugs are used in combination drug regimens for therapy of lung (small cell), prostate, and testicular carcinomas. The toxicities of etoposide and teniposide are similar.

Topotecan and Irinotecan

Topotecan inhibits the activity of topoisomerase I, the key enzyme responsible for cutting and religating (i.e., joining) single DNA strands, processes that are essential for normal DNA replication and repair. Inhibition of topoisomerase I results in DNA damage. Topotecan is indicated in the treatment of patients with advanced ovarian cancer and small cell lung cancer. The main route of elimination is renal excretion, and dosage reduction is required in patients with abnormal renal function. Irinotecan is a prodrug converted by the liver into an active metabolite that is also a potent inhibitor of topoisomerase I. Irinotecan is indicated in metastatic colorectal cancer. Diarrhea associated with irinotecan therapy can be severe, leading to significant electrolyte imbalance and dehydration.

Paclitaxel and Docetaxel

Although paclitaxel and docetaxel were originally extracted from the bark of the yew tree, these taxanes are now produced synthetically. Paclitaxel and docetaxel are given intravenously. The mechanism of action is interference with the mitotic spindle. In contrast to vinca alkaloids, taxanes prevent microtubule disassembly into tubulin monomers. Clinical uses include treatment for several solid tumors, including advanced breast and ovarian cancers. The toxicities of these drugs are not identical to each other (Table 31–4).

Antibiotics

This category of antineoplastic drugs comprises several structurally dissimilar agents, including **doxorubicin, daunorubicin, bleomycin, dactinomycin,** and **mitomycin.** A major mechanism of action of these antibiotics is binding to DNA through intercalation between specific bases. This results in blocking synthesis of RNA, DNA, or both and DNA strand scission, thus interfering with cell replication. Acute and delayed toxicities associated with these anticancer drugs are listed in Table 31–5.

Table 31–5.	Antibiotic cancer chemotherapy drugs and toxicities	
Drug	**Acute Toxicity**	**Delayed Toxicity**
Bleomycin	Allergic reactions, fever, hypotension	Skin toxicity, pulmonary fibrosis, mucositis, alopecia
Dactinomycin (actinomycin D)	Nausea and vomiting	Stomatitis, skin reactions, gastrointestinal tract upset, alopecia, bone marrow depression
Daunorubicin (daunomycin)	Nausea, fever, red urine (not hematuria)	Cardiotoxicity, alopecia, bone marrow depression
Doxorubicin	Nausea, red urine (not hematuria)	Cardiotoxicity, alopecia, bone marrow depression, stomatitis
Idarubicin	Nausea and vomiting	Bone marrow depression, mucositis, cardiotoxicity
Mitomycin	Nausea	Thrombocytopenia, anemia, leukopenia, mucositis

Bleomycin

Bleomycin is a mixture of glycopeptides that must be given parenterally. The drug is inactivated by tissue aminopeptidases, but some renal clearance of intact drug also occurs. Bleomycin generates free radicals that bind to DNA, causing strand breaks and inhibiting DNA replication. Bleomycin is a CCS drug active in the G_2 phase of the tumor cell cycle (Figure 31–2). Clinically, bleomycin is an important component of drug regimens for Hodgkin's disease and testicular cancer. The drug is also used for treatment of non-Hodgkin's lymphomas and for squamous cell carcinomas. Pulmonary fibrosis develops slowly, but is the dose-limiting toxicity. Hypersensitivity manifestations are common and include chills, fever, and anaphylaxis. Mucocutaneous reactions are also common and include alopecia, blister formation, and hyperkeratosis.

Doxorubicin, Daunorubicin, and Idarubicin

Doxorubicin and daunorubicin must be given intravenously. They are metabolized in the liver, and the products are excreted in the bile and urine. These anthracyclines have multiple mechanisms of action, including intercalation between base pairs in DNA, inhibition of topoisomerase II, and generation of free radicals. As a result, they block DNA and RNA synthesis and cause DNA strand scission. Membrane disruption also occurs. The anthracyclines are CCNS drugs. Clinically, doxorubicin is used in Hodgkin's disease, myelomas, sarcomas, and breast, endometrial, lung, ovarian, and thyroid cancers. The main use of daunorubicin is in the treatment of acute leukemias. Idarubicin, a newer anthracycline, is approved for use in acute myelogenous leukemia. These drugs demonstrate similar toxicities, including gastrointestinal distress and severe alopecia. Cardiotoxicity includes initial electrocardiographic abnormalities, with the possibility of arrhythmias, and a cumulative dose-dependent, slowly developing cardiomyopathy and congestive heart failure. Dexrazoxane, an inhibitor of iron-mediated free radical generation, may protect against cardiotoxicity. Liposomal formulations of doxorubicin may be less cardiotoxic.

Dactinomycin

Dactinomycin must be given parenterally. Intact drug and metabolites are excreted in the bile. Dactinomycin is a CCNS drug that binds to double-stranded DNA and inhibits DNA-dependent RNA synthesis. Clinically, dactinomycin is used in melanoma and Wilms' tumor.

Mitomycin

Mitomycin is given intravenously and is rapidly cleared via hepatic metabolism. The drug is a CCNS agent that is converted by liver enzymes to an alkylating agent that cross-links DNA. Mitomycin is used occasionally in combination regimens for adenocarcinomas of the cervix, stomach, pancreas, and lung. Myelosuppression is severe, and the drug is toxic to the heart, liver, lung, and kidney.

Hormonal Anticancer Agents

Many of these drugs are discussed in other chapters and are mentioned here only in relation to their clinical application in cancer chemotherapy. The toxicities associated with the hormonally active anticancer drugs are presented in Table 31–6.

Gonadal Hormone Antagonists

Breast cancer and prostate cancer, two common neoplasms, are usually present in a hormone dependent form. Agents that inhibit estrogen or progesterone synthesis or the receptors for these ligands are extremely useful in many patients with breast cancer. Similarly, antiandrogenic drugs have proven to be useful in men with advanced prostate cancer.

Tamoxifen, a selective estrogen receptor modulator (Chapter 22), acts as an estrogen antagonist in estrogen-sensitive breast cancer cells. It is used in estrogen receptor–positive breast carcinoma. Women with a strong family history of breast cancer are at high risk for breast cancer. Because tamoxifen appears to have a preventive effect in women at high risk for breast cancer, it is now approved as a chemopreventive agent in this population. **Toremifene** is a newer estrogen receptor antagonist that is used in advanced breast cancer.

Flutamide is an androgen receptor antagonist used in prostatic carcinoma. **Bicalutamide** and **nilutamide** are similar in mechanism and application. These drugs are often used in combination with the gonadotropin-releasing hormone (GnRH) analogs

Table 31–6.	Hormonally active drugs and toxicities

Drug	Acute Toxicity	Delayed Toxicity
Antiandrogens		
Flutamide, Bicalutamide, Nilutamide	Mild nausea	Hot flushes, transient elevations in liver function tests
Antiestrogen		
Tamoxifen	Transient flare of tumor symptoms	Menopausal symptoms, fluid retention and edema, thromboembolic events, increased incidence of endometrial hyperplasia and cancer
Progestins		
Megestrol acetate	None	Fluid retention
Adrenocorticosteroids		
Hydrocortisone	None	Fluid retention, hypertension, diabetes mellitus, increased susceptibility to infection, moon facies
Prednisone	None	
Gonadotropin-releasing hormone agonists		
Goserelin acetate	Transient flare of tumor symptoms, pain at injection site	Hot flushes, impotence, gynecomastia
Leuprolide	Transient flare of tumor symptoms, pain at injection site	Hot flushes, impotence, gynecomastia
Aromatase inhibitors		
Aminoglutethimide	Fatigue, mild nausea	Skin rash, adrenal insufficiency, myelosuppression (aminoglutethimide also blocks synthesis of other steroids)
Anastrozole	Mild nausea, headache	Fatigue, hot flushes, arthralgias
Exemestane	Mild nausea, headache	Fatigue, hot flushes
Letrozole	Mild nausea, headache	Fatigue, hot flushes, arthralgias

(see below) to prevent the initial tumor flare (i.e., short-lived increase in tumor growth and symptoms) caused by GnRH, and to prevent the action of androgens produced by extragonadal tissues. For additional information, see Chapter 22.

Gonadotropin-Releasing Hormone Analogs
Leuprolide, goserelin, and **nafarelin** are GnRH agonists (Chapter 22) that are effective in advanced prostatic carcinoma. When administered in constant doses to maintain stable blood levels, they inhibit release from the pituitary of luteinizing hormone (LH) and follicle-stimulating hormone (FSH). As a result,

androgen production drops to castration levels and tumor growth may be slowed.

Synthesis Inhibitors
Aminoglutethimide, anastrozole, exemestane, and **letrozole** inhibit steroid synthesis. Whereas aminoglutethimide inhibits synthesis of all steroid hormones, the other agents inhibit aromatase, the enzyme that converts precursor steroids into estrogens. Aromatase inhibitors are used commonly now in the treatment of estrogen receptor-positive breast cancer. Aminoglutethimide is used for some cases of metastatic breast cancer or advanced prostate cancer.

Glucocorticoids

Glucocorticoids are useful in the treatment of acute leukemia, lymphoma, multiple myeloma, and other hematologic malignancies as well as in advanced breast cancer. Anticancer actions probably involve multiple mechanisms. In addition, they are effective as supportive therapy in the management of cancer-related hypercalcemia. **Prednisone** is the most commonly used glucocorticoid in cancer chemotherapy. For additional information, see Chapter 23.

Miscellaneous Anticancer Agents

Additional anticancer drugs not associated with the previous drug classes are presented below, and their acute and delayed toxicities are listed in Table 31–7.

Asparaginase

Asparaginase is an enzyme that depletes serum asparagine by hydrolyzing circulating L-asparagine to aspartic acid and ammonia. The drug is used in the treatment of T-cell auxotrophic cancers (certain pediatric leukemias and lymphomas) that require exogenous asparagine for growth. Asparaginase is given intravenously.

Imatinib

Imatinib is an example of a selective anticancer drug whose development was guided by knowledge of a specific oncogene. Imatinib inhibits tyrosine kinase activity of the protein product of the *BCR-ABL* oncogene that is commonly expressed in chronic myelogenous leukemia (CML). Durable remissions and apparent cures have occurred in patients treated with this drug. Resistance may occur because of mutation of the *BCR-ABL* gene. Imatinib is also effective for treatment of gastrointestinal stromal tumors that express the c-kit tyrosine kinase.

Monoclonal Antibodies

Trastuzumab is a monoclonal antibody that binds to a surface growth factor receptor protein on cells that overexpress the human epidermal growth factor receptor-2 (*HER2*) gene in advanced breast cancers. Binding of trastuzumab to the HER2 receptor causes receptor uptake into the cell, thereby preventing receptors from being activated by the circulating ligand. Acute toxicity includes nausea and vomiting, chills, fevers, and headache. **Rituximab** is a monoclonal antibody with high affinity for a surface protein in non-Hodgkin's lymphoma cells. The drug is currently used with conventional anticancer drugs (e.g., cyclophosphamide plus vincristine plus prednisone) in some types of lymphomas. Use of rituximab is associated with hypersensitivity reactions and myelosuppression.

Interferons

The interferons are endogenous glycoproteins with antineoplastic, immunosuppressive, and antiviral actions. Alpha interferons (Chapter 32) are effective against a number of neoplasms, including hairy cell leukemia, early-stage CML, and T-cell lymphomas. Toxic effects of the interferons include myelosuppression and neurologic dysfunction.

Table 31–7.	Miscellaneous anticancer drugs and toxicities	
Drug	**Acute Toxicity**	**Delayed Toxicity**
Asparaginase	Nausea, fever, and allergic reactions	Hepatotoxicity, mental depression, acute pancreatitis, bleeding, and hypersensitivity reactions
Imatinib	Nausea and vomiting	Fluid retention with ankle and periorbital edema, diarrhea, myalgias
Trastuzumab	Nausea and vomiting, infusion-related hypersensitivity reaction	Cardiomyopathy, myelosuppression, pulmonary toxicity

STRATEGIES IN CANCER CHEMOTHERAPY

The Log-Kill Hypothesis

Patients with widespread cancer may have up to 10^{12} tumor cells throughout the body at the time of diagnosis (Figure 31–4). If an effective anticancer drug kills 10^3-fold (99.9%) of these tumor cells, treatment would induce a clinical remission associated with major symptomatic improvement and the number of tumor cells would be reduced 1,000-fold from 10^{12} to 10^9. Cytotoxic drugs act with *first-order kinetics*. That is, a given dose kills a constant proportion of a cell population rather than a constant number of cells. The log-kill hypothesis proposes that the magnitude of tumor cells killed by anticancer drugs is a logarithmic function. In the previous example, a 3-log-kill dose of an effective drug reduced the cancer cell population from 10^{12} cells to 10^9. This resulted from a total kill of 999×10^9 cells. The same dose would reduce a starting population of 10^6 cells to 10^3 cells. This would represent a kill of 999×10^3 cells. In both cases, the dose reduces the numbers of cells by 3 orders of magnitude, or "3 logs." The remaining cells might be inherently resistant to the drug, may reside in a pharmacologic sanctuary such as the central nervous system, or may have been in an insensitive stage of the cell cycle.

The relationship of the number of tumor cells to the time of diagnosis, symptoms, treatment, and death is presented in Figure 31–4. The value of repeated courses of anticancer treatment at intervals shorter than the time for tumor regrowth is indicated by comparing the middle treatment regimen to the upper treatment regimen. The middle treatment regimen also documents the value of earlier diagnosis, when there are fewer cancer cells. Finally, the lower treatment regimen illustrates the value of combining various therapeutic modalities such as surgery and anticancer drug regimens to decrease the number of neoplastic cells.

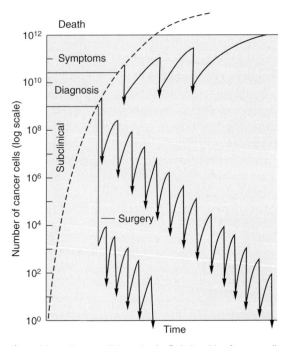

Figure 31–4. The log-kill hypothesis. Relationship of tumor cell number to time of diagnosis, symptoms, treatment, and death. Three approaches to drug treatment (*indicated by three lines with arrows*) are shown in comparison with the course of tumor growth when no treatment is given (*dashed line*). In the protocol diagrammed at the top, treatment is given infrequently (three times) and the result is increased survival, but with recurrence of symptoms between courses of treatment, and eventual death of the patient. For the protocol diagrammed in the middle section, the cancer is diagnosed and treatment begun earlier and given more frequently. Tumor cell kill exceeds regrowth, drug resistance does not develop, and "cure" results. In this middle example, treatment has been continued long after all clinical evidence of cancer has disappeared (1–3 years). This approach has been established as effective in the treatment of childhood acute leukemia, testicular cancers, and Hodgkin's disease. In the protocol diagrammed at the bottom of the graph, early surgery has been employed to remove the primary tumor, and intensive adjuvant chemotherapy has been administered long enough (up to 1 year) to eradicate remaining tumor cells that comprise the occult micrometastases.

Principles of Combination Therapy

Anticancer drugs found to be effective in various neoplasms are summarized in Table 31–8. Clinically, combinations of different anticancer drugs are often used.

Chemotherapy with combinations of anticancer drugs usually increases log-kill markedly, and in some cases synergistic effects are achieved. *Synergy* occurs when the effect of two different anticancer drugs is greater than

Table 31–8. Selected examples of effective cancer chemotherapy[1]

Diagnosis	Current Drug Therapy of Choice
Acute lymphocyte leukemia	Induction: vincristine plus prednisone
	Maintenance: mercaptopurine methotrexate and cyclophosphamide
Acute myelogenous leukemia	Cytarabine and daunorubicin or idarubicin
Breast carcinoma	Cyclophosphamide and doxorubicin, or hormonal therapy with tamoxifen, or an aromatase inhibitor (e.g., anastrozole)
Chronic myelogenous leukemia	Imatinib, busulfan, or interferon
Colon carcinoma	Fluorouracil, leucovorin, and irinotecan
Hodgkin's lymphoma	ABVD regimen: doxorubicin (Adriamycin) plus bleomycin plus vincristine plus dacarbazine
Non-Hodgkin's lymphoma	Cyclophosphamide, doxorubicin, vincristine, prednisone
Ovarian carcinoma	Paclitaxel and cisplatin or carboplatin
Prostate carcinoma	Leuprolide and androgen receptor antagonist (e.g., flutamide)
Lung carcinoma	Cisplatin plus paclitaxel or docetaxel
Testicular carcinoma	PEB regimen: cisplatin (Platinol), etoposide, and bleomycin

[1]Cancers that respond to chemotherapy with prolonged patient survival or cure.

the sum of the effects of each drug individually. Drug combinations are often cytotoxic to a heterogeneous population of cancer cells, and may prevent development of resistant clones. Drug combinations that include CCS and CCNS drugs may be cytotoxic to both dividing and resting cancer cells. Four principles are important for selecting appropriate drugs to use in combination chemotherapy. First, each drug should be active when used alone against the particular cancer. Second, the drugs should have different mechanisms of action. Third, cross-resistance between drugs should be minimal. Finally, the drugs should have different toxic effects.

Additional Strategies for Cancer Chemotherapy

Pulse Therapy

Pulse therapy involves intermittent treatment with high doses of an anticancer drug—doses that are too toxic to be used continuously. Intensive pulse therapy every 3 to 4 weeks allows for maximum effects on neoplastic cells, with hematologic and immunologic recovery between courses. This type of regimen is used

successfully in therapy of acute leukemias, testicular carcinomas, and Wilms' tumor.

Recruitment and Synchrony

The strategy of recruitment involves initial use of a CCNS drug to achieve a significant log-kill, which results in recruitment into cell division of cells previously resting in the G_0 phase of the cell cycle. Subsequent administration of a CCS drug that is active against dividing cells may then achieve maximal cell kill. A similar approach involves synchrony. One example is the use of vinca alkaloids to hold cancer cells in the M phase. Subsequent treatment with another CCS drug, such as the S phase–specific agent cytarabine, may result in a greater killing effect on the neoplastic cell population.

Rescue Therapy

Toxic effects of anticancer drugs can sometimes be alleviated by a rescue strategy. This involves the administration of essential metabolites to counteract the effects of anticancer drugs on normal (nonneoplastic) cells. For example, high doses of methotrexate may be given for 36 to 48 hours and terminated before severe toxicity occurs in cells of the gastrointestinal tract and bone marrow. **Leucovorin** (formyl tetrahydrofolate), which is accumulated more readily by normal than by neoplastic cells, is then administered. This results in rescue ("*leucovorin rescue*") of the normal cells because leucovorin bypasses the dihydrofolate reductase step in folic acid synthesis. **Mercaptoethanesulfonate** (mesna) "traps" acrolein released from cyclophosphamide and thus reduces the incidence of hemorrhagic cystitis. **Dexrazoxane** inhibits free radical formation and affords protection against the cardiac toxicity of anthracyclines (e.g., doxorubicin).

■ REHABILITATION FOCUS

The role of physical therapy and conditioning in patients undergoing chemotherapy has increased in importance in recent years. Rehabilitation programs are an integral component in the overall treatment regimen in this patient population. Research has documented that all patient populations benefit from these programs regardless of the type of cancer, gender, or age of the patients.

If possible, the rehabilitation program should begin prior to initiating cancer treatment. A reduced intensity program should occur during the "on phase" of cancer treatment. The on phase is when the patient is receiving chemotherapy, radiation, or surgical procedures. This phase of the program may occur in the hospital, outpatient clinic, or at home. During the "off phase" of the cancer treatment regimen, goals for increasing muscle force and aerobic capacity should be set to counteract the deterioration that often occurs during the on phase.

Although these rehabilitation programs require individualization, certain components should be included for optimal outcomes. First, the program should have both aerobic and resistive exercise components. Maintaining flexibility through active and passive range of motion and stretching is also critical. Range of motion is especially important when edema is a problem, such as in surgical or radiologic

procedures for breast cancer. These programs should be conducted every day or every other day during both on and off phases. They should be continued for 6 to 8 weeks following the last on phase of the regimen.

Rehabilitation programs have multiple benefits for cancer patients. They assist in maintaining cardiovascular and pulmonary function, as well as general aerobic capacity. Research indicates that moderate fatigue associated with rehabilitation programs improves patients' capacity to withstand pain, fatigue, and other adverse effects of anticancer regimens.

Patients participating in rehabilitation also receive psychologic benefits, as documented by improvements in various quality of life (QOL) surveys. In these patients, improvement in depression is proportional to improvement in QOL assessments and functional capacity.

Finally, careful evaluation of all patients should be conducted as pain and dysfunction associated with cancer may have musculoskeletal manifestations. For example, lung cancer with metastases to the lower thoracic or lumbar spine may present similarly to musculoskeletal low back pain.

■ CLINICAL RELEVANCE FOR REHABILITATION

Adverse Drug Reactions
- Nausea and vomiting
- Fatigue
- Decreased blood cell components (may include any or all of the following):
  - White blood cells (leukopenia)
  - Red blood cells (anemia)
  - Platelets (thrombocytopenia)

Effects Interfering with Rehabilitation
- Decreased wound healing
- Increased risk of infection
- Decreased exercise endurance

Possible Therapy Solutions
- Develop exercise regimen to increase endurance

PROBLEM-ORIENTED PATIENT STUDY

Brief History: The patient is a 42-year-old male with chronic myelogenous leukemia. He was referred to a major research hospital for full myeloablative (bone marrow–destroying) therapy and fractionated total body irradiation plus intravenous melphalan, followed by autologous hematopoietic cell transplantation. The on phase of the treatment was performed while the patient stayed at the hospital in an apartment provided onsite. The hospital has an established rehabilitation program to assist in maintaining function and overall health during this treatment regimen.

Current Medical Status and Drug Therapy: The patient completed the myeloablative therapy prior to receiving the autologous hematopoietic cells and cytokines to stimulate myelopoietic, erythrocyte, and platelet formation. Rehabilitation activities began at this time.

Rehabilitation Setting: The patient is complaining of nausea and vomiting and is receiving prednisolone for these adverse effects of the cancer regimen. He is also complaining of arthralgia and myalgia resulting from stimulation of hematopoietic activity. Owing to his decreased immunocompetence, the patient is treated individually. As immunocompetence improves, the patient will be allowed to interact with other individuals in the hospital.

Problem/Clinical Options: A rehabilitation program that incorporates maintaining functional capacity while relieving pain associated with the oncology treatment regimen is developed. Because of the patient's immunocompromised state, initial rehabilitation activities are conducted individually in the onsite apartment. Aerobic activities are limited to bed to chair and other transfers with limited ambulation on level surfaces with an ambulation device when required. The patient's hematocrit is also low, so he has minimal aerobic capacity. Active and passive range of motion (ROM) and stretching are conducted to maintain ROM. Modalities are incorporated to relieve pain. As immunocompetence and hematocrit improve, rehabilitation activities are continued in a common room where other patients undergoing cancer treatment are participating in conditioning programs. The rehabilitation program now includes active stretching to warm up, light weights for resistive training, followed by aerobic activity on a recumbent bicycle. At discharge, the patient is referred to a hospital-based outpatient clinic for supervision and progression of the rehabilitation program during the off phase of the cancer treatment regimen.

PREPARATIONS AVAILABLE

The reader is referred to the manufacturers' literature for the most recent information.

REFERENCES

Books and Monographs

Chabner BA, Longo DL: *Cancer Chemotherapy and Biotherapy: Principles and Practice*, 3rd ed. Philadelphia: Lippincott Williams & Wilkins, 2001.

Chu E, DeVita VT Jr: *Cancer Chemotherapy Drug Manual 2003*, 3rd ed. Sudbury, MA: Jones and Bartlett, 2002.

DeVita VT Jr, Hellman S, Rosenberg SA: *Cancer: Principles and Practice of Oncology*, 6th ed. Philadelphia: Lippincott Williams & Wilkins, 2001.

Holland JF, et al: *Cancer Medicine*, 4th ed. Hamilton, Ontario, Canada: BC Decker, 2000.

Pazdur R, et al (ed): *Cancer Management: A Multidisciplinary Approach*, 5th ed. PRR, 2001.

Perry MC: *The Chemotherapy Source Book*, 3rd ed. Philadelphia: Lippincott Williams & Wilkins, 2001.

Pizzo PA, Poplack AG: *Principles and Practice of Pediatric Oncology*, 4th ed. Philadelphia: Lippincott Williams & Wilkins, 2001.

Articles and Reviews

Abal M, et al: Taxanes: Microtubule and centrosome targets, and cell cycle dependent mechanisms of action. *Curr Cancer Drug Targets* 2003;3:193.

Kuwano M, et al: Multidrug resistance-associated protein subfamily transporters and drug resistance. *Anticancer Drug Des* 1999;14:123.

Skipper HE, et al: Implications of biochemical, pharmacologic, and toxicologic relationships in the design of optimal therapy. *Cancer Chemother Rep* 1970;54:431.

Smith IE, Dowsett M: Aromatase inhibitors in breast cancer. *N Engl J Med* 2003;348:2431.

Wu K, Brown P: Is low-dose tamoxifen useful for the treatment and prevention of breast cancer? *J Natl Cancer Inst* 2003;95:766.

Rehabilitation

Adamsen L, et al: Feasibility, physical capacity, and health benefits of a multidimensional exercise program for cancer patients undergoing chemotherapy. *Support Care Cancer* 2003;11:707.

Adamsen L, et al: The effect of a multidimensional exercise intervention on physical capacity, well-being and quality of life in cancer patients undergoing chemotherapy. *Support Care Cancer* 2006;14:116.

Adamsen L, et al: Transforming the nature of fatigue through exercise: Qualitative findings from a multidimensional exercise programme in cancer patients undergoing chemotherapy. *Eur J Cancer Care (Engl)* 2004;13:362.

Braith RW: Role of exercise in rehabilitation of cancer survivors. *Pediatr Blood Cancer* 2005;44:595.

Campbell A, et al: A pilot study of a supervised group exercise programme as a rehabilitation treatment for women with breast cancer receiving adjuvant treatment. *Eur J Oncol Nurs* 2005;9:56.

Coleman EA, et al: Facilitating exercise adherence for patients with multiple myeloma. *Clin J Oncol Nurs* 2003;7:529, 540.

Courneya KS, et al: Physical exercise and quality of life in cancer patients following high dose chemotherapy and autologous bone marrow transplantation. *Psychooncology* 2000;9:127.

Courneya KS, et al: Randomized controlled trial of exercise training in postmenopausal breast cancer survivors: Cardiopulmonary and quality of life outcomes. *J Clin Oncol* 2003;21:1660.

Dimeo FC, et al: Aerobic exercise in the rehabilitation of cancer patients after high dose chemotherapy and autologous peripheral stem cell transplantation. *Cancer* 1997;79:1717.

Gianni AM, et al: Durable and complete hematopoietic reconstitution after autografting of rhGM-CSF exposed peripheral blood progenitor cells. *Bone Marrow Transplant* 1990;6:143.

Gordon LG, et al: The impact of rehabilitation support services on health-related quality of life for women with breast cancer. *Breast Cancer Res Treat* 2005;93:217.

Headley JA, et al: The effect of seated exercise on fatigue and quality of life in women with advanced breast cancer. *Oncol Nurs Forum* 2004;31:977.

Jones LW, et al: Association between exercise and quality of life in multiple myeloma cancer survivors. *Support Care Cancer* 2004;12:780.

Kim CJ, et al: Cardiopulmonary responses and adherence to exercise in women newly diagnosed with breast cancer undergoing adjuvant therapy. *Cancer Nurs* 2006;29:156.

Marchese VG, et al: Effects of physical therapy intervention for children with acute lymphoblastic leukemia. *Pediatr Blood Cancer* 2004;42:127.

Midtgaard J, et al: The impact of a multidimensional exercise program on self-reported anxiety and depression in cancer patients undergoing chemotherapy: A phase II study. *Palliat Support Care* 2005;3:197.

Mock V, et al: Fatigue and quality of life outcomes of exercise during cancer treatment. *Cancer Pract* 2001;9:119.

Patriarca F, et al: Improvement of amyloid-related symptoms after autologous stem cell transplantation in a patient with hepatomegaly, macroglossia and purpura. *Bone Marrow Transplant* 1999;24:433.

Pinto BM, et al: Psychological and fitness changes associated with exercise participation among women with breast cancer. *Psychooncology* 2003;12:118.

Robb KA, et al: A pain management program for chronic cancer-treatment-related pain: A preliminary study. *J Pain* 2006;7:82–90.

Ross MD, Bayer E: Cancer as a cause of low back pain in a patient seen in a direct access physical therapy setting. *J Orthop Sports Phys Ther* 2005;35:651.

Schwartz AL, et al: Exercise reduces daily fatigue in women with breast cancer receiving chemotherapy. *Med Sci Sports Exerc* 2001;33:718.

Segal R, et al: Structured exercise improves physical functioning in women with stages I and II breast cancer: Results of a randomized controlled trial. *J Clin Oncol* 2001;19:657.

Segal RJ, et al: Resistance exercise in men receiving androgen deprivation therapy for prostate cancer. *J Clin Oncol* 2003;21:1653.

Thorsen L, et al: Effectiveness of physical activity on cardiorespiratory fitness and health-related quality of life in young and middle-aged cancer patients shortly after chemotherapy. *J Clin Oncol* 2005;23:2378.

Turner J, et al: Improving the physical status and quality of life of women treated for breast cancer: A pilot study of a structured exercise intervention. *J Surg Oncol* 2004;86:141.

Windsor PM, et al: A randomized, controlled trial of aerobic exercise for treatment-related fatigue in men receiving radical external beam radiotherapy for localized prostate carcinoma. *Cancer* 2004;101:550.

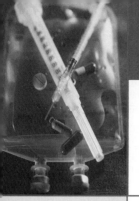

32

IMMUNOPHARMACOLOGY

Immunopharmacology concerns drugs that suppress, modulate, or stimulate immune functions (Figure 32–1). These agents include antibodies that have been developed for use in immune disorders. The drugs available comprise a wide variety of chemical and biopharmaceutical types. This chapter also describes the ways in which drugs activate the immune system and cause unwanted immunologic reactions.

IMMUNE MECHANISMS

The **innate** immune system is the first line of defense against an antigenic insult and includes physical (e.g., skin), biochemical (e.g., complement, lysozyme, interferons), and cellular (e.g., neutrophils, monocytes, macrophages) components. The innate immune system initiates defense against pathogens and antigenic insult. The system thus involves the concerted actions of complement components, lysozymes, macrophages, and neutrophils (Figure 32–2). If the innate response is inadequate, the **adaptive** immune response is mobilized. This culminates in the activation of B and T lymphocytes. The cell types involved in immune responses can be identified by specific cell surface components or **clusters of differentiation (CDs)**. Clusters of differentiation are molecules that can be used to characterize lymphocytes and other types of hematopoietic cells, including precursors of granulocytes, megakaryocytes, and erythrocytes. Thus a CD4 lymphocyte is one that carries the type 4 cluster of differentiation on its surface.

Antigen Recognition and Processing

This critical initial step in the adaptive immune response involves **antigen-presenting cells (APCs)**. Dendritic and Langerhans cells, macrophages, and B lymphocytes are examples of APCs. These cells process antigens into small peptides that can be recognized by **T-cell receptors (TCRs)** on **T helper (TH) cells** (Figure 32–3). T helper cells are lymphoid cells derived from the thymus that mediate cellular immunity and can modify serologic immunity. The main subclasses of T cells are helper (CD4) cells and cytotoxic (CD8) cells.

The most important antigen-presenting cell surface molecules are the **major histocompatibility complex (MHC)** class I and II antigens. When these cell surface molecules bind antigen fragments, they are recognized by TH cells. MHC class I molecules are expressed by all cells, whereas MHC class II molecules are expressed by APCs. T helper cell activation involves activation of TCRs and interaction of class II MHC molecules and specific co-stimulatory and adhesion molecules.

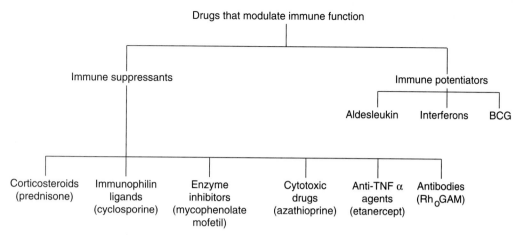

Figure 32–1. The initial division of drugs that affect the immune system is based on whether the drug suppresses or enhances immune function. Immune suppressants are divided into six classes. Immune potentiators are subsequently divided into three classes.

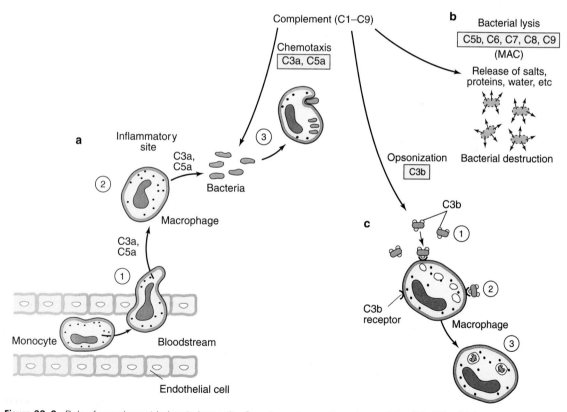

Figure 32–2. Role of complement in innate immunity. Complement comprises nine proteins (C1–C9), which are split into fragments during activation. (a) Complement components (C3a, C5a) attract phagocytes (1) to inflammatory sites (2), where they ingest and degrade pathogens (3). (b) Complement components C5b, C6, C7, C8, and C9 associate to form a membrane attack complex (MAC) that lyses bacteria, causing their destruction. (c) Complement component C3b is an opsonin that coats bacteria (1) and facilitates their ingestion (2) and digestion (3) by phagocytes.

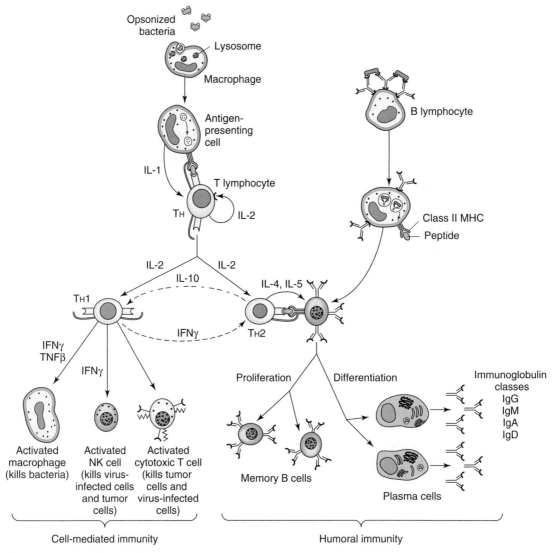

Figure 32–3. Scheme of cell-mediated and humoral immune responses. The cell-mediated arm of the immune response involves internalization and processing of antigen by APCs. The processed peptides bound to class II MHC surface proteins are recognized by the TCR on helper T cells, resulting in T-cell activation. Activated TH cells secrete cytokines such as IL-2, which cause proliferation and activation of TH1 and TH2 cell subsets. TH1 cells also produce IFN-γ and TNF-β, which can directly activate macrophages, cytotoxic T lymphocytes (CTLs), and natural killer (NK) cells. The humoral response is triggered when B lymphocytes bind antigen via their surface immunoglobulins. They are then induced by TH2-derived cytokines (e.g., IL-4, IL-5) to proliferate and differentiate into memory cells and antibody-secreting plasma cells.

Cell-Mediated Immunity

Activated TH cells secrete interleukin-2 (IL-2), a cytokine that causes proliferation and activation of two subsets of helper cells, TH1 and TH2 (Figure 32–3).

TH1 cells play a major role in cell-mediated immunity and delayed hypersensitivity reactions. They produce interferon-γ (INF-γ), IL-2, and tumor necrosis factor-β (TNF-β). These cytokines activate macrophages, cytotoxic T lymphocytes (CTLs), and natural killer (NK) cells. Activated CTLs recognize processed peptides bound to class I MHC molecules on the surface of virus-infected cells or tumor cells. The CTLs induce cell death via lytic enzymes, nitric oxide production, and stimulation of apoptosis pathways in the target cells. CTLs also play a role in autoimmune diseases by reacting against normal tissues, such as synovium in rheumatoid arthritis and myelin in multiple sclerosis. NK cells kill both virus-infected and neoplastic cells. They are also the main precursors of lymphokine-activated killer (LAK) cells, which are toxic to cells that do not express MHC. Lymphokines are cytokines that are capable of modulating lymphoid cell functions.

Humoral Immunity

B cells are lymphoid cells derived from the bone marrow that are capable of differentiating into antibody-forming cells. These cells are responsible for humoral immunity. The humoral response is triggered when B lymphocytes bind antigen via their surface immunoglobulins. The antigens are internalized, processed into peptides, and presented on the cell surface bound to MHC class II molecules. When T-cell receptors on TH2 cells are activated by complexes of MHC class II molecules bound to these peptides, they release interleukins IL-4, IL-5, and IL-6. These interleukins promote B-lymphocyte proliferation and differentiation into memory B cells and antibody-secreting plasma cells (Figure 32–3). Antibody–antigen interactions lead to precipitation of viruses and destruction of bacteria by phagocytic cells or lysis by the complement system (Figure 32–4). Proliferation and differentiation of both B and T lymphocytes is under the control of a complex interplay among the cytokines (Table 32–1) and other endogenous molecules, including amines, leukotrienes, and prostaglandins. For example, IL-10 and IFN-γ down-regulate TH1 and TH2 responses, respectively.

Immune Regulation

A less well-defined T-cell subset (TH3) has been described that produces transforming growth factor-β (TGF-β), whose numerous functions include decreasing proliferation and differentiation of T lymphocytes. Clinical pharmacologic regimens modulating TH3 cells are still under investigation.

Abnormal Immune Responses

Abnormal immune responses include hypersensitivity, autoimmunity, and immunodeficiency states. Immediate hypersensitivity is usually antibody mediated and includes *anaphylaxis* and hemolytic disease of the newborn. Delayed hypersensitivity, associated with extensive tissue damage, is cell mediated. Autoimmunity arises from lymphocytes that react to one's own molecules, or *self-antigens*. Examples of autoimmune diseases that are amenable to drug treatment include rheumatoid arthritis and systemic lupus erythematosus. Immunodeficiency states may be genetically acquired (e.g., DiGeorge syndrome) or result from extrinsic factors (e.g., HIV infection).

SITES OF ACTION OF IMMUNOSUPPRESSANT AGENTS

Sites of action of immunosuppressive agents are shown in Figure 32–5. Agents that interfere with antigen recognition (step 1) are antibodies and include **Rho(D) immune globulin, antilymphocyte globulin,** and **muromonab-CD3.** Inhibition of lymphoid proliferation (step 2) occurs with most immunosuppressants, including peptide antibiotics, anti-TNF-α agents, cytotoxic drugs, enzyme inhibitors, and glucocorticoids. Lymphoid differentiation (step 3) is partly inhibited by peptide antibiotics, **dactinomycin,** and **antilymphocyte globulin.** Glucocorticoids also modify tissue injury (step 6) via their anti-inflammatory properties.

IMMUNOSUPPRESSIVE AGENTS

Glucocorticoids

Mechanism of Action

Glucocorticoids act at multiple cellular sites to cause broad effects on inflammatory and immune processes. At the biochemical level, they modulate gene expression to decrease synthesis of enzymes that produce prostaglandins, leukotrienes, and cytokines.

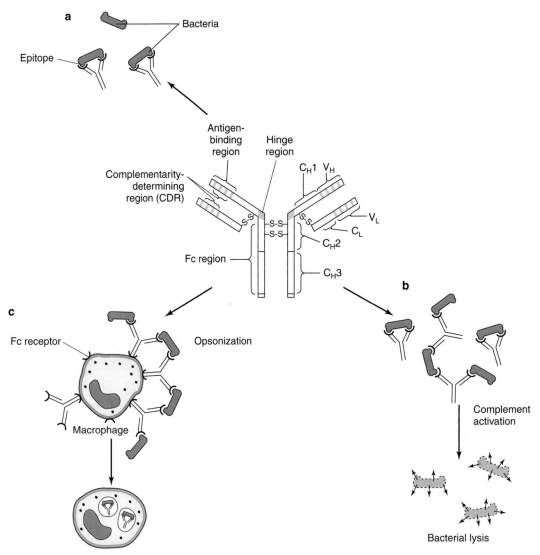

Figure 32–4. An antibody has multiple functions. The prototypical antibody consists of two heavy (H) and two light (L) chains, each subdivided into constant (CL, CH) and variable (VL, VH) domains. The structure is held together by intra- and interchain disulfide bridges. (a) The complementarity-determining region (CDR) of the antigen-binding portion of the antibody engages the antigenic determinant (epitope) in a lock and key fashion. (b) Antigen-antibody complexes activate complement to produce split complement components that cause bacterial lysis. (c) The Fc portion of antibodies binds to Fc receptors on phagocytes (e.g., macrophages, neutrophils) and facilitates uptake of bacteria (opsonization).

Glucocorticoids also reduce production of other signaling molecules that participate in immune responses (e.g., platelet-activating factor). At the cellular level, glucocorticoids suppress cell-mediated immunity by inhibiting T- lymphocyte proliferation and, to a lesser degree, dampen humoral immunity. At doses used for immunosuppression, the glucocorticoids are cytotoxic to certain subsets of T cells. Continuous therapy lowers immunoglobulin G (IgG) levels by increasing catabolism of this class of immunoglobulins.

Table 32–1. Cytokines that modulate immune responses

Cytokine	Characteristic Properties
Interferon-α (IFN-α)	Activates NK cells, antiviral, oncostatic
Interferon-β (IFN-β)	Activates NK cells, antiviral, oncostatic
Interferon-γ (IFN-γ)	Activates TH1, NK, cytotoxic T cells, and macrophages; antiviral, oncostatic
Interleukin-1 (IL-1)	T-cell activation, B-cell proliferation
Interleukin-2 (IL-2)	T-cell proliferation, activation of TH1, NK, and LAK cells
Interleukin-11 (IL-11)	B-cell differentiation (megakaryocyte proliferation)
Tumor necrosis factor-α (TNF-α)	Proinflammatory, macrophage activation, oncostatic
Tumor necrosis factor-β (TNF-β)	Proinflammatory, macrophage activation, oncostatic
Granulocyte colony-stimulating factor (G-CSF)	Granulocyte production
Granulocyte-macrophage colony-stimulating factor (GM-CSF)	Granulocyte, monocyte, eosinophil production
Macrophage colony-stimulating factor (M-CSF)	Monocyte production, macrophage activation

LAK = lymphokine-activated killer; NK = natural killer; TH1 = T helper 1.

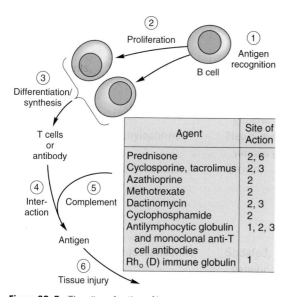

Figure 32–5. The sites of action of immunosuppressive agents.

Clinical Use and Toxicity

Glucocorticoids are used alone or in combination with other agents in a wide variety of medical conditions that have undesirable immunologic reactions. Because glucocorticoids induce apoptosis in immune cells, they are useful for treating several types of cancer (Chapter 31). Glucocorticoids are also used to suppress immunologic reactions in patients who undergo organ transplantation. Predictable adverse effects include adrenal suppression, growth inhibition, muscle wasting, osteoporosis, salt retention, impaired glucose regulation, and psychiatric disorders. Additional information on this drug class is presented in Chapter 23.

Cyclosporine, Tacrolimus, and Sirolimus

Mechanism of Action

These peptide antibiotics bind to *immunophilins*, which are small cytoplasmic proteins that play critical roles in the function of T and B cells. When these drugs bind to immunophilins, they interfere with the ability of T cells to respond to T-cell receptor (TCR) activation and to cytokines. Cyclosporine binds to cyclophilin and tacrolimus binds to FK-binding protein (FKBP). Both complexes inhibit calcineurin, a cytoplasmic phosphatase. Calcineurin regulates the ability of the nuclear factor of activated T cells (NF-AT) to translocate to the nucleus and regulate the production of cytokines. Thus, cyclosporin and tacrolimus inhibit cytokine production that normally occurs in response to TCR activation. Like tacrolimus, the immunosuppressant sirolimus also binds to FKBP. However, sirolimus does not inhibit calcineurin, but inhibits the response of T cells to cytokines without affecting cytokine production. Sirolimus is a potent inhibitor of T-cell proliferation, antibody production, and mononuclear cell responses to colony-stimulating factors.

Clinical Uses, Pharmacokinetics, and Toxicities

These immunosuppressants have been a major factor in the success of solid organ transplantation. Cyclosporine is used in solid organ transplantation and in graft-versus-host (GVH) disease in patients who have received stem cell transplantation. Tacrolimus is used for liver and kidney transplantation, and may be effective as rescue therapy in patients who fail standard therapy. Sirolimus is used alone or in combination with cyclosporine in kidney and heart transplantation. At lower doses, these agents (particularly cyclosporine) may also be effective in immune diseases, including rheumatoid arthritis, uveitis, psoriasis, asthma, and autoimmune versions of type 1 diabetes.

All three drugs can be used orally. However, because cyclosporine exhibits erratic bioavailability, serum levels should be monitored. Cyclosporine undergoes slow hepatic metabolism by the cytochrome P450 system and has a long half-life. The metabolism of cyclosporine is affected by a host of other drugs. Cyclosporine and tacrolimus have similar toxicity profiles. The most frequent adverse effects are renal dysfunction, hypertension, and neurotoxicity. They can also cause hyperglycemia, hyperlipidemia, and cholelithiasis. Sirolimus is more likely than the other agents to cause hypertriglyceridemia, hepatotoxicity, diarrhea, and myelosuppression.

Mycophenolate Mofetil

Mechanism of Action

Mycophenolate mofetil is rapidly converted into mycophenolic acid, which inhibits inosine monophosphate dehydrogenase, an enzyme in the de novo pathway of purine synthesis. This action suppresses both B- and T-lymphocyte activation. Lymphocytes are particularly susceptible to inhibitors of the de novo pathway because they lack necessary enzymes for the alternative salvage pathway for purine synthesis.

Clinical Use and Toxicity

Mycophenolate mofetil has been used successfully as a sole agent in kidney, liver, and heart transplants. In renal transplants, its use with low-dose cyclosporine has reduced cyclosporine-induced nephrotoxicity. Newer immunosuppressant applications for this drug include lupus nephritis, rheumatoid arthritis, and some dermatologic disorders. Mycophenolate mofetil can cause gastrointestinal disturbances and myelosuppression, especially neutropenia.

Azathioprine

Mechanism of Action

The prodrug azathioprine is transformed to the antimetabolite mercaptopurine, which on further metabolic conversion inhibits enzymes involved in purine metabolism. Azathioprine is cytotoxic in the early phase of lymphoid cell proliferation and has a greater effect on the activity of T cells than B cells. However, both cellular immunity and primary and secondary antibody responses can be blocked.

Clinical Use and Toxicity

Azathioprine is used in autoimmune diseases (e.g., systemic lupus erythematosus, rheumatoid arthritis) and for immunosuppression in renal transplantation. The drug has minimal effects on established graft rejections. The major toxic effect is bone marrow suppression, but gastrointestinal irritation, skin rashes, and liver dysfunction also occur. The use of azathioprine is associated with an increased incidence of cancer. The active metabolite of azathioprine, mercaptopurine, is metabolized by xanthine oxidase. Toxic effects may be exacerbated by concomitant administration of allopurinol, a drug used in the treatment of gout (Chapter 34).

Cyclophosphamide

Mechanism of Action

This orally active prodrug is transformed by liver enzymes to an alkylating agent that is cytotoxic to proliferating lymphoid cells. Cyclophosphamide has a greater effect on B cells than T cells, and inhibits an established immune response. Other cytotoxic drugs that similarly suppress proliferating lymphoid cells, and which are sometimes used as immunosuppressants, include cytarabine, dactinomycin, methotrexate, and vincristine (Chapter 31).

Clinical Use and Toxicity

Cyclophosphamide is effective in autoimmune diseases (including hemolytic anemia), antibody-induced red cell aplasia, bone marrow transplants, and possibly other organ transplant procedures. Cyclophosphamide does not prevent the GVH reaction in bone marrow transplantation. The large doses usually needed for immunosuppression cause pancytopenia, gastrointestinal distress, hemorrhagic cystitis, and alopecia. Cyclophosphamide (and other alkylating agents) may cause sterility.

NEWER IMMUNOSUPPRESSANTS

Etanercept

This chimeric protein is a recombinant form of a portion of the human TNF receptor combined with a fragment of an IgG immunoglobulin. Etanercept binds TNF-α, a proinflammatory cytokine, and thereby prevents TNF-α from stimulating the formation of interleukins and adhesion molecules that activate leukocytes. Etanercept is used in rheumatoid arthritis and is being investigated in other inflammatory diseases. Injection site reactions and hypersensitivity may occur. **Infliximab** and **adalimumab** are monoclonal antibodies that also block the actions of TNF-α (discussed below).

Leflunomide

This drug inhibits dihydroorotic acid dehydrogenase, an enzyme involved in ribonucleotide synthesis. Leflunomide arrests lymphocytes in the G_1 phase of the cell cycle. Leflunomide is used in rheumatoid arthritis. The drug can cause alopecia, rash, and diarrhea.

Thalidomide

This sedative drug, notorious for its teratogenic effects, has immunosuppressant actions that appear to be due to suppression of TNF-α production. Thalidomide also inhibits angiogenesis and is being investigated as an anticancer drug. Thalidomide is used for some forms of leprosy reactions and for immunologic diseases (e.g., systemic lupus erythematosus). The drug is also effective in treating aphthous ulcers and HIV-associated wasting syndrome. Because of its teratogenic action, it is absolutely contraindicated in pregnancy.

Alefacept

This engineered protein targets the CD2 receptor found on the surface of T cells. The natural ligand for the CD2 receptor is lymphocyte-associated antigen 3 (LFA-3), a protein expressed on the surface of many cells. Alefacept contains the CD2-binding region of LFA-3 fused to a human IgG Fc region. Alefacept inhibits T-cell activation and causes a dose-dependent reduction in circulating T cells, so T-cell counts must be monitored in patients treated with the drug. Alefacept is approved for treatment of psoriasis.

ANTIBODIES AS IMMUNOSUPPRESSANTS

Antilymphocyte Globulin and Antithymocyte Globulin

Mechanism of Action

Two types of antisera directed against lymphocytes are available. Antilymphocyte globulin (ALG) and antithymocyte globulin (ATG) are produced in horses or sheep by immunization against human lymphoid cells. Antibodies in these preparations bind to T cells involved in antigen recognition and initiate their destruction by activation of the complement cascade. These antibodies selectively block cell-mediated immunity rather than humoral immunity, which accounts for their ability to suppress organ graft rejection, a cell-mediated process.

Clinical Use and Toxicity

Both ALG and ATG are used before bone marrow transplantation to prevent the GVH reaction. They are also used in combination with cyclosporine or cytotoxic drugs (or both) for maintenance after bone marrow, heart, and renal transplantations. Because serologic (i.e., humoral) immunity may remain intact, injection of ALG or ATG can cause hypersensitivity reactions, including serum sickness and anaphylaxis. Pain and erythema occur at injection sites, and lymphoma has been noted as a late complication.

Rh$_0$(D) Immune Globulin

This formulation is a human IgG preparation that contains antibodies against red cell Rh$_0$(D) antigens. Administration of this antibody to Rh$_0$(D)-negative, D^u-negative mothers at time of antigen exposure (i.e., birth of an Rh$_0$(D)-positive or a D^u-positive child) blocks the mother's primary immune response to the foreign cells and prevents her from forming antibodies against Rh$_0$(D) antigens that could cause hemolytic anemia in a subsequent pregnancy with a Rh$_0$(D)-positive fetus.

Monoclonal Antibodies

Monoclonal antibodies (MAbs) have the potential advantage of high specificity because they can be developed to interact with a single molecule. "Humanization" of murine monoclonal antibodies has reduced the likelihood of forming neutralizing antibodies and

of immune reactions. Characteristics of some currently available MAbs are shown in Table 32–2.

Abatacept

Abatacept is a fusion protein that binds to receptors on macrophages or other antigen-processing cells. This binding suppresses the immune response by preventing activation of T cells and subsequent cytokine release. Clinical application is in the treatment of patients with rheumatoid arthritis who have failed other disease-modifying antirheumatic drugs.

Muromonab-CD3

This MAb binds to the CD3 antigen on the surface of human thymocytes (immature T cells) and mature T cells. The antibody blocks the killing action of cytotoxic T cells and probably interferes with other T-cell functions. Muromonab-CD3 is used to manage renal transplant rejection crises. First-dose effects include fever, chills, dyspnea, and pulmonary edema. Hypersensitivity reactions may also occur.

Daclizumab

Daclizumab is a highly specific MAb that binds to the alpha subunit of the IL-2 receptor expressed on T cells and prevents its activation by IL-2. Although it facilitates

Table 32–2.	Characteristics of selected monoclonal antibodies (MAbs)
MAb	**Characteristics and Clinical Uses**
Abatacept	Binds to the antigen-processing cell CD80 or CD86 receptors, blocking the activation of T cells and cytokine release.
Abciximab	Antagonist of glycoprotein IIb/IIIa receptor, preventing cross-linking reaction in platelet aggregation. Used postangioplasty and in acute coronary syndromes. (Chapter 11)
Daclizumab	Binds to the alpha subunit of the IL-2 receptor, preventing lymphocyte activation. Used in renal transplants.
Infliximab	Antibody targeted against TNF-α. Used in Crohn's disease and rheumatoid arthritis.
Muromonab	Antibody to the T3 (CD3) antigen on thymocytes. Used in acute renal allograft rejection.
Rituximab	Binds to the CD20 antigen of B lymphocytes and recruits immune effector functions to mediate lysis. Used in B-cell non-Hodgkin's lymphoma. (Chapter 31)
Trastuzumab	Binds to the HER2 protein on the surface of tumor cells. Cytotoxic for breast tumors that overexpress HER2 protein. (Chapter 31)

HER2 = human epidermal growth factor receptor-2; TNF = tumor necrosis factor.

the actions of other immunosuppressants in renal transplants, daclizumab is not used for acute rejection episodes. In contrast to cyclosporine, tacrolimus, or cytotoxic immunosuppressants, the adverse effects of daclizumab are equivalent to those of placebo. **Basiliximab** is a chimeric human-mouse IgG with an action that is equivalent to that of daclizumab.

Infliximab

This humanized MAb has a mechanism similar to that of etanercept because it is targeted against TNF-α. Infliximab induces remissions in treatment-resistant Crohn's disease, but long-term efficacy has not been established. In combination with methotrexate, infliximab improves symptoms in patients with rheumatoid arthritis. Infusion reactions and an increased rate of infection may occur. **Adalimumab** is a completely human IgG monoclonal antibody that binds to TNF-α and is approved for treatment of rheumatoid arthritis.

■ CLINICAL USES OF IMMUNOSUPPRESSIVE DRUGS

As discussed, immunosuppressive agents are commonly used in two clinical circumstances: transplantation and autoimmune disorders (Table 32–3). Because autoimmune disorders are very complex, optimal treatment schedules have yet to be established in many clinical situations.

■ IMMUNOMODULATING AGENTS

Agents that *stimulate* immune responses represent a newer area in immunopharmacology with potential for use in the treatment of immune deficiency diseases, chronic infectious diseases, and cancer. Interest in pharmacologic treatment of immune deficiency diseases has increased with the AIDS epidemic. The cytokines are a large and heterogeneous group of proteins with diverse functions, including immunomodulation. **Cytokines** may be broadly classified as interleukins, interferons, tumor necrosis factor, and colony-stimulating factors. Interferons and other cytokines are finding increasing clinical application as adjuvants to vaccines.

Aldesleukin

Aldesleukin is recombinant **interleukin-2** (IL-2), an endogenous lymphokine that promotes the production of cytotoxic T cells and activates NK cells (Table 32–1). Aldesleukin is indicated for the adjunctive treatment of renal cell carcinoma and malignant melanoma. Recombinant IL-2 is being investigated for possible efficacy in restoring immune function in AIDS and other immune deficiency disorders.

Interferons

Interferon-α-2a inhibits cell proliferation. This interferon is used in hairy cell leukemia, chronic myelogenous leukemia, malignant melanoma, Kaposi sarcoma, and hepatitis B and C. **Interferon-β-1b** has some beneficial effects in relapsing multiple sclerosis. **Interferon-γ-1b** has greater immune-enhancing actions than the other interferons and appears to act by increasing TNF-α synthesis. The recombinant form is used to decrease the incidence and severity of infections in patients with chronic granulomatous disease.

Thymosin

Thymosin is a protein hormone from the thymus gland that stimulates the maturation of pre-T cells (thymocytes) and promotes the formation of T cells from ordinary lymphoid stem cells. Thymosin-containing preparations have been used in DiGeorge syndrome (thymic aplasia), but their efficacy in other immune deficiency states has not been established.

■ MECHANISMS OF DRUG ALLERGY

Drugs can activate the immune system in undesirable ways: these hypersensitivity reactions are known as "drug allergies." Four major types of hypersensitivity reactions have been identified on the basis of their underlying molecular mechanisms. Types I, II, and III are mediated by antibodies, whereas type IV is cell mediated. Any of the four major types of hypersensitivity can be associated with allergic drug reactions.

Table 32–3.   Clinical uses of immunosuppressive agents

Autoimmune Diseases	Immunosuppressive Agents Used	Response
Idiopathic thrombocytopenic purpura	Prednisone,[1] vincristine, occasionally cyclophosphamide, mercaptopurine, or azathioprine; commonly high-dose gamma globulin, plasma immunoadsorption or plasma exchange	Usually good
Autoimmune hemolytic anemia	Prednisone,[1] cyclophosphamide, chlorambucil, mercaptopurine, azathioprine, high-dose gamma globulin	Usually good
Acute glomerulonephritis	Prednisone,[1] mercaptopurine, cyclophosphamide	Usually good
Acquired factor XIII antibodies	Cyclophosphamide plus factor XIII	Usually good
Autoreactive tissue disorders (autoimmune diseases)[2]	Prednisone, cyclophosphamide, methotrexate, interferon-α and interferon-β, azathioprine, cyclosporine, infliximab, etanercept, adalimumab	Often good, variable
Isoimmune Disease		
Hemolytic disease of the newborn	$Rh_0(D)$ immune globulin	Excellent
Organ Transplantation		
Renal	Cyclosporine, azathioprine, prednisone, ALG, OKT3, tacrolimus, basiliximab,[3] daclizumab[3]	Very good
Heart	Cyclosporine, azathioprine, prednisone, ALG, OKT3, tacrolimus, basiliximab,[3] daclizumab[3]	Good
Liver	Cyclosporine, prednisone, azathioprine, tacrolimus	Fair
Bone marrow	Cyclosporine, cyclophosphamide, prednisone, methotrexate, ALG	Good

ALG = antilymhocytic globulin; OKT3 = muromonab.
[1]Drug of choice.
[2]Including systemic lupus erythematosus, rheumatoid arthritis, scleroderma, dermatomyositis, mixed tissue disorder, multiple sclerosis, Wegener's granulomatosis, chronic active hepatitis, lipoid nephrosis, inflammatory bowel disease.
[3]Basiliximab and daclizumab are approved for renal transplant only.

Type I (Immediate) Drug Allergy

In this form of drug allergy, a drug links covalently to a host protein (hapten) and the drug-hapten complex induces the production of IgE antibodies (generally fixed to tissue mast cells and blood basophils) specific for the drug-hapten complex. When the offending drug is reintroduced into the body, it binds the cell-surface IgE and signals the explosive release of mediators such as histamine, prostaglandins, leukotrienes, kinins, and proteases. These mediators cause the clinical symptoms of itchy skin rash with wheals (urticaria), fever, and possibly anaphylaxis. In severe anaphylactic reactions, the life-threatening events commonly involve airway obstruction, laryngeal edema, and vascular collapse resulting from peripheral vasodilation and reduction in blood volume. Hypoxemia can contribute to cardiac events, including arrhythmias and myocardial infarction. Anaphylaxis is treated emergently with epinephrine, which relaxes bronchial smooth muscle and supports blood pressure (Chapter 6) and inhibits further mediator release. Glucocorticoids and antihistamines are also used as supportive therapy. Bee sting is the most common cause of serious type I allergy in the United States. Drugs that commonly cause type I reactions include penicillins and sulfonamides.

Type II (Cytotoxic) Drug Allergy

Type II, or cytotoxic hypersensitivity, occurs when IgG or IgM antibodies directed at antigens of the cell membrane activate complement and generate an attack that damages the cell membrane. In addition to causing cell lysis, complement activation attracts phagocytic cells to the site and induces them to release enzymes that further damage cells. Drugs can induce autoimmune antibodies by attaching to surface proteins. When drugs such as penicillins, methyldopa, and quinidine induce autoimmune antibodies after binding to the surface of red blood cells, hemolytic anemia can result. Quinidine and other drugs can attach to platelets and the resulting autoimmune antibodies can cause thrombocytopenia with subsequent increased risk of bleeding. Many drugs can bind to granulocytes and cause agranulocytosis. The vasodilator hydralazine is an example of a drug that modifies host tissue and induces the production of autoantibodies directed at cellular DNA. These autoantibodies underlie a syndrome resembling systemic lupus erythematosus. Autoimmune reactions to drugs usually subside within several months after the inciting drug is discontinued. Immunosuppressive therapy is only warranted when the reaction is severe.

Type III (Immune Complex) Drug Allergy

Type III, or immune-complex hypersensitivity, occurs when antigen-antibody complexes induce an inflammatory response in tissues. If immune complexes are not promptly removed by the reticuloendothelial system, they can build up in tissues, where they initiate a cascade of inflammation and tissue damage by activating the complement system and attracting polymorphonuclear cells. In drug-induced serum sickness (so named because it can be induced by the injection of foreign serum, not because the reaction is restricted to the blood), immune complexes are deposited in many tissues and cause a syndrome of fever, itchy rash, arthralgia, lymphadenopathy, and peripheral edema. Drug-induced vasculitis, which results from inflammatory reactions to immune complexes within blood vessels, also involves type III mechanisms. Drug-induced vasculitis appears to underlie dermatologic hypersensitivity reactions such as erythema multiforme and the severe Stevens-Johnson reaction, which consists of erythema multiforme, arthritis, nephritis, central nervous system abnormalities, and myocarditis. Severe type III hypersensitivity reactions can sometimes be attenuated by glucocorticoids.

Type IV (Delayed) Drug Allergy

Type IV allergy is a cell-mediated reaction that can occur from topical application of drugs. Contact dermatitis is an example of type IV allergy.

▎ REHABILITATION FOCUS

While immunosuppressant therapy has significantly reduced the morbidity and mortality associated with organ transplantation, the adverse effects associated with these drug classes may limit the rate of rehabilitation or the quality of life after transplantation. In addition to causing organ dysfunction, these drugs have significant detrimental effects on musculoskeletal function. Glucocorticoids such as prednisone cause both muscle atrophy and osteoporosis. Calcineurin antagonists such as cyclosporine decrease the concentration of oxidative enzymes in skeletal muscle. These pharmacologic changes, in combination with the deconditioned state of the patient, adversely affect rehabilitation outcomes.

Instituting a rehabilitation program prior to transplantation delays the decrement in pulmonary, cardiovascular, and skeletal muscle function. Challenges specific to posttransplant rehabilitation are related to surgical procedure, previously deconditioned state of the patient, pharmacologic regimen, and specific organ transplanted. For example, heart transplant patients have limited chronotropic and inotropic responses to exercise. This is due to, in part, organ denervation, but also to immunosuppressants and the use of other drugs to control cardiovascular dynamics. These patients require an extended warm-up phase, several minutes between resistive exercise sets, and 5-minute cool-down periods to prevent hypotension.

Evidence clearly demonstrates that posttransplant rehabilitation programs reduce morbidity and mortality in heart transplant patients. For patients who begin rehabilitation programs that include both aerobic and resistive exercises immediately posttransplant, long-term outcomes approach 95% of the functional parameters for age-matched norms. Additionally, even at 5 years posttransplant, a 1-year rehabilitation program begun immediately after transplant improves cardiovascular and skeletal muscle function.

Most research in rehabilitation prior to and following transplantation has focused on heart transplantation. Initial investigations suggest that rehabilitation programs for patients receiving other types of transplanted organs may also reduce morbidity and mortality. This beneficial effect is not limited to the geriatric population because pediatric patients who receive transplants also appear to benefit.

CLINICAL RELEVANCE FOR REHABILITATION

Adverse Drug Reactions
- Nausea and vomiting
- Fatigue
- Decreased blood cell components caused by immunosuppressants (may include any or all of the following)
  - White blood cells (leukopenia)
  - Red blood cells (anemia)
  - Platelets (thrombocytopenia)

Effects Interfering with Rehabilitation
- Increased risk of infection
- Decreased exercise endurance

Possible Therapy Solutions
- Except during periods of acute phase rejection, develop exercise programs to increase cardiovascular, pulmonary, and musculoskeletal functions.

PROBLEM-ORIENTED PATIENT STUDY

Brief History: The patient is 66-year-old male with a medical history of three myocardial infarctions within the last decade. Over that time, he demonstrated symptom-limited exercise tests with a decline in sustainable workload to approximately 4 metabolic equivalents (METs). He was enrolled in the precardiac transplant program on an outpatient basis. As part of the program, he began a pretransplant rehabilitation to delay further decrements in function. Two months ago, he underwent a heart transplant.

Current Medical Status and Drug Therapy: The maintenance immunosuppressant posttransplant is tacrolimus. In addition, he is taking other drugs to maintain cardiovascular hemodynamics.

Rehabilitation Setting: After surgery, he spent 7 days in the cardiac care unit, was then transferred to the cardiac floor for an additional 7 days, and finally was discharged on day 14. On day 18, he was evaluated for a 12-week phase two cardiac rehabilitation program in an outpatient setting. On day 21, he began aerobic training with 5 minutes of warm-up, followed by treadmill ambulation for 20 minutes at 7 METs with a Borg Rating of Perceived Exertion (RPE) of 12. The session was completed with 5 minutes of cool-down exercise. By day 28, he progressed to the target RPE of 11 at 8 METS for aerobic activities. At 42 days posttransplant, resistance training was incorporated into the program with alternating

PROBLEM-ORIENTED PATIENT STUDY (*Continued*)

upper and lower body exercises and 2 minutes of walking between exercises to prevent hypotension. On day 48, a week ago, his participation in the rehabilitation program decreased because of complaints of chest pain and fatigue. A medical diagnosis of rejection-induced coronary artery vasculitis was made. Tacrolimus was discontinued and the patient was placed on muromonab-CD3 and bolus intravenous methylprednisolone.

Problem/Clinical Options: During the period of rejection, resistive activities should be completely eliminated and aerobic activities should be significantly reduced and based on the patient's tolerance. Resistive activities should be eliminated for two reasons. First, there is an increased risk of a coronary event during bolus administration of corticosteroids. Second, the potential benefits of resistive activities are overwhelmed by the catabolic influence of corticosteroids on muscle and bone. When the acute rejection phase passes, the patient may return toward achieving target aerobic activities and begin resistive activities again.

PREPARATIONS AVAILABLE[1]

Abciximab (ReoPro)
Parenteral: 2 mg/mL solution for IV injection

Adalimumab (Humira)
Parenteral: 40 mg/vial for IV injection

Alefacept (Amevive)
Parenteral: 7.5, 15 mg for IV injection

Alemtuzumab (Campath)
Parenteral: 30 mg/3 mL vial for IV injection

Anti-Thymocyte Globulin (Thymoglobulin)
Parenteral: 25 mg/vial for IV injection

Azathioprine (generic, Imuran)
Oral: 50-mg tablets
Parenteral: 100 mg/vial for IV injection

Basiliximab (Simulect)
Parenteral: 20-mg powder for IV injection

BCG (Bacillus Calmette-Guérin) (Tice BCG)
Parenteral: 30 mg, 1 × 108 organism/vial for percutaneous vaccination

Cyclophosphamide (Cytoxan, Neosar)
Oral: 25-, 50-mg tablets
Parenteral: 100 mg/mL for injection

Cyclosporine (Sandimmune, Neoral, SangCya)
Oral: 25-, 50-, 100-mg capsules; 100 mg/mL solution
Parenteral: 50 mg/mL for IV administration

Daclizumab (Zenapax)
Parenteral: 25 mg/5 mL vial for IV infusion

Etanercept (Enbrel)
Parenteral: 25-mg lyophilized powder for subcutaneous injection

Gemtuzumab (Mylotarg)
Parenteral: 5-mg powder for injection

Glatiramer (Copaxone)
Parenteral: 20 mg for SC injection

Ibritumomab tiuxetan (Cevalin)
Parenteral: 3.2 mg/2 mL for injection

Immune Globulin Intravenous (IGIV) (Gamimune, Gammagard, Iveegam, Polygam, others)
Parenteral: 5, 10% solutions; 2.5-, 5-, 6-, 10-, 12-g powder for injection

Infliximab (Remicade)
Parenteral: 100-mg lyophilized powder for IV injection

Interferon alfa-2a (Roferon-A)
Parenteral: 3–36 million units in vials or prefilled single-use syringes

Interferon alfa-2b (Intron-A)
Parenteral: 3–50 million units in vials or multi-dose pens

Interferon beta-1a (Avonex, Rebif)
Parenteral: 22-, 33-, 44-mcg powder for IV injection

Interferon beta-1b (Betaseron)
Parenteral: 0.3-mg powder for SC injection

Interferon gamma-1b (Actimmune)
Parenteral: 100-mcg vials

Interleukin-2, IL-2, aldesleukin (Proleukin)
Parenteral: 22-million unit vials

Leflunomide (Arava)
Oral: 10-, 20-, 100-mg tablets

Levamisole (Ergamisol)
Oral: 50-mg tablets

Lymphocyte immune globulin (Atgam)
Parenteral: 50 mg/mL for injection (in 5 mL ampules)

Methylprednisolone sodium succinate (Solu-Medrol, others)
Parenteral: 40-, 125-, 500-, 1000-, 2000-mg powder for injection

Muromonab-CD3 (OKT3) (Orthoclone OKT3)
Parenteral: 5 mg/5 mL ampule for injection

Mycophenolate mofetil (CellCept)
Oral: 250-mg capsules; 500-mg tablets; 200-mg powder for suspension
Parenteral: 500-mg powder for injection

Pegademase Bovine (Adagen)
Parenteral: 250 units/mL for IM injection
Note: Pegademase is bovine adenosine deaminase

Peginterferon alfa-2a (Pegasys)
Parenteral: 180 mcg/mL

Peginterferon alfa-2b (PEG-Intron)
Parenteral: 50, 80, 120, 150 mcg/0.5 mL

Prednisone (generic)
Oral: 1-, 2.5-, 10-, 20-, 50-mg tablets; 1, 5 mg/mL solution

Rh$_0$(D) Immune Globulin Micro-dose (BayRho-D, BayRho-D Mini-Dose, MICRhoGAM, RhoGam, WinRho)
Parenteral: in single-dose and micro-dose vials

Rituximab (Rituxan)
Parenteral: 10 mg/mL for IV infusion

Sirolimus (Rapamune)
Oral: 1-mg tablets; 1 mg/mL solution

Tacrolimus [FK506] (Prograf)
Oral: 0.5-, 1-, 5-mg capsules
Parenteral: 5 mg/mL
Topical (Protopic): 0.03%, 0.1% ointment

Thalidomide (Thalomid)
Oral: 50-mg capsules
Note: Thalidomide is labeled for use only in erythema nodosum leprosum in the United States.

Trastuzumab (Herceptin)
Parenteral: 440-mg powder for IV infusion

[1]Several drugs discussed in this chapter are available as orphan drugs but are not listed here. Other drugs not listed here will be found in other chapters.

REFERENCES

Ballow M: Primary immunodeficiency disorders: Antibody deficiency. *J Allergy Clin Immunol* 2002; 109:581.

Benito AI, et al: Sirolimus (rapamycin) for the treatment of steroid-refractory acute graft-versus-disease. *Transplantation* 2001;72:1924.

Brogan BL, Olsen NJ: Drug-induced rheumatic syndromes. *Curr Opin Rheumatol* 2003;15:76.

Gallin JI, Goldstein IM, Snyderman R: *Inflammation—Basic Principles and Clinical Correlates,* 3rd ed. New York: Raven Press, 1999.

Gerards AH, et al: Cyclosporine A monotherapy versus cyclosporine A and methotrexate combination therapy in patients with early rheumatoid arthritis: A double blind randomized placebo controlled trial. *Ann Rheum Dis* 2003;62:291.

Goldsby RA, et al: *Immunology 3,* 5th ed. New York: Freeman, 2003.

Janeway C, et al: *Immunobiology: The Immune System in Health and Disease,* 6th ed. Current Biology Publications, 2005.

Ju C, Uetrecht JP: Mechanism of idiosyncratic drug reactions: Reactive metabolite formation, protein binding and the regulation of the immune system. *Curr Drug Metab* 2002;3:367.

Matthews SJ, McCoy C: Thalidomide: A review of approved and investigational uses. *Clin Ther* 2003;25:342.

Moder KG: Mycophenolate mofetil: New applications for this immunosuppressant. *Ann Allergy Asthma Immunol* 2003;90:15.

Radovancevic B, Vrtovec B: Sirolimus therapy in cardiac transplantation. *Transplant Proc* 2003;35(3 Suppl):S171.

Reichert JM: Therapeutic monoclonal antibodies: Trends in development and approval in the US. *Curr Opin Mol Ther* 2002;4:110.

Rosenberg SA. Progress in the development of immunotherapy for the treatment of patients with cancer. *J Intern Med* 2001; 250:462.

Shlomchik MJ, et al: From T to B and back again: Positive feedback in systemic autoimmune disease. *Nat Rev Immunol* 2001;1:147.

Tutuncu Z, Morgan GJ Jr, Kavanaugh A: Anti-TNF therapy for other inflammatory conditions. *Clin Exp Rheumatol* 2002;20(6 Suppl 28):S146.

Umetsu DT, et al: Asthma: an epidemic of dysregulated immunity. *Nat Immunol* 2002;3:715.

Wall WJ: Use of antilymphocyte induction therapy in liver transplantation. *Liver Transpl Surg* 1999;5(4 Suppl 1): S64.

Rehabilitation

Arena R, et al: Safety and efficacy of exercise training in a patient awaiting heart transplantation while on positive intravenous inotropic support. *J Cardiopulm Rehabil* 2000;20:259.

Ballester M, et al: Reversal of rejection-induced coronary vasculitis detected early after heart transplantation with increased immunosuppression. *J Heart Transplant* 1989;8:413.

Baran DA, et al: Calcineurin inhibitor-associated early renal insufficiency in cardiac transplant recipients: Risk factors and strategies for prevention and treatment. *Am J Cardiovasc Drugs* 2004;4:21.

Braith RW, Edwards DG: Exercise following heart transplantation. *Sports Med* 2000;30:171.

Cahalin LP: Preoperative and postoperative conditioning for lung transplantation and volume-reduction surgery. *Crit Care Nurs Clin North Am* 1996;8:305.

Cantarovich M, et al: Treatment of steroid-resistant and recurrent acute cardiac transplant rejection with a short course of antibody therapy. *Clin Transplant* 1997;11:316.

Costanzo-Nordin MR, et al: Long-term follow-up of heart transplant recipients treated with murine antihuman mature T cell monoclonal antibody (OKT3): The Loyola experience. *J Heart Transplant* 1989;8:288.

Downs AM: Physical therapy in lung transplantation. *Phys Ther* 1996;76:626.

Emery RW, et al: Cardiac transplant patient at one year. Cyclosporine vs conventional immunosuppression. *Chest* 1986;90:29.

Grimm M, et al : Superior prevention of acute rejection by tacrolimus vs. cyclosporine in heart transplant recipients—a large European trial. *Am J Transplant* 2006;6:1387.

Haykowsky M, et al: Effect of exercise training on VO2peak and left ventricular systolic function in recent cardiac transplant recipients. *Am J Cardiol* 2005;95:1002.

Kavanagh T: Exercise rehabilitation in cardiac transplantation patients: A comprehensive review. *Eura Medicophys* 2005;41:67.

Maher C, Williams M: Factors influencing the use of outcome measures in physiotherapy management of lung transplant patients in Australia and New Zealand. *Physiother Theory Pract* 2005;21:201.

Marconi C, Marzorati M: Exercise after heart transplantation. *Eur J Appl Physiol* 2003;90:250.

Sadowsky HS: Cardiac transplantation: A review. *Phys Ther* 1996;76:498.

Shore S, Shepard RJ: Immune responses to exercise in children treated for cancer. *J Sports Med Phys Fitness* 1999;39:240.

Takaoka ST, Weinacker AB: The value of preoperative pulmonary rehabilitation. *Thorac Surg Clin* 2005;15:203.

Tegtbur U, et al: Time course of physical reconditioning during exercise rehabilitation late after heart transplantation. *J Heart Lung Transplant* 2005;24:270.

Vintro AQ, et al: Roles of nutrition and physical activity in musculoskeletal complications before and after liver transplantation. *AACN Clin Issues* 2002; 13:333.

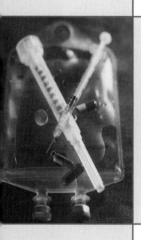

DRUGS AFFECTING
THE MUSCULOSKELETAL
SYSTEM

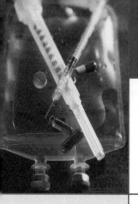

33

SKELETAL MUSCLE RELAXANTS

Drugs that affect skeletal muscles fall into two major therapeutic groups: those used during surgical procedures and in intensive care units to cause paralysis (i.e., **neuromuscular blockers**), and those used to reduce spasticity in a variety of neurologic conditions or to reduce muscle spasm following muscle injury or inflammation (i.e., **spasmolytics**) (Figure 33–1). Neuromuscular blocking drugs interfere with transmission at the neuromuscular end plate and lack central nervous system activity. These compounds are used primarily as adjuncts to general anesthesia. Drugs in the spasmolytic group have traditionally been called "centrally acting" muscle relaxants because most of them act at multiple sites in the central nervous system (CNS) rather than at the neuromuscular end plate. However, two spasmolytic drugs—**dantrolene** and **botulinum toxin**—act in or near skeletal muscle with no significant central effects. Spasmolytic drugs (with one exception) do not prevent muscle contraction but rather decrease neuronal excitability. For basic and clinical pharmacology of neuromuscular blocking drugs, see Chapter 5.

PATHOPHYSIOLOGY OF SPASTICITY AND MUSCLE SPASM

Spasticity is characterized by an increase in tonic stretch reflexes and flexor muscle spasms (i.e., increased basal muscle tone), together with muscle weakness and a reduction in viscoelastic muscle properties. It is often associated with cerebral palsy, multiple sclerosis, spinal cord injury, and stroke. These conditions often involve abnormal function of the bowel and bladder as well as skeletal muscle. The mechanisms underlying spasticity in these types of neurologic injury appear to involve not only the stretch reflex arc itself but also higher centers in the CNS (upper motor neuron lesions), with damage to descending pathways in the spinal cord, resulting in loss of supraspinal inhibition to the alpha and gamma motor neurons in the anterior horn of the spinal cord. With damage to descending pathways, upper motor neurons from the cerebral cortex and brain stem nuclei no longer modulate spinal reflexes, and no longer activate the spinal cord inhibitory interneuron pools. The decrease in activity in the inhibitory interneurons results in increased excitability of alpha motor neurons in the cord. Some of the components involved in these descending inhibitory pathways are shown in Figure 33–2.

Pharmacologic therapy can ameliorate some of the signs and symptoms of neurologic injury spasticity by modifying the stretch reflex arc or, in the case of dantrolene, by interfering directly with skeletal muscle (i.e., excitation-contraction coupling). The important components involved in these processes are shown in Figure 33–3. Drugs that modify the reflex arc may modulate excitatory or inhibitory synapses (Chapter 12). To reduce the hyperactive stretch reflex, it is desirable to reduce the activity of the Ia fibers providing afferent information from

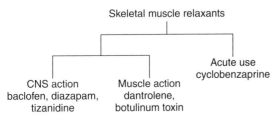

Figure 33–1. Skeletal muscle relaxants in this chapter may be initially divided into those used acutely to reduce muscle spasms, and those used chronically to treat central nervous system (CNS) associated spasticity. The latter group are subsequently divided into those which act within the CNS, and those that act at the muscle.

the muscle spindle that excites the primary motor neuron, or to enhance the activity of the inhibitory internuncial neurons. These structures are shown in greater detail in Figure 33–4.

In contrast to spasticity, muscle spasms are characterized by an increase in skeletal muscle tension associated with musculoskeletal injuries and inflammation secondary, for example, to nerve impingement, muscle strains, or muscle overuse. Muscle injury spasms may also result from chemical or mechanical stimuli in the peripheral nervous system. These noxious stimuli set in

motion a negative pain-tension-pain cycle that can be interrupted by enhancing the activity of inhibitory internuncial neurons.

A variety of pharmacologic agents described as depressants of the spinal "polysynaptic" reflex arc (e.g., barbiturates [phenobarbital] and glycerol ethers [mephenesin]) have been used to treat these conditions of excess skeletal muscle tone. Drugs used to treat neurologic injury spasticity are classified as antispasticity drugs, whereas drugs used to treat muscle injury spasms are typically classified as antispasm drugs. Regardless of the origin of excess skeletal muscle tone, nonspecific depression of all synapses involved in the stretch reflex by such drugs would reduce the desired inhibitory activity as well as the undesirable excitatory transmission, as illustrated in Figure 33–4. Also, excessive depression of synapses at the level of the spinal cord segments can result in a loss of voluntary muscle activity. Thus, selective *enhancement* of inhibitory or selective *depression* of excitatory transmission is needed.

Unfortunately, the lack of convenient and quantifiable measures of clinical response and of appropriate experimental models has hampered development of better agents for this heterogeneous group of medical conditions. Furthermore, while currently available

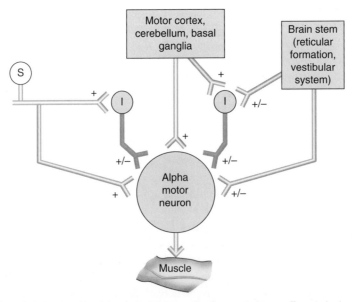

Figure 33–2. Input to alpha motor neurons. *S* = sensory primary afferent; *I* = brain stem interneuron; + = excitatory synapse; – = inhibitory synapse.

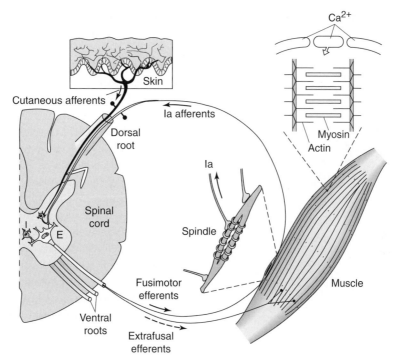

Figure 33–3. Diagram of the structures involved in the stretch reflex arc. *I* = inhibitory presynaptic terminal; *E* = excitatory presynaptic terminal; *Ia* = primary intrafusal afferent fiber; Ca²⁺ = activator calcium stored in the sarcoplasmic reticulum of skeletal muscle. (Reproduced, with permission, from Young RR, Delwaide PJ: Drug therapy: Spasticity. *N Engl J Med* 1981;304:28.)

drugs provide significant relief from neurologic injury spasticity (antispasticity drugs) as well as painful muscle injury spasms (antispasm drugs), they are all less effective in improving meaningful function (e.g., mobility, functional activity, and return to work). Table 33–1 lists the half-lives and clinical uses for several skeletal muscle relaxants from different drug classes.

■ SPASMOLYTIC (ANTISPASTICITY) DRUGS

Diazepam

As described in Chapter 13, benzodiazepines facilitate the action of gamma-aminobutyric acid (GABA) in the CNS. Diazepam, the benzodiazepine most commonly used as a spasmolytic agent, acts at all GABA$_A$ synapses, but its action in reducing neurologic injury spasticity is at least partly mediated in the spinal cord (Figure 33–4). Diazepam is somewhat effective in treating spasticity resulting from cord transection and spasticity due to cerebral palsy. It can also be used in patients with muscle injury spasm of almost any origin, including local muscle trauma. However, it produces sedation in most patients at the dose required to significantly reduce muscle tone. Other benzodiazepines have been used as spasmolytics, but experience with them is much more limited.

Baclofen

Baclofen (*p*-chlorophenyl-GABA) is an orally active GABAmimetic agent and exerts its spasmolytic activity at GABA$_B$ receptors. Activation of central GABA$_B$ receptors by baclofen results in hyperpolarization, probably by increased K⁺ conductance. It has been suggested that hyperpolarization causes presynaptic inhibition by reducing calcium influx which reduces the release of excitatory transmitters in both the brain and the spinal cord. Baclofen may

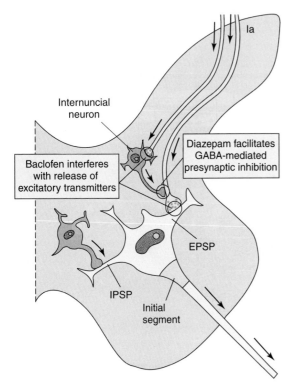

Figure 33–4. Postulated sites of spasmolytic drug action in the spinal cord. EPSP = excitatory postsynaptic potential; IPSP = inhibitory postsynaptic potential. (Reproduced, with permission, from Young RR, Delwaide PJ: Drug therapy: Spasticity. *N Engl J Med* 1981;304:28.)

also reduce pain in patients with excessive skeletal tone, perhaps by inhibiting the release of substance P in the spinal cord.

Baclofen is at least as effective as diazepam in reducing spasticity due to neurologic injury and it produces much less sedation. In addition, although baclofen reduces overall muscle strength, the degree of induced weakness is not as severe as with other classes of centrally acting skeletal muscle relaxants such as diazepam. Baclofen is rapidly and completely absorbed after oral administration. Adverse effects of this drug include drowsiness, to which the patient may become tolerant with chronic administration, and generalized muscle weakness at higher doses. Increased seizure activity has been reported in epileptic patients, especially upon withdrawal of the drug. Therefore, withdrawal of baclofen must be done very slowly.

Studies show that intrathecal administration of baclofen can control severe spasticity and muscle pain that is not responsive to medication by other routes of administration. Owing to the poor egress of baclofen from the spinal cord, peripheral symptoms are rare. Therefore, higher central concentrations of baclofen may be tolerated. Partial tolerance to the effect of the drug may occur after several months of therapy but can be overcome by upward dosage adjustments to maintain the beneficial effect. Several cases of excessive somnolence, respiratory depression, and even coma have been reported. Although a major disadvantage of this therapeutic approach is the difficulty of maintaining

		Clinical Uses		
Generic Name	**Elimination Half-life (h)**	**Spasticity**	**Muscle Spasm**	**Other Uses**
Diazepam	43 ± 13	Yes	Yes	Sedative-hypnotic
Baclofen	4.9 ± 1.9	Yes	No	
Dantrolene	8.7	Yes	No	Succinylcholine-induced malignant hyperthermia
Gabapentin	6 ± 1	Yes	No	Neuropathic pain Antiepileptic
Cyclobenzaprine	18 ± 9.1	Yes	Yes	Fibrositis
Tizanidine	~2	Yes	No	Cluster headache

Table 33–1. Characteristics of several skeletal muscle relaxants

the drug-delivery catheter in the subarachnoid space, long-term intrathecal baclofen therapy can improve the quality of life for patients with severe spasticity associated with multiple sclerosis, stroke, and cerebral palsy. This route of administration is becoming more widely used due to the specificity of delivery and the reduced occurrence of systemic adverse drug reactions.

Oral baclofen has been studied in several other medical conditions. Preliminary studies suggest that it may be effective in reducing craving in recovering alcoholics. It has also been found effective in preventing migraine attacks in some patients.

Tizanidine

As noted in Chapter 6, alpha adrenoceptor agonists such as clonidine and other imidazoline compounds have a variety of effects on the CNS that are not fully understood. Among these effects is the ability to reduce muscle spasm. Tizanidine has significant alpha$_2$-adrenoceptor agonist effects, but it reduces spasticity in experimental models at doses that cause fewer cardiovascular effects than clonidine. Studies in animals and humans suggest that tizanidine reinforces both presynaptic and postsynaptic inhibition in the spinal cord. Tizanidine also inhibits nociceptive transmission in the spinal dorsal horn.

Clinical trials with tizanidine report comparable efficacy to that of diazepam, baclofen, and dantrolene in relieving spasticity due to neurological injury. For this reason, tizanidine may be a better choice for reducing spasticity while maintaining adequate muscle strength for transfers, ambulation, and general activity. However, tizanidine produces a different spectrum of adverse effects, including drowsiness, hypotension, dry mouth, and asthenia. The dosage requirements vary markedly among patients, suggesting that individual dosage titration is necessary to achieve an optimal effect.

Other Centrally Acting Spasmolytic Drugs

Gabapentin is an antiepileptic drug (Chapter 14) that has shown considerable promise as a spasmolytic agent in several studies involving patients with multiple sclerosis and spinal cord injury. However, this drug has been approved by the Food and Drug Administration only for use in epilepsy and postherpetic neuralgia.

Although the exact mechanism of action is not known, it is thought that gabapentin enhances the inhibitory effects of GABA by stimulating GABA-like receptors on spinal neurons or increasing GABA release in the spinal cord. It is very effective when used in combination with more typical antispasticity drugs such as baclofen. Gabapentin has also been reported to be useful in the treatment of chronic pain. Additional research is needed to fully understand its role in controlling spasticity and muscle spasms due to various injuries. **Progabide** and **glycine** have also been found in preliminary studies to reduce spasticity. Progabide is a GABA$_A$ and GABA$_B$ agonist and has active metabolites, including GABA itself. Glycine is another inhibitory amino acid neurotransmitter (Chapter 12). It appears to possess pharmacologic activity when given orally and readily passes the blood-brain barrier. **Idrocilamide** and **riluzole** are newer drugs for the treatment of amyotrophic lateral sclerosis that appear to have spasm-reducing effects, possibly through inhibition of glutamatergic transmission in the CNS.

Dantrolene

Dantrolene is a hydantoin derivative related to phenytoin that has a unique mechanism of spasmolytic activity. In contrast to the centrally active drugs, dantrolene reduces skeletal muscle strength by interfering with excitation-contraction coupling in the muscle fibers. The normal contractile response involves release of calcium from its stores in the sarcoplasmic reticulum (Figures 33–3 and 33–5).

Dantrolene interferes with the release of activator calcium through the sarcoplasmic reticulum calcium channel. Because more effective drugs, such as diazepam, baclofen, and the polysynaptic inhibitors, are currently available for providing significant relief from painful spasms and injury spasticity, dantrolene is rarely prescribed by physicians for outpatient use. It is usually given to treat severe spasticity due to neurological injury when other agents have been deemed ineffective. It is not advocated for use in the treatment of muscle injury spasms. The most common side effect is pronounced generalized muscle weakness. It may also cause severe hepatotoxicity, and for this reason it is not a first-choice drug.

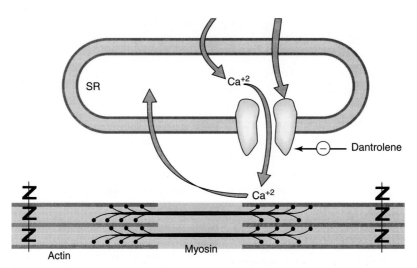

Figure 33–5. Mechanism of action of dantrolene. Dantrolene blocks the calcium release channels in the sarcoplasmic reticulum (SR). The sarcomere boundary is shown by the Z lines (Z).

A special inpatient application of dantrolene is in the treatment of malignant hyperthermia, a rare heritable disorder characterized by often fatal hyperthermia due to a sudden and prolonged release of calcium, with massive muscle contraction, lactic acid production, and increased body temperature. Dantrolene inhibits skeletal muscle contraction throughout the body, thus reducing excessive body temperature generated by massive, repetitive muscle contractions.

Botulinum Toxin

The therapeutic use of botulinum toxin for local muscle spasm was discussed in Chapter 5. Local injection of botulinum toxin has become popular for the treatment of generalized spastic disorders (e.g., cerebral palsy) as well as more localized spastic disorders (e.g., stroke). Most clinical studies to date have involved administration in one or two limbs or in specific muscle groups, and the benefits appear to persist for weeks to several months after a single treatment. Two forms of the toxin, type A and type B, are available for clinical use. The degree of lasting improvement in functional ability appears to be extremely variable and must be assessed on a case by case basis.

Local facial injections of botulinum toxin are widely used for the short-term treatment (1 to 3 months per treatment) of wrinkles around the eyes, mouth, and forehead.

ANTISPASM DRUGS

Polysynaptic Inhibitors

A large number of drugs (e.g., **carisoprodol, chlorphenesin, chlorzoxazone, cyclobenzaprine, metaxalone, methocarbamol,** and **orphenadrine**) are promoted for the relief of acute muscle spasm caused by local tissue trauma or muscular strains. It has been suggested that these drugs act primarily at the levels of the brain stem and spinal cord. Although their mechanisms of action are not well understood, animal research suggest that some of these drugs interfere with the polysynaptic transmission of neuronal impulses within the spinal cord, thus reducing alpha motor neuron excitability and activity. Table 33–2 describes the onset and duration of action, and common adverse effects of these drugs.

The major adverse effects of these drugs are generalized sedation, confusion, headache, and nausea and vomiting. They are often used as adjuncts to rest and physical therapy for relief of muscle spasm associated with acute, painful musculoskeletal injuries. They are often prescribed in combination with nonsteroidal anti-inflammatory agents or analgesics. Some formulations

Table 33–2. Polysynaptic inhibitors used as antispasm agents

Drug	Onset of Action (min)	Duration of Action (h)	Most Common Adverse Reactions
Carisoprodol	30	4–6	Drowsiness
Chlorphenesin carbamate	–	–	Drowsiness, dizziness
Chlorzoxazone	<60	3–4	Drowsiness, dizziness
Cyclobenzaprine	<60	12–24	Drowsiness, dizziness
Metaxalone	<60	4–6	Drowsiness, dizziness, headache, nausea, and vomiting
Methocarbamol	<30	24	Drowsiness, dizziness
Orphenadrine citrate	<60	12	Drowsiness, headache

are available that incorporate an analgesic such as aspirin or acetaminophen (e.g., orphenadrine combined with aspirin). They are ineffective in treating spasticity caused by cerebral palsy, multiple sclerosis, or spinal cord injury. A listing of muscle relaxants used in the treatment of muscle spasms and spasticity is presented in Table 33–3.

REHABILITATION FOCUS

Skeletal muscle relaxants are prescribed for many patients involved in rehabilitation programs. These drugs are used for both neurologic injury spasticity and for muscle injury spasms. When these drugs are used as primary agents to treat spasticity, simultaneous physical therapy and occupational therapy interventions are very important to improve the overall functional status of the patient. Weakness complications, because they affect functional outcomes, must be monitored with functional or quality of life assessment tools. Intense therapy to facilitate more normal physiologic motor control and functioning is necessary to replace previously used spastic tone. Successful use of these agents decreases spasticity, resulting in improved self-care or nursing care, and reduced spastic contractures. The latter are often very painful and

Table 33–3. Skeletal muscle relaxants used as antispasm versus antispasticity agents

Antispasticity Agents	Antispasm Agents
Baclofen	Carisoprodol
Botulinum toxin type A	Chlorphenesin
Botulinum toxin type B	Chlorzoxazone
Dantrolene	Cyclobenzaprine
Diazepam	Diazepam
Gabapentin	Metaxalone
Note: This drug is labeled for use only in epilepsy.	Methocarbamol
	Orphenadrine
Riluzole	
Note: This drug is labeled only for use in amyotrophic lateral sclerosis.	
Tizanidine	

detrimental to overall functional outcomes. Similarly, when antispasm agents are used to reduce muscle spasm following muscle strains or nerve root impingement, they will complement many nonpharmacologic interventions. These interventions include thermal agents, electrotherapy, manual therapy, and treatment based on biomechanical analysis. Overall, the patient benefits from pain relief and improved functional status. Used alone these drugs have no anti-inflammatory activity, and must therefore be used in conjunction with other medications if such an effect is desired. To minimize additional muscular injury, other therapeutic interventions must be implemented.

■ CLINICAL RELEVANCE FOR REHABILITATION

Adverse Drug Reactions
• Generalized muscle weakness
• Decreased muscle tone
• Sedation
• Dizziness
• Ataxia

Effects Interfering with Rehabilitation
• Motor control problems
• Functional decline for daily activities
• Decreased alertness
• Weakness
• Tolerance and physical dependence (not associated with all types of skeletal muscle relaxants)

Possible Therapy Solutions
• Schedule physical therapy at a time of day when sedative effects are less marked.
• Discuss with the prescribing physician the generalized weakness implications as they affect functional outcomes.
• In the case of patients with spasticity due to neurological injury, use intensive physical therapy to promote normal physiologic motor control for previously used spastic tone.
• In the case of patients with muscle spasm, use intensive physical therapy to improve muscle strength, posture, and flexibility including proper body mechanics to decrease the need for the drugs by decreasing the incidence of spasms.

PROBLEM-ORIENTED PATIENT STUDY

Brief History: The patient is a 54-year-old male with a primary diagnosis of relapsing remitting multiple sclerosis (RR-MS). He was diagnosed approximately 12 years ago. He lives at home with his wife and teenage children. His major mode of mobility is an electric wheelchair; however, he states that he would like to stand and walk more if possible. He is self-employed and works approximately 30 hours a week.

Current Medical Status and Drug Therapy: He is slightly overweight. His cholesterol and blood glucose levels are within normal ranges. The patient has no history of heart disease or other medical conditions. He is currently taking oral baclofen and tizanidine for bilateral lower extremity spasticity.

Rehabilitation Setting: The patient was referred to physical therapy for evaluation of assistive devices during ambulation. Upon initial evaluation, the patient had limited movement and volitional activity of his lower extremities but his upper extremity strength was normal. He had significant functional strength as he was able to lift himself into and out of his vehicle. He was initially fitted with custom molded ankle-foot orthotics and began a neuromuscular re-education program to improve his ambulatory skills.

Problem and Clinical Options: This patient had significant neurologic injury spasticity in his lower extremities. He would suffer significant lower extremity spasticity with transfers and with any weight-bearing activity in his lower extremities. This spasticity was limiting his ability to gain functional strength and improve his functional abilities. The patient's baclofen was increased to a

PROBLEM-ORIENTED PATIENT STUDY (*Continued*)

maximum tolerated oral dose along with a slight increase in his oral dose of tizanidine. It was apparent that after this increase in his oral medications, the patient was suffering from significant upper extremity weakness. He was now experiencing difficulty transferring into and out of his vehicle as well as increased difficulty in ambulation. Although his spasticity was now well controlled, it left him with limited functional ability. The patient, physician, and rehabilitation team decided that a baclofen pump might make it possible to control his spasticity without reducing his upper extremity strength. The patient received a baclofen pump. After recovery from the surgery and titration of the intrathecal baclofen dose, he returned to therapy. The patient was well maintained with this drug-delivery system and was able to improve his ambulatory ability.

PREPARATIONS AVAILABLE

Muscle Relaxants (Spasmolytics)

Baclofen (generic, Lioresal)
Oral: 10-, 20-mg tablets
Intrathecal: 0.05, 0.5, 2 mg/mL

Botulinum toxin type A (Botox)
Parenteral: Powder for solution, 100 units/vial

Botulinum toxin type B (Myobloc)
Parenteral: 5000 units/mL for injection

Carisoprodol (generic, Soma)
Oral: 350-mg tablets

Chlorphenesin (Maolate)
Oral: 400-mg tablets

Chlorzoxazone (generic, Paraflex)
Oral: 250-, 500-mg tablets, caplets

Cyclobenzaprine (generic, Flexeril)
Oral: 10-mg tablets

Dantrolene (Dantrium)
Oral: 25-, 50-, 100-mg capsules
Parenteral: 20 mg per vial powder to reconstitute for injection

Diazepam (generic, Valium)
Oral: 2-, 5-, 10-mg tablets; 5 mg/5 mL, 5 mg/mL solutions
Parenteral: 5 mg/mL for injection

Gabapentin (Neurontin)
Oral: 100-, 300-, 400-mg capsules; 600-, 800-mg tablets
Note: This drug is labeled for use only in epilepsy and postherpetic neuralgia.

Metaxalone (Skelaxin)
Oral: 400-mg tablets

Methocarbamol (generic, Robaxin)
Oral: 500-, 750-mg tablets
Parenteral: 100 mg/mL for IM, IV injection

Orphenadrine (generic, Norflex)
Oral: 100-mg tablets; 100-mg sustained-release tablets
Parenteral: 30 mg/mL for IM, IV injection

Riluzole (Rilutek)
Oral: 50-mg tablets
Note: This drug is labeled only for use in amyotrophic lateral sclerosis.

Tizanidine (Zanaflex)
Oral: 4-mg tablets

REFERENCES

Addolorato G, et al: Ability of baclofen in reducing alcohol craving and intake: II. Preliminary clinical evidence. *Alcohol Clin Exp Res* 2000;24:67.

Cutter NC, et al: Gabapentin effect on spasticity in multiple sclerosis: A placebo-controlled, randomized trial. *Arch Phys Med Rehabil* 2000;81:164.

Davidoff RA: Antispasticity drugs: Mechanisms of action. *Ann Neurol* 1985;17:107.

Gracies JM, et al: Traditional pharmacological treatments for spasticity. Part II: General and regional treatments. *Muscle Nerve Suppl* 1997;6:S92.

Groves L, et al: Tizanidine treatment of spasticity: A meta-analysis of controlled, double-blind, comparative studies with baclofen and diazepam. *Adv Ther* 1998;15:241.

Hunskaar S, Donnell D: Clinical and pharmacological review of the efficacy of orphenadrine and its combination with paracetamol in painful conditions. *J Int Med Res* 1991;19:71.

Koman LA, et al: Botulinum toxin type A neuromuscular blockade in the treatment of lower extremity spasticity in cerebral palsy: A randomized, double-blind, placebo-controlled trial. BOTOX study group. *J Pediatr Orthop* 2000;20:108.

Lopez JR, et al: Effects of dantrolene on myoplasmic free [Ca^{2+}] measured in vivo in patients susceptible to malignant hyperthermia. *Anesthesiology* 1992;76:711.

Pierson SH, et al: Botulinum toxin in the treatment of spasticity: Functional implications and patient selection. *Arch Phys Med Rehab* 1996;77:717.

Simpson DM, et al: Botulinum toxin type A in the treatment of upper extremity spasticity: A randomized, double-blind, placebo-controlled trial. *Neurology* 1996;46:1306.

Stanko JR: Review of oral skeletal muscle relaxants for the craniomandibular disorder (CMD) practioner. *Cranio* 1990;8:234.

Wagstaff AJ, Bryson HM: Tizanidine: A review of its pharmacology, clinical efficacy and tolerability in the management of spasticity associated with cerebral and spinal disorders. *Drugs* 1997;53:435.

Young RR (ed): Symposium: Role of tizanidine in the treatment of spasticity. *Neurology* 1994;44(Suppl 9):1. [Entire issue.]

Young RR, Wiegner AW: Spasticity. *Clin Orthop* 1987;219:50.

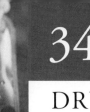

34

DRUGS AFFECTING EICOSANOID METABOLISM, DISEASE-MODIFYING ANTIRHEUMATIC DRUGS, AND DRUGS USED IN GOUT

Eicosanoids are 20-carbon fatty acids (eicosa- means 20) found in many tissues of the body. These compounds are extremely important in multiple physiologic responses, such as gastric mucosal protection and controlling resistance in various vascular beds. They are also significant mediators of pain and inflammation. Thus, both eicosanoid agonists and antagonists are important, but the antagonists are more commonly used clinically.

Inflammation and pain are common manifestations in rheumatic diseases, and eicosanoid antagonists are heavily prescribed to reduce symptoms. Other drugs modify the cellular- and humoral-immune responses in some autoimmune-mediated rheumatic diseases. These drugs are classified as disease-modifying antirheumatic drugs (DMARDs).

Gout is a disease that results from crystallization of a nucleic acid metabolite—uric acid, in the body. In the joints, this crystallization results in inflammation and pain. Patients with gout are treated with anti-inflammatory drugs, and drugs that either decrease formation of these metabolites or increase their excretion. Drug classes discussed in this chapter are reviewed in Figure 34–1.

■ EICOSANOID METABOLISM

The eicosanoids are an important group of endogenous fatty acid derivatives that are produced from arachidonic acid, a normal constituent of cell membranes.

Synthesis

Eicosanoids are synthesized in response to a variety of stimuli (e.g., physical injury, immune reactions). These stimuli activate phospholipases in the cell membrane or cytoplasm, and arachidonic acid is released from membrane phospholipids (Figure 34–2). Arachidonic acid is then metabolized by one of several mechanisms. Metabolism to straight-chain products is performed by *lipoxygenase* (LOX), ultimately producing **leukotrienes** (LTs). Alternatively, cyclization by the enzyme *cyclooxygenase* (COX) results in the production of three major subgroups: **prostacyclin** (PGI), **prostaglandins** (PGs), and **thromboxane** (TX). There are several series for most of the principal cyclized subgroups based on different substituents (indicated by letters A, B, etc.) and different numbers of double bonds (indicated by a subscript number) in the molecule.

The COX enzyme exists in at least two forms. COX-1 is found in many tissues; the prostaglandins produced in these tissues by COX-1 appear to be important for a variety of normal

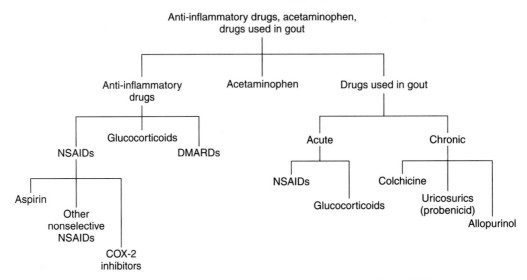

Figure 34–1. Drug classes used in the treatment of inflammation and associated pain. Anti-inflammatory drugs are divided into nonsteroidal anti-inflammatory drugs (NSAIDs), glucocorticoids, and disease-modifying antirheumatic drugs (DMARDs). The NSAIDs are further divided based on their mechanism of action. Acetaminophen is in a drug class alone because of its mechanism of action. The drugs used in the treatment of gout are classified as acute or chronic therapies. In the acute phase, NSAIDs and glucocorticoids are used to decrease inflammation and associated pain. In the chronic phase, drugs are classified based on whether they inhibit inflammatory cell function (colchicine), increase the excretion of uric acid (uricosurics), or inhibit the formation of uric acid (allopurinol).

physiologic processes (especially gastrointestinal function). In contrast, COX-2 is primarily expressed in activated lymphocytes, polymorphonuclear cells, and other inflammatory cells. The results of its actions play a major role in tissue injury (e.g., inflammation). A third form of the enzyme has been hypothesized, COX-3; evidence is inconclusive as to the significance of this enzyme in humans compared to other animal species. Thromboxane is preferentially synthesized in platelets by COX-1, whereas prostacyclin is synthesized in the endothelial cells of vessels by COX-2. Naturally occurring eicosanoids have very short half-lives (seconds to minutes) and are inactive when given orally.

Mechanism of Action and Physiologic Effects

Most eicosanoid effects appear to be brought about by activation of cell surface receptors that are coupled by G proteins to adenylyl cyclase, producing the second-messenger cyclic adenosine monophosphate (cAMP); or the phosphatidylinositol cascade, producing inositol 1,4,5-trisphosphate (IP_3) and diacylglycerol (DAG) second messengers.

Eicosanoids produce a vast array of physiologic effects in smooth muscle, platelets, the central nervous system (CNS), and other tissues. Some of the most important effects are summarized in Table 34–1. Exogenous $PGF_{2\alpha}$ reduces intraocular pressure, but it is not known whether this is a physiologic effect of the endogenous substance. PGE_1 and its derivatives have significant protective effects on the gastric mucosa. This mechanism may involve increased secretion of bicarbonate and mucus, decreased acid secretion, or both. PGE_1, PGE_2, and PGI_2 may play important roles as endogenous vasodilators. PGE_2 appears to be the natural vasodilator that maintains patency of the ductus arteriosus during fetal development. PGI_2 is formed in response to an increase in wall shear stress in vascular endothelial cells. PGE_1

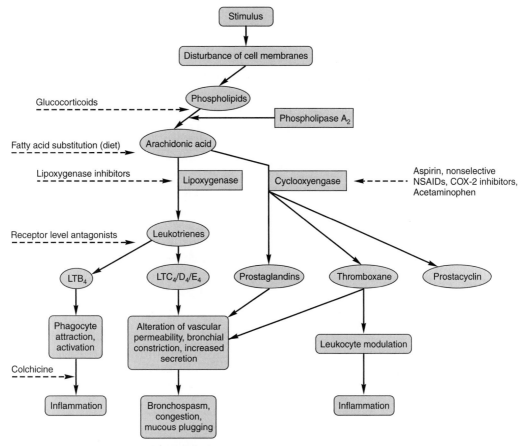

Figure 34–2. Scheme for mediators of inflammation derived from arachidonic acid via the cyclooxygenase (COX) or lipoxygenase pathways. Inhibitory sites of action are presented with dashed arrows. Aspirin and the nonselective NSAIDs inhibit, to varying degrees, all COX isozymes. The COX-2 inhibitors preferentially inhibit COX-2. Acetaminophen inhibits a COX isozyme present in the CNS. The lipoxygenase pathway may be inhibited at an enzymatic level or receptor level. Fatty acid substitution from the diet, with eicosapentaenoic acid for example, results in less potent eicosanoid products.

Table 34–1.	Effects of some important eicosanoids						
Effect	**PGE$_2$**	**PGF$_{2\alpha}$**	**PGI$_2$**	**TXA$_2$**	**LTB$_4$**	**LTC$_4$**	**LTD$_4$**
Vascular tone	↓	↑ or ↓	↓↓	↑↑↑	?	↑ or ↓	↑ or ↓
Bronchial tone	↓↓	↑	↓	↑↑↑	?	↑↑↑	↑↑↑↑
Uterine tone	↑↑	↑↑↑	↓	↑↑	?	?	?
Platelet aggregation	↑ or ↓	?	↓↓↓	↑↑↑	?	?	?
Leukocyte chemotaxis	?	?	?	?	↑↑↑↑	?	?

PG = prostaglandin; TX = thromboxane; LT leukotriene; ? = unknown effect.

and PGE_2 also relax nonvascular smooth muscle. PGE_2 and $PGF_{2\alpha}$ are released in large amounts from the endometrium during menstruation and may play a physiologic role in labor. PGE_2 also appears to be involved in the physiologic changes of the cervix at term. $PGF_{2\alpha}$ and TXA_2 are the two eicosanoid products from the COX cascade most directly involved in pathologic processes. Dysmenorrhea is associated with uterine contractions induced by prostaglandins, especially $PGF_{2\alpha}$. Platelet aggregation is strongly activated by TXA_2.

Eicosanoid products involved in pathologic processes from the LOX cascade include the leukotrienes LTC_4 and LTD_4, which compose an important mediator of bronchoconstriction, *slow-reacting substance of anaphylaxis* (SRS-A). Leukotriene LTB_4 is a chemotactic factor and it is also important in inflammation. These LOX metabolites are mediators of dysfunction in asthma and other pulmonary diseases and are discussed in Chapter 35.

Inflammation and Pain

Inflammation is a common nonspecific manifestation of many diseases, and may be acute or chronic in form; the acute and chronic forms may occur independently or simultaneously. The primary initial manifestations of inflammation are vasodilation with subsequent redness (*rubor*) and heat (*calor*) in the area, swelling (*tumor*), and pain (*dolor*).

Inflammation also involves the activation and proliferation of the immune system. Immune responses are regulated in part by cytokines (Chapter 32) and in part by eicosanoids. Inflammation and the immune response may benefit the host if they cause invading organisms to be phagocytosed or neutralized. On the other hand, these processes may be deleterious if they lead to chronic inflammation without resolution of the underlying injurious process.

The pain associated with inflammation is also mediated in part by eicosanoids in both peripheral tissues at inflammatory sites and within the CNS. In the peripheral tissues, PGE_2 and PGI_2 sensitize nociceptive nerve endings to painful stimuli. Centrally, both COX and LOX metabolites, PGE_2 and LTB_4, may modulate nociceptive transmission.

■ EICOSANOID AGONISTS

Clinical Uses

Obstetrics

PGE_2 and $PGF_{2\alpha}$ are involved in contraction of the uterus. PGE_2 (**dinoprostone**) is approved for use to ripen the cervix at term before induction of labor with oxytocin (Chapter 22). Both PGE_2 and $PGF_{2\alpha}$ have been used as abortifacients in the second trimester of pregnancy. Although effective in inducing labor at term, they produce more adverse effects (nausea, vomiting, diarrhea) than oxytocin, which is used for this application. In Europe, and more recently in the United States, the PGE_1 analog (**misoprostol**) has been used with the progesterone antagonist **mifepristone** (RU-486) as an extremely effective and safe abortifacient combination (Chapter 22).

Pediatrics

PGE_1 (**alprostadil**) is given as an infusion to maintain patency of the ductus arteriosus in infants with transposition of the great vessels until surgical correction can be undertaken.

Pulmonary Hypertension and Dialysis

PGI_2 (**epoprostenol**) is approved for use in severe pulmonary hypertension and to prevent platelet aggregation in dialysis machines.

Gastrointestinal Dysfunction

Peptic ulceration is a common adverse effect associated with nonsteroidal anti-inflammatory drug (NSAID) use. Misoprostol is approved in the United States for the prevention of peptic ulcers in patients who must take high doses of NSAIDs for arthritis, and who have a history of gastric ulcers associated with this use.

Urology

Alprostadil (PGE_1) is used in the treatment of impotence. Preparations are available for injection into the penile tissue as well as an intraurethral minisuppository.

Ophthalmology

Latanoprost, a $PGF_{2\alpha}$ derivative, is used for the treatment of glaucoma. **Bimatoprost, travoprost,** and **unoprostone**

are newer, related drugs. These agents reduce intraocular pressure, apparently by increasing the outflow of aqueous humor.

◾ EICOSANOID ANTAGONISTS

These drugs decrease the effects of eicosanoids, mainly by blocking the enzymatic activities of phospholipase A_2, COX, or LOX (Figure 34–2). A few drugs decrease the physiologic effects of eicosanoids by inhibiting the binding of eicosanoids with LT receptors. Aspirin, NSAIDs (including COX-2 inhibitors), and acetaminophen are used to inhibit the formation of eicosanoids by inhibiting COX activity. Glucocorticoids inhibit the formation of all eicosanoid products by several mechanisms, including inhibition of phospholipase A_2 activity. Glucocorticoids are discussed in Chapter 23, and are briefly reviewed under rheumatic diseases later in this chapter. Inhibitors of LOX activity or LT receptors are used in the treatment of pulmonary dysfunction, and are discussed in Chapter 35.

Aspirin and Nonselective NSAIDS

Aspirin (acetylsalicylic acid) is the prototype of the salicylates. The other "traditional" nonselective NSAIDs (ibuprofen, indomethacin, and many others) vary primarily in their potency and duration of action (Table 34–2).

Mechanism of Action
Aspirin and the older nonselective NSAIDs inhibit all forms of COX, and thereby decrease prostaglandin, prostacyclin, and thromboxane synthesis throughout the body. Synthesis of prostaglandins necessary for homeostatic function is disrupted, as is release of prostaglandins involved in inflammation. The major difference between the mechanisms of action of aspirin and other NSAIDs is that aspirin acetylates and thereby *irreversibly* inhibits COX. The other NSAIDs *reversibly* inhibit COX. Salicylate is a metabolite of aspirin.

Pharmacokinetics
The pharmacokinetics of these drugs along with recommended anti-inflammatory dosages are listed in Table 34–2.

ASPIRIN. Aspirin is readily absorbed and is hydrolyzed in blood and tissues to acetate and salicylic acid. The half-life is 0.25 hour. Salicylate is a reversible nonselective inhibitor of COX. Elimination of salicylate is first order at low doses, with a half-life of 3 to 5 hours. At high (anti-inflammatory) doses, half-life increases to 15 hours or more and elimination becomes zero order. Excretion is via the kidney.

OTHER NONSELECTIVE NSAIDS. The other NSAIDs are well absorbed after oral administration. **Ibuprofen** has a half-life of about 2 hours, is relatively safe, and is the least expensive of the older, nonselective NSAIDs. **Naproxen** is similar, with a half-life of about 12 hours. **Indomethacin** is a potent NSAID with increased toxicity. **Oxaprozin** and **piroxicam** are noteworthy because of their longer half-lives (>50 hours), which permit less frequent dosing.

Physiologic Effects
COX inhibitors reduce the manifestations of inflammation (their *anti-inflammatory* effect), although they have no effect on underlying tissue damage or immunologic reactions. Prostaglandin synthesis in the CNS is stimulated by pyrogens. NSAIDs suppress this CNS prostaglandin synthesis, thus reducing fever (*antipyretic* effect). The pain relief mechanism (*analgesic* effect) of these agents is less well understood. Activation of peripheral nociceptors may be diminished as a result of reduced production of prostaglandins in injured tissue. In addition, a central COX mechanism is operative which provides analgesia. Ibuprofen and naproxen have moderate anti-inflammatory and analgesic efficacy. Other NSAIDs such as indomethacin have greater anti-inflammatory effectiveness, whereas **ketorolac** has greater analgesic efficacy. Aspirin and the nonselective NSAIDs all have antiplatelet action (*antithrombotic* effect). The prolonged antiplatelet action of aspirin, compared to the other nonselective NSAIDs, results from the irreversible inhibition of platelet COX-1. Thus, inhibition of thromboxane synthesis by aspirin is essentially permanent in platelets because they lack the machinery for new COX-1 synthesis. In contrast, in vascular endothelium, aspirin-mediated inhibition of COX-2 and prostacyclin synthesis is temporary because these cells can synthesize

Table 34–2.	Properties of aspirin and some nonsteroidal anti-inflammatory drugs	
Drug	Half-life (h)	Urinary Excretion of Unchanged Drug (%)
Aspirin	0.25	<2
Salicylate[1,2]	2–19	2–30
Celecoxib	11	27[3]
Diclofenac	1.1	<1
Diflunisal	13	3–9
Etodolac	6.5	<1
Fenoprofen	2.5	30
Flurbiprofen	3.8	<1
Ibuprofen	2	<1
Indomethacin	4–5	16
Ketoprofen	1.8	<1
Ketorolac[4]	4–10	58
Meclofenamate	3	2–4
Meloxicam	20	Data not found
Nabumetone[5]	26[6]	1
Naproxen	14	<1
Oxaprozin	58[6]	1–4
Piroxicam	57[6]	4–10
Sulindac	8	7
Tolmetin	1	7

[1]Major anti-inflammatory metabolite of aspirin.
[2]Salicylate is usually given in the form of aspirin.
[3]Total urinary excretion including metabolites.
[4]Recommended for treatment of acute (e.g., surgical) pain only.
[5]Nabumetone is a prodrug; the half-life and urinary excretion are for its active metabolite.
[6]A single daily dose is sufficient because of the long half-life.

new COX-2. The irreversible platelet action of aspirin results in a longer duration of its antiplatelet effect compared to other NSAIDs. Aspirin and the nonselective NSAIDs also interfere with the homeostatic functions of prostaglandins. Most importantly, they reduce prostaglandin-mediated cytoprotection in the gastrointestinal tract and autoregulation of renal function.

Clinical Uses
Aspirin and the nonselective NSAIDs have four main therapeutic effects: anti-inflammatory, analgesic,

antipyretic, and antithrombotic. Aspirin has three oral optimal therapeutic dose ranges: The low range (<300 mg/day) is effective in reducing platelet aggregation; intermediate doses (600 to 650 mg/day) have antipyretic and analgesic effects; and high doses (45 mg/kg/day in divided doses) are used for the anti-inflammatory effect. Aspirin and other NSAIDs are used to treat mild to moderate pain. This includes musculoskeletal pain associated with inflammatory arthropathies (rheumatoid arthritis, gout, and others) and pain associated with osteoarthritis and musculoskeletal overuse injuries. Use of these drugs for treatment of pain associated with osteoarthritis and musculoskeletal overuse injuries exceeds use for inflammatory arthropathies. The more frequent use of these drugs for osteoarthritis and musculoskeletal overuse injuries is the result of their availability as over-the-counter (OTC; i.e., without a prescription) products.

Aspirin and certain NSAIDs are also commonly used to treat nonmusculoskeletal conditions such as dysmenorrhea, dental pain, and headache. For severe pain, these drugs are often combined with opioid analgesics (Chapter 20). In infants with patent ductus arteriosus, closure of a patent ductus arteriosus in an otherwise normal infant can be accelerated with an NSAID such as indomethacin or ibuprofen. Owing to aspirin's irreversible inhibition of COX and its effects on platelet function, it is the optimal antithrombotic drug to minimize the risk of coronary occlusion and heart attacks (Chapter 11). Long-term use of NSAIDs also reduces the risk of colon cancer.

Ketorolac is used mainly as a systemic analgesic and not as an anti-inflammatory drug (although it has typical nonselective NSAID properties).

Adverse Effects

ASPIRIN. The most common adverse effect from therapeutic anti-inflammatory doses of aspirin is gastric upset. Chronic use can result in gastric ulceration, upper gastrointestinal bleeding, and renal effects, including acute tubular necrosis and interstitial nephritis. Aspirin increases the bleeding time owing to its antiplatelet effect. When prostaglandin synthesis is inhibited by even small doses of aspirin, persons with aspirin hypersensitivity may experience asthma. Research suggests that some cases of aspirin allergy result from diversion of arachidonic acid to the leukotriene pathway when the cyclooxygenase-catalyzed prostaglandin pathway is blocked. The resulting increase in leukotriene synthesis causes the bronchoconstriction that is typical of aspirin allergy. For unknown reasons, this form of aspirin allergy is more common in individuals with nasal polyps. This type of hypersensitivity to aspirin precludes treatment with any NSAID.

At higher doses of aspirin, tinnitus, vertigo, hyperventilation, and respiratory alkalosis are observed. At very high doses, the drug causes metabolic acidosis, dehydration, hyperthermia, collapse, coma, and death. Children with viral infections are at increased risk for Reye's syndrome (hepatic fatty degeneration and encephalopathy) if they are given aspirin.

Concomitant administration of nonselective NSAIDs with aspirin may diminish the irreversible platelet inhibition induced by aspirin. This is because both drugs compete for COX-1 in the platelet. Binding of the reversible NSAID to COX-1 prevents aspirin from binding and irreversibly inhibiting the enzymatic site. To avoid this interaction between aspirin and the other NSAIDs, dosing recommendations are to take the aspirin, for its antiplatelet effect, a minimum of 1 hour prior to taking any of the other nonselective NSAIDs.

OTHER NONSELECTIVE NSAIDS. Like aspirin, these agents are associated with significant gastrointestinal disturbance, but the incidence is lower than with aspirin. There is a risk of renal damage with any of the NSAIDs, especially in patients with preexisting renal disease. Because these drugs are cleared by the kidney, renal damage results in higher, more toxic serum concentrations. Use of parenteral ketorolac is generally restricted to 72 hours because of the risk of gastrointestinal and renal damage with longer administration. Serious hematologic reactions have been noted with indomethacin. In 2005, the Food and Drug Administration (FDA) requested that all prescriptions of NSAIDs contain a warning about the increased risk of serious adverse cardiovascular events associated with these drugs. The OTC use of these drugs was not required to have a similar warning because OTC dosages are lower.

COX-2 Inhibitors

Celecoxib, rofecoxib, and **valdecoxib** are members of the COX-2–selective inhibitors class. Theoretically, COX-2–selective inhibitors should have less effect on the prostaglandins involved in homeostatic function, particularly those in the gastrointestinal tract. These drugs have analgesic, antipyretic, and anti-inflammatory effects similar to those of the nonselective NSAIDs. Celecoxib is the only COX-2 inhibitor currently available in the

United States (Table 34–2) because increased cardio-vascular risks were reported for rofecoxib (see below under toxicity).

Clinical Use

COX-2 inhibitors are primarily used in inflammatory disorders. Nonselective NSAIDs and COX-2–selective drugs also reduce polyp formation in the colon in patients with primary familial adenomatous polyposis.

Adverse Effects

The COX-2–selective inhibitors have demonstrated a reduced risk of gastrointestinal effects, including gastric ulcers and serious gastrointestinal bleeding. They are not recommended in renal dysfunction because COX-2 is constitutively active in the kidney. Celecoxib is a sulfonamide and may cause a hypersensitivity reaction in patients who are allergic to other sulfonamides. In contrast to nonselective COX inhibitors (aspirin and nonselective NSAIDs), COX-2 inhibitors do not reduce platelet aggregation and they lack antithrombotic activity. Thus, COX-2 inhibitors offer no protection in patients at high-risk of myocardial infarction or stroke. Clinical investigations have documented an *increased* risk of adverse cardiovascular events in patients medicated with certain COX-2 inhibitors. This increased risk is not equivalent across the spectrum of COX-2 inhibitors and resulted in two of these COX-2 inhibitors (rofecoxib and valdecoxib) being voluntarily withdrawn from the market in the United States by their manufacturers.

COX Inhibition Selectivity

The inhibition of COX-1 compared to COX-2 by aspirin, nonselective NSAIDs, and COX-2 inhibitors is relative and varies with the drug. Celecoxib selectivity for inhibiting COX-2 is 10 to 20 times that for COX-1. Meloxicam and etodolac are included with the nonselective NSAIDs in this chapter (Table 34–2); however, both of these NSAIDs have a slightly higher selectivity for COX-2 compared to COX-1. In contrast, a number of the nonselective NSAIDs inhibit both COX-1 and COX-2 equally (diclofenac, flurbiprofen, ibuprofen, indomethacin, ketoprofen, meclofenamate, piroxicam, tenoxicam, and tolmetin).

Acetaminophen

Acetaminophen does not fall into any of the previous drug classifications, and is available in the United States without prescription. Phenacetin is a toxic prodrug that is metabolized to acetaminophen, and is still available in some other countries.

Mechanism of Action and Physiologic Effects

Acetaminophen is an analgesic and antipyretic agent lacking anti-inflammatory or antithrombotic effects. The mechanism of analgesic action of acetaminophen is unclear. The drug is only a weak COX-1 and COX-2 inhibitor in peripheral tissues, which accounts for its lack of anti-inflammatory effect. Some evidence suggests that acetaminophen inhibits a CNS COX isozyme that accounts for its analgesic and antipyretic properties.

Pharmacokinetics and Clinical Use

Acetaminophen is effective for the same indications as intermediate-dose aspirin. Acetaminophen is, therefore, useful as an aspirin substitute, especially in children with viral infections and in individuals with any type of aspirin intolerance. Acetaminophen is well absorbed orally and metabolized in the liver. The half-life is 2 to 3 hours in persons with normal hepatic function and the half-life is unaffected by renal disease.

Adverse Effects

In therapeutic dosages, acetaminophen has negligible toxicity in most individuals. However, when taken in overdose or by patients with severe liver impairment, the drug is a dangerous hepatotoxin. The mechanism of toxicity requires oxidation to cytotoxic intermediates by phase I cytochrome P450 enzymes. This occurs if substrates for phase II conjugation reactions (acetate and glucuronide) are lacking (Chapter 3). People who regularly consume three or more alcoholic drinks per day are at increased risk of acetaminophen-induced hepatotoxicity (Chapters 3 and 21).

ARTHRITIS-ASSOCIATED DISEASES

Arthritis refers to any type of inflammation and damage to a joint. The term is applied to more than 100 rheumatic diseases, oversimplifying the nature of the various disease processes. **Rheumatic disease** describes a disease process associated with connective tissues, muscles, bursae, and ligaments. The etiologies of arthritis and musculoskeletal disorders may be classified into three broad categories: those associated with immune complex disorders, those associated with degeneration of the joints, and those associated with metabolic disorders and crystal deposition in joints.

Chronic autoimmune-mediated inflammation is the underlying mechanism of tissue damage in several idiopathic diseases (e.g., rheumatoid arthritis, ankylosing spondylitis, systemic lupus erythematosus). Arthropathies are also associated with infectious immune complexes. In **rheumatoid arthritis,** the main sites of tissue damage are the diarthrodial joints. In contrast, in **ankylosing spondylitis,** the attachments of tendons and ligaments at bones are the sites of chronic inflammation. In **systemic lupus erythematosus,** a multitude of tissue sites (skin, joints, and kidneys) are potential sites of inflammation and tissue damage. In infectious arthropathies, the inflammation is the result of the immune response when infective agents are concentrated in connective tissues. The development and the roles of cell- and humoral-mediated immune responses in these processes are discussed in Chapter 32.

Mechanical overloading of joints results in subsequent loss of hyaline cartilage and bone deformation in affected joints. Clinically, this process is described as **osteoarthritis;** also previously known as degenerative joint disease. This is the most prevalent arthritic disease. Causes of osteoarthritis include previous trauma or infection at the affected joint, obesity, and genetic predisposition, but some cases are of unknown etiology. Osteoarthritis is a major cause of morbidity in the geriatric population, and becoming an increasing cause of morbidity in the younger obese population as well.

Gout is typified by metabolic dysfunction with arthritis, the arthritic component resulting from crystal-induced synovial joint inflammation. Gout is associated with the excessive production or reduced elimination of uric acid. Concentrations of uric acid increase in bodily fluids, ultimately resulting in monosodium urate crystal precipitation, especially in the peripheral tissues where both blood flow and tissue temperature may be reduced. Crystal formation in joints results in a painful acute inflammatory response that over time can result in joint damage.

Therapeutic Strategies

The treatment of patients with rheumatic and other joint diseases involves two primary goals. The first goal is relief of pain, which is often the presenting symptom and the major complaint of the patient. The second goal is the slowing or, if possible, arrest of any tissue-damaging process.

Anti-inflammatory drugs used in the treatment of arthritic diseases are shown in Figure 34–1. Some of these treatment strategies involve inhibiting the formation of eicosanoid products with glucocorticoids or NSAIDs. Reduction of inflammation with NSAIDs or glucocorticoids often results in relief of pain for significant periods. Acetaminophen may relieve pain associated with rheumatic diseases, but does not affect the underlying inflammatory process initiating the pain. In contrast cellular proliferation and activation of cell- and humoral-mediated immune processes may be inhibited by disease-modifying antirheumatic drugs. These drugs slow the tissue damage associated with inflammation, and are thought to affect more basic inflammatory mechanisms than do the NSAIDs. Unfortunately, they are also more toxic. In gout, several drug classes are used to inhibit the inflammatory process (colchicine, NSAIDs, or glucocorticoids). Other drugs are used in gout to prevent formation of uric acid (allopurinol), or increase its excretion (uricosurics).

NSAIDs and Glucocorticoids

The use of NSAIDs in relieving inflammation and associated pain in rheumatic diseases has been discussed. Glucocorticoids (Chapter 23) inhibit the release of arachidonic acid by phospholipases in the membrane (Figure 34–2). This effect is mediated by intracellular steroid receptors that, when activated by an appropriate steroid, increase expression of specific proteins capable of inhibiting phospholipase. Steroids also inhibit the synthesis of COX-2. These actions are thought to be the major mechanisms of the important anti-inflammatory action of glucocorticoids. Both oral administration and local injection can be used in treatment. Intra-articular injections to alleviate painful joint symptoms are helpful and often preferable to increased systemic dosage of the drugs. When first introduced, glucocorticoids were considered to be the ultimate answer to the treatment of inflammatory arthritis because of their powerful anti-inflammatory effects. Unfortunately, the toxicity associated with chronic glucocorticoid therapy restricts their use to the control of acute severe exacerbations and long-term low-dose use in patients with severe disease not controlled by other agents. Therefore, the NSAIDs have assumed a major role in the long-term treatment of arthritis.

Disease-Modifying Antirheumatic Drugs

The disease-modifying antirheumatic drugs (DMARDs) are a heterogeneous group of agents (Table 34–3) that have anti-inflammatory actions in autoimmune-mediated rheumatic diseases. These agents are called disease-modifying drugs because some evidence shows slowing or even reversal of damage to cartilage and bone in rheumatoid arthritis, an effect never seen with NSAIDs. They are also called slow-acting because it may take 6 weeks to 6 months for their benefits to become apparent. Glucocorticoids may be considered anti-inflammatory drugs with an intermediate rate of action; that is, slower than NSAIDs but faster than the DMARDs.

Table 34–3. Some disease-modifying antirheumatic drugs

Drug	Other Clinical Uses	Toxicity When Used for Rheumatoid Arthritis
Abatacept		Increased risk of infection
Chlorambucil	SLE and other autoimmune disorders	Bone marrow suppression, infertility in both males and females, increased risk of neoplasia
Chloroquine and hydroxychloroquine	Antimalarial,[1] SLE	Rash, gastrointestinal disturbance, ototoxicity, myopathy, peripheral neuropathy, ocular toxicity (higher dosages)
Cyclosporine	Tissue transplantation	Nephrotoxicity, hypertension, peripheral neuropathy
Etanercept		Activation of latent TB and general increased risk of infections, injection site reactions
Gold Compounds Aurothiomalate, auranofin, and aurothioglucose		Many adverse effects, including diarrhea, dermatitis, hematologic abnormalities (including aplastic anemia)
Infliximab	Inflammatory bowel disease	Upper respiratory infection, activation of latent TB
Leflunomide		Teratogen, hepatotoxicity, gastrointestinal disturbance, skin reactions
Methotrexate	Anticancer	Nausea, mucosal ulcers, hematotoxicity, teratogenicity
Penicillamine	Chelating agent	Many adverse effects, including proteinuria, dermatitis, gastrointestinal disturbance, hematologic abnormalities (including aplastic anemia)
Sulfasalazine	Inflammatory bowel disease	Rash, gastrointestinal disturbance, dizziness, headache, leukopenia

SLE = systemic lupus erythematosus; TB = tuberculosis.
[1]See Chapter 29.

Mechanisms of Action

DMARDs have multiple mechanisms of action; for many drugs the mechanism is unknown. Anticancer drugs such as **methotrexate** and **cyclophosphamide** probably act by reducing the numbers of immune cells available to maintain the inflammatory response (Chapters 31 and 32). The efficacy of **cyclosporine** is probably related to its immunosuppressive action (Chapter 32). The action of **sulfasalazine** as an antirheumatic drug appears to differ from its action in ulcerative colitis (Chapter 36). Both sulfasalazine and one of its metabolites, **sulfapyridine**, may provide immunomodulatory and anti-inflammatory effects. For sulfasalazine and sulfapyridine, the following have been postulated as providing the clinical benefits: inhibition of the formation and release of both cytokines and antibodies (IgA and IgM) and preferential suppression of B-cell function compared to T cells. **Chloroquine** and **hydroxychloroquine** may interfere with the activity of T lymphocytes, decrease leukocyte chemotaxis, stabilize lysosomal membranes, interfere with DNA and RNA synthesis in immune cells, and trap free radicals. **Penicillamine** appears to have anti-inflammatory effects similar to those of hydroxychloroquine. Organic gold compounds (**gold sodium thiomalate, aurothioglucose, auranofin**) alter the activity of macrophages. These cells play a central role in inflammation, especially that of rheumatoid arthritis. Organic gold compounds also suppress phagocytic activity by polymorphonuclear leukocytes.

Several new DMARDs have been introduced in recent years. **Leflunomide** is a prodrug that is rapidly metabolized to a compound that inhibits dihydroorotate dehydrogenase, an enzyme required by activated lymphocytes for synthesis of the pyrimidines that are needed for RNA synthesis. In lymphocytes, inhibition of this enzyme results in cell cycle arrest. Other cell types are not affected to the same degree because they can use other biochemical pathways to synthesize pyrimidines. **Infliximab** and **adalimumab** are monoclonal antibodies that bind to and prevent the action of **tumor necrosis factor-α** (TNF-α). TNF-α is a cytokine that appears to play a key role in chronic inflammation in several different disease processes. **Etanercept** is a recombinant fusion protein comprising two TNF receptors linked to immunoglobulin; it acts as a decoy binding site, decreasing the cellular actions of TNF-α.

Pharmacokinetics and Clinical Use

Sulfasalazine, hydroxychloroquine, methotrexate, cyclosporine, penicillamine, and leflunomide are given orally. Anti–TNF-α drugs are given by injection. Gold sodium thiomalate and aurothioglucose are available for parenteral use and auranofin for oral administration. DMARDs are used in patients with various rheumatic joint and other pathophysiologies in which an autoimmune component is thought to be key to the disease process. These diseases include rheumatoid arthritis, lupus erythematosus, arthritis associated with Sjögren's syndrome, juvenile rheumatoid arthritis, and others. Of these drugs, methotrexate is now considered to be the initial treatment of choice, although used at lower doses than as an anticancer drug, and it is often the "background therapy" to which other DMARDs are added.

Adverse Effects

All disease-modifying agents can cause severe or fatal toxicities. Careful monitoring of patients who take these drugs is mandatory. Their major adverse effects are listed in Table 34–3, and these are discussed in greater detail elsewhere (Chapters 31 and 32).

Combination Therapy with DMARDs

Combinations of DMARDs can be designed rationally on the basis of complementary mechanisms of action, different pharmacokinetics, and nonoverlapping toxicities. When added to methotrexate background therapy, cyclosporine, chloroquine, leflunomide, infliximab, adalimumab, and etanercept have all shown improved efficacy. A triple-therapy regimen (methotrexate, sulfasalazine, and hydroxychloroquine) was recently documented to be clinically more efficacious than any combination of only two of the medications. While it might be anticipated that combination therapy might result in more toxicity, this is often not the case. Combination therapy for patients not responding adequately to monotherapy is becoming the rule in the treatment of rheumatoid arthritis.

DIETARY MANIPULATION OF INFLAMMATION

Dietary manipulation that substitutes different unsaturated fatty acids, such as eicosapentaenoic acid (found in marine fish), causes these alternative fatty acids to be metabolized by COX and LOX (Figure 34–2), changing the final prostaglandin and leukotriene products of the process. These products of eicosapentaenoic acid metabolism are less potent than the corresponding eicosatetraenoic mediators derived from arachidonic acid, sometimes by several orders of magnitude. Eicosapentaenoic acid metabolites diminish the activities of the eicosatetraenoic mediators by competing with them for shared target-cell receptors.

Clinical studies suggest that therapy with dietary eicosapentaenoic acid decreases both morning stiffness and the number of tender joints in patients with rheumatoid arthritis as well as erythema associated with psoriasis. The efficacy of dietary eicosapentaenoic acid approximates that of the NSAIDs. These preliminary results and the near absence of significant adverse effects suggest that dietary alteration or supplementation to provide 1 to 4 g per day of eicosapentaenoic acid may be a beneficial addition to conventional treatment of rheumatoid arthritis.

DRUGS USED IN GOUT

Gout is associated with increased serum concentrations of uric acid, and usually an increase in total body uric acid. Uric acid is very insoluble and readily precipitates, especially in the peripheral tissues. Treatment strategies are twofold. First, reduce inflammation during acute attacks. NSAIDs, or glucocorticoids may be used to decrease inflammation during the acute episode. In the past, colchicine was used for this purpose. Second, once the acute episode is controlled, pharmacotherapy is used to accelerate renal excretion of uric acid with uricosuric drugs, or to reduce the conversion of purines to uric acid by inhibiting xanthine oxidase with allopurinol. Allopurinol is the preferred and standard therapy. Uricosuric drugs are used when allopurinol is contraindicated or when tophi appear.

Anti-Inflammatory Drugs Used for Gout

Mechanisms of Action and Physiologic Effects
Potent NSAIDs, such as **indomethacin,** and **glucocorticoids** are effective inhibitors of inflammation in acute gouty arthritis. These agents act through the reduction of prostaglandin formation and the inhibition of crystal phagocytosis by inflammatory cells (Figure 34–3). Similarly, **colchicine** reduces inflammation by inhibiting leukocyte migration and phagocytosis. The drug reacts with tubulin and interferes with microtubule assembly. Tubulin is necessary for normal cell division, motility, and many other cellular processes. Colchicine is considered a general mitotic poison. The drug may also reduce production of leukotriene LTB_4 and decrease free radical formation (Figure 34–2).

Clinical Uses
Indomethacin, some glucocorticoids, and colchicine are used orally; parenteral preparations of glucocorticoids and colchicine are also available. Because of toxicity, colchicine is now used only for prophylaxis; indomethacin or other NSAIDs are the preferred treatment in acute gouty arthritis. All NSAIDs (except aspirin, salicylate, and tolmetin) have been used with clinical success in the treatment of acute gouty episodes. For monoarticular attacks, intra-articular glucocorticoids are effective and less toxic than systemic steroids. A glucocorticoid may be used if high doses of NSAIDs fail to provide analgesia and minimize inflammation. Lower doses of colchicine are used for prophylaxis to prevent attacks of gout in patients with a history of multiple acute attacks. Colchicine is also of value in the management of Mediterranean fever, a disease of unknown cause characterized by fever, hepatitis, peritonitis, pleuritis, arthritis, and, occasionally, amyloidosis.

Adverse Effects
Indomethacin may cause renal damage or bone marrow depression, so other NSAIDs are being increasingly used in acute gout. Intensive courses of glucocorticoids can cause behavioral changes and are diabetogenic. Although colchicine can be used for acute attacks, the doses required cause significant gastrointestinal disturbance, particularly diarrhea. Owing to these adverse

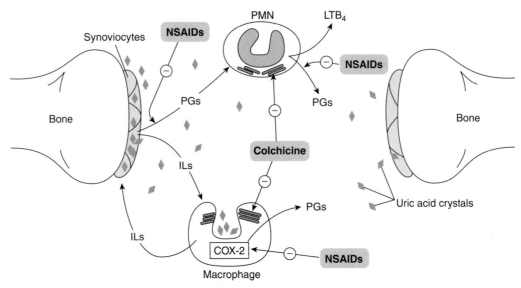

Figure 34–3. Sites of action of some anti-inflammatory drugs in a gouty joint. Synoviocytes damaged by uric acid crystals release prostaglandins (PGs), interleukins (ILs), and other mediators of inflammation. Polymorphonuclear leukocytes (PMNs), macrophages, and other inflammatory cells enter the joint and also release inflammatory substances, including leukotrienes (e.g., LTB_4), that attract additional inflammatory cells. Colchicine acts on microtubules in the inflammatory cells. NSAIDs act on cyclooxygenase-2 (COX-2) in all of the cells of the joint.

effects of colchicine, NSAIDs have replaced it for acute gout. Additionally, colchicine can severely damage the liver and kidney, and the dosage must be carefully limited and monitored. Overdose can be fatal.

Allopurinol

Mechanism of Action
Allopurinol is converted to oxypurinol (alloxanthine) by xanthine oxidase, the enzyme that converts hypoxanthine to xanthine and xanthine to uric acid. Allopurinol and oxypurinol are irreversible inhibitors of this enzyme.

Physiologic Effects
Inhibition of xanthine oxidase increases the concentrations of the more soluble hypoxanthine and xanthine and decreases the concentration of the less soluble uric acid. As a result, there is less likelihood of precipitation of uric acid crystals in joints and tissues.

Clinical Use
Allopurinol is given orally in the management of chronic gout. The drug is usually withheld for 1 to 2 weeks after

an acute episode of gouty arthritis. Allopurinol is also used as an adjunct to cancer chemotherapy to slow the formation of uric acid from purines released by the death of large numbers of neoplastic cells.

Adverse Effects and Drug Interactions
Allopurinol can precipitate acute attacks of gout during the early phase of treatment. The drug can also cause gastrointestinal upset and cutaneous rash. Allopurinol can rarely cause peripheral neuritis, vasculitis, or bone marrow dysfunction (including aplastic anemia). Allopurinol inhibits the metabolism of mercaptopurine and azathioprine, drugs that depend on xanthine oxidase for elimination. This drug-drug interaction increases the risk of adverse effects when these drugs are used concomitantly.

Uricosuric Agents

Mechanism of Action
Uricosuric agents (**probenecid, sulfinpyrazone**) are weak acids that compete with uric acid for reabsorption by the weak acid transport mechanism in the proximal

tubules of the kidney. At low doses, these agents may also compete with uric acid for secretion by the tubule and, occasionally, can even elevate serum uric acid concentration. Elevation of uric acid levels by this mechanism occurs with aspirin (another weak acid) over much of its dose range.

Physiologic Effects and Clinical Use

Uricosuric drugs act primarily in the kidney and inhibit the secretion of a large number of other weak acids (e.g., penicillin, methotrexate) in addition to inhibiting the reabsorption of uric acid. Inhibition of renal secretion of these weakly acidic drugs by uricosuric drugs may increase the plasma levels and half-life of these weak acids. These drugs are of no value in acute gouty arthritis and are best withheld for 1 to 2 weeks after an acute episode. Once the acute episode subsides, these drugs may be initiated prophylactically during the chronic phase.

Adverse Effects

Like allopurinol, uricosuric drugs may precipitate an attack of acute gouty arthritis during the early phase of their action. This can be avoided by simultaneously administering colchicine or indomethacin. Because they are sulfonamides, the uricosuric drugs may share allergenicity with other classes of sulfonamide drugs (diuretics, antimicrobials, oral hypoglycemic drugs).

◼ REHABILITATION FOCUS

The drug classes discussed in this chapter have a high impact and strong association with the practice of the physical therapist. Several facts account for this. Most patients attending treatment with physical therapists are taking drugs discussed in this chapter. These drugs increase functional activities of daily living by reducing musculoskeletal pain. Their effects are maximal at peak plasma levels. Thus, the clinician should be familiar with the pharmacokinetic profiles of these drugs and set appointment times for treatment to occur at peak plasma levels to improve function and decrease pain during the therapy. In addition, clinical investigations demonstrate that combining drug therapy with rehabilitation therapy optimizes functional improvements

in patients and decreases perceived pain. These functional improvements may shorten the time for return to work, or delay disability in patients with chronic rheumatic autoimmune-mediated pathophysiologies. These drugs have some of the highest potential for improving rehabilitation outcomes. No other drug classes are likely to have as significant an influence on musculoskeletal function.

◼ CLINICAL RELEVANCE FOR REHABILITATION

Adverse Drug Reactions
- Glucocorticoids can increase insulin resistance, immunosuppression, sodium and water retention, and catabolic metabolic effects.
- Aspirin and the other nonselective NSAIDs may increase bleeding.
- Different COX-2 inhibitors have varying increased cardiovascular risk.
- DMARDs can cause peripheral neuropathy, myopathy, immunosuppression, nephrotoxicity, and hypertension.

Effects Interfering with Rehabilitation
Clinical effects of glucocorticoids include:
  - Type 2 diabetes mellitus
  - Increased risk of infection
  - Hypertension
  - Chronic use can result in muscle wasting.
- Hemorrhage into muscles and joints as a result of aerobic activities may present as muscle and joint soreness at the next therapy session.
- COX-2 inhibition can predispose patients to deep vein thrombosis, myocardial infarction, and ischemic stroke.
- Peripheral neuropathy and myopathy in both upper and lower extremities can affect all aspects of rehabilitation.
- Nephropathy can lead to electrolyte imbalances and hypertension.
- Aerobic activities in rehabilitation can exacerbate hypertension.
- Immunosuppression can increase the risk of infection.

Possible Therapy Solutions

- Check a patient's heart rate and blood pressure prior to, during, and after aerobic activities.
- Have diabetic patients check glucose prior to aerobic activities.
- Adjust aerobic activities to account for muscle wasting.
- Differentiate clinical presentation of delayed-onset muscle soreness from pain-associated arthropathy and myopathy due to hemorrhage.
- Recognize the clinical manifestations of deep vein thrombosis, myocardial infarction, and ischemic stroke.

Potentiation of Functional Outcomes Secondary to Drug Therapy

- Nonselective NSAIDs, COX-2 inhibitors, and acetaminophen decrease musculoskeletal pain and allow increased patient participation in rehabilitation.
- Nonselective NSAIDs and COX-2 inhibitors decrease inflammation that may result from the aerobic activities associated with rehabilitation.
- DMARDs delay the destructive inflammatory processes associated with autoimmune rheumatic disease. Rehabilitation activities should be coordinated with periods of drug-induced remission for these patients to help them accomplish functional activities.

PROBLEM-ORIENTED PATIENT STUDY

Brief History: The patient is a 24-year-old female with a diagnosis of severe primary dysmenorrhea, which began with menses at age 13. Pain usually begins 3 to 4 days prior to menstruation, and often results in her being unable to leave the bed, missing several days of work with some episodes. During previous years, the patient has attempted to control the pain with opioid analgesics, traditional NSAIDs, and oral contraceptives. Even with these pharmacologic treatments, the patient still presents to the emergency room several times per year.

Current Medical Status and Drug Therapy: The patient arrived the previous evening at the emergency room of the local hospital complaining of severe pelvic, abdominal, and low back pain preventing her from standing erect. She also complains of hot flushes, headaches, nausea, and vomiting. The patient was given promethazine as an antiemetic and sedative. The patient was sent home with a recommendation to continue taking Percodan (aspirin and oxycodone) four times daily, and she was referred to physical therapy the next day for additional pain relief treatments as needed.

Rehabilitation Setting: The patient arrives at the physical therapy clinic with the previous manifestations, stating that her current pain level is 8/10 on a visual analog scale, even with her continued use of the Percodan. The therapist decides to use pulsed-shortwave diathermy over the anterior pelvic region, as a deep heat modality for symptomatic pain relief. Following the treatment, the patient states that her pain level is 4/10, and requests to return the next day for another treatment. The subsequent day the patient arrives for another diathermy treatment. She notes her continued use of the Percodan as prescribed and that her pain level today is 6/10. Following the treatment, the patient states that her pain is 0/10. She notes that this is the first time in the last several days that she has been pain-free. She again requests another treatment the next day, stating that her menstrual cycle should begin in a day or so. The patient returns the third day. When questioned about her cycle condition, she states that her pain level is down significantly at 3/10 and that her cycle has begun. However, she is concerned because the menstrual blood flow this time appears to be heavier than what she has previously experienced.

(*continued*)

PROBLEM-ORIENTED PATIENT STUDY (*Continued*)

Problem/Clinical Options: The concern is whether the increased blood flow during menstruation was related to the diathermy treatment. The diathermy utilizes electromagnetic radiation in an alternating field to heat subcutaneous tissues. The increased tissue temperatures would increase blood flow as a response. Percodan contains oxycodone, an opioid analgesic, and aspirin. The concentration of aspirin in each tablet is 325 mg, and when taken four times a day, the total aspirin dose would be 1,300 mg. This dosage would provide an analgesic effect, but would also inhibit platelet function, increasing bleeding time. With the combined effects of increased blood flow to the pelvic area resulting from the thermal effect of the diathermy and the inhibition of platelet activity, increased blood flow during menstruation may occur. The therapist should inform the patient that the increased blood flow during menstruation may occur with the combined use of diathermy and Percodan and explain the mechanisms.

PREPARATIONS AVAILABLE

Eicosanoid Agonists

Alprostadil
Penile injection (Caverject, Edex): 5-, 10-, 20, 40-mcg sterile powder for reconstitution
Penile pellet (Muse): 125, 250, 500, 1000 mcg
Parenteral (Prostin VR Pediatric): 500 mcg/mL ampules

Bimatoprost (Lumigan)
Ophthalmic drops: 0.03% solution

Carboprost tromethamine (Hemabate)
Parenteral: 250 mcg carboprost and 83 mcg tromethamine per mL ampules

Dinoprostone (prostaglandin E2) (Prostin E2, Prepidil, Cervidil)
Vaginal: 20-mg suppositories, 0.5-mg gel, 10-mg controlled-release system

Epoprostenol (prostacyclin) (Flolan)
Intravenous: powder to make 3, 5, 10, 15 mcg/mL

Latanoprost (Xalatan)
Topical: 50 mcg/mL ophthalmic solution

Misoprostol (Cytotec)
Oral: 100- and 200-mcg tablets

Travoprost (Travatan)
Ophthalmic solution: 0.0004%

Treprostinil (Remodulin)
Parenteral: 1, 2.5, 5, 10 mg/mL for continuous subcutaneous infusion

Unoprostone (Rescula)
Ophthalmic solution 0.15%

NSAIDs

Aspirin, acetylsalicylic acid (generic, Easprin, others)
Oral (regular, enteric-coated, buffered): 81-, 165-, 325-, 500-, 650-, 800-, 975-mg tablets; 81-, 650-, 800-mg timed- or extended-release tablets
Rectal: 120-, 200-, 300-, 600-mg suppositories

Choline salicylate (Arthropan)
Oral: 870 mg/5 mL liquid

Diclofenac (generic, Cataflam, Voltaren)
Oral: 50-mg tablets; 25-, 50-, 75-mg delayed-release tablets; 100-mg extended-release tablets
Ophthalmic: 0.1% solution

Diflunisal (generic, Dolobid)
Oral: 250-, 500-mg tablets

Etodolac (generic, Lodine)
Oral: 200-, 300-mg capsules; 400-, 500-mg tablets; 400-, 500-, 600-mg extended-release tablets

Fenoprofen (generic, Nalfon)
Oral: 200-, 300-mg capsules; 600-mg tablets

Flurbiprofen (generic, Ansaid)
Oral: 50-, 100-mg tablets
Ophthalmic (generic, Ocufen): 0.03% solution

Ibuprofen (generic, Motrin, Rufen, Advil [OTC], Nuprin [OTC], others)
Oral: 100-, 200-, 400-, 600-, 800-mg tablets; 50-, 100-mg chewable tablets; 200-mg capsules; 100 mg/2.5 mL suspension, 100 mg/5 mL suspension; 40 mg/mL drops

Indomethacin (generic, Indocin, others)
Oral: 25-, 50-mg capsules; 75-mg sustained-release capsules; 25 mg/5 mL suspension
Rectal: 50-mg suppositories

Ketoprofen (generic, Orudis, others)
Oral: 12.5-mg tablets; 25-, 50-, 75-mg capsules; 100-, 150-, 200-mg extended-release capsules

Ketorolac tromethamine (generic, Toradol)
Oral: 10-mg tablets
Parenteral: 15, 30 mg/mL for IM injection
Ophthalmic: 0.5% solution

Magnesium salicylate (Doan's Pills, Magan, Mobidin)
Oral: 545-, 600-mg tablets; 467-, 500-, 580-mg caplets

Meclofenamate sodium (generic)
Oral: 50-, 100-mg capsules

Mefenamic acid (Ponstel)
Oral: 250-mg capsules

Meloxicam (Mobic)
Oral: 7.5-mg tablets

Nabumetone (Relafen)
Oral: 500-, 750-mg tablets

Naproxen (generic, Naprosyn, Anaprox, Aleve [otc])
Oral: 200-, 250-, 375-, 500-mg tablets; 375-, 550-mg sustained-release tablets; 375-, 500-mg delayed-release tablets; 125 mg/5 mL suspension

Oxaprozin (Daypro)
Oral: 600-mg tablets

Piroxicam (generic, Feldene)
Oral: 10-, 20-mg capsules

Salsalate, salicylsalicylic acid (generic, Disalcid)
Oral: 500-, 750-mg tablets; 500-mg capsules

Sodium salicylate (generic)
Oral: 325-, 650-mg enteric-coated tablets

Sodium thiosalicylate (generic, Rexolate)
Parenteral: 50 mg/mL for IM injection

Sulindac (generic, Clinoril)
Oral: 150-, 200-mg tablets

Suprofen (Profenal)
Topical: 1% ophthalmic solution

Tolmetin (Tolectin, generic [400 mg only])
Oral: 200-, 600-mg tablets; 400-mg capsules

COX-2 Inhibitors

Celecoxib (Celebrex)
Oral: 100-, 200-mg capsules

Disease-Modifying Antirheumatic Drugs

Adalimumab (Humira)
Parenteral: 40 mg/0.8 mL for SC injection

Auranofin (Ridaura)
Oral: 3-mg capsules

Aurothioglucose (Solganal)
Parenteral: 50 mg/mL suspension for injection

Chloroquin (Aralen)
Oral: 50-, 250-mg tablets

Etanercept (Enbrel)
Parenteral: 25-mg powder for subcutaneous injection

Gold sodium thiomalate (generic, Aurolate)
Parenteral: 50 mg/mL for injection

Hydroxychloroquine (Plaquenil)
Oral: 200-mg tablets

Infliximab (Remicade)
Parenteral: 100-mg powder for IV infusion

Leflunomide (Arava)
Oral: 10-, 20-, 100-mg tablets

Methotrexate (generic, Rheumatrex)
Oral: 2.5-mg tablets

Penicillamine (Cuprimine, Depen)
Oral: 125-, 250-mg capsules; 250-mg tablets

Sulfasalazine (Azulfidine)
Oral: 500-mg tablets; 500-mg delayed-release tablets

Acetaminophen

Acetaminophen (generic, Tylenol, Tempra, Panadol, Acephen, others)
Oral: 160-, 325-, 500-, 650-mg tablets; 80-mg chewable tablets; 160-, 500-, 650-mg caplets; 325-, 500-mg capsules; 80, 120, 160 mg/5 mL elixir; 500 mg/15 mL elixir; 100 mg/mL solution

Rectal: 80-, 120-, 125-, 300-, 325-, 650-mg suppositories

Drugs Used in Gout

Allopurinol (generic, Zyloprim, others)
Oral: 100-, 300-mg tablets

Colchicine (generic)
Oral: 0.5-, 0.6-mg tablets
Parenteral: 0.5 mg/mL for injection

Probenecid (generic)
Oral: 500-mg tablets

Sulfinpyrazone (generic, Anturane)
Oral: 100-mg tablets; 200-mg capsules

REFERENCES

Greidinger EL, Rosen A: Inflammatory Rheumatic Diseases. In *Pathophysiology of Disease*, 4th ed. McPhee SL, Lingappa VR, Ganong WF, eds. New York: McGraw-Hill, 2003.

Hellman DB, Stone JH: Arthritis and musculoskeletal disorders. In *Current Medical Diagnosis & Treatment 2007*. McPhee ST, Papadakis MA, eds. New York: McGraw-Hill, 2007.

Rizzo DB. Disorders of skeletal function: Rheumatic disorders. In *Pathophysiology: Concepts of Altered Health States*. 7th ed, C. M. Porth, ed. Philadelphia: Lippincott Williams & Wilkins, 2005.

Singh G, et al: Toxicity profiles of disease modifying antirheumatic drugs in rheumatoid arthritis. *J Rheumatol* 1991;18:188.

Vane J, Botting R: Inflammation and the mechanism of action of anti-inflammatory drugs. *FASEB J* 1987;1:89.

NSAIDs

Barthel T, et al: Prophylaxis of heterotopic ossification after total hip arthroplasty: A prospective randomized study comparing indomethacin and meloxicam. *Acta Orthop Scand* 2002;73:611.

Bombardier C: An evidence-based evaluation of the gastrointestinal safety of coxibs. *Am J Cardiol* 2002; 89(Suppl 6A):3D.

Bombardier C, et al: Comparison of upper gastrointestinal toxicity of rofecoxib and naproxen in patients with rheumatoid arthritis. VIGOR Study Group. *N Engl J Med* 2000;343:1520.

Chan FK, et al: Celecoxib versus diclofenac and omeprazole in reducing the risk of recurrent ulcer bleeding in patients with arthritis. *N Engl J Med* 2002; 347:2104.

Deeks JJ, et al: Efficacy, tolerability, and upper gastrointestinal safety of celecoxib for treatment of osteoarthritis and rheumatoid arthritis: Systematic review of randomised controlled trials. *BMJ* 2002;325:619.

Grosser T, et al: Biological basis for the cardiovascular consequences of COX-2 inhibition: Therapeutic challenges and opportunities. *J Clin Invest* 2006;116:4.

Jones SC. Relative thromboembolic risks associated with COX-2 inhibitors. *Ann Pharmacother* 2005;39:1249.

Kivitz A, et al: Randomized placebo-controlled trial comparing efficacy and safety of valdecoxib with naproxen in patients with osteoarthritis. *J Fam Pract* 2002;51:530.

Lago P, et al: Safety and efficacy of ibuprofen versus indomethacin in preterm infants treated for patent ductus arteriosus: A randomized controlled trial. *Eur J Pediatr* 2002;161:202.

Laine L, et al: Serious lower gastrointestinal clinical events with nonselective NSAID or coxib use. *Gastroenterology* 2003;124:288.

Makarowski W, et al: Efficacy and safety of the COX-2 specific inhibitor valdecoxib in the management of osteoarthritis of the hip: A randomized, double-blind, placebo-controlled comparison with naproxen. *Osteoarthritis Cartilage* 2002;10:290.

Niccoli L, et al: Renal tolerability of three commonly employed non-steroidal anti-inflammatory drugs in elderly patients with osteoarthritis. *Clin Exp Rheumatol* 2002;20:201.

Reicin AS, et al: Comparison of cardiovascular thrombotic events in patients with osteoarthritis treated with rofecoxib versus nonselective nonsteroidal anti-inflammatory drugs (ibuprofen, diclofenac, and nabumetone). *Am J Cardiol* 2002;89:204.

Rovensky J, et al: Treatment of knee osteoarthritis with a topical non-steroidal anti-inflammatory drug. Results of a randomized, double-blind, placebo-controlled study on the efficacy and safety of a 5% ibuprofen cream. *Drugs Exp Clin Res* 2001;27:209.

Disease-Modifying Antirheumatic Drugs and Glucocorticoids

Genovese MC, et al: Abatacept for rheumatoid arthritis refractory to tumor necrosis factor α inhibition. *N Engl J Med* 2005;353:1114.

Mease PJ, et al: Adalimumab for the treatment of patients with moderately to severely active psoriatic arthritis. *Arthritis Rheum* 2005;52:3279.

Moreland LW, et al: Etanercept therapy in rheumatoid arthritis. A randomized, controlled trial. *Ann Intern Med* 1999;130:478.

Plosker GL, Croom KF. Sulfasalazine: A review of its use in the management of rheumatoid arthritis. *Drugs* 2005; 65:1825.

Teng GG, et al: Abatacept: A costimulatory inhibitor for treatment of rheumatoid arthritis. *Expert Opin Biol Ther* 2005;5:1245.

Other Analgesics

Linden CH, Rumack BH: Acetaminophen overdose. *Emerg Med Clin North Am* 1984;2:103.

Styrt B, Sugarman B: Antipyresis and fever. *Arch Intern Med* 1990;150:1589.

Drugs Used in Gout

Becker MA, et al: Febuxostat compared with allopurinol in patients with hyperuricemia and gout. *N Engl J Med* 2005;353:2450.

Emmerson BT: The management of gout. *N Engl J Med* 1996;334:445.

Schumacher HR: Febuxostat: A non-purine, selective inhibitor of xanthine oxidase for the management of hyperuricaemia in patients with gout. *Expert Opin Invest Drugs* 2005;14:893.

Rehabilitation

Arslan S, Celiker R: Comparison of the efficacy of local corticosteroid injection and physical therapy for the treatment of adhesive capsulitis. *Rheumatol Int* 2001;21:20.

Benson CJ, et al: The role of Army physical therapists as nonphysician health care providers who prescribe certain medications: Observations and experiences. *Phys Ther* 1995;75:380.

Biederman RE: Pharmacology in rehabilitation: Nonsteroidal anti-inflammatory agents. *J Orthop Sports Phys Ther* 2005;35:356.

de Jong Z, et al: Long term high intensity exercise and damage of small joints in rheumatoid arthritis. *Ann Rheum Dis* 2004;63:1399.

Draper DO, et al: Temperature change in human muscle during and after pulsed short-wave diathermy. *J Orthop Sports Phys Ther* 1999;29:13.

Field CS: Dysfunctional uterine bleeding. *Prim Care* 1988; 15:561.

Grimmer K, et al: Non-steroidal anti-inflammatory drugs (NSAIDs): Physiotherapists' use, knowledge and attitudes. *Aust J Physiother* 2002;48:82.

Jan MH, et al: Effects of repetitive shortwave diathermy for reducing synovitis in patients with knee osteoarthritis: An ultrasonographic study. *Phys Ther* 2006; 86:236.

Morrison DS, et al: Non-operative treatment of subacromial impingement syndrome. *J Bone Joint Surg Am* 1997; 79:732.

van Baar ME, et al: The effectiveness of exercise therapy in patients with osteoarthritis of the hip or knee: A randomized clinical trial. *J Rheumatol* 1998;25:2432.

Vance AR, et al: Microwave diathermy treatment for primary dysmenorrhea. *Phys Ther* 1996;76:1003.

Zuckerman JD, et al: The painful shoulder: Part II. Intrinsic disorders and impingement syndrome. *Am Fam Physician* 1991;43:497.

SPECIAL TOPICS

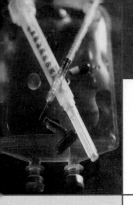

35

DRUGS AFFECTING THE RESPIRATORY SYSTEM

The respiratory tract may be divided into upper and lower portions. The upper portion consists of the nose, sinuses, oropharynx, and larynx. The lower portion comprises the trachea and lungs with their associated airways. Disorders and drug therapy of the upper respiratory system differ from those of the lower respiratory tract.

Disorders of the upper respiratory tract are those associated with infections (most commonly uncomplicated viral rhinotracheitis) and seasonal allergies (allergic rhinoconjunctivitis and rhinotracheitis). For the most part, these dysfunctions are self-limiting, and the drug classes used to treat them may be obtained without a prescription (over-the-counter, OTC). Disorders of the lower respiratory tract may be broadly classified as parenchymal infections (e.g., pneumonia) and obstructive airway (bronchial) conditions. In general, the latter disorders limit expiratory airflow. They are divided into bronchial asthma, which is characterized by acute episodes, and chronic obstructive airway disorders. Chronic obstructive airway disorders are further subdivided into chronic bronchitis, emphysema, bronchiectasis, and cystic fibrosis. The treatment of infections in all parts of the respiratory tract is discussed in Chapter 27.

DISORDERS OF THE UPPER RESPIRATORY TRACT

Manifestations of upper respiratory tract dysfunctions include mucous and watery discharges and vasodilation, mediated in part through histamine and other substances released from mast cells. Mast cells are important "gate-keeper" cells that are concentrated in the skin and other tissues near external body surfaces.

Histamine is produced from the amino acid histidine and is stored in vesicles. The four histamine receptor subtypes characterized to date are designated H_1 to H_4. H_1 receptors mediate mucous discharge and vasodilation, H_2 receptors are important in gastric acid secretion (Chapter 36), H_3 receptors are found in the central nervous system (CNS), and H_4 receptors may modulate inflammatory reactions by chemotactic effects on eosinophils and mast cells. Secretion of histamine and other mast cell mediators causes vasodilation of the nasal vasculature, leading to the nasal congestion and "runny nose" commonly associated with seasonal allergies and viral infections. Drugs used to decrease these manifestations include H_1 receptor antagonists (antihistamines) to decrease mucus production and vasodilation, nasal decongestants to decrease vasodilation, and mast cell stabilizers.

Bronchial congestion with cough and excessive mucus production are also associated with viral infections. These manifestations may be relieved with drugs that suppress coughing (antitussives)

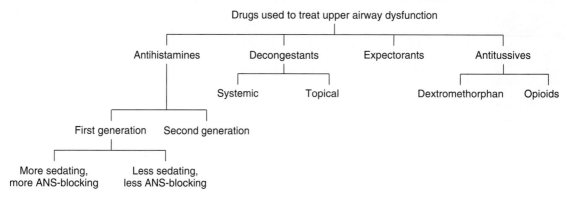

Figure 35–1. Drug classes used to treat upper airway dysfunction. Initially the drug classes are divided into histamine type 1 receptor antagonists (antihistamines), decongestants, expectorants, and antitussives. Antihistamines are divided into first and second generations. Decongestants are divided into those taken systemically and those applied topically to the nasal mucosa. Antitussives are divided into opioids with weakly addictive properties and dextromethorphan.

or assist in clearance of mucus from larger airways in the lungs (expectorants). The various drug classes used in therapy of the upper respiratory tract are outlined in Figure 35–1. Many of the OTC drugs are presented in Table 35–1. Mast cell stabilizers are discussed in connection with lower respiratory tract conditions.

DRUGS USED IN UPPER RESPIRATORY TRACT DISORDERS

H_1-Blocking Antihistamines

Classification and Prototypes

A wide variety of H_1 blockers are available (Table 35–1). Two major subgroups or "generations" have been developed. The older members of the first-generation agents, typified by **diphenhydramine** and **doxylamine,** are highly sedating agents with significant autonomic receptor-blocking effects. A newer subgroup of first-generation agents is less sedating and has fewer autonomic effects. **Chlorpheniramine** and **cyclizine** may be considered prototypes of this newer subgroup. The second-generation H_1 blockers, typified by **fexofenadine, loratadine,** and **cetirizine,** are far less lipid soluble than first-generation agents, and are largely free of sedative and autonomic effects. Because they have been developed for use in chronic conditions, all H_1 blockers are active by the oral route. Most are metabolized

extensively in the liver. Half-lives of the older H_1 blockers vary from 4 to 12 hours. Most newer agents (e.g., fexofenadine, cetirizine, loratadine) have half-lives of 12 to 24 hours.

Mechanisms and Physiologic Effects

H_1 blockers are competitive antagonists at the H_1 receptor. Therefore, these drugs have no effect on histamine release from storage sites and are more effective if given before histamine release occurs. Because their structure closely resembles that of muscarinic blockers and alpha (α)-adrenoceptor blockers, many of the first-generation agents are potent pharmacologic antagonists at these autonomic receptors. A few agents also block serotonin receptors. Most of the older first-generation agents are sedating, and some first-generation agents have antimotion sickness effects. Many H_1 blockers are potent local anesthetics. H_1-blocking drugs have negligible effects at H_2 receptors (Chapter 36).

Clinical Uses

H_1 blockers have major applications in type 1 allergic responses as well as additional clinical uses. Immediate allergic responses, which include **hay fever** and **urticaria,** are caused by antigens acting on immunoglobulin E (IgE) antibody-sensitized mast cells. H_1 blockers are often formulated into OTC combination preparations, and are listed in Table 35–1 under "Allergy and Cold

Table 35–1. Ingredients of known efficacy for selected over-the-counter (OTC) drug classes

OTC Category	Ingredients	Product Examples	Comments
Allergy and Cold Preparations	Chlorpheniramine	Chlor-Trimeton Allergy 4-Hour, Chlor-Trimeton Allergy 12-Hour, various generic	Antihistamines alone relieve most symptoms associated with allergic rhinitis or hay fever. Chlorpheniramine, brompheniramine, and clemastine cause less drowsiness than diphenhydramine and doxylamine. Several second-generation antihistamines have been approved for OTC use; they are therapeutically comparable to first-generation agents but have a much lower incidence of sedation. Occasionally, symptoms unrelieved by the antihistamine respond to the addition of a sympathomimetic.
	Brompheniramine	Dimetapp Cold and Allergy, various generic	
	Clemastine	Tavist Allergy	
	Diphenhydramine	Benadryl Allergy, Allergy, various generic	
	Loratadine	Alavert, Claritin, Tavist ND	
	Chlorpheniramine + pseudoephedrine	Allerest Maximum Strength, Sudafed Cold and Allergy, various generic	
	Triprolidine + pseudoephedrine	Sudafed Maximum Strength Sinus Nighttime, various generic	
Decongestants, Topical	Oxymetazoline	Afrin, Dristan 12-Hour Nasal, Neo-Synephrine 12-Hour, various generic	Topical sympathomimetics are effective for the temporary acute management of rhinorrhea associated with common colds and allergies. Long-acting agents (oxymetazoline and xylometazoline) are generally preferred, although phenylephrine is equally effective. Topical decongestants should not be used for longer than 3 days to prevent rebound nasal congestion.
	Phenylephrine	Neo-Synephrine, various generic	
	Xylometazoline	Otrivin	
Decongestants, Systemic	Pseudoephedrine	Sudafed, various generic	Orally administered decongestants are often combined with other drugs in OTC cold and seasonal allergy formulations. Systemic administration often results in longer duration of action, but also increases the incidence of adverse effects.
	Phenylephrine	Sudafed PE, various generic	

(continued)

Table 35–1.	Ingredients of known efficacy for selected over-the-counter (OTC) drug classes (*Continued*)		
OTC Category	**Ingredients**	**Product Examples**	**Comments**
Antitussives	Codeine	Mytussin A-C, Guiatuss AC, various generic	Act centrally to increase the cough threshold. In doses required for cough suppression, the addictive liability associated with codeine is low. Many codeine-containing antitussive combinations are schedule V narcotics, and OTC sale is restricted in some states.
	Dextromethorphan	Cold DM, Vicks 44 Cough Relief, various generic	Dextromethorphan is a nonanalgesic nonaddicting congener of levorphanol. It is often used with antihistamines, decongestants, and expectorants in combination products.
Expectorants	Guaifenesin	Guiatuss, Robitussin, various generic	The only OTC expectorant recognized as safe and effective by the Food and Drug Administration. Often used with antihistamines, decongestants, and antitussives in combination products.

Preparations." An additional clinical use of **diphenhydramine, dimenhydrinate, cyclizine, meclizine,** and **promethazine** is as antimotion sickness drugs. Diphenhydramine is also used for management of chemotherapy-induced vomiting.

Adverse Effects

Sedation and antimuscarinic effects such as dry mouth and blurred vision occur with some first-generation drugs, especially with diphenhydramine, doxylamine, and promethazine. Sedation is much less common with second-generation agents, which do not readily enter the CNS (Table 35–2). Drugs with α-adrenoceptor–blocking actions may cause orthostatic hypotension.

Interactions occur between older antihistamines and other drugs with sedative effects (e.g., benzodiazepines and alcohol). Drugs that inhibit hepatic metabolism may result in dangerously high levels of certain antihistamines if they are taken concurrently. For example, azole antifungal drugs and certain other P450 inhibitors interfere with the metabolism of **astemizole** and **terfenadine,** second-generation antihistamines that were withdrawn from the US market because high plasma concentrations of either can precipitate lethal arrhythmias. Some adverse effects can be exploited therapeutically (e.g., they are often used as hypnotics in institutions and in OTC sleep aids).

Decongestants

Classification and Prototypes

Nasal decongestants are agonists at α adrenoceptors and may be classified as systemic or topical (Figure 35–1). Several available OTC formulations are listed in Table 35–1. Despite its long history of use, **ephedrine** has not been extensively studied in humans. Ephedrine is one of the active components of "ma-huang," a popular herbal supplement taken for appetite suppression and weight reduction. Significant safety concerns have been associated with ingestion of ephedrine contained in ma-huang, including hypertension,

Table 35–2. Some H$_1$ antihistaminergic drugs in current clinical use

Drugs	Anticholinergic Activity	Comments
First-Generation Antihistamines		
Ethanolamines		
Dimenhydrinate (salt of diphenhydramine, e.g., Dramamine)	+++	Marked sedation; antimotion sickness activity
Diphenhydramine (e.g., Benadryl)	+++	Marked sedation, antimotion sickness activity
Piperazine derivatives		
Hydroxyzine (e.g., Atarax)	ND	Marked sedation
Cyclizine (e.g., Marezine)	–	Slight sedation; antimotion sickness activity
Meclizine (e.g., Bonine)	–	Slight sedation, antimotion sickness activity
Alkylamines		
Brompheniramine (e.g., Dimetane)	+	Slight sedation
Chlorpheniramine (e.g., Chlor-trimeton)	+	Slight sedation; common component of OTC cold medications
Phenothiazine derivatives		
Promethazine (e.g., Phenergan)	+++	Marked sedation; antiemetic
Miscellaneous		
Cyproheptadine (e.g., Periactin)	+	Moderate sedation; also has antiserotonin activity
Second-Generation Antihistamines		
Piperidines		
Fexofenadine (Allegra)	–	Lower risk of arrhythmia
Miscellaneous		
Loratadine (Claritin)	–	Longer action
Cetirizine (Zyrtec)	–	

ND = no data found; OTC = over-the-counter.

arrhythmias, myocardial infarction, and stroke. **Pseudoephedrine** is one of four ephedrine enantiomers, and is used in orally administered nasal decongestants. The convenience of oral administration and longer duration of action come at the cost of lower local concentrations of the drug in the nasal mucosa and greater potential for cardiac and nervous system adverse effects. **Xylometazoline** and **oxymetazoline** are classified as long-acting topical decongestants. **Phenylephrine** is formulated in both in topical and systemic decongestant nasal sprays. All of these mucous membrane decongestants are available as OTC products.

Physiologic Effects

The classification of α receptors, mechanisms of action of drugs stimulating α receptors, and general physiologic effects of α receptor stimulation were discussed in Chapters 4 and 6. Blood vessels of the upper respiratory tract mucosa contain α$_1$ and α$_2$ receptors. Stimulation of these receptors decreases blood flow and thus volume of the nasal mucosa. Ephedrine, phenylephrine, pseudoephedrine, xylometazoline, and oxymetazoline are all direct-acting α agonists and ephedrine and pseudoephedrine also have indirect sympathomimetic effects. Ephedrine also activates β receptors, which probably accounts for its earlier use in asthma. Because ephedrine gains access to the central nervous system (CNS), it is a mild stimulant. The duration of action of these drugs is dependent on the individual compound and the route of administration. These sympathomimetics are not inactivated by catechol-*O*-methyltransferase; as such they have durations of action of 30 minutes to several hours.

Clinical Use

Mucous membrane decongestants are α agonists that reduce the discomfort of hay fever and, to a lesser extent, the common cold.

Adverse Effects

The adverse effects of adrenoceptor agonists are primarily extensions of their pharmacologic effects in the cardiovascular system and CNS (Chapter 6). Rebound hyperemia—an increase in blood flow to the mucous membranes—may follow the use of these agents. Repeated topical use of high drug concentrations may result in ischemic changes in the mucous membranes, probably as a result of vasoconstriction of nutrient arteries. Cardiovascular effects include an elevation in blood pressure and increased cardiac workload. The latter may evoke manifestations of cardiac ischemia such as angina pectoris. Stimulatory CNS effects may present as insomnia, nervousness, tremor, and anxiety. When taken in large doses, oxymetazoline may cause hypotension.

Antitussives and Expectorants

Classification and Prototypes

Codeine and **hydrocodone** are opioids that may be included in antitussive formulations. **Dextromethorphan** is an opioid derivative that lacks analgesic and addictive properties. This drug has recently received attention as a drug of abuse among adolescents because of its hallucinogenic effects. **Guaifenesin** is the most commonly formulated expectorant in both OTC and prescription medications.

Physiologic Effects and Clinical Use

Natural opioids and their derivatives, such as dextromethorphan, suppress the cough center in the medulla oblongata. This suppression increases the stimulatory threshold required to initiate the cough reflex.

Guaifenesin assists in expectoration of respiratory mucus by stimulating respiratory tract secretions, resulting in increased airway fluid volumes and decreased mucus viscosity.

These drugs may be formulated alone, with each other, or in combinations with decongestants or antihistamines (Table 35–1). Except for the opioid drugs, many are available OTC.

Adverse Effects

Opioids can decrease respiratory drive by inhibiting brainstem respiratory mechanisms. This may result in hypercapnia, which may not be tolerated in patients with obstructive airway disorders. For additional adverse effects of opioids on other systems, see Chapter 20. Dextromethorphan can also cause gastrointestinal (GI) distress. When taken in massive overdosage (e.g., when used as a drug of abuse), hallucinogenic effects may result from noncompetitive inhibition of central *N*-methyl-D-aspartate receptors. These are the receptors antagonized by phencyclidine (PCP, Chapter 21). Additional toxic manifestations include tachycardia, hypertension, lethargy, psychomotor delay, and seizures. Dextromethorphan has weak serotonergie effects and may interact with MAO inhibitors (Chapter 19). Guaifenesin may cause GI distress, dizziness, and drowsiness.

■ DRUGS USED IN OBSTRUCTIVE AIRWAY DISORDERS

Pathogenesis

Bronchial asthma is a chronic episodic bronchospastic disorder characterized by an early-phase response beginning immediately following exposure to a trigger stimulus and a late-phase response which begins 6 to 8 hours later. In the classic immunologic model, the early phase is initiated by the stimulus (often an allergen) binding to IgE bound to mast cells in the airway mucosa (Figure 35–2). Subsequent release of eicosanoids and other mediators result in the initial bronchospasm and influx of additional inflammatory cells. Bronchospasm decreases the airway diameter and limits expiratory airflow. The hallmark of the late-phase response is airway inflammation with interstitial airway edema, invasion

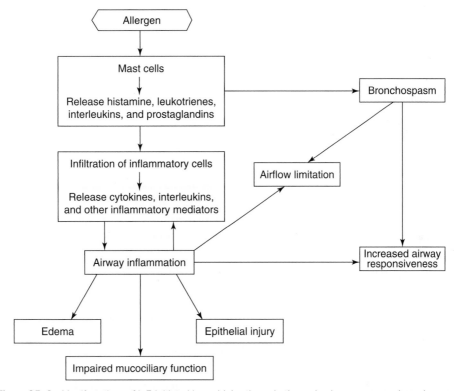

Figure 35–2. Manifestations of IgE-initiated bronchial asthma. In the early-phase response, bronchospasm predominates resulting in decreased expiratory airflow. In the late-phase response, airway inflammation, edema, increased mucus production, and impaired mucociliary function decrease expiratory airflow. Both early- and late-phase responses are also associated with increased airway responsiveness to subsequent allergic triggers. (Reproduced, with permission, from Porth CM: *Pathophysiology: Concept of Altered Health States*, 7th ed. Philadelphia: Lippincott Williams & Wilkins, 2005:696.)

of white blood cells, epithelial injury with decreased mucociliary function, and sustained bronchoconstriction. This combination of factors during the late-phase response also decreases airway diameter and limits expiratory airflow. Both the early and late phases are associated with increased airway responsiveness to subsequent allergen challenges. Examples of allergen triggers that initiate the immunologic response include house dust mites and cockroach detritus, animal dander, pollens, and molds. Nonallergen triggers that provoke asthmatic responses include viral respiratory tract infections, inhaled irritants (e.g., smoke), strong emotions, exercise, and cold air.

Chronic obstructive airway disease (or chronic obstructive pulmonary disease, COPD) includes chronic bronchitis, emphysema, and bronchiectasis. Common characteristics of COPD include chronic and repeated airway obstruction and inflammation. The most common cause of COPD is smoking. Emphysema is a loss of elasticity of the parenchyma (alveoli and interstitial tissue) and breakdown of the alveolar walls. The former inhibits expiratory airflow and the latter results in a loss of surface area available for gas diffusion. In contrast, chronic bronchitis is caused by inflammation that results in submucosal hyperplasia and edema, along with excessive mucous secretion. Airway narrowing and mucous plugs inhibit expiratory airflow. Bronchiectasis is a form of COPD that results from cycles of bacterial infection and subsequent inflammation. This process destroys the elastic support of the airways and forms mucous plugs that decrease expiratory airflow. Cystic fibrosis is a genetic disorder that affects many organs. In the pulmonary system, it results in production of abnormally viscous mucus and blockage of airways with inhibition of expiratory airflow and repeated bacterial infections.

Therapeutic Strategies for Obstructive Lung Diseases

The drug classes used in the treatment of asthma and other obstructive airway disorders are presented in Figure 35–3. Therapeutic interventions may be divided into two categories: "short-term relievers" and "long-term controllers." The former drugs relieve acute bronchospasm associated with obstructive airway diseases, and the latter drugs minimize the associated inflammation or prevent subsequent acute bronchospastic attacks.

Acute bronchospasm can usually be treated promptly and effectively with bronchodilators. Beta$_2$ (β_2)–selective agonists, muscarinic antagonists, and theophylline and its derivatives are available for this indication. Late response inflammation and bronchial hyperreactivity can be treated with corticosteroids, cromolyn or nedocromil, and leukotriene antagonists. These drugs inhibit release of mediators from mast cells and other inflammatory cells or block their effects. The

leukotriene antagonists may have inhibitory effects on both bronchoconstriction and inflammation. Anti-IgE antibodies also appear promising for chronic therapy in some cases. A review of these drug classes and their clinical use in asthma is presented in Figure 35–4. Many of these drug classes are used clinically for other obstructive airway disorders.

Bronchodilator Drugs

β-ADRENOCEPTOR AGONISTS

Prototypes and Pharmacokinetics. The β_2-selective agonists are the most important drugs used to reverse asthmatic bronchoconstriction. **Epinephrine** and **isoproterenol** are still used occasionally even though they are not selective for β_2 receptors. **Albuterol, terbutaline,** and **metaproterenol** are the most important short-acting β_2 agonists in the United States. **Salmeterol** and **formoterol** are long-acting β_2 agonists. Beta-receptor agonists are given almost exclusively by inhalation, usually from pressurized aerosol canisters, but occasionally by nebulizer. The inhalational route decreases the systemic dose (and adverse effects), while delivering an effective dose locally to the airway smooth muscle. The older drugs have durations of action of 6 hours or less; salmeterol and formoterol act for 12 hours or more.

Mechanism and Physiologic Effects. The classification of β receptors, mechanisms of action of drugs stimulating

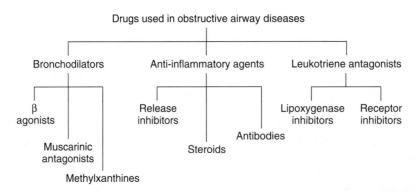

Figure 35–3. Drug classes useful in obstructive airway disorders include bronchodilators (smooth muscle relaxants) and anti-inflammatory drugs. Bronchodilators include β_2-selective agonists, muscarinic antagonists, and methylxanthines. Anti-inflammatory drugs include mast cell release inhibitors, corticosteroids, and an anti-IgE antibody. Leukotriene antagonists have both bronchodilator and anti-inflammatory mechanisms of action.

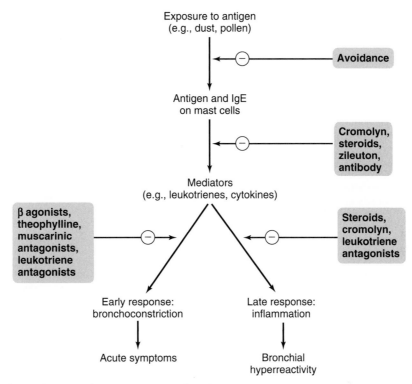

Figure 35–4. Summary of treatment strategies in asthma. (Reproduced, with permission, from Cockcroft DW: The bronchial late response in the pathogenesis of asthma and its modulation by therapy. *Ann Allergy* 1985;55:857.)

these receptors, and general physiologic effects of β receptor stimulation are discussed in Chapters 4 and 6. Activation of β receptors stimulates adenylyl cyclase, and increases intracellular cyclic adenosine monophosphate (cAMP) in smooth muscle cells. This causes a decrease in smooth muscle tone and a powerful bronchodilator response (Figure 35–5).

Clinical Use. These drugs are used extensively in asthma. Shorter-acting β_2 agonists (albuterol, metaproterenol, terbutaline) should be used only for acute episodes of bronchospasm (not for prophylaxis). The long-acting agents (salmeterol, formoterol) should be used for prophylaxis, not for acute episodes, because they are effective in improving asthmatic control when taken regularly but have a slow onset of action. In almost all patients, the shorter-acting β agonists are the most effective bronchodilators available and therefore the drugs of choice for acute asthma. Some patients with chronic COPD also benefit,

although the incidence of adverse effects is increased in this condition.

Adverse Effects. Skeletal muscle tremor is a common adverse β_2 effect of these drugs. The β_2 selectivity of these drugs is not complete. At high dosage, these agents have significant β_1 cardiac effects. Even when they are given by inhalation, tachycardia is common. When the agents are used excessively, arrhythmias may occur. Loss of responsiveness (tolerance, tachyphylaxis) can occur with excessive use of short-acting β_2 agonists. Patients with COPD often have concurrent cardiac disease and may have arrhythmias even at normal dosage.

METHYLXANTHINES

Prototypes and Pharmacokinetics. The methylxanthines are purine derivatives. Three major methylxanthines are found in plants and provide the stimulant effects of three common beverages: **caffeine** (in coffee), **theophylline**

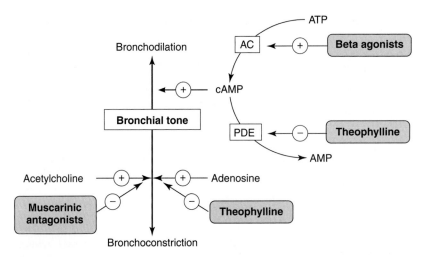

Figure 35–5. Bronchodilation is promoted by cyclic adenosine monophosphate (cAMP). Intracellular levels of cAMP can be increased by β-adrenoceptor agonists, which increase the rate of cAMP synthesis by adenylyl cyclase (AC); or by phosphodiesterase (PDE) inhibitors such as theophylline, which slow the rate of cAMP degradation. Bronchoconstriction can also be inhibited by muscarinic antagonists and possibly by adenosine antagonists.

(in tea), and **theobromine** (in cocoa). Theophylline is the only member of this group important in the treatment of asthma.

Theophylline and several analogs are orally active and available as a base and as various salts. The drug is available in both prompt-release and slow-release forms, and is eliminated by P450 drug-metabolizing enzymes in the liver. Clearance varies with age (highest in young adolescents), smoking status (higher in smokers), and concurrent use of other drugs that inhibit or induce hepatic enzymes.

Mechanism and Physiologic Effects. The methylxanthines inhibit phosphodiesterase (PDE), the enzyme that degrades cAMP to adenosine monophosphate (AMP) (Figure 35–5), and thus increase cAMP levels. This anti-PDE effect, however, requires high concentrations of the drug. Methylxanthines also block adenosine receptors in the CNS and elsewhere, but a relationship between this action and the bronchodilating effect has not been clearly established. Finally, the possibility exists that bronchodilation is caused by an unrecognized action.

In asthma, bronchodilation is the most important therapeutic action. Increased diaphragm contraction strength has also been demonstrated in some patients. Other effects of therapeutic doses include CNS stimulation, cardiac stimulation, vasodilation, a slight increase in blood pressure (probably caused by release of norepinephrine from adrenergic nerve endings), and increased GI motility.

Clinical Use. The major clinical indication for the use of methylxanthines is asthma, but none of these drugs are as safe or effective as the β$_2$ agonists. Slow-release theophylline (for control of nocturnal asthma) is the most important methylxanthine in clinical use. Another methylxanthine derivative, **pentoxifylline**, is promoted as a remedy for intermittent claudication; this effect is said to result from decreased blood viscosity. Nonmedical use of methylxanthines in coffee, tea, and cocoa is far greater, in total quantities consumed, than their medical uses.

Adverse Effects. These drugs have a narrow therapeutic window. Therapeutic plasma concentrations range from 5 to 20 mg/L, whereas adverse effects begin to occur in some patients when plasma concentrations reach 15 to 20 mg/L. Common adverse effects include GI distress, tremor, and insomnia. Severe nausea and vomiting, hypotension, cardiac arrhythmias, and convulsions may result from overdosage. Very large overdoses (e.g., in suicide attempts) are potentially lethal because of arrhythmias and convulsions. Beta-receptor antagonists are useful antidotes for severe cardiovascular toxicity from theophylline.

MUSCARINIC ANTAGONISTS

Prototypes and Pharmacokinetics. Atropine and other naturally occurring belladonna alkaloids were used for many years in the treatment of asthma but have been replaced by **ipratropium**, a quaternary antimuscarinic agent. Ipratropium is delivered to the airways by pressurized aerosol and has little systemic action. **Tiotropium** is a newer, longer-acting analog.

Mechanism and Physiologic Effect. When given as an aerosol, ipratropium competitively blocks muscarinic receptors in the airways and effectively prevents bronchoconstriction mediated by vagal discharge (Figure 35–5). If given systemically (not an approved use), the drug is indistinguishable from other short-acting muscarinic blockers. Ipratropium reverses bronchoconstriction in some asthma patients (especially children) and in many patients with COPD. The drug has no effect on the inflammatory aspects of asthma.

Clinical Use. Ipratropium is only useful in one-third to two-thirds of asthmatic patients; β_2 agonists are effective in almost all. Therefore, β_2 agonists are usually preferred for acute bronchospasm. However, in patients with COPD, which is often associated with acute episodes of bronchospasm, antimuscarinic agents may be more effective and less toxic than β_2 agonists.

Adverse Effects. Because ipratropium is delivered directly to the airway and minimally absorbed, there are few systemic effects. When given in excessive dosage, minor atropine-like toxic effects may occur (Chapter 5). In contrast to β_2 agonists, ipratropium does not cause tremors or arrhythmias.

Anti-Inflammatory Drugs

CORTICOSTEROIDS

Prototypes and Pharmacokinetics. For an expanded discussion of the mechanisms of action, clinical uses, and adverse effects of corticosteroids (glucocorticoids), see Chapter 23. All of the corticosteroids are potentially beneficial in severe asthma. However, because of their toxicity, systemic (oral) corticosteroids are used chronically only if other drug delivery options are unsuccessful. In contrast, local aerosol administration of surface-active corticosteroids (e.g., **beclomethasone, budesonide, dexamethasone, flunisolide, fluticasone, mometasone**) is relatively safe. Inhaled corticosteroids have become common first-line therapy for individuals with moderate to severe asthma. Important intravenous corticosteroids for status asthmaticus (acute severe bronchospasm unresponsive to usual bronchodilator medications) include **prednisolone** (the active metabolite of **prednisone**) and **hydrocortisone**.

Mechanism and Physiologic Effects. Corticosteroids inhibit phospholipase A_2 and reduce eicosanoid synthesis. Excessive activity of phospholipase A_2 is thought to be particularly important in asthma because the leukotrienes that result from eicosanoid synthesis are extremely potent bronchoconstrictors, and also participate in the late inflammatory response (Figure 35–6). Corticosteroids reduce the release of arachidonic acid by phospholipase A_2 and inhibit the expression of type 2 cyclooxygenase (COX-2, Chapter 34), the inducible form of cyclooxygenase. Corticosteroids may also increase the responsiveness of β_2 adrenoceptors in the airway. Corticosteroids bind intracellular receptors and activate glucocorticoid response elements in the nucleus, resulting in synthesis of substances that prevent the full expression of inflammation and allergy (Chapter 23).

Clinical Use. Inhaled corticosteroids are now considered appropriate (even for children) in most cases of moderate asthma that are not fully responsive to aerosol β_2 agonists. Early use of corticosteroids may prevent the severe, progressive inflammatory changes characteristic of long-standing asthma. This is a shift from earlier beliefs that steroids should be used only in severe refractory asthma. In such cases of severe asthma, patients are usually hospitalized and stabilized on daily systemic prednisone and then switched to inhaled or alternate-day oral therapy before discharge. In status asthmaticus, parenteral steroids are lifesaving and apparently act more promptly than in ordinary asthma. Their mechanism of action in this condition is not fully understood.

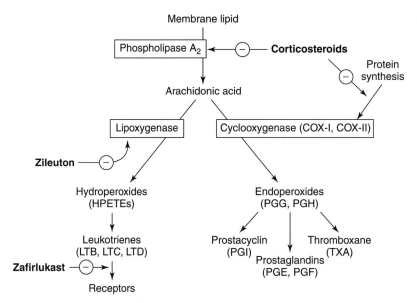

Figure 35–6. Flow diagram of the eicosanoid cascade and the mechanisms of action of different anti-inflammatory drugs. Corticosteroids inhibit the release of arachidonic acid, the substrate for lipoxygenase and cyclooxygenase. Other leukotriene pathway antagonists either inhibit the lipoxygenase enzyme directly, or inhibit the receptors for lipoxygenase products (leukotrienes B, C, or D).

Adverse Effects. Local aerosol administration can occasionally result in a very small degree of adrenal suppression, but this is rarely significant. More commonly, changes in oropharyngeal flora result in candidiasis. This adverse effect can be minimized by gargling with water following drug administration. If oral (systemic) therapy is required, adrenal suppression can be reduced by using alternate-day therapy (i.e., giving the drug in slightly higher dosage every other day rather than smaller doses every day). The major systemic toxicities of these drugs (Chapter 23) are much more likely to occur if systemic treatment is required for more than 2 weeks, as in severe refractory asthma. Regular use of inhaled steroids causes mild growth retardation in children, but these children eventually reach predicted adult stature.

Leukotriene Antagonists

These drugs interfere with leukotriene synthesis or their receptor interactions. They reduce the frequency of exacerbations but are not as effective as corticosteroids in severe asthma and are not useful in acute episodes.

LIPOXYGENASE INHIBITORS. **Zileuton** is an orally active drug that selectively inhibits 5-lipoxygenase, a key enzyme in the conversion of arachidonic acid to leukotrienes. The drug is effective in preventing both exercise- and antigen-induced bronchospasm. Zileuton is also effective against "aspirin allergy," the bronchospasm that results from ingestion of aspirin by individuals who apparently divert all eicosanoid production to leukotrienes when the cyclooxygenase pathway is blocked (Figure 35–6). The toxicity of zileuton includes occasional elevation of liver enzymes. Therefore, this drug is less popular than the leukotriene receptor blockers.

LEUKOTRIENE RECEPTOR BLOCKERS. **Zafirlukast** and **montelukast** are antagonists at the LTD_4 leukotriene receptor (Figure 35–6). The LTE_4 receptor is also blocked. These drugs are orally active and are used for prophylaxis. They have been shown to be effective in preventing exercise-, antigen-, and aspirin-induced bronchospastic attacks. They are not recommended for acute episodes of asthma. Toxicity is generally low, but rare reports of Churg-Strauss syndrome (allergic granulomatous angiitis) have appeared. Evidence of a causal association is lacking.

Anti-IgE Antibody

Omalizumab is a humanized murine monoclonal antibody to human IgE. The antibody binds to the IgE antibody on sensitized mast cells and prevents mast cell activation and subsequent release of inflammatory mediators by asthma triggers. This very expensive therapy is approved for prophylaxis in asthma and it must be administered parenterally.

Cromolyn and Nedocromil

PROTOTYPES AND PHARMACOKINETICS. Cromolyn (disodium cromoglycate) and nedocromil are unusual chemicals. They are extremely insoluble, so that even massive doses given orally or by aerosol result in minimal systemic blood levels. Because they are not absorbed from the site of administration, cromolyn and nedocromil have only local effects. When administered orally, cromolyn has some efficacy in preventing food allergy. Similar actions have been demonstrated after local application in the conjunctivae and the nasopharyngeal tract. When used in the nasopharyngeal tract (for hay fever) or in the bronchi (for asthma), these drugs are delivered by aerosol.

MECHANISM AND EFFECTS. The mechanism of action of these drugs is poorly understood but appears to involve a decrease in the release of mediators (such as leukotrienes and histamine) from mast cells. Although these drugs have no bronchodilator action, they can prevent bronchoconstriction caused by a challenge with antigen to which the patient is allergic. Cromolyn and nedocromil are capable of preventing both early and late responses to challenge.

CLINICAL USES. Asthma (especially in children) is the most important use for cromolyn and nedocromil and requires inhalation of the drugs. Nasal and eye drop formulations of cromolyn are available for hay fever, and an oral formulation is used for food allergy.

ADVERSE EFFECTS. These drugs may cause cough and airway irritation when given by aerosol. Rare instances of drug allergy have been reported.

REHABILITATION FOCUS

Patients may be taking OTC drugs for respiratory disorders without consulting health-care professionals, and some of these drugs can have significant interactions with rehabilitation therapy. Decongestants can increase blood pressure and cardiac workload. Cardiac effects may be manifested as exertional angina or tachycardia during aerobic activities or painful procedures during wound care. Orthostatic hypotension may also occur when a patient is taking oxymetazoline, but is more common with opioid antitussives and antihistamines. Antitussives can also depress respiratory drive, resulting in hypercapnia during aerobic activities. Finally, antihistamines and antitussives can cause sedation.

Patients with obstructive airway disorders will often be in rehabilitation. Some of these patients will be in rehabilitation for nonpulmonary therapy, but their pulmonary disorders and the drugs used to treat these disorders can have significant effects on rehabilitation outcomes. Other patients will be in pulmonary rehabilitation for these same obstructive airway disorders. Exercise therapy has proven beneficial in patients with COPD and cystic fibrosis. There is less clear evidence for the benefits of exercise therapy in patients with asthma and bronchiectasis. In some asthmatics, bronchospasm is precipitated by exercise. These patients may also benefit from resistive exercises to improve aerobic conditioning.

Patients should be educated regarding the benefits of maintaining their respiratory prescription regimens for rehabilitation activities. Drugs used to treat obstructive airway disorders will reduce the effort of respiration and improve aerobic capacity during the treatment sessions.

Optimal pulmonary rehabilitation programs include exercise therapy, patient education, and psychosocial-behavioral training. The same drugs that benefit the patient with obstructive airway disorder may also precipitate adverse effects during the treatment process. Bronchodilators such as β_2 agonists and methylxanthines can cause cardiac disturbances, which are exacerbated during aerobic activities in rehabilitation. The corticosteroid drugs, when administered systemically for prolonged periods, can result in osteoporosis and insulin resistance.

CLINICAL RELEVANCE FOR REHABILITATION

Adverse Drug Reactions

Drugs used to treat upper airway dysfunction

- Antihistamines cause sedation and orthostatic hypotension.
- Nasal decongestants may increase blood pressure or cause headaches.
- All antitussives decrease respiratory drive.

Drugs used to treat lower airway dysfunction

- Beta$_2$ agonists may cause tachycardia with ordinary use, and excessive use is associated with cardiac arrhythmias.
- Methylxanthines may cause cardiac arrhythmias and convulsions.
- Antimuscarinic drugs when taken in excessive doses may result in hyperthermia or tachycardia. (See Chapter 5 for more information.)
- Chronic systemic administration of corticosteroids may result in insulin resistance, hyperglycemia, and osteoporosis. (See Chapter 23 for more information.)

Effects Interfering with Rehabilitation

- Drugs that cause sedation and orthostatic hypotension may increase the risk of falls.
- Nasal decongestants that increase blood pressure or heart rate may precipitate angina in patients during rehabilitation as a result of increased cardiac workload.
- Opioid drugs that decrease respiratory drive may precipitate hypercapnia in patients during aerobic activities.
- Antimuscarinic drugs that inhibit perspiration may result in hyperthermia in patients during aerobic activities.
- Patients taking corticosteroids and those with poor glucose control associated with diabetes mellitus may have short-term plasma glucose elevations exacerbated by aerobic activities.

Possible Therapy Solutions

- Monitor heart rate (may not be elevated if β blockers are present) or relative perceived exertion during rehabilitation activities.
- Monitor plasma glucose levels prior to rehabilitation.
- Monitor for signs of hyperthermia during aerobic activities.

Potentiation of Functional Outcomes Secondary to Drug Therapy

- Patients with obstructive airway diseases may benefit from the use of bronchodilators prior to beginning rehabilitation:
  - If exercise has been documented to initiate an asthmatic attack in a patient where aerobic activities are a component of the treatment.
  - If the treatment includes lumbar traction or aquatic therapy, and this activity results in dyspnea.

PROBLEM-ORIENTED PATIENT STUDY

Brief History: The patient is a 54-year-old male who works in the shipping and receiving department at a state university. His job entails transporting mail and other objects to and from various locations around the university. Two days ago, he hurt his back while moving several boxes. The pain prevents him from walking and from moving objects, thus preventing him from completing his job. He was referred to the university-associated rehabilitation clinic.

Current Medical Status and Drug Therapy: The patient's medical chart states that he had asthma in childhood, and that he currently smokes and

PROBLEM-ORIENTED PATIENT STUDY (*Continued*)

has a 30-plus pack-year history of smoking. He has a prescription for ipratropium and albuterol (Combivent) to take as needed for dyspnea. He also has essential hypertension and takes nadolol combined with bendroflumethiazide (Corzide) as an antihypertensive medication. His current blood pressure and heart rate are 138/82 mm Hg and 79 bpm, respectively.

Rehabilitation Setting: The patient's diagnosis was documented as severe low back strain. Initial treatment was for pain relief and initiation of pain-free functional movement. The rehabilitation clinic does not have a traction table, but instead uses aquatherapy at the university pool. A small pool to the side of the main pool has a shallow end at 2 to 4 feet and a deeper end at 6 to 10 feet. This pool is kept at 34°C, and is used by both the rehabilitation clinic and athletics programs at the university. The patient is sent from the rehabilitation clinic to the pool. He is observed smoking a cigarette along the way. In the shallow end of the pool, a float is attached to the upper chest of the patient under the axillas; this keeps his head out of the water. Then a 4-kg weight is attached to each ankle. The patient is guided to the deep end of the pool so that his feet do not touch the bottom. The patient is told to relax and see if the pain begins to decrease. After 10 minutes, the patient states that the pain begins to decrease. The patient is then instructed to begin slowly walking in place. Approximately 4 minutes into this part of the therapy, the patient begins to complain of shortness of breath. He is pale and frantically attempts to reach the shallow end of the pool. He is assisted to the side of the pool and out of the water. His blood pressure and heart rate are 154/90 mm Hg and 89 bpm, respectively.

Problem/Clinical Options: During the aerobic part of the aquatherapy to provide analgesia and pain-free function, the patient developed exertional dyspnea as the result of a combination of factors. Although not diagnosed with COPD, the patient currently smokes, has a significant smoking history, had asthma in childhood, and uses prescribed bronchodilators as needed (ipratropium and albuterol). This information strongly suggests a diminished pulmonary reserve. Nadolol in his combination antihypertensive medication (nadolol and bendroflumethiazide) is a nonselective beta-receptor antagonist. Therefore, this drug would block both β_1 receptors on the heart and β_2 receptors in the airways. The latter blockade would cause bronchoconstriction and make breathing more difficult. With the patient in the pool up to his neck, the hydrostatic pressure on the thorax increases. This increased external pressure diminishes ventilation and thus reduces gas exchange. Weights on the lower extremities would also diminish the elevation of the rib cage during inspiration. This combination of factors exceeded the patient's pulmonary reserve during the aerobic portion of therapy, and he became dyspneic. Finally, smoking a cigarette prior to the therapy session decreased the oxygen-carrying capacity of his red blood cells. Incomplete combustion of organic matter (smoking) results in the formation of carbon monoxide. Carbon monoxide binds to hemoglobin in red blood cells forming carboxyhemoglobin. Carboxyhemoglobin prevents the binding of oxygen to hemoglobin, leading to hypoxemia and peripheral tissue hypoxia. Patients should be strongly advised not to smoke prior to performing aerobic activities because the oxygen-carrying potential of the blood is diminished.

PREPARATIONS AVAILABLE

Sympathomimetics Used in Asthma (see also Chapter 6)

Albuterol (generic, Proventil, Ventolin, others)
Inhalant: 90 mcg/puff aerosol; 0.083, 0.5% solution for nebulization
Oral: 2-, 4-mg tablets; 2 mg/5 mL syrup
Oral sustained-release: 4-, 8-mg tablets

Albuterol/Ipratropium (Combivent, DuoNeb)
Inhalant: 103 mcg albuterol + 18 mcg ipratropium/puff; 3 mg albuterol + 0.5 mg ipratropium/3 mL solution for nebulization

Bitolterol (Tornalate)
Inhalant: 0.2% solution for nebulization

Ephedrine (generic)
Oral: 25-mg capsules
Parenteral: 50 mg/mL for injection

Epinephrine (generic, Adrenalin, others)
Inhalant: 1, 10 mg/mL for nebulization; 0.22 mg epinephrine base aerosol
Parenteral: 1:10,000 (0.1 mg/mL), 1:1000 (1 mg/mL)

Formoterol (Foradil)
Inhalant: 12 mcg/puff aerosol; 12 mcg/unit inhalant powder

Isoetharine (generic)
Inhalant: 1% solution for nebulization

Isoproterenol (generic, Isuprel, others)
Inhalant: 0.5, 1% for nebulization; 80, 131 mcg/puff aerosols
Parenteral: 0.02, 0.2 mg/mL for injection

Levalbuterol (Xenopex)
Inhalant: 0.31, 0.63, 1.25 mg/3-mL solution

Metaproterenol (Alupent, generic)
Inhalant: 0.65 mg/puff aerosol in 7-, 14-g containers; 0.4, 0.6, 5% for nebulization

Pirbuterol (Maxair)
Inhalant: 0.2 mg/puff aerosol in 80- and 300-dose containers

Salmeterol (Serevent)
Inhalant aerosol: 25 mcg salmeterol base/puff in 60- and 120-dose containers
Inhalant powder: 50 mcg/unit

Salmeterol/Fluticasone (Advair Diskus)
Inhalant: 100, 250, 500 mcg fluticasone + 50 mcg salmeterol/unit

Terbutaline (Brethine, Bricanyl)
Inhalant: 0.2 mg/puff aerosol
Oral: 2.5-, 5-mg tablets
Parenteral: 1 mg/mL for injection

Aerosol Corticosteroids (see also Chapter 23)

Beclomethasone (QVAR, Vanceril)
Aerosol: 40, 80 mcg/puff in 20-dose containers

Budesonide (Pulmicort)
Aerosol powder: 160 mcg/activation

Flunisolide (AeroBid)
Aerosol: 250 mcg/puff in 100-dose container

Fluticasone (Flovent)
Aerosol: 44, 110, and 220 mcg/puff in 120-dose container; powder, 50, 100, 250 mcg/activation

Fluticasone/Salmeterol (Advair Diskus)
Inhalant: 100, 250, 500 mcg fluticasone + 50 mcg salmeterol/unit

Triamcinolone (Azmacort)
Aerosol: 100 mcg/puff in 240-dose container

Leukotriene Antagonists

Montelukast (Singulair)
Oral: 10-mg tablets; 4-, 5-mg chewable tablets; 4 mg/packet granules

Zafirlukast (Accolate)
Oral: 10-, 20-mg tablets

Zileuton (Zyflo)
Oral: 600-mg tablets

Cromolyn Sodium and Nedocromil Sodium

Cromolyn sodium
Pulmonary aerosol (generic, Intal): 800 mcg/puff in 200-dose container; 20 mg/2 mL for nebulization (for asthma)
Nasal aerosol (Nasalcrom)[1]: 5.2 mg/puff (for hay fever)
Oral (Gastrocrom): 100 mg/5 mL concentrate (for gastrointestinal allergy)

Nedocromil sodium (Tilade)
Pulmonary aerosol: 1.75 mg/puff in 112–metered-dose container

Methylxanthines: Theophylline and Derivatives

Aminophylline (theophylline ethylenediamine, 79% theophylline) (generic, others)
Oral: 105 mg/5 mL liquid; 100-, 200-mg tablets
Oral sustained-release: 225-mg tablets
Rectal: 250-, 500-mg suppositories
Parenteral: 250 mg/10 mL for injection

Theophylline (generic, Elixophyllin, Slo-Phyllin, Uniphyl, Theo-Dur, Theo-24, others)
Oral: 100-, 125-, 200-, 250-, 300-mg tablets; 100-, 200-mg capsules; 26.7, 50 mg/5 mL elixirs, syrups, and solutions
Oral sustained-release, 8–12 hours: 50-, 60-, 75-, 100-, 125-, 130-, 200-, 250-, 260-, 300-mg capsules
Oral sustained-release, 8–24 hours: 100-, 200-, 300-, 450-mg tablets

Oral sustained-release, 12 hours: 100-, 125-, 130-, 200-, 250-, 260-, 300-mg capsules
Oral sustained-release, 12–24 hours: 100-, 200-, 300-tablets
Oral sustained-release, 24 hours: 100-, 200-, 300-mg tablets and capsules; 400-, 600-mg tablets
Parenteral: 200-, 400-, 800-mg/container, theophylline and 5% dextrose for injection

Other Methylxanthines

Dyphylline (generic, other)
Oral: 200-, 400-mg tablets; 33.3, 53.3 mg/5 mL elixir
Parenteral: 250 mg/mL for injection

Oxtriphylline (generic, Choledyl)
Oral: equivalent to 64, 127, 254, 382 mg theophylline tablets; 32, 64 mg/5 mL syrup

Pentoxifylline (generic, Trental)
Oral: 400-mg tablets and controlled-release tablets
Note: Pentoxifylline is labeled for use in intermittent claudication only.

Antimuscarinic Drugs Used in Asthma

Ipratropium (generic, Atrovent)
Aerosol: 18 mcg/puff in 200–metered-dose inhaler; 0.02% (500 mcg/vial) for nebulization
Nasal spray: 21, 42 mcg/spray

Antibody

Omalizumab (Xolair)
Powder for SC injection, 202.5 mg

[1]OTC preparation.

REFERENCES

Pathophysiology of Airway Disease
James A, Carroll N: Airway smooth muscle in health and disease: Methods of measurement and relation to function. *Eur Respir J* 2000;15:782.

Jeffery PK: Remodeling in asthma and chronic obstructive lung disease. *Am J Respir Crit Care Med* 2001; 164:S28.
Mazzone SB, Canning BJ: Central nervous system control of the airways: Pharmacological implications. *Curr Opin Pharmacol* 2002;2:220.

McPhee SJ, Papadakis MA, Tierney LM Jr: *Current Medical Diagnosis and Therapy 2007*. New York: McGraw-Hill, 2007.

Ryu JH, et al: Bronchiolar disorders. *Am J Respir Crit Care Med* 2003;168:1277.

Spina D, Page CP: Pharmacology of airway irritability. *Curr Opin Pharmacol* 2002;2:264.

Methylxanthines

Murciano D, et al: Effects of theophylline on diaphragmatic strength and fatigue in patients with chronic obstructive pulmonary disease. *N Engl J Med* 1984;311:349.

Page CP: Recent advances in our understanding of the use of theophylline in the treatment of asthma. *J Clin Pharmacol* 1999; 39:237.

Cromolyn and Nedocromil

Barnes PJ, et al: Asthma mechanisms, determinants of severity and treatment: The role of nedocromil sodium. *Clin Exp Allergy* 1995;25:771.

Corticosteroids

Dinwiddie R: Anti-inflammatory therapy in cystic fibrosis. *J Cyst Fibros* 2005;4(Suppl 2):45.

Robinson DS, Geddes DM: Inhaled corticosteroids: Benefits and risks. *J Asthma* 1996;33:5.

Suissa S, et al: Low-dose inhaled corticosteroids and the prevention of death from asthma. *N Engl J Med* 2000; 343:332.

Beta Agonists

Colombo JL: Long-acting bronchodilators in cystic fibrosis. *Curr Opin Pulm Med* 2003;9:504.

Ullman A, Svedmyr N: Salmeterol, a new long acting inhaled β_2-adrenoceptor agonist: Comparison with salbutamol in adult asthmatic patients. *Thorax* 1988;43:674.

Antimuscarinic Drugs

Lee AM, et al: Selective muscarinic receptor antagonists for airway diseases. *Curr Opin Pharmacol* 2001;1:223.

Leukotriene Pathway Inhibitors

Calhoun WJ: Anti-leukotrienes for asthma. *Curr Opin Pharmacol* 2001;1:230.

Krawiec ME, Wenzel SE: Leukotriene inhibitors and non-steroidal therapies in the treatment of asthma. *Exp Opin Invest Drugs* 2001;2:47.

Malmstrom K, et al: Oral montelukast, inhaled beclomethasone, and placebo for chronic asthma. A randomized, controlled trial. Montelukast/Beclomethasone Study Group. *Ann Intern Med* 1999;130:487.

Other Drugs for Asthma

Leckie MJ, et al: Effects of an interleukin-5 blocking monoclonal antibody on eosinophils, airway hyper-responsiveness, and the late asthmatic response. *Lancet* 2000;456:2144.

Patacchini R, Maggi CA: Peripheral tachykinin receptors as targets for new drugs. *Eur J Pharmacol* 2001;429:13.

Smyth A: Prophylactic antibiotics in cystic fibrosis: A conviction without evidence? *Pediatr Pulmonol* 2005;40:471.

Pharmacotherapy of Upper Airway Diseases

Ferguson BJ: Cost-effective pharmacotherapy for allergic rhinitis. *Otolaryngol Clin North Am* 1998;31:91.

Katcher ML: Cold, cough, and allergy medications: Uses and abuses. *Pediatr Rev* 1996;17:12.

Kelly LF: Pediatric cough and cold preparations. *Pediatr Rev* 2004;25:115.

Mabry RL: Therapeutic agents in the medical management of sinusitis. *Otolaryngol Clin North Am* 1993;26:561.

Schwartz RH: Adolescent abuse of dextromethorphan. *Clin Pediatr (Phila)* 2005;44:565.

Rehabilitation

Anderson SD, Brannan JD: Long-acting beta$_2$-adrenoceptor agonists and exercise-induced asthma: lessons to guide us in the future. *Paediatr Drugs* 2004;6:161.

Bradley J, et al: Physical training for bronchiectasis. *Cochrane Database Syst Rev* 2002;CD002166.

Darnley GM, et al: Effects of resistive breathing on exercise capacity and diaphragm function in patients with ischaemic heart disease. *Eur J Heart Fail* 1999;1:297.

Hill NS: Pulmonary rehabilitation. *Proc Am Thorac Soc* 2006;3:66.

Satta A: Exercise training in asthma. *J Sports Med Phys Fitness* 2000;40:277.

Schmitt-Grohe S, Zielen S: Leukotriene receptor antagonists in children with cystic fibrosis lung disease: Anti-inflammatory and clinical effects. *Paediatr Drugs* 2005; 7:353.

Smidt N, et al: Effectiveness of exercise therapy: A best-evidence summary of systematic reviews. *Aust J Physiother* 2005;51:71.

Taylor NF, et al: Progressive resistance exercise in physical therapy: A summary of systematic reviews. *Phys Ther* 2005;85:1208.

van Helvoort HA, et al: Systemic immunological response to exercise in patients with chronic obstructive pulmonary disease: What does it mean? *Respiration* 2006; 73:255.

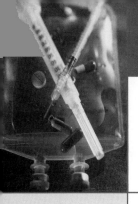

36

DRUGS USED TO TREAT GASTROINTESTINAL DISORDERS

The various components of the gastrointestinal (GI) tract serve several functions, including digestive, excretory, endocrine, and exocrine. Control of these functions requires neuronal activity from both local and higher centers.

NEURONAL CONTROL

The GI system has a complex collection of highly organized neurons called the **enteric nervous system (ENS)** located in the intestinal walls (Figure 36–1). The ENS may be considered a third division of the autonomic nervous system, and includes the myenteric plexus and the submucosal plexus. These neuronal networks receive preganglionic fibers from the parasympathetic system as well as postganglionic sympathetic axons. They also receive sensory input from within the wall of the gut. Fibers from the cell bodies in these plexuses travel to the smooth muscle of the gut to control motility. Other motor fibers go to the secretory cells. Sensory fibers transmit information from the mucosa and from stretch receptors to motor neurons in the plexuses and to postganglionic neurons in the sympathetic ganglia. The parasympathetic and sympathetic fibers that synapse on enteric plexus neurons appear to play a modulatory role.

Multiple neurotransmitters, neuromodulators, and autocrine factors are present in the GI system. Autacoids are endogenous molecules that have powerful physiologic and pharmacologic effects but do not fall into traditional autonomic or hormonal groups. Two important amine-autacoids, histamine (H) and serotonin (5-hydroxytryptamine, 5-HT), and numerous peptide autacoids are present. Both of these amine-autacoids are discussed in previous chapters; histamine in the respiratory system (Chapter 35) and 5-HT in the central nervous system (Chapter 19). Other well-documented autacoids are cytokines (Chapter 32) and prostaglandins (Chapter 34).

As previously discussed (Chapter 35), stimulation of histamine type 1 receptors results in mucous secretion in the respiratory system and contraction of several types of smooth muscle. In contrast, stimulation of histamine type 2 (H_2) receptors results in gastric acid secretion in the stomach. Serotonin is produced from the amino acid tryptophan and stored in vesicles in the enterochromaffin cells of the gut as well as neurons in the ENS. In addition to its activity as a central nervous system neurotransmitter (Chapters 12 and 19), 5-HT has a physiologic role as a neurotransmitter in the ENS and perhaps a role as a local hormone that modulates gastrointestinal smooth muscle activity. Fourteen 5-HT receptor subtypes have been characterized, and subtypes 2, 3, and 4 play roles in GI function or emesis. After release, both histamine and 5-HT may be metabolized by monoamine oxidase. Finally, dopamine (D), which has been previously

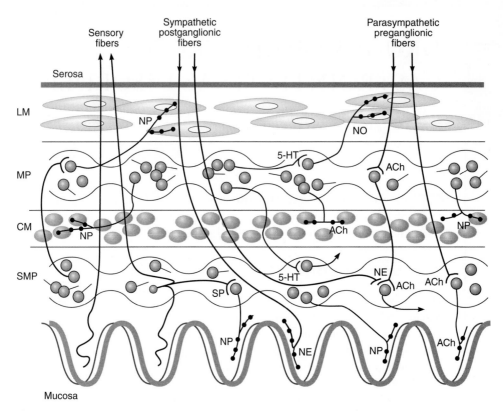

Figure 36–1. A highly simplified diagram of the intestinal wall and some of the circuitry of the enteric nervous system (ENS). The ENS receives input from both the sympathetic and the parasympathetic systems and sends afferent impulses to sympathetic ganglia and to the central nervous system. Many transmitter or neuromodulator substances have been identified in the ENS. These agents include acetylcholine (ACh), norepinephrine (NE), nitric oxide (NO), neuropeptides (NP), substance P (SP), and serotonin (5-HT). Additional abbreviations: longitudinal muscle layer (LM), myenteric plexus (MP), circular muscle layer (CM), and submucosal plexus (SMP).

discussed (Chapters 4, 12, 17, and 18), indirectly modulates gastric motility. Stimulation of dopamine type 2 (D_2) receptors located on cholinergic neurons in the ENS has an inhibitory effect on acetylcholine (ACh) release, and thus decreases peristalsis.

These transmitters, modulators, and their receptors provide numerous important drug targets, and many of the drugs used in gastrointestinal disease have been discussed in earlier chapters of this book. Those drugs will be reviewed briefly in this chapter. Drugs used in GI disorders may be divided into those for acid-peptic disorders, motility promoters (*prokinetics*), those used to prevent vomiting (*antiemetics*), drugs

used for treatment of inflammatory bowel disease, and other miscellaneous agents (Figure 36–2).

PHYSIOLOGY OF ACID SECRETION

Ulceration and erosion of the lining of the gastrointestinal tract are common problems. Mucosal erosions or ulcerations arise when the caustic effects of pepsin, acid, or bile overwhelm the defensive factors such as mucus, prostaglandins, and bicarbonate. Cells lining the stomach include mucus-producing cells, parietal cells, and gastrin-containing cells. Parietal cells contain receptors for gastrin, histamine, and

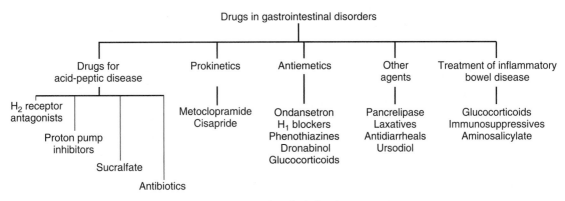

Figure 36–2. Drugs classes used in the treatment of gastrointestinal disorders.

acetylcholine (Figure 36–3). When ACh or gastrin bind to parietal cell receptors, they cause an increase in cytosolic calcium, which in turn activates protein kinases that stimulate acid secretion from a H^+/K^+–ATPase (proton pump) on the canalicular surface. This proton pump exchanges intracellular H^+ for K^+ present in the lumen of the stomach. In close proximity to the parietal cells are gut endocrine cells called enterochromaffin-like cells. These cells have receptors for gastrin, ACh, and neuropeptides, and are

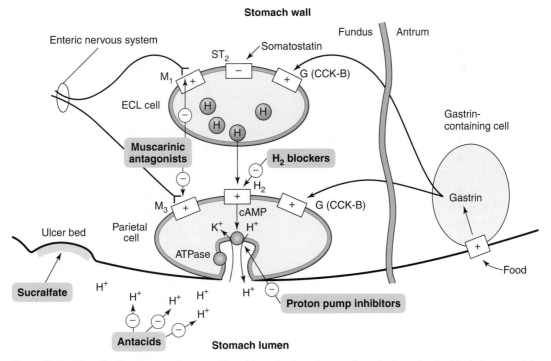

Figure 36–3. Sites of action of some drugs used in acid-peptic ulcer disease. Receptor types involved include muscarinic receptors (M_1, M_3), which bind acetylcholine, histamine type 2 (H_2), and peptide (somatostatin [ST], gastrin [G]) receptors. The site of action of misoprostol is not shown; it is thought to reduce acid secretion and increase protective factors such as mucus and bicarbonate. ECL, enterochromaffin-like; CCK, cholecystokinin.

the major source for histamine release. Histamine binds to the H_2 receptor on the parietal cell, resulting in activation of adenylyl cyclase, which increases intracellular cyclic adenosine monophosphate (cAMP). The cAMP activates protein kinases that stimulate H^+ secretion by the proton pump. Research suggests that the major effect of gastrin upon acid secretion is mediated indirectly through the release of histamine rather than through direct parietal cell stimulation.

DRUGS USED IN ACID-PEPTIC DISEASE

Acid-peptic diseases include **gastroesophageal reflux (GERD)**, gastric and duodenal ulcers, and stress-related mucosal injuries. In all of these conditions, mucosal erosions or ulcerations occur. Several drug classes are used in the treatment of peptic disease. Antimuscarinic drugs (Chapter 5) and the eicosanoid analog misoprostol (Chapter 34) have been previously discussed. Other drugs used in peptic disease include H_2 antihistamines, antacids, sucralfate, proton pump inhibitors, and antibiotics. Figure 36–3 shows the sites of action of most of the drugs used in the treatment of acid-peptic ulcer disease.

H_2 Antihistamines

Four H_2 blockers are available; **cimetidine** is the prototype. **Ranitidine, famotidine,** and **nizatidine** differ only in having fewer drug interactions than cimetidine. They are orally active, with half-lives of 1 to 3 hours. Because they are relatively nontoxic, they can be given in large doses. The duration of action of a single dose may be from 12 to 24 hours.

Mechanism and Effects

These drugs produce a reversible pharmacologic blockade of H_2 receptors. They are relatively selective and have no significant blocking actions at H_1 or autonomic receptors. The only therapeutic effect of clinical importance is the reduction of gastric acid secretion. Blockade of cardiovascular and mast cell H_2 receptor–mediated effects can be demonstrated but has no clinical significance when they are used in ulcer treatment.

Clinical Use

In acid-peptic disease, especially duodenal ulcers, these drugs reduce symptoms, accelerate healing, and prevent recurrences. An acute ulcer is usually treated with two or more doses per day, whereas recurrence of ulcers can often be prevented with a single bedtime dose. These antihistamines are also effective in accelerating healing and preventing recurrences of gastric peptic ulcers. In Zollinger-Ellison syndrome, which is characterized by acid hypersecretion, severe recurrent peptic ulceration, gastrointestinal bleeding, and diarrhea, these drugs are helpful but large doses are required. Similarly, the H_2 blockers have been used in GERD. In these latter two clinical uses, antihistamines are not as effective as proton pump inhibitors (discussed later). All of the H_2 blockers are available over-the-counter.

Toxicity

Cimetidine is a potent inhibitor of some hepatic drug-metabolizing enzymes and may also reduce hepatic blood flow. In high doses, cimetidine also has significant antiandrogen effects. Ranitidine has a weaker inhibitory effect on hepatic drug metabolism; neither it nor the other H_2 blockers appear to have any endocrine effects.

Antacids

Antacids are simple physical agents that react with protons (H^+) in the lumen of the gut. Aluminum-containing antacids may also stimulate the protective functions of the gastric mucosa. The antacids effectively reduce the recurrence rate of peptic ulcers when used regularly in the large doses needed significantly to raise the stomach pH.

The antacids differ mainly in their absorption and effects on stool consistency. The most popular antacids used in the United States are **magnesium hydroxide** ($Mg[OH]_2$) and **aluminum hydroxide** ($Al[OH]_3$). Neither of these weak bases is significantly absorbed from the bowel. Magnesium hydroxide has a strong laxative effect, whereas aluminum hydroxide has a constipating action. These drugs are available as single-ingredient products and as combined preparations. The combination products are usually preferred because they balance the laxative and constipating effects of either single formulation. Calcium carbonate and sodium bicarbonate are also weak bases, but they differ from aluminum and magnesium hydroxides in that they are absorbed from the gut. Because of their systemic effects, calcium carbonate and sodium bicarbonate salts are less popular as antacids than magnesium and aluminum compounds.

Sucralfate

Sucralfate is aluminum sucrose sulfate, a small, poorly soluble molecule that polymerizes in the acid environment of the stomach. This polymer binds to injured tissue and forms a protective coating over ulcer beds. The drug accelerates the healing of peptic ulcers and reduces the recurrence rate. Unfortunately, sucralfate must be taken four times daily. Sucralfate is too insoluble to have significant systemic effects when taken by the oral route; toxicity is very low. Sucralfate is also occasionally used in open wounds as a protective barrier and to minimize excessive exudate.

Proton Pump Inhibitors

Omeprazole is the prototype of the class of inhibitors of the proton pump of gastric parietal cells. Other agents in the group include **esomeprazole, lansoprazole, pantoprazole**, and **rabeprazole**. Oral formulations of these drugs are enteric coated to prevent acid inactivation in the stomach. They are rapidly metabolized in the liver, with half-lives of 1 to 2 hours. However, their durations of action are approximately 24 hours, and they may require 3 to 4 days of treatment to achieve their full effectiveness.

Mechanism of Action

These drugs are lipophilic weak bases that diffuse into the parietal cell canaliculi where they become protonated and concentrated more than 1,000-fold. There they undergo conversion to sulfenamides, which react covalently with the proton pump and irreversibly inactivate the enzyme. Proton pump inhibitors are very effective in peptic ulcer disease associated with the bacterium *Helicobacter pylori* and with nonsteroidal anti-inflammatory drug (NSAID) treatment. They are also useful in the treatment of GERD and Zollinger-Ellison syndrome, the latter a condition usually associated with a gastrin-secreting tumor.

Adverse Effects

The adverse effects of proton pump inhibitors occur infrequently and include diarrhea, abdominal pain, and headache. Chronic treatment with proton pump inhibitors may result in hypergastrinemia. Proton pump inhibitors may decrease the oral bioavailability of vitamin B_{12} and certain drugs (e.g., digoxin, ketoconazole) that require acidity for their gastrointestinal absorption. *Note:* Because gastric acid is a major barrier to the colonization and infection of the gut, chronic use of proton pump inhibitors can increase the risk of enteric infections.

Antibiotics

Chronic infection with *H pylori* is present in the majority of patients with recurrent non-NSAID-induced peptic ulcers, and eradication of this organism greatly reduces the rate of recurrence of ulcers in these patients. The regimens of choice consist of a proton pump inhibitor plus a course of bismuth (Pepto-Bismol), tetracycline, and metronidazole or a course of amoxicillin plus clarithromycin.

■ DRUGS THAT PROMOTE UPPER GASTROINTESTINAL MOTILITY

Diabetes and other diseases that damage nerves to the viscera frequently cause a marked loss of motility in the esophagus and stomach, resulting in gastric paralysis (gastroparesis). Gastroparesis is associated with delayed stomach emptying, nausea, and severe bloating. **Metoclopramide** and **cisapride** are prokinetic drugs; that is, they stimulate motility in the upper GI tract and emptying of the stomach by indirectly stimulating cholinergic activity in the gut wall. Metoclopramide probably acts as an ACh facilitator by antagonizing D_2 receptors. Cisapride appears to act as a 5-HT_4 agonist, facilitating the release of ACh from cholinergic nerve endings. Adverse effects of metoclopramide with chronic use include symptoms of pseudoparkinsonism and other extrapyramidal effects and hyperprolactinemia. In high doses, cisapride is associated with a long QT syndrome and has caused fatal cardiac arrhythmias. For this reason, cisapride is now available only on a limited basis.

DRUGS WITH ANTIEMETIC ACTIONS

A variety of drugs are valuable in the prevention and treatment of vomiting during cancer chemotherapy and following general anesthesia. Glucocorticoids (Chapter 23) have been discussed previously. Dopamine receptor antagonists such as **metoclopramide** and **prochlorperazine**, a phenothiazine (Chapter 18), prevent emesis by inhibiting D_2 receptors in the postrema area of the medulla.

H$_1$ ANTAGONISTS: Some previously discussed antihistamines (H$_1$ receptor antagonists; Chapter 35), such as **diphenhydramine** and **meclizine**, have antiemetic properties and prevent motion sickness. Sedation is a common adverse effect of all of these older (first-generation) antihistamines, as is dry mouth and other anticholinergic effects. Orthostatic hypotension may also occur as a result of α_1-receptor antagonism when taking these drugs.

5-HT$_3$ RECEPTOR ANTAGONISTS: The drugs **ondansetron**, **granisetron**, and **dolasetron** are extremely useful in preventing nausea and vomiting associated with chemotherapy and with surgical anesthesia but not motion sickness. These 5-HT$_3$ receptor antagonists have a central antiemetic action in the area postrema of the medulla and also on peripheral sensory and enteric nerves. **Alosetron**, another 5-HT$_3$ antagonist, is used in the treatment of women with diarrhea associated with irritable bowel syndrome. The adverse effects of ondansetron, granisetron, and dolasetron include diarrhea and headache. Dolasetron has been associated with QRS and QTc prolongation in the electrocardiogram and should not be used in patients with heart disease. Alosetron causes significant constipation in some patients and has been associated with fatal bowel complications.

MARIJUANA DERIVATIVES: Antiemetic properties have also been demonstrated in the active ingredient in marijuana and its derivative, **dronabinol** (Δ^9-tetrahydrocannabinol) and **nabilone** (Chapter 21).

PANCREATIC ENZYME REPLACEMENTS

Steatorrhea, a condition of decreased fat absorption coupled with increased fat excretion in the stool results from inadequate pancreatic secretion of lipase. The abnormality of fat absorption can be significantly relieved by oral administration of pancreatic lipase (**pancrelipase**) obtained from pigs. Pancreatic lipase is inactivated at a pH below 4; thus, up to 90% of an administered dose will be destroyed in the stomach unless the pH is raised with antacids or drugs that reduce acid secretion.

LAXATIVES

Laxatives increase the probability of a bowel movement by several mechanisms: an irritant or stimulant action on the bowel wall, a bulk-forming action on the stool that evokes reflex contraction of the bowel, a softening action on hard or impacted stool, or a lubricating action that eases passage of stool through the rectum. Examples of drugs that act by these mechanisms are in Table 36–1.

Table 36–1.	The major laxative mechanisms and some representative laxative drugs
Mechanism	**Examples**
Irritant	Castor oil, cascara, senna, phenolphthalein
Bulk-forming	Saline cathartics (e.g., Mg[OH]$_2$, psyllium)
Stool-softening	Dioctyl sodium sulfosuccinate (docusate)
Lubricating	Mineral oil, glycerin

ANTIDIARRHEAL AGENTS

The most effective antidiarrheal drugs are the opioids and their derivatives that have been selected for maximal antidiarrheal and minimal central nervous system effects. Of the latter group, the most important are **diphenoxylate** and **loperamide**, meperidine analogs with very weak or no analgesic effects. Diphenoxylate is formulated with antimuscarinic alkaloids (e.g., atropine) to reduce the likelihood of abuse; loperamide is formulated alone and sold over-the-counter (OTC) as such. **Difenoxin**, the active metabolite of diphenoxylate, is also available as a prescription medication. **Kaolin** is hydrated magnesium aluminum silicate, and **pectin** is an indigestible carbohydrate from apples. Available in combination as Kaopectate, both kaolin and pectin act as absorbents of bacterial toxins and fluid. Finally, **cholestyramine** and **colestipol**, bile salt–binding resins previously discussed in Chapter 26, may decrease diarrhea associated with increased bile acids. Common adverse effects associated with these drugs include constipation. The absorbents and the bile salt resins may decrease the absorption of some drugs, and the resins may also reduce the absorption of lipid-soluble vitamins.

DRUGS THAT INHIBIT THE FORMATION OF GALLSTONES

The formation of cholesterol gallstones can be inhibited by several drugs, although none is dramatically effective. Such drugs include the bile acid derivatives **chenodiol** and **ursodiol**. Chenodiol appears to reduce the secretion of bile acids by the liver, whereas the mechanism of action of ursodiol is unknown.

DRUGS USED IN INFLAMMATORY BOWEL DISEASE

Inflammatory bowel disease may be divided into two related conditions: ulcerative colitis and Crohn's disease. Ulcerative colitis is a nonspecific inflammation of the colon with mucosal damage & bleeding. Crohn's disease is a recurrent granulomatous inflammation that may affect any part of the small or large bowel. **Glucocorticoids** (Chapter 23) are used in the treatment of ulcerative colitis and Crohn's disease. Immunosuppressive agents such as **azathioprine**, **6-mercaptopurine**, **methotrexate**, and **infliximab** (Chapter 32) are also used in the treatment of these diseases. These drugs have been discussed in other chapters. Aminosalicylates (e.g., **sulfasalazine, balsalazide, mesalamine**) also used in the treatment of inflammatory bowel disease. These drugs are not absorbed significantly after oral administration and are designed to release **5-aminosalicylic acid** (5-ASA) into various parts of the distal segment of the small bowel and colon. 5-ASA inhibits the synthesis of both prostaglandins and inflammatory leukotrienes. Sulfasalazine (a combination of 5-ASA and sulfapyridine) has a high incidence of adverse effects, which are attributable to the systemic absorption of the sulfapyridine. These effects are dose related and include nausea, gastrointestinal upset, headaches, arthralgia, myalgia, bone marrow suppression, malaise, and severe hypersensitivity reactions. Other aminosalicylates, which do not contain sulfapyridine, are well tolerated.

REHABILITATION FOCUS

Drugs that are swallowed pass through parts of the GI system prior to reaching the systemic circulation. Thus, drugs used to treat GI conditions have the potential to interfere with other orally administered drugs, and cause drug-drug interactions. These adverse effects may range from decreased absorption of some drugs resulting in undermedication to decreased biotransformation of other drugs resulting in overmedication. Many drugs used in treating GI dysfunction may be obtained without prescription. The use of these OTC drugs by the patient further complicates the assessment of the drug history. The patient may not consider including such OTC drugs when asked by the health-care provider about "medications." Examples of such drugs are the antihistamines used in acid-peptic disease.

Nonpharmacologic treatments for emesis are also being investigated. Unconventional types of transcutaneous electrical nerve stimulation (TENS) on acupuncture points are being investigated to prevent emesis following chemotherapy and surgical procedures. Optimal therapy may be a combination of antiemetic drugs together with TENS.

■ CLINICAL RELEVANCE FOR REHABILITATION

Adverse Drug Reactions

Acid-peptic drugs
- Cimetidine inhibits biotransformation of some drugs.
- Antacids may decrease the absorption of some drugs.
- Proton pump inhibitors may cause GI distress, decrease B_{12} absorption, possibly increase GI bacterial infections, and decrease absorption of some drugs.

Prokinetic drugs
- D_2 antagonists can cause extrapyramidal effects. Some drugs that modulate 5-HT receptors cause cardiac dysrhythmias.

- Long-term use of some laxatives can decrease absorption of fat-soluble vitamins.
- Several antidiarrheal drugs can decrease absorption of some drugs.

Effects Interfering with Rehabilitation
- Decreased absorption of drugs can result in reduced blood drug levels and increase the risk of an inadequate clinical effect.
- Decreased biotransformation of drugs can result in increased blood drug levels and increase the risk of overmedication toxicity.
- Extrapyramidal motor effects of prokinetic drugs can interfere with functional performance in the clinic.

Possible Therapy Solutions
- If the patient demonstrates manifestations of undermedication or overmedication, contact the referring health-care provider. A complete drug history of the patient may assist in this determination.
- If extrapyramidal effects occur with prokinetic drugs, contact the referring health-care provider.

PROBLEM-ORIENTED PATIENT STUDY

Brief History: The patient is a 63-year-old African American female with a 20-year history of type 2 diabetes mellitus. The patient has hyperglycemia, hypertension, and hyperlipidemia. The patient previously had neuropathic ulcers at the first metatarsal head on the plantar surfaces of both feet.

Current Medical Status and Drug Therapy: The patient is on multiple medications for treatment of her diseases. Two weeks ago, the patient was diagnosed with gastroparesis and she was prescribed metoclopramide as a prokinetic. The patient's neuropathic ulcer on the plantar surface at the first

metatarsal head on the left foot reulcerated last week. She was referred for evaluation and possible foot orthotics to prevent further wound progression.

Rehabilitation Setting: The patient has been seen by the physical therapist on previous occasions for evaluation and treatment of previous neuropathic ulcerations. She arrives today as scheduled for the evaluation. The patient is first observed in the waiting room; She has difficulty initiating sit-to-stand activity and is assisted by her spouse. When the patient finally stands, she has a wide base of support with her upper extremities in low guard position, suggesting decreased initial stability in

PROBLEM-ORIENTED PATIENT STUDY (*Continued*)

standing. The patient also has difficulty initiating ambulation, and is again assisted by her spouse. During ambulation, she has a decreased step length resulting in a slow shuffling gait. The patient is finally seated in the treatment area. When asked during the evaluation, she and her spouse suggest that the changes in function observed in the waiting room are recent, although they cannot provide a specific time frame.

Problem/Clinical Options: Multiple antihypertensive and cardiovascular medications may cause orthostatic hypotension, which presents during

standing. However, the instability during standing, the difficulty initiating movement, and the slow shuffling ambulation are manifestations of parkinsonism. These manifestations are recent as was the prescription for metoclopramide as a prokinetic. This drug inhibits dopaminergic receptors in the GI system. An adverse effect of this drug is parkinsonism resulting from inhibition of dopamine receptors in the motor areas of the brain. The health-care professional prescribing the metoclopramide should be immediately informed of these adverse effects.

PREPARATIONS AVAILABLE

Antacids

Aluminum hydroxide gel[1] (Amphojel, ALternaGEL, others)
Oral: 300-, 500-, 600-mg tablets; 400-, 500-mg capsules; 320, 450, 675 mg/5 mL suspension

Aluminum hydroxide and magnesium hydroxide combination preparations[1] (Maalox, Mylanta, Gaviscon, Gelusil, others)
Oral: 400- to 800-mg combined hydroxides per tablet, capsule, or 5 mL suspension

Calcium carbonate[1] (Tums, others)
Oral: 350-, 420-, 500-, 600-, 650-, 750-, 1000-, 1250-mg chewable tablets; 1250 mg/5 mL suspension

H₂ Histamine Receptor Blockers

Cimetidine (generic, Tagamet, Tagamet HB[1])
Oral: 100-,[1] 200-, 300-, 400-, 800-mg tablets; 300 mg/5 mL liquid

Parenteral: 300 mg/2 mL, 300 mg/50 mL for injection

Famotidine (generic, Pepcid, Pepcid AC[1])
Oral: 10-mg tablets,[1] gelcaps[1]; 20-, 40-mg tablets; powder to reconstitute for 40 mg/5 mL suspension
Parenteral: 10 mg/mL for injection

Nizatidine (Axid, Axid AR[1])
Oral: 75-mg tablets[1]; 150-, 300-mg capsules

Ranitidine (generic, Zantac, Zantac 75[1])
Oral: 75,[1] 150-, 300-mg tablets; 150-mg effervescent tablets; 150-, 300-mg capsules; 15 mg/mL syrup
Parenteral: 1-, 25- mg/mL for injection

Selected Anticholinergic Drugs

Atropine (generic)
Oral: 0.4-mg tablets
Parenteral: 0.05, 0.1, 0.3, 0.4, 0.5, 0.8, 1 mg/mL for injection

Belladonna alkaloids tincture (generic)
Oral: 0.27–0.33 mg/mL liquid

Dicyclomine (generic, Bentyl, others)
Oral: 10-, 20-mg capsules; 20-mg tablets; 10 mg/5 mL syrup
Parenteral: 10 mg/mL for injection

Glycopyrrolate (generic, Robinul)
Oral: 1-, 2-mg tablets
Parenteral: 0.2 mg/mL for injection

l-Hyoscyamine (Anaspaz, others)
Oral: 0.125-, 0.15-mg tablets; 0.375-mg timed-release capsules; 0.125 mg/5 mL oral elixir and solution
Parenteral: 0.5 mg/mL for injection

Methscopolamine (Pamine)
Oral: 2.5-mg tablets

Propantheline (generic, Pro-Banthine)
Oral: 7.5-, 15-mg tablets

Scopolamine (generic)
Oral: 0.4-mg tablets
Parenteral: 0.3, 0.4, 0.86, 1 mg/mL for injection

Tridihexethyl (Pathilon)
Oral: 25-mg tablets

Proton Pump Inhibitors

Esomeprazole (Nexium)
Oral: 20-, 40-mg delayed-release capsules

Lansoprazole (Prevacid)
Oral: 15-, 30-mg delayed-release capsules; 15-, 30-mg enteric-coated granules for oral suspension

Omeprazole (Prilosec)
Oral: 10-, 20-, 40-mg delayed-release capsules

Pantoprazole (Protonix)
Oral: 20-, 40-mg delayed release tablets
Parenteral: 40 mg/vial powder for IV injection

Rabeprazole (Aciphex)
Oral: 20-mg delayed-release tablets

Mucosal Protective Agents

Misoprostol (Cytotec)
Oral: 100-, 200-mcg tablets

Sucralfate (generic, Carafate)
Oral: 1-g tablets; 1 g/10 mL suspension

Digestive Enzymes

Pancrelipase (Cotazym, Pancrease, Viokase, others)
Oral: Capsules, tablets, or powder containing lipase, protease, and amylase activity. See manufacturers' literature for details.

Drugs for Motility Disorders and Selected Antiemetics

Alosetron (Lotronex)
Oral: 1-mg tablets

Cisapride (Propulsid)
Oral 10-, 20-mg tablets, 1 mg/ml suspension

Dolasetron (Anzemet)
Oral: 50-, 100-mg tablets
Parenteral: 20 mg/mL for injection

Dronabinol (Marinol)
Oral: 2.5-, 5-, 10-mg capsules

Granisetron (Kytril)
Oral: 1-mg tablets
Parenteral: 1 mg/mL for injection

Metoclopramide (generic, Reglan, others)
Oral: 5-, 10-mg tablets; 5 mg/5 mL syrup, 10 mg/mL concentrated solution
Parenteral: 5 mg/mL for injection

Ondansetron (Zofran)
Oral: 4-, 8-, 24-mg tablets; 4 mg/5 mL solution
Parenteral: 2 mg/mL for IV injection

Prochlorperazine (Compazine)
Oral: 5-, 10-, 25-mg tablets; 10-, 15-, 30-mg capsules; 1 mg/mL solution
Rectal: 2.5-, 5-, 25-mg suppositories
Parenteral: 5 mg/mL for injection

Tegaserod (Zelnorm)
Oral: 2-, 6-mg tablets

Selected Anti-Inflammatory Drugs Used in Gastrointestinal Disease

Balsalazide (Colazal)
Oral: 750-mg capsules

Budesonide (Entocort)
Oral: 3-mg capsules

Hydrocortisone (Cortenema, Cortifoam)
Rectal: 100 mg/60 mL unit retention enema;
90 mg/applicatorful intrarectal foam

Infliximab (Remicade)
Parenteral: 100-mg powder for injection

Mesalamine (5-ASA)
Oral: Asacol: 400-mg delayed-release tablets;
  Pentasa: 250-mg controlled-release capsules
Rectal: Rowasa: 4 g/60 mL suspension;
500-mg suppositories

Methylprednisolone (Medrol Enpack)
Rectal: 40 mg/bottle retention enema

Olsalazine (Dipentum)
Oral: 250-mg capsules

Sulfasalazine (generic, Azulfidine, others)
Oral: 500-mg tablets and enteric-coated tablets

Selected Antidiarrheal Drugs

Bismuth subsalicylate[1] (Pepto-Bismol, others)
Oral: 262-mg caplets, chewable tablets; 130,
262, 524 mg/15 mL suspension

Difenoxin (Motofen)
Oral: 1-mg (with 0.025 mg atropine sulfate)
tablets

Diphenoxylate (generic, Lomotil, others)
Oral: 2.5-mg (with 0.025 mg atropine sulfate)
tablets and liquid

Kaolin/pectin[1] (generic, Kaopectate, others)
Oral (typical): 5.85 g kaolin and 260 mg pectin
per 30 mL suspension

Loperamide[1] (generic, Imodium, others)
Oral: 2-mg tablets, capsules; 1 mg/5 mL liquid

Selected Laxative Drugs[1]

Bisacodyl (generic, Dulcolax, others)
Oral: 5-mg enteric-coated tablets
Rectal: 10-mg suppositories

Cascara sagrada (generic)
Oral: 325-mg tablets; 5 mL per dose fluid extract
(approximately 18% alcohol)

Castor oil (generic, others)
Oral: liquid or liquid emulsion

Docusate (generic, Colace, others)
Oral: 50-, 100-, 250-mg capsules; 100-mg
tablets; 20, 50, 60, 150 mg/15 mL syrup

Glycerin liquid (Fleet Babylax)
Rectal liquid: 4 mL per applicator

Glycerin suppository (generic, Sani-Supp)

Lactulose (Chronulac, Cephulac)
Oral: 10 g/15 mL syrup

Magnesium hydroxide [milk of magnesia, Epsom Salt]
(generic)
Oral: 400, 800 mg/5 mL aqueous suspension

Methylcellulose
Oral: bulk powder

Mineral oil (generic, others)
Oral: liquid or emulsion

Polycarbophil (Equalactin, Mitrolan, FiberCon,
Fiber-Lax)
Oral: 500-, 625-mg tablets; 500-mg chewable
tablets

Polyethylene glycol electrolyte solution (CoLyte,
GoLYTELY, others)
Oral: Powder for oral solution, makes 1 gallon
(approximately 4 L)

Psyllium (generic, Serutan, Metamucil, others)
Oral: 3.3-, 3.4-, 3.5-, 4.03-, 6-g psyllium granules
or powder per packet

Senna (Senokot, Ex•Lax, others)
Oral: 8.6-, 15-, 17-, 25-mg tablets; 8.8,
15 mg/mL liquid

Drugs That Dissolve Gallstones

Ursodiol (Actigall)
Oral: 300-mg (Actigall) capsules

[1]Over-the-counter formulations.

REFERENCES

Acid-Peptic Diseases

Chan FK, Leung WK: Peptic-ulcer disease. *Lancet* 2002; 360:933.

Davies NM, et al: Misoprostol therapeutics revisited. *Pharmacotherapy* 2001;21:60.

Feldman M, Burton ME: Histamine 2-receptor antagonists. Standard therapy for acid-peptic disorders. 1. *N Engl J Med* 1990;323:1672.

Gisbert J, et al: Proton pump inhibitors versus H2-antagonists: A meta-analysis of their efficacy in treating bleeding peptic ulcer. *Aliment Pharmacol Ther* 2001; 15:917.

Laine L, et al: Potential gastrointestinal effects of long-term acid suppression with proton pump inhibitors. *Aliment Pharmacol Ther* 2000;14:651.

Laine L: Approaches to nonsteroidal anti-inflammatory drug use in the high-risk patient. *Gastroenterology* 2001; 120:594.

Scott LJ, et al: Esomeprazole: A review of its use in the management of acid-related disorders. *Drugs* 2002;62:1503.

Stedman CA, Barclay ML: Comparison of the pharmacokinetics, acid suppression and efficacy of proton pump inhibitors. *Aliment Pharmacol Ther* 2000;14:963.

Suerbaum S, Michetti P: Helicobacter pylori infection. *N Engl J Med* 2002;347:1175.

Wolfe WM, Sachs G: Acid suppression: Optimizing therapy for gastroduodenal ulcer healing, gastroesophageal reflux disease, and stress-related erosive syndrome. *Gastroenterology* 2000;118(2 Suppl 1):S9.

Motility Disorders

Booth CM, et al: Gastrointestinal promotility drugs in the critical care setting: A systemic review of the evidence. *Crit Care Med* 2002;30:1429.

Bytzer P: H(2) receptor antagonists and prokinetics in dyspepsia: A critical review. *Gut* 2002;50(Suppl 4):58.

De Giorgio R, et al: The pharmacological treatment of acute colonic pseudo-obstruction. *Aliment Pharmacol Ther* 2001;15:1717.

Holte K, Kehlet H: Postoperative ileus: Progress towards effective management. *Drugs* 2002;62:2603.

Quigley EM: Pharmacotherapy of gastroparesis. *Expert Opin Pharmacother* 2000;1:881.

Laxatives

Schiller LR: The therapy of constipation. *Aliment Pharmacol Ther* 2001;15:749.

Toledo TK, DiPalma JA: Colon cleansing preparation for gastrointestinal procedures. *Aliment Pharmacol Ther* 2001;15:605.

van Gorkom BA, et al: Anthranoid laxatives and their potential carcinogenic effects. *Aliment Pharmacol Ther* 1999;13:443.

Xing JH, Soffer EE: Adverse effects of laxatives. *Dis Colon Rectum* 2001;44:1201.

Antidiarrheal Agents

Farthing MG: Novel targets for the control of secretory diarrhea. *Gut* 2002;50(Suppl 3):III15.

Ramzan NN: Traveler's diarrhea. *Gastroenterol Clin North Am* 2001;30:665.

Ung KA, et al: Role of bile acids and bile acid binding agents in patients with collagenous colitis. *Gut* 2000;46:170.

Wingate D, et al: Guidelines for adults on self-medication for the treatment of acute diarrhoea. *Aliment Pharmacol Ther* 2001;15:773.

Drugs Used for Irritable Bowel Syndrome

American College of Gastroenterology Functional Gastrointestinal Task Force: An evidence-based position statement on the management of irritable bowel syndrome in North America. *Am J Gastroenterol* 2002;97:S1.

Camilleri M: Tegaserod. *Aliment Pharmacol Ther* 2001; 15:277.

Drossman DA, et al: AGA technical review on irritable bowel syndrome. *Gastroenterology* 2002;123:2108.

Gunput MD: Clinical pharmacology of alosetron. *Aliment Pharmacol Ther* 1999;13(Suppl 2):70.

Kamm MA: The complexity of drug development for irritable bowel syndrome. *Aliment Pharmacol Ther* 2002; 16:343.

Antiemetic Agents

Goodin S, Cunningham R: 5-HT3–receptor antagonists for the treatment of nausea and vomiting: A reappraisal of their side-effect profile. *Oncologist* 2002;7:424.

Gralla RJ: New agents, new treatment, and antiemetic therapy. *Semin Oncol* 2002;29(Suppl 4):119.

Hesketh PJ: Comparative review of 5-HT3 receptor antagonists in the treatment of acute chemotherapy-induced nausea and vomiting. *Cancer Invest* 2000;18:163.

Magee LA, et al: Evidence-based view of safety and effectiveness of pharmacologic therapy for nausea and vomiting of pregnancy (NVP). *Am J Obstet Gynecol* 2002;185(Suppl):S256.

Tramer MR, et al: Cannabinoids for control of chemotherapy-induced nausea and vomiting: Quantitative systematic review. *BMJ* 2001;323:16.

Tramer MR: A rational approach to the control of postoperative nausea and vomiting: Evidence from systematic reviews. Part I. Efficacy and harm of antiemetic interventions, and methodological issues. *Acta Anaesthesiol Scand* 2001;45:4.

Tramer MR: A rational approach to the control of postoperative nausea and vomiting: Evidence from systematic reviews. Part II. Recommendations for prevention and treatment, and research agenda. *Acta Anaesthesiol Scand* 2001;45:14.

Drugs Used for Inflammatory Bowel Disease

Blam ME, et al: Integrating anti-tumor necrosis factor therapy in inflammatory bowel disease: Current and future perspectives. *Am J Gastroenterol* 2001;96:1977.

De Vos M: Clinical pharmacokinetics of slow release mesalazine. *Clin Pharmacokinet* 2000;39:85.

Gionchetti P, et al: Treatment of mild to moderate ulcerative colitis and pouchitis. *Aliment Pharmacol Ther* 2002; 16(Suppl 4):13.

Kane SV, et al: The effectiveness of budesonide therapy for Crohn's disease. *Aliment Pharmacol Ther* 2002;16:1509.

Klotz U: The role of aminosalicylates at the beginning of the new millennium in the treatment of chronic inflammatory bowel disease. *Eur J Clin Pharmacol* 2000;56:353.

Muijsers RB, Goa KL: Balsalazide: A review of its therapeutic use in mild-to-moderate ulcerative colitis. *Drugs* 2002;62:1689.

Nielsen OH, et al: The treatment of inflammatory bowel disease with 6-mercaptopurine or azathioprine. *Aliment Pharmacol Ther* 2001;15:1699.

Plevy SE: Corticosteroid-sparing treatments in patients with Crohn's disease. *Am J Gastroenterol* 2002;97:1607.

Schwab M, Klotz U: Pharmacokinetic considerations in the treatment of inflammatory bowel disease. *Clin Pharmacokinet* 2001;40:723.

Vandell AG, DiPiro JT: Low-dosage methotrexate for treatment and maintenance of remission in patients with inflammatory bowel disease. *Pharmacotherapy* 2002; 22:613.

Pancreatic Enzyme Supplements

Greenberger NJ: Enzymatic therapy in patients with chronic pancreatitis. *Gastroenterol Clin North Am* 1999;28:687.

Stern RC, et al: A comparison of the efficacy and tolerance of pancrelipase and placebo in the treatment of steatorrhea in cystic fibrosis patients with clinical exocrine pancreatic insufficiency. *Am J Gastroenterol* 2000;95:1932.

Bile Acids for Gallstone Therapy

Crosignani A, et al: Clinical pharmacokinetics of therapeutic bile acids. *Clin Pharmacokinet* 1996;30:333.

Paumgartner G, Beuers U: Ursodeoxycholic acid in cholestatic liver disease: Mechanisms of action and therapeutic use revisited. *Hepatology* 2002;36:525.

Rehabilitation

Coloma M, et al: Comparison of acustimulation and ondansetron for the treatment of established postoperative nausea and vomiting. *Anesthesiology* 2002; 97:1387.

Kabalak AA, et al: Transcutaneous electrical acupoint stimulation versus ondansetron in the prevention of postoperative vomiting following pediatric tonsillectomy. *J Altern Complement Med* 2005;11:407.

Ozgur Tan M, et al: Combination of transcutaneous electrical nerve stimulation and ondansetron in preventing cisplatin-induced emesis. *Urol Int* 2001;67:54.

GLOSSARY

Absence seizures: generalized seizure disorder characterized by brief interruptions of awareness and activity.

Accommodation: ability of the eye to focus on objects at different distances from the eye.

Acetylcholinesterase (AChE): enzyme that inactivates acetylcholine.

Acidosis: plasma pH less than 7.35.

Acromegaly: syndrome of growth hormone excess in adulthood.

Action potential: temporary positive deflection of the voltage potential across a cell plasma membrane, associated with the opening and closing of cation channels.

Activated partial thromboplastin time (aPTT): plasma coagulation assay; used to monitor effects of heparin.

Active immunization: inoculation with a vaccine that triggers the immune system to produce antibodies and cell-mediated immunity against a particular virus.

Addiction: previously defined as "psychological dependence," is the compulsive and relapsing use of a drug despite the negative consequences of such use.

Addisonian crisis: acute onset of adrenocortical insufficiency; if untreated, can lead to severe hypotension, shock, and death.

Adjunctive agent: secondary drug used in addition to a primary drug.

Afterload: pressure against which the ventricles of the heart work to pump blood into the arterial system.

Agonist: a drug that binds to a receptor and /activates the receptor's function.

Agranulocytosis: decrease in number of granulocyte white blood cells.

Alcohol dehydrogenase (ADH): cytosolic enzyme found mainly in liver and gut that metabolizes low to moderate doses of ethanol.

Aldosterone: steroid hormone produced by the adrenal gland that stimulates sodium (and water) retention and potassium excretion.

Alkylation: transfer of an alkyl group (general formula C_nH_{2n+1}) from one molecule to another.

Allergic rhinoconjunctivitis: allergic inflammation of ocular conjunctiva and nasal mucosa.

Allergic rhinosinusitis: allergic inflammation of nasal mucosa and paranasal sinuses.

Allogeneic: transfer of biological products (e.g., blood, bone marrow) from a person other than the recipient.

Alopecia: hair loss.

Amebiasis: intestinal infection with amebae, often characterized by diarrhea that contains blood or mucus.

Amebic dysentery: severe diarrhea due to inflammation of intestinal lining caused by *E histolytica*; usually acquired by ingesting food or water contaminated with feces.

Amnesia: loss of memory.

Anaphylaxis: immediate, life-threatening allergic reaction (type I hypersensitivity reaction) to drug or other substance.

Anemia: lower than normal number of red blood cells (erythrocytes).

Angina: severe pain; angina pectoris when associated with cardiac ischemia.

Anorexia: loss of appetite.

Antagonist: a drug that prevents receptor stimulation, in that it has an affinity for a receptor and by binding to it prevents the receptor from responding to an agonist.

Antegrade: normal or forward propagation of conduction or flow.

Antithrombin III (ATIII): endogenous anticlotting protease.

Aphthous: white, painful lesions found on lips or inside mouth.

Aplastic anemia: decreased ability of the bone marrow to generate red blood cells, white blood cells, and platelets.

Apoferritin: protein found in intestinal mucosal cells that binds and stores iron by forming ferritin.

Apoptosis: programmed cell death.

Aqueous: a water-based system.

Aprotinin: is a serine protease inhibitor that inhibits fibrinolysis by plasmin and by plasmin-streptokinase complex.

Ascariasis: infection caused by parasitic roundworms.

Aspergillosis: infection caused by *Aspergillus* fungus; most commonly affected tissues include lungs, bronchi, sinuses, ears, and eyes; occurs more frequently in immunosuppressed individual.

Asplenia: absence of a spleen.

Asthenia: a decrease or absence of skeletal muscle force.

Atherosclerosis: disease process in which lipids and products resulting from inflammatory responses accumulate in arterial walls.

Autacoid: substance formed and released having localized effects.

Autologous: transfer of biological products (e.g., blood, bone marrow) utilizing person's own tissues.

Autolytic: self-digestion.

Auxotrophic: inability of a cell type or organism to synthesize a compound required for its growth, thus requiring its uptake from the environment for survival.

"Bad" cholesterol: atherogenic lipoproteins, such as low density lipoproteins (LDLs).

Balanced anesthesia: the modern practice of anesthesiology involving the use of combinations of intravenous and inhaled drugs, taking advantage of their individual favorable properties while attempting to minimize adverse reactions.

Bioactivation: metabolic activation.

Bioavailability: percentage of a drug that is actually available at particular sites in the body.

Bioequivalence: a measure of the ability of two drug formulations with identical active ingredients or two different dosage forms to demonstrate the same bioavailability and therapeutic effect.

Bipolar affective (manic-depressive) disorder: mood disorder characterized by manic, mixed, or hypomanic episodes, usually with a history of major depressive episodes.

Bleeding diathesis: tendency to bleed due to defective coagulation processes.

Bradycardia: heart rate less than 60 beats per minute.

Bronchoconstriction: decreased diameter of the airways in the lungs.

Bronchospasm: difficulty in breathing resulting from involuntary spasmodic contraction of smooth muscles in the airway.

Buccal transmucosal: alternative to parenteral route of drug administration.

Cachexia: severe loss of lean body mass commonly seen in patients with AIDS, cancer, or other diseases; also called wasting.

Capsid: protein shell surrounding a virus.

Catabolism: metabolic breakdown.

Catechol-*O*-methyltransferase (COMT): enzyme that inactivates several monoamine neurotransmitters by addition of a methyl group.

Cell cycle—nonspecific drugs (CCNS): anticancer drugs insensitive to the phase of the cell cycle.

Cell cycle—specific drugs (CCS): anticancer drugs most effective in a particular phase of the cell cycle.

Cestodes: parasitic flatworms of class *Cestoda*; commonly known as tapeworms.

Chimeric: hybrid; a chimeric molecule is comprised of two dissimilar molecular fragments that are not normally found together; often found in mouse-human antibodies used in therapy or autoimmune disease.

Cholelithiasis: gallstones.

Cholestasis: impaired or blocked bile flow from liver through the bile ducts.

Cholinomimetics: drugs that mimic the effects of acetylcholine.

Chronotropic: changes in cardiac pacemaker activity.

Cinchonism: adverse effects due to excessive or long-term use of quinine; also known as quinism.

Cobalamin: vitamin B_{12}; water-soluble vitamin required for nerve cells, blood cells, and DNA synthesis.

Complex partial seizures: seizure disorder that is characterized by impaired consciousness that is preceded, accompanied, or followed by psychological symptoms.

Congener: drug that shares similar chemical structures and characteristics with another.

Conscious sedation: monitored anesthesia care employing oral or parenteral sedatives, often in conjunction with local anesthetics.

Contractility: mechanical performance of muscles (ability to shorten or exert force).

Cortisol: primary glucocorticoid hormone produced by human adrenal gland; also called hydrocortisone.

Covalent bonds: chemical structure in which electron pairs are shared between two atoms.

Cross-linking: covalent bonds linking one structure to another.

Cyanocobalamin: form of vitamin B_{12}.

Cyclooxygenase (COX): enzyme required for formation of prostanoids; many anti-inflammatory drugs (e.g., NSAIDs) act by inhibiting this enzyme .

Cycloplegia: paralysis of the eye's ciliary muscle.

Cystitis: bladder inflammation.

Cytochrome P450 (CYP450) system: class of enzymes responsible for drug metabolism; drugs metabolized by this system increase the likelihood of drug-drug adverse interactions.

Cytokine: nonantibody protein that acts as an extracellular mediator of immune responses.

Date rape: criminal activity involving forcing someone to submit to sexual acts; potent rapid-onset benzodiazepines or sedative-hypnotics such as GHB, are sometimes used to aid this crime.

Deep vein thrombosis (DVT): formation of blood clots (thromboses) in deep veins, usually in the lower extremities.

Dehydrogenase: enzyme that transfers hydrogen to an acceptor (e.g., NAD).

Delirium: acute disorder of confusion, disordered speech, and hallucinations.

Delirium tremens (DTs): acute, severe form of alcohol withdrawal that includes mental or neurological changes.

Dependence: previously defined as "physical dependence"; state in which withdrawal of a drug produces symptoms and signs that are frequently opposite of those caused by the drug.

Depolarization: positive deflection of the voltage potential across a cell membrane resulting from the influx of cations.

Designer drugs: drugs that are modified by illicit manufacturers so as not to be specifically listed as controlled substances.

Diacylglycerol: an intracellular second messenger consisting of a glycerol backbone and fatty acids in positions SN-1 and SN-2.

Diarthrodial joint: a synovium-containing joint.

Diastole: time period in the cardiac cycle during which ventricular filling occurs.

Diastolic blood pressure: blood pressure during the relaxation phase of the cardiac cycle.

Dipeptidase: an enzyme that cleaves a dipeptide from the C-terminal end of peptides.

Direct acting: molecule affecting synaptic activity at the post-synaptic receptor.

Dissemination: spreading of a pathogen throughout the body.

Diuresis: renal loss of water (usually with sodium).

DNA polymerase: enzyme that assists in DNA replication.

Dopamine (DA): one of several monoamine neurotransmitters.

Down-regulation: decrease in the number of available receptors.

Dromotropic: changes in electrical conduction through cardiac tissue.

Drug: a substance that affects a biologic system through chemical effects.

Drug abuse: drugs used in ways that are not medically approved.

Dyscrasias: a synonym for disease, especially hematologic disease.

Dysmenorrhea: severe pain associated with menstrual cycle.

Efficacy: the ability of a molecule to activate a receptor complex.

Ejection fraction: the blood volume ejected by ventricles divided by the volume in the ventricles at the end of diastole.

Electrostatic bonds: attraction between oppositely charged atoms.

Emesis: vomiting.

Empyema: pus in a body cavity, especially in the pleural space.

Endogenous opioid peptides: small proteins that have opioid-like pharmacologic properties.

Endometriosis: endometrial tissue (uterine lining) located outside the uterus (e.g., fallopian tubes, ovaries, peritoneum).

Enterocolitis: inflammation of small and large intestine.

Enterohepatic cycling: occurs with a few drugs that are eliminated in the bile, reabsorbed from the intestine, returned by the circulation to the liver, and again eliminated in the bile.

Enuresis: involuntary loss of urine while asleep; "bed wetting."

Envelope: glycoprotein coat surrounding some viruses.

Enzymopathy: genetic metabolic disorder consisting of defective or absent enzymes.

Epilepsy: a disease marked by recurrent seizures.

Erythema: skin redness due to increased blood flow, often caused by inflammation.

Erythromelalgia: episodic burning, throbbing, and redness of the extremities caused by local dilation of blood vessels.

Esterase: an enzyme that degrades ester bonds and splits esters into their constituent alcohols and acids.

Euphoria: exaggerated feeling of well-being, characteristic of amphetamines and cocaine; sometimes an initial side effect of exogenous glucocorticoid use (i.e., "steroid high").

Exophthalmos: excessive bulging of eyes; often associated with Graves' disease, a form of hyperthyroidism.

Ferric ion (Fe^{3+}): oxidized form of iron in intestinal mucosal cells.

Ferritin: iron-protein complex found mainly in liver that serves to store iron.

Ferrous ion (Fe^{2+}): form of free iron that is absorbed from iron supplements and from complexes in food; required for oxygen binding by hemoglobin.

Filariasis: parasitic disease caused by nematodes and transmitted by mosquito bites; when lymphatics infected, lymphedema and elephantiasis result.

First-order kinetics: process in which the rate of change is proportional to the amount of material; in zero-order kinetics, the rate is fixed, regardless of the amount present.

First-pass metabolism: also known as first-pass effect; enzymatic or chemical modofication of a drug by gastrointestinal or liver cells that limits drug concentration in the blood.

Flatulence: excessive intestinal gas.

Flukes: another name for trematode worms; different types can infect liver, blood, or lung.

Functional tolerance: type of tolerance due to compensatory changes in receptors, effector enzymes, or membrane actions of a drug.

Gamma-aminobutyric acid (GABA): the major inhibitory neurotransmitter.

Gastroparesis: decreased gastric emptying.

Generalized seizures: seizure disorder that results from electrical discharges that affect both hemispheres of the brain.

Glaucoma: elevated intraocular pressure.

Glucocorticoid: class of steroid hormones produced by adrenal gland that has profound influence on macronutrient metabolism and immune function.

Gluconeogenesis: biosynthesis of new glucose (i.e., not glucose from glycogen).

Glutathione: tripeptide comprised of glutamic acid, cysteine, and glycine; nonspecific reducing agent found within cells.

"Good" cholesterol: high density lipoproteins (**HDL**) that remove cholesterol from atheromas in blood vessels and return it the liver.

Graft-versus-host disease: a sometimes serious complication of transplanted tissue in which white blood cells from a donor attack tissues of the recipient.

Graves' disease: autoimmune disorder resulting in hyperthyroidism during the early phase; can progress to hypothyroidism if the thyroid gland is destroyed in later phases.

Gynecomastia: excessive, abnormal breast enlargement in males.

Half-life: time required for half the amount of a drug (or other substance, such as a hormone) to be metabolized or eliminated by the body.

Hallucination: a sensory perception experienced without appropriate external stimuli.

Hematopoiesis: formation and development of formed elements of blood (e.g., blood cells and platelets).

Heme: essential nonprotein, iron-containing constituent of hemoglobin and myoglobin.

Hemochromatosis: metabolic disease in which body absorbs too much iron, which is deposited in tissues and results in toxicity.

Hemoglobin: iron-containing, oxygen-carrying heme-protein complex in erythrocytes.

Hemolytic anemia: type of anemia characterized by premature destruction of erythrocytes.

Hemophilia: group of hereditary bleeding disorders due to inability to form effective blood clots; usually caused by inadequate synthesis of Factors VIII or IX.

Hemostasis: process of blood clotting.

Hepatic steatosis: fatty liver.

Herb: a plant or plant component valued for its properties (medicinal, culinary, or aromatic).

Herpes varicella: chickenpox.

Herpes zoster: shingles.

Highly active antiretroviral therapy (HAART): combination drug therapy used in treatment of HIV infection.

Hirsutism: excessive growth of thick, dark hair in places where hair is usually minimal or absent.

Homeostatic: maintenance of the internal physiologic function.

Humanization: technique for reducing immunogenicity of monoclonal antibodies from nonhuman (usually mouse) sources; antibodies are modified by using human frameworks and substituting residues from mouse monoclonal antibody into human framework regions.

Hydrophilic: associated with an affinity for water.

Hydrophobic: lacking an affinity for water.

Hydroxocobalamin: form of vitamin B_{12}.

Hydroxyapatite: mineral form of calcium phosphate present in bone salts and teeth.

Hypercalcemia: calcium in the blood exceeding 10.5 mg/dL.

Hypercalciuria: excessive calcium concentration in urine.

Hypercapnia: greater than 29 mEq/L of carbon dioxide in blood.

Hyperglycemia: a plasma glucose level greater than 109 mg/dL fasting, or greater than 140 mg/dL 2 hours after a 75-gram glucose challenge.

Hyperkalemia: plasma potassium concentration greater than 5 mEq/L.

Hyperkeratosis: thickening of outermost layer of the epidermis.

Hyperlipidemia: high level of fats (triglycerides, cholesterol, or lipoproteins) in the blood; significant risk factor for heart disease.

Hypernatremia: plasma sodium level of greater than 145 mEq/L.

Hyperuricemia: greater than 7.4 mg/dL of uric acid in the blood; a metabolic by product due to increased purine metabolism or decreased renal function.

Hypoglycemia: plasma glucose levels less than 60 mg/dL.

Hypokalemia: plasma potassium level of less than 3.5 mEq/L.

Hyponatremia: plasma sodium level of less than 135 mEq/L.

Hypoprothrombinemia: decreased levels of prothrombin, a critical protein in hemostasis (i.e., blood clotting).

Hypotension: abnormal decrease in blood pressure resulting in functional deficit or symptoms: orthostatic hypotension—hypotension with positional change).

Immunoglobulin: antibody.

Immunosuppression: reduced function of the immune system.

Impotence: male inability to initiate or maintain an erection for sexual performance.

Indirect acting: molecule affecting synaptic activity at a site other than the post-synaptic receptor.

Inoculation: injection.

Inotropic: pertaining to changes in muscle force independent of the Frank-Starling mechanism.

Insomnia: inability to fall asleep or obtain adequate sleep.

Integrase: enzyme that integrates newly formed double-stranded viral DNA into (human) host genome.

Interleukin-2: cytokine produced by certain immune cells; exogenous recombinant form used in treatment of some cancers.

Interleukin-3: cytokine produced by certain immune cells that stimulates proliferation of hematopoietic pluripotent progenitor cells.

Intranasal: an alternative means of drug administration that avoids repeated parenteral drug injections and the first-pass metabolism of orally administered drugs.

Intrinsic factor: protein product of stomach parietal cells necessary for absorption of vitamin B_{12}.

Ionotropic receptors: receptors on ion channels that directly regulate the channel permeability.

Ischemia: insufficient blood flow due to obstruction or contraction of a blood vessel.

Jaundice: yellowing of skin, eyes, and mucous membranes due to increased concentration of bilirubin in blood; associated with liver dysfunction.

Kernicterus: brain damage due to abnormal accumulation of bilirubin in severe newborn jaundice.

Kinase: enzyme that catalyzes transfer of a high energy phosphate group from a donor (such as ADP or ATP) to a protein substrate.

Kininase: enzyme in the blood that inactivates kinins.

Lacrimation: production of tears in the eye.

Leptospirosis: rare bacterial infection with *Leptospira interrogans* that is transmitted through contact with food, water, or soil contaminated from an infected animal.

Ligand-gated channel: ion channel that by the binding of a chemical, usually a neurotransmitter.

Lipogenesis: formation of fat.

Lipolysis: catabolism of triglycerides stored in adipocytes into triglycerides and glycerol.

Lipoprotein: molecular complex containing fat (including cholesterol and triglycerides) and proteins that serves to transport fats in the blood.

Liposomal: method of drug preparation in which active drug is encapsulated within very small fat particles to enhance distribution.

Livedo reticularis: semi-permanent bluish mottling of the skin of the legs and hands.

Log-kill hypothesis: concept used in cancer chemotherapy to indicate that anticancer drugs kill a fixed proportion of a tumor cell population, not a fixed number of tumor cells (i.e., a 1-log-kill will decrease tumor cell population by one order of magnitude).

Macrolide antibiotic: named after presence of macrolide ring, which is a large lactone ring (alcohols linked with carboxylic acid groups) with one or more deoxy sugars (hydroxyl group replaced with a hydrogen) attached.

Malignant hyperthermia: a rare heritable disorder characterized by often fatal hyperthermia due to a sudden and prolonged release of calcium in muscle, with massive contraction, lactic acid production, and increased body temperature.

Mannitol: naturally occurring sugar in fruits and vegetables that is also used as an osmotic diuretic.

MDR1: multidrug resistance gene that codes for a cell surface P-glycoprotein, a transport protein normally present in cells throughout the body and responsible for pumping many drugs and toxins out of cells.

Mean arterial pressure: average pressure of the systemic circulation and equal to (diastolic + [systolic-diastolic]/3).

Median effective dose (ED_{50}): dosage at which 50% of the population respond.

Median lethal dose (LD_{50}): dosage at which 50% of the population die.

Median toxic dose (TD_{50}): dosage at which 50% of the population demonstrate an adverse effect.

Megaloblastic anemia: anemia characterized by presence of megaloblasts (immature erythrocytes) due to deficiency of either folic acid or vitamin B_{12}.

Merozoite: daughter cell arising from asexual division of protozoan parasite.

Metabolic tolerance: drug tolerance due to increased drug disposition.

Metabotropic receptors: G protein-coupled receptors that alter second messenger levels, which secondarily regulate ion channels.

Metastasis: migration of cancer cells from original site to other sites in the body.

Methemoglobinemia: condition in which blood contains large amounts of methemoglobin, an altered form of hemoglobin that cannot carry oxygen; generally affects infants who have consumed formula mixed in water with high nitrate levels or adults who have consumed a large dose of a nitrite salt or drug.

Micrometastasis: small metatases usually not detected in diagnostic tests, but must be detected microscopically.

Microsomal ethanol-oxidizing system (MEOS): liver microsomal mixed-function oxidase system that metabolizes ethanol at blood ethanol levels >100 mg/dL.

Micturition: the act of passing urine.

Mineralocorticoid: class of steroid hormones produced by adrenal gland that influences sodium, potassium, and water metabolism.

Minimal effective dose (MED): dosage below which no clinical benefit is observed.

Minimal toxic dose (MTD): lowest dosage at which adverse effect(s) are first documented.

Minimum alveolar anesthetic concentration (MAC): the alveolar concentration of an inhaled anesthetic that is required to eliminate the response to a standardized painful stimulus in 50% of patients. It is used to measure the potency of inhaled anesthetics. The higher the MAC of a given anesthetic, the lower its potency.

Miosis: constriction of the pupil of the eye.

Monoamine: substance that contains an amino ($-NH_2$) group; includes: norepinephrine, epinephrine, dopamine, serotonin, and histamine.

Monoamine oxidase (MAO): enzyme that inactivates several monoamine neurotransmitters by oxidation of the carbon-amine bond.

Mucocutaneous: skin and mucous membranes.

Murine: material derived from rodents, especially mice.

Muscle injury spasms: an increase in skeletal muscle tension associated with musculoskeletal injuries and inflammation secondary to nerve impingement, muscle strains, muscle overuse, etc.

Mycobacteria: rod-shaped bacteria that cause tuberculosis and leprosy and a few other less common infections.

Mydriasis: dilation of the pupil of the eye.

Myelosuppression: decreased ability of bone marrow to produce blood cells, including leukocytes, erythrocytes, and platelets.

Myoclonic seizures: single or multiple myoclonic jerks.

Myoglobin: oxygen-carrying heme-protein complex in muscle cells.

Nematodes: worms that usually lack specialized attachment structures; commonly known as roundworms; parasitic forms include pinworms, whipworms, hookworms, and threadworms.

Neoplastic: abnormal, uncontrolled, and disorganized growth of cells.

Nephrolithiasis: kidney stones.

Nephrotic syndrome: disease of basement membrane of glomeruli of the kidney, characterized by edema and proteinuria.

Neuraminidase: viral enzyme that cleaves attachments between viral proteins and surface proteins of infected cells, allowing for virion release.

Neuroleptanesthesia: a state of analgesia and amnesia produced when fentanyl is used with droperidol and nitrous oxide.

Neurological injury spasticity: an increase in tonic stretch reflexes and flexor muscle spasms (i.e., increased basal muscle tone), together with muscle weakness and a reduction in viscoelastic muscle properties. This spasticity is often associated with upper motor neuron lesions such as cerebral palsy, multiple sclerosis, spinal cord injury, and stroke.

Nitric oxide (NO): endogenous gas that serves important signalling functions in many cell types.

N-methyl-D-aspartate (NMDA): type of glutamate receptor.

Nociceptive: having to do with detection, transmission, and modulation of pain.

Nonrapid eye movement (NREM): phase of sleep during which rapid eye movements are absent.

Nonsteroidal anti-inflammatory drugs (NSAIDs): major group of non-narcotic analgesic and anti-inflammatory drugs that. The NSAIDs have a significantly lower maximal analgesic efficacy than the opioids but no addiction liability. They are available with an ordinary prescription and over the counter.

Norepinephrine (NE): neurotransmitter and hormone.

Nosocomial: acquired in health-care setting, or resulting from medical attention.

Nutritional rickets: childhood disease of the skeletal system due to vitamin D deficiency, leading to softening and deformation of bones.

Onchocerciasis: insect-borne disease caused by *Onchocerca volvulus* and transmitted by bites of certain flies; commonly called river blindness.

Oncogene: mutant form of normal gene that is found in naturally occurring tumors, and when expressed in previously noncancerous cells, causes them to behave like cancer cells.

Oropharyngeal candidiasis: opportunistic mucosal infection caused, in most cases, by *Candida albicans*.

Ostealgia: bone pain.

Osteoblast: cells that form bone.

Osteoclast: cells whose primary function is bone resorption.

Osteopetrosis: genetic condition characterized by excessive calcification of bones, leading to spontaneous fractures.

Ototoxicity: adverse effects to nerves or organs associated with balance or hearing.

Pancytopenia: decreased number of all cell types in the blood (e.g., RBCs, WBCs, and platelets).

Papillomatosis: disease characterized by multiple papillomas, or warts (benign tumors).

Parasite: organism that lives in or on a host, obtaining its nourishment from host without providing benefit to host.

Parenchymal: belonging to the functional tissue of an organ, as distinguished from connective tissue.

Partial seizures: seizure disorder that typically begins with focal or local discharges in one part of the brain. Consciousness is usually preserved.

Partial thromboplastin time (PTT): plasma coagulation assay; used to monitor effects of heparin.

Passive immunization: inoculation with preformed antibodies to an individual to prevent disease; immunity is temporary.

Patient-controlled analgesia (PCA): a type of continuous pain control used to treat breakthrough pain in which the patient controls a parenteral infusion device by depressing a button to deliver a preprogrammed dose of the desired analgesic.

Pegylated: attachment of polyethylene glycol to a compound; usually provides a longer half-life.

Pernicious anemia: type of anemia due to inability to absorb vitamin B_{12}; more common in elderly due to decreased production of intrinsic factor.

Pharmacodynamics: effect of a substance on the biologic system.

Pharmacokinetics: study of how a substance is absorbed, distributed, and eliminated.

Pharmacology: the science of how substances influence biologic systems through chemical interactions.

Pharmacotherapeutics: the investigation of how substances may be used to diagnose, treat, or prevent disease.

Phosphatase: enzyme that catalyzes removal of phosphate groups from proteins.

Phosphatidylinositol: a phospholipid consisting of a glycerol backbone, fatty acids in positions SN-1 and SN-2, and a phosphorylated hexahydric alcohol at SN-3.

Phospholipase: an enzyme that hydrolyzes (breaks) the ester bond in phospholipids releasing either fatty acids or phosphatidyl derivatives.

pKa: pH at which a compound is 50% ionized.

Platelet activating factor: lipid mediator released by mast cells after stimulation by antigen binding to IgE (during allergic reactions); one of many actions is contraction of airway smooth muscle.

Pneumocystosis: pneumonia caused by atypical fungus *Pneumocystosis jiroveci;* generally found only in immuno-compromised individuals.

Polyene: chemical having many double bonds.

Polymerase: enzyme that catalyzes synthesis of nucleic acid polymers (e.g., an enzyme that transcribes DNA into messenger RNA).

Porphyrias: abnormalities in enzymes in the heme biosynthetic pathways that produce skin and nervous system symptoms.

Postcoital: after sexual intercourse.

Precipitated withdrawal: a more intense state of withdrawal that results when a drug antagonist is administered to a physically dependent individual.

Precocious puberty: early onset of puberty.

Preload: volume and pressure of blood in the ventricles at the end of diastole.

Priapism: abnormal, painful, and continuous erection of the penis, occurring usually without sexual desire.

Prodrug: inactive precursor of a drug that is converted by the body's metabolism to an active drug molecule.

Prolactinoma: anterior pituitary tumor that produces prolactin; usually benign.

Properdin: serum protein that, in conjunction with magnesium ions and complement proteins, helps destroy some bacteria and viruses.

Prothrombin time (PT): plasma coagulation assay; used to monitor effects of warfarin.

Protozoa: simplest single-celled organisms of the animal kingdom.

Pruritus: intense itching.

Pseudomembranous colitis: severe colon irritation caused by *Clostridium difficile* bacteri.

Psychologic dependence: compulsive drug-seeking behavior in which an individual uses a drug repetitively, often despite known health risks.

Psychosis: a severe mental disorder in which there is a severe loss of contact with reality, evidenced by hallucinations, delusions, disorganized speech, and bizarre behaviors.

Psychotomimetic: drug that produces effects that mimic psychosis; psychedelic drugs.

Pulse pressure: the difference between the systolic and the diastolic arterial pressures.

RAFT: mnemonic for rigidity of skeletal muscles, akinesia (or bradykinesia), flat facies, and tremor at rest seen in parkinsonism.

Rapid eye movement (REM): phase of sleep during which rapid eye movements are present.

RAVE drugs: MDMA ("ecstasy") and similar substances grouped together as drugs of abuse used during all-night music and dance parties.

Receptor: the three dimensional structure with which a drug interacts.

Receptor uncoupling: a dysfunction of interactions between receptors and G proteins, second messenger systems, and their target effector systems. The phenomenon is thought to be one reason for the development of tolerance with extended use of some drugs.

Rectal suppositories: a alternative means of drug administration when oral and parenteral routes are undesirable.

Reductase: enzyme that catalyzes reduction, the addition of electrons or hydrogen, to a substance.

Refractory period: time required for ion channels to open and recover to permit a new action potential.

Repolarization: negative deflection of the voltage potential across a cell membrane resulting from the efflux of cations.

Resting membrane potential: voltage potential between the inside and outside of a plasma cell membrane.

Retrograde: occurring in a direction opposite to normal or forward conduction or flow.

Retrovirus: enveloped virus with single-stranded RNA genome (e.g., HIV).

Reverse transcriptase: enzyme that transcribes viral genome from RNA into DNA.

Rhabdomyolysis: breakdown and necrosis of skeletal muscle due to muscle injury; manifested by severe pain and dark urine (due to excretion of intracellular muscle constituents that leak out of damaged cells).

Rhinotracheitis: allergic inflammation of nasal and tracheal mucosa.

Ribonuclease: enzyme that catalyzes breakdown of RNA to nucleotides.

Rosacea: inflammatory skin disease that causes facial redness and mostly affect adults with fair skin.

Schistosomiasis: disease caused by parasitic flatworms that occurs after contact with water containing certain types of snails that carry the worms.

Schizophrenia: a common thought disorder marked by delusions, hallucinations, and disorganized speech and behaviour and by flat affect, social withdrawal, and absence of violence.

Second messenger: an intracellularly acting molecule that communicates the activation of a receptor to an effector molecule, for example, an enzyme or ion channel. Important second messengers include cAMP, IP_3, DAG, and others.

Seizures: repetitive abnormal electrical discharges within the brain. Seizures are characterized as partial, generalized, or unclassified.

Serotonin (5-HT): 5-hydroxytryptamine, a neurotransmitter.

Side chain: in biochemistry, the variable part of amino acids or amino acid residues that are attached to the peptide backbone.

Sodium pump: a cell membrane protein pump that transports both sodium (out) and potassium (in) against concentration gradients and requires dephosphorylation of adenosine triphosphate to adenosine diphosphate.

Spinal action: effects of a drug acting directly on the spinal cord.

Splanchnic: associated with the viscera, that is, gastrointestinal system, spleen.

Sporozoites: protozoan cells, for example, malaria, that infect new hosts.

Status epilepticus: continuous seizure activity without an intervening period of normal brain function; a medical emergency.

Steatorrhea: excessive fats in the stool caused by malabsorption.

Stevens-Johnson syndrome: life-threatening hypersensitivity reaction (type III allergy) affecting skin and mucous membranes.

Supraspinal actions: effects of a drug from interacting with receptors above the spinal cord in areas such as the brain stem, limbic structures, etc.

Synergy: use of a drug combination that results in an effect greater than that achieved with a single drug, and greater than the sum of the effects of each drug individually.

Systole: time period in the cardiac cycle during which ventricular contraction occurs.

Systolic blood pressure: peak blood pressure during the contraction phase of the cardiac cycle.

Tachycardia: heart rate faster than 100 beats per minute.

Tapeworms: parasitic worms in class *Cestoda* that have specialized structures to secure attachment to host's intestine or blood vessels.

Tardive dyskinesia: a neurological syndrome marked by slow, rhythmical, automatic stereotyped movements, either generalized or in single muscle groups.

Teratogen: substance that causes severe birth defects.

Thrombocytopenia: decrease in number of circulating thrombocytes (platelets).

Thromboembolism: obstruction of blood vessel by a blood clot (thrombus) that has broken away from another site.

Thrombosis: excessive clotting.

Thyrotoxicosis: syndrome caused by excess thyroid hormone.

Tinnitus: a ringing or roar perception in the ear without external stimulus.

Titer: strength per volume of a solution; usually refers to amount of antibodies in a given volume of serum.

Tolerance: a condition that arises with frequently repeated administration of therapeutic doses of certain drugs, and is characterized by a gradual loss in effectiveness. To reproduce the original response, a larger dose must be administered.

Tonic-clonic seizures: generalized seizure disorder that is characterized by loss of consciousness with violent movements of the extremities.

Toxic epidermal necrolysis: typically drug-induced life-threatening condition in which epidermal cells die and separate from underlying dermis.

Toxicology: the study of adverse effects of substances on biologic systems, from a single organism to an ecosystem.

Transdermal patch: a method of drug administration that provides stable blood levels of drug while avoiding the need for repeated parenteral injections. Avoids the first-pass effect.

Transferrin: iron-transporting protein found in plasma.

Trematodes: parasitic worms in class *Trematoda,* commonly referred to as flukes.

Trichomoniasis: protozoan infection usually transmitted during sexual contact.

Tularemia: commonly called "rabbit fever"; bacterial infection characterized by fever, weight loss, and myalgias that is transmitted to humans by ticks, fleas, flies, or by handling infected animals.

Tumor flare: short-lived increase in tumor growth and symptoms due to an increase in drug agonist concentrations that stimulate the tumor.

Up regulation: increase in the number of available receptors.

Urinary hesitancy: difficulty in initiating urine flow.

Urticaria: itchy skin rash with wheals.

Vaccine: infectious particle (or part of one) given to an individual for purpose of establishing immunity or resistance to disease caused by that particular agent (e.g., virus).

Vasculitis: inflammation of blood vessels.

Vasodilator: an agent capable of dilating blood vessels.

Vector: delivery vehicle.

Vertigo: a vestibular dysfunction in which there is a perception of motion.

Virion: virus particle consisting of nucleic acids surrounded by a protein shell.

Voltage-gated ion channel: ion channel that is activated by changes in electrical potential difference near the channel.

INDEX

Page numbers followed by *f* or *t* indicate figures or tables, respectively.